HOMEOSTASIS OF PHOSPHATE AND OTHER MINERALS

THIRD INTERNATIONAL WORKSHOP ON PHOSPHATE AND OTHER MINERALS MADRID, SPAIN, JULY 15–18, 1977

ADVANCES IN EXPERIMENTAL MEDICINE AND BIOLOGY

Recent Volumes in this Series

Volume 98
IMMUNOBIOLOGY OF PROTEINS AND PEPTIDES • I
Edited by M. Z. Atassi and A. B. Stavitsky

Volume 99
THE REGULATION OF RESPIRATION DURING SLEEP AND ANESTHESIA
Edited by Robert S. Fitzgerald, Henry Gautier, and Sukhamay Lahiri

Volume 100
MYELINATION AND DEMYELINATION
Edited by Jorma Palo

Volume 101
ENZYMES OF LIPID METABOLISM
Edited by Shimon Gatt, Louis Freysz, and Paul Mandel

Volume 102
THROMBOSIS: Animal and Clinical Models
Edited by H. James Day, Basil A. Molony, Edward E. Nishizawa, and Ronald H. Rynbrandt

Volume 103
HOMEOSTASIS OF PHOSPHATE AND OTHER MINERALS
Edited by Shaul G. Massry, Eberhard Ritz, and Aurelio Rapado

Volume 104
THE THROMBOTIC PROCESS IN ATHEROGENESIS
Edited by A. Bleakley Chandler, Karl Eurenius, Gardner C. McMillan, Curtis B. Nelson, Colin J. Schwartz, and Stanford Wessler

Volume 105
NUTRITIONAL IMPROVEMENT OF FOOD PROTEINS
Edited by Mendel Friedman

Volume 106
GASTROINTESTINAL HORMONES AND PATHOLOGY OF THE DIGESTIVE SYSTEM
Edited by Morton Grossman, V. Speranza, N. Basso, and E. Lezoche

Volume 107
SECRETORY IMMUNITY AND INFECTION
Edited by Jerry R. McGhee, Jiri Mestecky, and James L. Babb

HOMEOSTASIS OF PHOSPHATE AND OTHER MINERALS

Edited by

Shaul G. Massry
University of Southern California
Los Angeles, California

Eberhard Ritz
University of Heidelberg
Heidelberg, Germany

and

Aurelio Rapado
Fundación Jiménez Díaz
Madrid, Spain

PLENUM PRESS • NEW YORK AND LONDON

Library of Congress Cataloging in Publication Data

International Workshop on Phosphate and Other Minerals, 3d, Madrid, 1977.
Homeostasis of phosphate and other minerals.

(Advances in experimental medicine and biology; v. 103)
Includes index.
1. Phosphorus metabolism disorders–Congresses. 2. Phosphorus metabolism–Congresses. 3. Mineral metabolism–Congresses. 4. Homeostasis–Congresses. I. Massry, Shaul G. II. Ritz, Eberhard. III. Rapado, A. IV. Fundación Jiménez Díaz. [DNLM: 1. Phosphates–Metabolism–Congresses. 2. Homeostasis–Congresses. W3 IN9327G 3d 1977h/QV285 I61 1977h]
RC632.P56I57 1977 616.3'9 78-5709

DOI 10.1007/978-1-4684-7758-0

Proceedings of the Third International Workshop
on Phosphate and Other Minerals
held at the Fundación Jiménez Díaz, Madrid, Spain,
July 15–18, 1977

MyCopy version of the original edition 1978
A Division of Plenum Publishing Corporation
227 West 17th Street, New York, N.Y. 10011

To our teachers
who taught us the art of medicine
and the scientific approach to research

Preface

We are pleased to present to our readers the Proceedings of the Third International Workshop on Phosphate and Other Minerals which was held in Madrid, during July 15-18, 1977. It was hosted by Dr. Aurelio Rapado, Head of the Metabolic Unit at the Fundacion Jimenez Diaz.

The Third International Workshop was organized in the tradition of the previous two Workshops. Scientists from 15 countries attended the meeting which provided a forum for formal presentations and informal discussions of topics of current interest in the field of phosphate metabolism, and that of the homeostasis of other minerals. One day of the Workshop was devoted to the subject of Phosphate Depletion. The latest information on the various aspects of the metabolic consequences of phosphate depletion were brought into focus.

In the preface of the Proceedings of the Second International Workshop on Phosphate, we indicated that the enthusiasm with which these Workshops were received generated the idea for the creation of a Journal which will publish research endeavors related to mineral and electrolyte metabolism. These efforts were brought into fruition, and the first issue of the new Journal, *Mineral and Electrolyte Metabolism* has already appeared in November, 1977. It is published by Karger of Basel, Switzerland under the Editorship of Dr. Shaul G. Massry of Los Angeles, with Dr. Louis V. Avioli of St. Louis and Dr. Eberhard Ritz of Heidelberg, serving as Associate Editors. The Journal is supported by an Editorial Board of 44 distinguished scientists from all over the world. It is designed to be a scientific forum which will provide for the dissemination of information in the broad field of mineral and electrolyte metabolism. Its content will be of interest to the biochemist, endocrinologist, nephrologist, nutritionist and internist involved in investigation of the clinical disorders and in the basic research of mineral and electrolyte homeostasis.

The Fourth International Workshop on Phosphate and Other Minerals will be held during the month of June, 1979 in Strassbourg,

France. It will be hosted by Professor H. Jahn, of the University of Strassbourg. The theme of this coming Workshop will continue to focus on the pathophysiology of phosphate homeostasis and the metabolism of other minerals.

We would like to express our deepest appreciation for all those who have stimulated, encouraged, and supported us to hold the Third Workshop in Madrid. This endeavor could not have been possible without the generous financial support of the Direccion General de Relaciones Culturales del Minesterio de Asuntos Exteriores, Excmo Ayuntamiento de Madrid, Bellco, A. Christianes, Hoffman-LaRoche (USA, Proctor and Gamble Co (USA), Upjohn Co (USA), and Plenum Publishing Corporation (USA).

A special thanks goes to Ms. Maria Ramon, Ms. Carla Schoenmakers and Ms. Gracy Fick for their invaluable and tireless efforts in the organization of the Third International Workshop on Phosphate and Other Minerals.

Shaul G. Massry, M.D.
Eberhard Ritz, M.D.
Aurelio Rapado, M.D.

Contents

I. RENAL HANDLING OF PHOSPHATE, CALCIUM, AND MAGNESIUM

II. INTESTINAL TRANSPORT OF PHOSPHATE

III. METABOLISM OF PHOSPHATE AND OTHER MINERALS IN DISEASE STATES

V. TOPICS ON BONE

VI. TOPICS ON VITAMIN D

VII. TOPICS ON PARATHYROID HORMONE

Renal Handling of Phosphate, Calcium, and Magnesium

RECENT PROGRESS IN RENAL HANDLING OF PHOSPHATE

Henri Kuntziger and Claude Amiel

INSERM U.64, Hôpital Tenon, Paris, and Lab. Physiologie

Hôpital Louis Mourier, Colombes, France

In mammals inorganic phosphate (Pi) is filtered at the glomerulus and reabsorbed in the tubules (1).

Filtered load of Pi is adequately calculated as plasma Pi times glomerular filtration rate. Glomerular micropuncture studies in the Munich strain of the Wistar rat have shown that in vivo Pi is almost completely ultrafiltrable (2, 3).

Pi is reabsorbed in the proximal convoluted tubule (4) and in the pars recta (5, 6). No Pi transport occurs in other segments of the loop of Henle as has been shown in the rabbit (7). Free flow distal micropuncture and ^{32}P distal microinjection studies have given rise to controversy concerning terminal ^{32}P reabsorption (8, 9). In intact animals the amount of phosphate in the superficial distal tubule was significantly greater than that found in the final urine (8). These findings have been interpreted as evidence for Pi reabsorption in distal convoluted tubules and/or collecting ducts (8, 10, 11). Such an interpretation has been criticized, because of a possible nephron heterogeneity for Pi transport (9). This criticism deserves comment. Indeed the difference between Pi distal delivery and urinary excretion increases in chronic parathyroidectomized rats (CPTX) (8). Assuming no terminal reabsorption of Pi then implies an increase in the deep nephron fraction of glomerular filtrate in CPTX as compared to intact animals. Such an increase has not been found however (Table 1). But distal ^{32}P microinjection and stationary microperfusion studies did not show ^{32}P reabsorption by terminal nephron (12, 13, 14, 15), with the exception of one study which found that in terminal nephron the unidirectional ^{32}P reabsorptive flux was 17.4% of delivered load (16). ^{32}P distal microinjections are open to criticism, because all of its variables are not always controlled, such as

Table 1. Glomerular filtration Data, (mean ± SEM) normal (NRL) and CPTX Rats. (H. Kuntziger and C. Amiel, unpublished data)

	NRL N=6 (31)	CPTX N=7 (34)	P
GFR, $ml.min^{-1}$	1.3 ± 0.08	1.2 ± 0.03	N.S.
Distal SNGFR, $nl.min^{-1}$	49.0 ± 2.3	49.0 ± 2.0	N.S.
Number of nephrons (GFR/distal SNGFR)	27900 ± 1465	25100 ± 635	N.S.

tracer conditions, contact time, pH, physico-chemical characteristics of tracer ... Recent findings might end the controversy (17). Superficial distal ^{32}P microinjection studies have shown a terminal ^{32}P reabsorption in some strains of Wistar rats, but not in the Munich one. In the Munich strain Pi terminal reabsorption occurs only in deep nephrons, which are not accessible to micropuncture. In these Munich rats unidirectional ^{32}P flux measured for all the nephrons, by renal artery injection of the tracer, is the same as the whole kidney fractional Pi reabsorption. But unidirectional ^{32}P flux measured for the superficial nephrons alone, by glomerular injection of the tracer, is significantly less than the whole kidney fractional Pi reabsorption. As suggested by Poujeol et al. (18) terminal reabsorption of Pi in deep nephrons might occur in the granular portions of distal convoluted tubules and cortical collecting ducts. These structures form arcades, where a parathyroid-hormone-sensitive adenylate cyclase is located, as studies in the rabbit have shown (19, 20).

Bidirectional tubular flux of Pi in mammals remains controversial. Free flow micropuncture studies have demonstrated its occurence in early proximal tubule and in terminal nephron, under conditions of Pi loading with and without parathyroid hormone administration (21). Bidirectional Pi flux has also been found in proximal split droplet (22) and microperfusion experiments in the rat (21) as well as ^{32}P renal artery injection and renal surface application studies in the dog (23). Other microperfusion experiments did not show any Pi flux into the tubular lumen (24, 25). An in vitro microperfusion study of isolated rabbit proximal convoluted tubule and pars recta also did not find any bath to lumen transport of Pi (6). No information is available concerning the pathway of the elusive blood and/or cell to lumen flux of Pi, paracellular across the tight junctions and/or transcellular. Study of the hypophosphatemic mutant mouse, model for human vitamin D-resistant rickets, should help to clarify these issues (26,27). Data favouring bidirectional tubular flux of Pi have indeed been reported in a study of human X - linked hypophosphatemic rickets (28).

Recent progress in the understanding of cellular and subcellular mechanisms of renal tubular Pi transport has been achieved by several methods : in vivo stopped flow microperfusion of proximal tubule with peritubular capillary perfusion (29) separation and isolation of proximal tubular brush border and basal-lateral membrane fractions (30) and in vitro microperfusion of isolated proximal convoluted tubule and pars recta of the rabbit (6). Since a lecture of the present Workshop is devoted to this topic (29), it will not be analyzed here.

Among the factors which influence tubular transport of Pi, two are of major physiological importance, parathyroid hormone (PTH) and dietary phosphorus. PTH decreases Pi reabsorption in the proximal convoluted tubule and in the pars recta (13, 31, 32, 33). An effect on terminal nephron handling of Pi is very probable, yet not definitely established (9, 11, 33). The effect of PTH on Pi tubular transport is mediated through cAMP (34). Tentatively, the sequence of events might be the following one. The peritubular capillary borne hormone interacts with adenylate cyclase located at the contraluminal cell membrane (35). Intracellular cAMP rises and stimulates a protein kinase located at the luminal brush border membrane (36). The cAMP dependent protein kinase activates by phosphorylation a protein involved in the active Pi transport across the brush border membrane (36). The effect of PTH on Pi tubular transport is terminated by dephosphorylation of the specific phosphoprotein brought about by a brush-border associated phospho protein phosphatase (36). cAMP dissociates from its brush border receptor and is inactivated by tubular cell phosphodiesterases (37). A fraction of cAMP escapes inactivation and is added to tubular fluid (34, 38). Net tubular addition of cAMP occurs in superficial proximal tubule, but not in Henle's loop and in the terminal nephron (39). Increasing extracellular cAMP concentration - by glucagon (38) or calcitonin (40) administration or by cAMP infusion (31, 33, 38, 41) - has the same effect on tubular Pi handling than PTH, which primarily increases intratubular cell cAMP. This effect of cAMP exists in the proximal convoluted tubule and in the loop (pars recta) (33). cAMP probably also influences terminal nephron transport of Pi (33). In the rabbit PTH stimulates adenylate cyclase in the proximal convoluted tubule and in the pars recta, as well as in the thick ascending cortical limb of Henle's loop and of the granular, confluent segments of distal convoluted tubules and cortical collecting ducts (19, 20). The PTH responsive segments of the terminal nephron form arcades, which are especially well developped in deep nephrons (20). If PTH and cAMP influence terminal Pi transport at the level of these arcades, their effect predominantly occurs in deep nephrons. The mechanism of the effect of extracellular cAMP on Pi tubular transport is not understood.

Controversy exists concerning the cellular permeability to cAMP (42, 43). A rapid breakdown of extracellular cAMP to nucleosides and nucleotides has been demonstrated on the outer surface of liver, adipose tissue and kidney cells (44). Despite the poor cellular permeability and/or the rapid extracellular metabolism of cAMP, the effect of extracellular cAMP on Pi tubular transport is identical to that of PTH (31, 33, 38, 41). Recent findings might solve this problem. cAMP binds to brush border membranes (45). This apical cAMP receptor might be associated with the apical Pi transport system, through regulation of the brush-border cAMP-dependent protein kinase (36, 46). The apical cAMP receptor might then be accessible to cAMP, not only from the cell interior but also from the tubular lumen. This hypothesis has received experimental support. Indeed PTH inhibited isotonic fluid reabsorption in proximal tubules preferentially when applied from the contraluminal cell side and cAMP inhibited preferentially, when applied from the luminal cell side (47). It has also been reported that the brush-border bound cAMP is resistant to hydrolysis by phosphodiesterases (45). After dissociation from its brush border receptor, the fraction of cAMP bound towards the cell interior is inactivated by brush-border and/or cell phosphodiesterases. The fraction of cAMP bound towards the lumen is carried away by tubular fluid before inactivation occurs.

Variations in dietary Pi strikingly modulate the tubular Pi transport capacity (48, 49, 50). In animals fed a low Pi diet, Pi urinary excretion is low. In animals fed a high Pi diet, Pi urinary excretion is high. The influence of dietary Pi is not mediated by PTH, since it occurs in parathyroidectomized animals. It is also independent of filtered load of Pi, extracellular volume, acid-base status, extracellular calcium and vitamin D. Tubular adaptation of Pi transport can be demonstrated 72 hours after changing Pi dietary level. The site in the nephron, where this adaptation occurs could be the early proximal tubule and the terminal nephron (51). The mechanism of this tubular adaptation is not known. Renal tubules can change their capacity to transport Pi according to homeostatic requirements. They adjust to the needs of the organism. Variations in the needs of Pi result from changes in dietary Pi, in intestinal Pi reabsorption and in bone accretion of Pi and calcium. Tentatively tubular Pi transport, capable to adapt to fluctuating entry of Pi into extracellular fluid, might derive from phylogenetically archaic membrane systems of Pi transport. Such systems have been described for many different plant and animal cells (30). The addition of a second regulatory mechanism, triggered by PTH, would then be a phylogenetically recent event, appearing in vertebrates with the emergence of the tetrapods (52).

REFERENCES

1. MUDGE, G.H., BERNDT, W.O., and VALTIN, H. : Tubular transport of urea, glucose, phosphate, uric acid, sulfate, and thiosulfate. In : Handbook of Physiology, Orloff, J. and Berliner, R. W. (eds). American Physiological Society, Washington, pp. 587-652, 1973.
2. HARRIS, C.A., BAER, P.G., CHIRITO, E., and DIRKS, J.H. : Composition of mammalian glomerular filtrate. Am. J. Physiol. 227: 972, 1974.
3. LE GRIMELLEC, C., POUJEOL, P., and de ROUFFIGNAC, C. : ^{3}H-inulin and electrolyte concentration in Bowman's capsule in rat kidney. Pflügers Arch. 354 : 117, 1975.
4. STRICKLER, J.C., THOMPSON, D.D., KLOSE, R.M., and GIEBISCH, G. : Micropuncture study of inorganic phosphate excretion in the rat. J. clin. Invest. 43 : 1596, 1964.
5. KUNTZIGER, H., AMIEL, C., and GAUDEBOUT, C. : Phosphate handling by the rat nephron during saline diuresis. Kidney Intern. 2 : 318, 1972.
6. DENNIS, V.W., WOODHALL, P.B., and ROBINSON, R.R. : Characteristics of phosphate transport in isolated proximal tubule. Am. J. Physiol. 231 : 979, 1976.
7. ROCHA, A.S., MAGALDI, J.B., and KOKKO, J.P. : Calcium and phosphate transport in isolated segments of rabbit Henle's loop. J. clin. Invest. 59 : 975, 1977.
8. AMIEL, C., KUNTZIGER, H., and RICHET, G. : Micropuncture study of handling of phosphate by proximal and distal nephron in normal and parathyroidectomized rat. Evidence for distal reabsorption. Pflügers Arch. 317 : 93, 1970.
9. KNOX, F.G., GREGER, R.F., LANG, F.C., and MARCHAND, G.R. : Renal handling of phosphate : Update. 2nd International Workshop on Phosphate, Heidelberg 1976, Plenum Press, page 3, 1977.
10. LE GRIMELLEC, C., ROINEL, N., and MOREL, F. : Simultaneous Mg, Ca, P, K, Na and Cl analysis in rat tubules fluid. I- During perfusion of either inulin or ferrocyanide. Pflügers Arch. 340 : 181, 1973.
11. GOLDBERG, M. : Renal handling of phosphate : an overview. 1st International Workshop, Phosphate Metabolism, Kidney and Bone, Paris, 1975.
12. STAUM, B.B., HAMBURGER, R.J., and GOLDBERG, M. : Tracer microinjection study of renal tubular phosphate reabsorption in the rat. J. clin. Invest. 51 : 2271, 1972.
13. BRUNETTE, M.G., TAÏEB, L., and CARRIERE, S. : Effect of parathyroid hormone on phosphate reabsorption along the nephron of the rat. Am. J. Physiol. 225 : 1076, 1973.
14. GREGER, R., LANG, F., MARCHAND, G.R., and KNOX, F.G. : Nephron site of phosphate reabsorption in thyroparathyroidectomized rat. Fed. Proc. 35 : 466, 1976.

15. LANG, F., GREGER, R., MARCHAND, G.R., and KNOX, F.G. : Stationary microperfusion study of phosphate reabsorption in proximal and distal nephron segments. Pflügers Arch. 368 : 45, 1977.
16. POUJEOL, P., and de ROUFFIGNAC, C. : Microinjection studies of phosphate permeability in rats during mild saline diuresis : influence of acute thyroparathyroidectomy and parathormone administration. 1st International Workshop, Phosphate Metabolism, Kidney and Bone, Paris 1975.
17. POUJEOL, P., CORMAN, B., TOUVAY, C., and de ROUFFIGNAC, C. : Renal reabsorption of phosphate (P) by the rat nephron. Intrarenal heterogeneity and strain differences. XXVIIth International Congress of Physiological Sciences, Paris, 1977.
18. POUJEOL, P., CHABARDES, D., ROINEL, N., and de ROUFFIGNAC, C. : Influence of extracellular fluid volume expansion on magnesium, calcium and phosphate handling along the rat nephron. Pflügers Arch. 365 : 203, 1976.
19. CHABARDES, D., IMBERT, M., CLIQUE, A., MONTEGUT, M., and MOREL, F. : PTH sensitive Adenyl cyclase activity in different segments of the rabbit nephron. Pflügers Arch. 354 : 229, 1975.
20. MOREL, F., CHABARDES, D., and IMBERT, M. : Functional segmentation of the rabbit distal tubule by microdetermination of hormone-dependent adenylate cyclase activity. Kidney Intern. 9 : 264, 1976.
21. BOUDRY, J.F., TROEHLER, V., TOUABI, M., FLEISCH, H., and BONJOUR, J.P. : Secretion of inorganic phosphate in the rat nephron. Clin. Sci. mol. Med. 48 : 475, 1975.
22. SHIRLEY, D.G., POUJEOL, P., and LE GRIMELLEC, C.: Phosphate, calcium and magnesium fluxes into the lumen of the rat proximal convoluted tubule. Pflügers Arch. 362 : 247, 1976.
23. SCHNEIDER, E.G., and Mc LANE, L.A. : Evidence for a peritubular-to-luminal flux of phosphate in the dog kidney. Am. J. Physiol. 232 : F 159, 1977.
24. MURAYAMA, Y., MOREL, F., and LE GRIMELLEC, C. : Phosphate, calcium and magnesium transfers in proximal tubules and loops of Henle, as measured by single nephron microperfusion experiments in the rat. Pflügers Arch. 333 : 1, 1972.
25. GREGER, R.F., LANG, F.C., KNOX, F.G., and LECHENE, C.P. : Absence of significant secretory flux of phosphate in the proximal convoluted tubule. Am. J. Physiol. 232 : F 235, 1977.
26. EICHER, E.M., SOUTHARD, J.L., SCRIVER, C.R., and GLORIEUX, F.H. : Hypophosphatemia : Mouse model for human familial hypophosphatemic (vitamin D-resistant) rickets. Proc. natl. Acad. Sci. USA 73 : 4667, 1976.
27. BRUNETTE, M.G., GIASSON-DESJARDINS, S., VIGNEAULT, N., and CARRIERE, S. : Micropuncture study of phosphorus transport in genetic hypophosphatemic mice. 3rd International Workshop on phosphate and other minerals, Madrid 1977.

28. GLORIEUX, F., and SCRIVER, C.R. : Loss of a parathyroid hormone sensitive component of phosphate transport in X-linked hypophosphatemia. Science 175 : 997, 1972.
29. ULLRICH, K.J. : Mechanisms of cellular and subcellular transport of phosphate. 3rd International Workshop on phosphate and other minerals, Madrid, 1977.
30. HOFFMANN, N., THEES, M., and KINNE, R. : Phosphate transport by isolated brush border vesicles. Pflügers Arch. 362 : 147, 1976.
31. AGUS, Z.S., PUSCHETT, J.B., SENESKY, D., and GOLDBERG, M. : Mode of action of parathyroid hormone and cyclic adenosine 3',5'-monophosphate on renal tubular phosphate reabsorption in the dog. J. clin. Invest. 50 : 617, 1971.
32. GEKLE, D. : Der Einfluss von Parathormon auf die Nierenfunktion. Pflügers Arch. 323 : 96, 1971.
33. KUNTZIGER, H., AMIEL, C., ROINEL, N., and MOREL, F. : Effects of parathyroidectomy and cyclic AMP on renal transport of phosphate, calcium, and magnesium. Am. J. Physiol. 227 : 905, 1974.
34. CHASE, L.R., and AURBACH, G.D. : Parathyroid function and the renal excretion of 3',5'-adenylic acid. Proc. Natl. Acad. Sci. USA 58 : 518, 1967.
35. SHLATZ, L.J., SCHWARTZ, I.L., KINNE-SAFFRAN, E., and KINNE, R.: Distribution of parathyroid hormone-stimulated adenylate cyclase in plasma membranes of cells of the kidney cortex. J. Membrane Biol. 24 : 131, 1975.
36. KINNE, R., SHLATZ, L.J., KINNE-SAFFRAN, E., and SCHWARTZ, I.L.: Distribution of membrane - bound cyclic AMP - dependent protein kinase in plasma membranes of cells of the kidney cortex. J. Membrane Biol. 24 : 145, 1975.
37. FILBURN, C.R. and SACKTOR, B. : Cyclic nucleotide phosphodiesterases of rabbit renal cortex. Characterization of brush border membrane activities. Arch. Biochem. Biophys. 174 : 249, 1976.
38. BUTLEN, D., and JARD, S. : Renal handling of 3',5'-cyclic AMP in the rat : the possible role of luminal 3',5'-cyclic AMP in the tubular reabsorption of phosphate. Pflügers Arch. 331 : 172, 1972.
39. KUNTZIGER, H., CAILLA, H.L., AMIEL, C., and DELAAGE, M.A. : Renal tubular handling of 3',5'-cAMP in normal and parathyroidectomized rats. 2nd International Workshop on Phosphate, Heidelberg 1976, Plenum Press, page 75, 1977.
40. ARDAILLOU, R., ISAAC, R., NIVEZ, M.P., KUHN, J.M., CAZOR, J.L., and FILLASTRE, J.P. : Effect of salmon calcitonin on renal excretion of adenosine 3',5'-monophosphate in man. Horm. Metab. Res. 8 : 136, 1976.
41. RASMUSSEN, H., PECHET, M., and FAST, D. : Effect of dibutyryl cyclic adenosine 3',5'-monophosphate, theophylline, and other nucleotides upon calcium and phosphate metabolism. J. clin. Invest. 47 : 1843, 1968.

42. ROBINSON, G.A., BUTCHER, and SUTHERLAND, E.W. : in Cyclic AMP, Chapter 5, page 91, Academic Press, New York, 1971.
43. COULSON, R. : Metabolism and excretion of exogenous adenosine 3',5'-monophosphate and guanosine 3',5'-monophosphate. Studies in the isolated perfused rat kidney and in the intact rat. J. biol. Chem. 251 : 4958, 1976.
44. GORIN, E., and BRENNER, T. : Extracellular metabolism of cyclic AMP. Biochim. Biophys. Acta 451 : 20, 1976.
45. INSEL, P., BALAKIR, R., and SACKTOR, B. : The binding of cyclic AMP to renal brush border membranes. J. Cyclic Nucleotide Research 1 : 107, 1975.
46. WALKENBACH, R.J., and FORTE, C.R. : Solubilization and photoaffinity labeling of renal membrane cyclic AMP receptors. Biochim. Biophys. Acta 464 : 165, 1977.
47. BAUMANN, K., CHAN, Y.L. , BODE, F., and PAPAVASSILIOU, F. : Effect of parathyroid hormone and cyclic adenosine 3',5'-monophosphate on isotonic fluid reabsorption : Polarity of proximal tubular cells. Kidney Intern. 11 : 77, 1977.
48. STEELE, T.H., ENGLE, J.E., TANAKA, Y., LORENC, R.S., DUDGEON, K.L., and DE LUCA, H.F. : Phosphatemic action of 1,25 - dihydroxy-vitamin D3. Am. J. Physiol. 229 : 489, 1975.
49. TRÖHLER, U., BONJOUR, J.P., and FLEISCH, H. : Inorganic phosphate homeostasis : Renal adaptation to the dietary intake in intact and thyroparathyroidectomized rats. J. clin. Invest. 57 : 264, 1976.
50. STEELE, T.H., and DE LUCA, H.F. : Influence of the dietary phosphorus on renal phosphate reabsorption in the parathyroidectomized rat. J. clin. Invest. 57 : 867, 1976.
51. BONJOUR, J.P., TRÖHLER U., MÜHLBAUER, R., PRESTON, C., and FLEISCH, H. : Is there a bone-kidney link in the homeostasis of inorganic phosphate (Pi) ? 2nd International Workshop on Phosphate, Heidelberg 1976, Plenum Press, page 319, 1977.
52. GORBMAN, A. : Endocrinology of the amphibia. In : Physiology of the Amphibia, Moore, J.A. (ed.) Academic Press, pp. 391-393, 1964.

INTERACTIONS BETWEEN PTH, VITAMIN D METABOLITES, AND OTHER FACTORS IN TUBULAR REABSORPTION OF PHOSPHATE

M.M.Popovtzer, S.Mehandru, D.Saghafi, and M.S.Blum

Temple University School of Medicine, Dept. of Medicine

Philadelphia, Pennsylvania 19140, USA

The direct effect of calcium on renal handling of phosphorus, has been the subject of numerous investigations which for the most part have produced discrepant results (1-5). This incongruity at least partly could be explained by the lack of consistency in the experimental designs and the species of experimental animals.

To further examine the effect of serum calcium level on the phosphaturic action of parathyroid hormone (PTH) hypercalcemia was induced in parathyroidectomized (PTX) hydropenic rats (6). Intravenous administration of calcium was started either before, or after the beginning of a continuous infusion of PTH. In both experimental settings hypercalcemia failed to alter the tubular reabsorption of phosphorus and the urinary excretion of cyclic AMP(cAMP). In contrast to the hydropenic PTH-infused PTX rats, in PTX volume expanded rats hypercalcemia consistently produced a fall in the urinary excretion of phosphorus (6). These observations suggested that hypercalcemia blocks the mechanism by which extracellular volume expansion produces phosphaturia, but does not affect the mechanism by which PTH produces the same response. However, the administration of calcium ionophore (Eli Lilly A 23187) that presumably increases the cytoplasmic calcium concentration by facilitating its passive entry into the cell, produced a significant decrease in the excretion rates of phosphorus and cAMP in PTX hydropenic rats undergoing PTH infusion (7). These results could be interpreted by reference to previous studies that suggested that increases in intracellular, but not extracellular calcium can inhibit the PTH-induced activation of adenyl cyclase/cAMP system which mediates the phosphaturic effect of PTH (6,8,9).

Vitamin D has been variously reported to increase or decrease tubular reabsorption of phosphorus (10-12). The interpretation of these observations has been complicated by the multifaceted actions of the vitamin and its derivatives. In intact rats 25(OH)vitamin D_3 produced a prompt increase in tubular reabsorption of phosphorus (13). This response became noticeable with 1 unit/100g per h of 25(OH)vitamin D_3, which may be considered as a physiological dose. Even though this response was not associated with a measurable increase in serum calcium concentration it was not possible to exclude that suppression of endogenous PTH secretion produced the fall in urinary phosphorus excretion. The latter possibility was further reinforced by the proposed direct suppression of PTH-secretion by vitamin D and its derivatives, which may be independent of serum calcium level (14,15). To further examine the role of PTH, experiments were conducted in chronically PTX rats. In these animals neither 25(OH)vitamin D_3, nor $1,25(OH)_2$ vitamin D_3 effected an increase in tubular reabsorption of phosphorus (13). These findings demonstrated not only that the presence of PTH is necessary for the response to occur, but also that the absence of antiphosphaturic action cannot be accounted for by a failure of the conversion of 25(OH)vitD_3 into $1,25(OH)_2$vitD_3. Furthermore, infusion of serum obtained from intact 25(OH)vitD_3-loaded rats to PTX animals also failed to alter tubular reabsorption of phosphorus (16). Similarly the correction of hypocalcemia to a normal serum calcium level by oral and parenteral administration of calcium did not restore the response to 25(OH)vitaminD_3 (13).

Since PTX rats exhibit very low basal excretion rates of phosphorus that might obscure the antiphosphaturic effect of 25(OH) vitamin D_3, the same experiments were conducted after that the urinary excretion of phosphorus was deliberately augmented by various phosphaturic challenges. Intravenous administration of sodium phosphate, and extracellular volume expansion with normal saline were associated with sustained phosphaturia which was not altered by 25(OH)vitD_3 (13). Likewise the phosphaturia that followed the administration of two diuretic agents, acetazolamide and chlorothiazide was not affected by 25(OH)vitaminD_3.

By contrast to the lack of response during the administration of sodium phosphate, normal saline, acetazolamide and chlorothiazide, 25(OH)vitD_3 appeared to suppress the phosphaturia induced by exogenous PTH (13). This finding suggested that the action of the vitamin is in some way linked with a transport mechanism which is responsive to PTH. It has been proposed that the phosphaturic effect of PTH is mediated by the adenyl cyclase/cAMP mechanism in the following sequence. First the hormone binds to a specific membrane-bound receptor complex on the contraluminal side of the cell (17, 18). This activates the receptor-linked enzyme adenyl cyclase and increases the formation of cAMP. The nucleotide exerts its effect at the luminal portion of the cell by activating a protein kinase which subsequently induces phosphorylation of certain elements that are located in the brush border (19). The latter step is believed to produce the physiologic response, either by blocking the active reabsorption of phosphorus, or by increasing its passive efflux (20). Theoretically, 25(OH)vitD_3 could exert its effect by interfering with one or more steps of this chain reaction. To further characterize this response urinary excretion of cAMP was measured in PTX PTH-infused rats before and after the administration of 25(OH)vit D_3. A significant decrease in the urinary excretion of cAMP occurred during the administration of 25(OH)vitD_3 and it paralleled the decrease in the urinary excretion of phosphorus (21). The fall in urinary cAMP could be explained either by a decreased formation or an increased degradation of cAMP or both. In addition it could reflect a decrease in cellular permeability to both, inorganic phosphorus and cAMP.

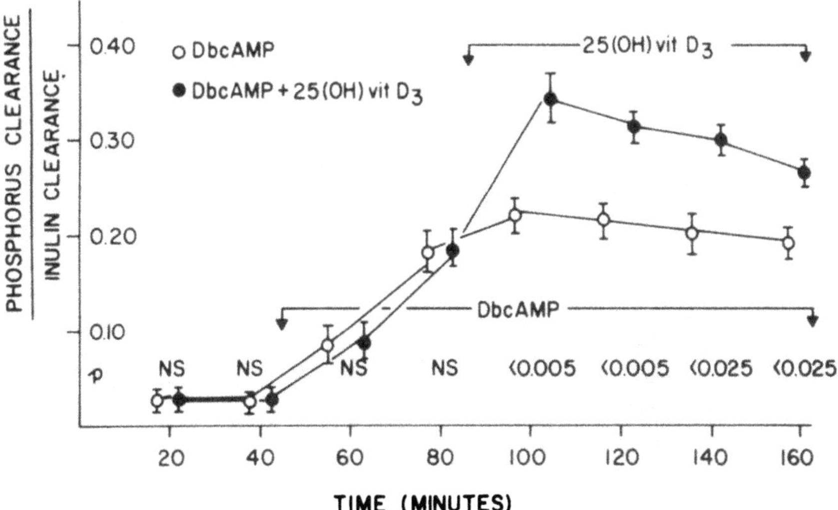

Figure 1. The effect of 25(OH)vitD_3 on renal handling of phosphorus in PTX rats receiving continuous infusion of dibutyryl cyclic AMP(dbcAMP). p refers to the difference between the control animals (open circles) and the experimental animals (closed circles).

To further explore above alternatives the effect of 25(OH) vitaminD_3 on the phosphaturic action of exogenous nucleotide was examined (Figure 1). 25(OH)vitaminD_3 enhanced the phosphaturic action of dbcAMP as opposed to its suppressive effect on the phosphaturic response to PTH. The observed enhancement of dbcAMP-induced phosphaturia neither supported the possibility that 25(OH)vitD_3 accelerates the degradation of the nucleotide nor that it reduces the cellular permeability to it, and obviously it ruled out the possibility that the vitamin blocks the action of the nucleotide to produce phosphaturia. However, it was consistent with an interference of 25(OH)vitD_3 with the first step in the cascade, namely suppression of the hormone binding,the activation of the enzyme and the formation of cAMP.

In an attempt to further define the effect of 25(OH)vitD_3 we raised the question whether the response was specific to PTH or could it reflect a more general effect comprising additional phosphaturic hormones that act through the adenyl cyclase/cAMP axis.

The phosphaturic action of calcitonin similarly to that of PTH has been attributed to activation of adenyl cyclase/cAMP system even though its receptors are distinct from those of PTH (18,22). When 25(OH)vitD_3 was given to PTX rats receiving constant infusion of calcitonin urinary excretion of phosphorus decreased (23). Furthermore, the fall in the urinary excretion of phosphorus was paralleled by a commensurate decline in urinary excretion of cAMP. This observation suggested that the response to 25(OH)vitD_3 is not limited to an interaction with PTH only but it may also involve other hormones.

The exact nature of the response to 25(OH)vitD_3 cannot be defined by the present experiments. Previous studies by Borle indicated that in a state of vitamin D deficiency the administration of the vitamin increases the pool of calcium in the cytoplasm (24). If a similar rise in cytoplasmic calcium occurred in the present experiments it could suppress the activity of adenylate cyclase resulting in a decreased formation of cAMP and a fall in urinary excretion of phosphorus.

The results of the foregoing experiments can be fitted into a hypothetical model which proposes the existence of two major components of phosphorus transport. This model does not pretend to present a physiological delineation of renal handling of phosphorus, it is merely shown for the purpose of summary (Figure 2). Phosphorus may be transported actively against an electrochemical gradient from the lumen into the cell. Experimental evidence suggests that this system is located in the vesicles of the brush border (25). There is also experimental evidence that implies indirectly that phosphorus may exit and enter the cell in a passive fashion (20,26-28). The balance of these two cellular processes is the net cellular absorption of phosphorus. At least theoretically phosphorus may move in and out of the lumen without crossing the cell membrane by being routed through the paracellular pathway via the tight junctions. The work of Boulpaep provides experimental support to the possibility that during extracellular volume expansion the natriuresis could be entirely accounted for by a backflux of sodium through the tight junctions (29,30).

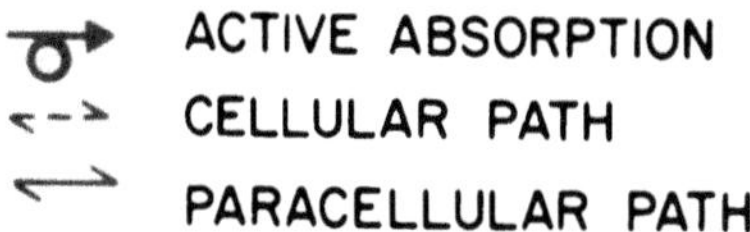

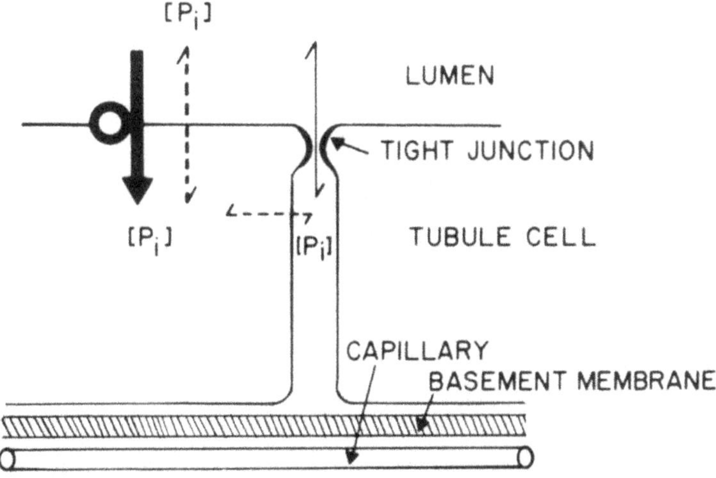

Figure 2. Schematic presentation of renal handling of phosphorus. Two components of tubular absorption of inorganic phosphorus (Pi).

Assuming that phosphorus is present in the intercellular fluid, the backflux could equally facilitate the translocation of phosphorus into the tubular lumen leading to both, natriuresis and phosphaturia (Figure 3).

Net paracellular Pi back-leak is augmented by extracellular volume expansion with saline and is inhibited by hypercalcemia but not by 25(OH)vit D_3

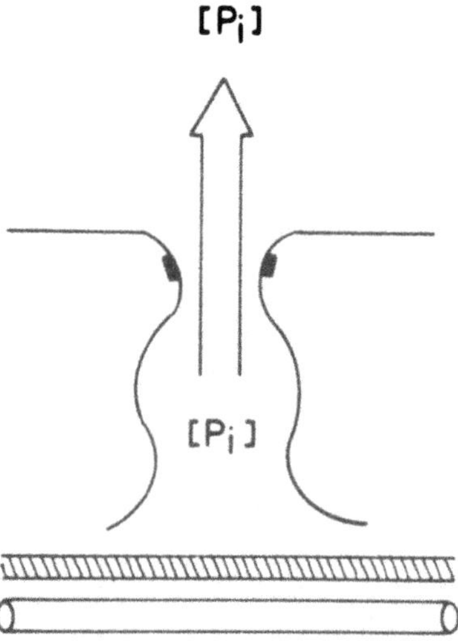

Figure 3. Schematic presentation of the paracellular component of renal handling of phosphorus during extracellular volume expansion when the tight junction becomes leaky.

As already stated the phosphaturia associated with volume expansion is not affected by 25(OH)vitD_3 but is blunted by hypercalcemia. The mechanism by which hypercalcemia acts in this instance is unknown but two considerations are worth comment. First, even in the absence of changes in glomerular filtration hypercalcemia could alter the balance of the peritubular Starling forces by its effect on renal hemodynamics. Second, hypercalcemia could reduce directly the permeability of the tight junctions. A blocking effect of calcium on the ionic selectivity of the tight junctions in mammalian kidney, has been demonstrated by Fromter et al (31).

The second component of the proposed model consists of the cellular transport pathway. The diagram (Figure 4) depicts receptors which differ one from another by their distinct specificity relative to the hormone that their interact with. However, the receptors have one common feature, the presence of adenyl cyclase in close juxtaposition. This enzyme increases the formation of cAMP that exerts its effect on the opposite side of the cell. The present

Renal Interactions of parathyroid hormone (PTH) calcitonin (CT), cyclic AMP (cAMP) and 25(OH) vit D_3

⇒ **Net P_i absorption, ⊖ blocking effect**

A is inhibited by 25(OH) vit D_3 and by Ca-ionophore but not by hypercalcemia

B is enhanced by 25(OH) vit D_3

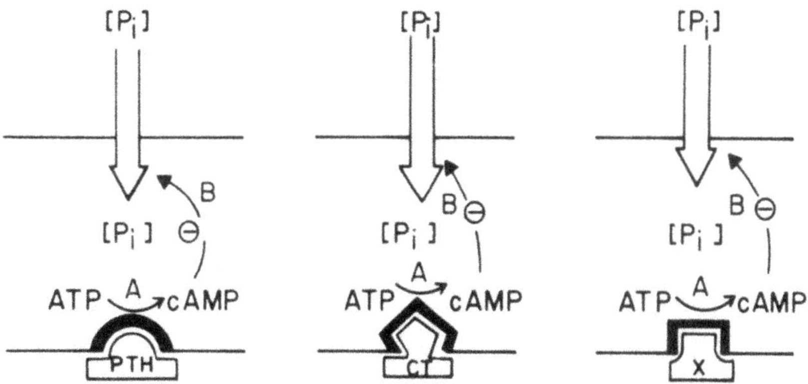

Figure 4. Schematic presentation of the cellular component of tubular absorption of inorganic phosphorus. X refers to additional unknown hormones that act in the same way as PTH and CT.

data are consistent with a dual action of 25(OH)vitD_3 on that system. On one hand the steroid inhibits step A, and thus diminishes the formation of cAMP and the excretion of phosphorus, on the other hand it enhances step B which is associated with increased urinary excretion of phosphorus.

The physiological importance of these opposing effects of 25(OH)vitD_3 is not well understood but perhaps it may help explain why vitamin D has been reported to exert variable effects on tubular reabsorption of phosphorus in different experimental and clinical situations.

REFERENCES

1. Lavender, A.R., and Pullman, T.N.: Changes in inorganic phosphate excretion induced by renal arterial infusion of calcium. Am. J. Physiol. 205: 1025, 1963.
2. Beck, N., Singh, H., Reed, S.W., and Davis, B.B.: Direct inhibitory effect of hypercalcemia on renal actions of parathyroid hormone. J. Clin. Invest. 53: 717, 1974.
3. Wen, S.F.: Micropuncture studies of phosphate transport in the proximal tubule of the dog. J. Clin. Invest. 53: 143, 1974.
4. Amiel, C., Kuntziger, H., Coutte, S., Coureau, C., and Bergounioux, N.: Evidence for parathyroid hormone-independent calcium modulation of phosphate transport along the nephron. J. Clin. Invest. 57: 256, 1976.
5. Cuche, J.L., Ott, C.E., Marchand, G.R., Diaz-Buxo, J.A., and Knox, F.G.: Intrarenal calcium in phosphate handling. Am. J. Physiol. 230: 790, 1976.
6. Popovtzer, M.M., Robinette, J.B., McDonald, K.M., and Kuruvila, C.K.: Effect of Ca^{++} on renal handling of PO_4: Evidence for two reabsorptive mechanisms. Am. J. Physiol. 229: 901, 1975.
7. Popovtzer, M.M., Flis, R.S., and Blum, M.S.: The effect of calcium ionophore on renal handling of phosphorus. Kidney International. In press.
8. Nagata, N., and Rasmussen, H.: Parathyroid hormone, 3',5' AMP, Ca^{++} and renal gluconeogenesis. Proc. Natl. Acad. Sci. US 65: 368, 1970.
9. Biddulph, D.M., and Wrenn, R.W.: Effects of parathyroid hormone on cyclic AMP, cyclic GMP, and efflux of calcium in isolated renal tubules. J. Cyclic Nucleotide Res. 3: 129, 1977.
10. Harrison, E.E., and Harrison, H.C.: The renal excretion of inorganic phosphate in relation to the action of vitamin D and the parathyroid hormone, J. Clin. Invest. 20: 47, 1941.
11. Crawford, J.D., Gribetz, D. and Talbot, N.B.: Mechanism of renal tubular phosphate reabsorption and the influence thereon of vitamin D in completely parathyroidectomized rats. Am. J. Physiol 180: 156, 1955.
12. Ney, R.L., Kelly, G., and Bartter, F.C.: Actions of vitamin D independent of parathyroid glands. Endocrinology 82: 760, 1968.
13. Popovtzer, M.M., Robinette, J.B., DeLuca, H.F., and Holick, M.F.: The acute effect of 25-hydroxycholecalciferol on renal handling of phosphorus. J. Clin. Invest. 53: 913, 1974.
14. Lumb, G.A., and Stanbury, S.W.: Parathyroid function in human vitamin D deficiency and vitamin D deficiency in primary hyperparathyroidism. Am. J. Med. 56: 833, 1974.
15. Chertow, B.S., Baylink, D.J., Wergedal, J.E., Su, M.H.H., and Norman, A.W.: Decrease in serum immunoreactive parathyroid hormone in rats and in parathyroid hormone secretion in vitro by 1,25-dihydrocholecalciferol. J. Clin. Invest. 56: 668, 1975.
16. Popovtzer, M.M., and Robinette, J.B.: Unpublished observations.

17. Marx, S.J. Fedak, S.A., and Aurbach,G.D.: Preparation and characterization of a hormone-responsive renal plasma membrane fraction. J. Biol. Chem. 247: 6913, 1972.
18. Aurbach, G.D., and Heath, D.A.: Parathyroid hormone and calcitonin regulation of renal function. Kidney Int. 6: 331, 1974.
19. Kinne, R., Shlatz, L., Kinne-Safran, E., and Schwartz, I.L.: Distribution of membrane bound cyclic AMP-dependent protein Kinase in plasma membranes of cells of kidney cortex. J. Membrane Biol. 24: 145, 1975.
20. Mudge, G.H., William, O.B., and Valtin, H.: Tubular transport of urea, glucose, phosphate, uric acid, sulfate, and thiosulfate. In: Handbook of Physiology, Section 8, Renal Physiology. Editors: J. Orloff and R.W. Berliner. American Physiological Society, Washington, D.C. 1973. p 618.
21.Popovtzer, M.M., and Robinette, J.B.: Effect of 25(OH)vitaminD_3 on urinary excretion of cyclic adenosine monophosphate. Am. J. Physiol. 229: 907, 1975.
22. Kurokawa, K., Nagata, N., Sasaki, M., and Nakane, N.: Effects of calcitonin and parathyroid hormone and adenyl cyclase-cyclic AMP system in rat kidney. Endocrinology 94: 1514, 1974.
23. Popovtzer, M.M., Blum, M.S., and Flis, R.S.: Evidence for interference of 25(OH)vitaminD_3 with phosphaturic action of calcitonin. Am. J. Physiol. 232: 515, 1977.
24. Borle, A.B.: Calcium metabolism at the cellular level. Federation Proc. 32: 1944, 1973.
25. Hoffmann, N., Thees, M., and Kinne, R.: Phosphate transport by isolated renal brush border vesicles. Pflugers. Arch. 362: 147, 1976.
26. Egawa, J., and Neuman, W.F.: Effect of parathyroid extract on the metabolism of radioactive phosphate in Kidney. Endocrinology 74: 90, 1964.
27. Shirley, D.G., Poujeol, P., and LeGrimellec, C.: Phosphate, calcium, and magnesium fluxes into the lumen of the rat proximal convoluted tubule. Pflugers Arch. 362: 247, 1976.
28. Schneider, E.G., and McLane, L.A.: Evidence for a peritubular-to-luminal flux of phosphate in the dog Kidney. Am. J. Physiol. 232: 159, 1977.
29. Boulpaep, E.L.: Permeability changes of the proximal tubule of Necturus during saline loading. Am. J. Physiol. 222: 517, 1972.
30. Grandchamp, A., and Boulpaep, E.L.: Pressure control of sodium reabsorption and intercellular backflux across proximal kidney tubule. J. Clin. Invest. 54: 69, 1974.
31. Fromter, E., Muller, C.W., and Knauf, H.: Fixe negative Wandlaudungen im proximalen Konvolut der Rattenniere und ihre Beeinflussung durch Calciumionen in Vlth Symp der Ges f Nephrologie, edited by Watschinger B, Wien, Verlag der Wiener Med. Akademie, 1969, p 61.

MECHANISMS OF CELLULAR PHOSPHATE TRANSPORT IN RAT KIDNEY PROXIMAL TUBULE

K.J. Ullrich

Max-Planck-Institut für Biophysik

6000 Frankfurt/Main, Germany

This review is an extension of those which Knox et al. (1) and Kinne et al. (2) gave during the last year meeting on "Phosphate Metabolism" in Heidelberg. The data and discussion presented by them can be considered to be the starting point of the experiments which were performed during the past year and which I will present here.

Since more data are available on the P_i transport on cellular rather than on subcellular level I will briefly outline the respective method, namely that of the doubly perfused proximal tubule where the tubular lumen as well as the peritubular capillaries were perfused, and the change of luminal phosphate concentration relative to the capillary phosphate concentration was measured. The tubules were equilibrated with ^{32}P for 4 1/2 minutes so that the radioactivity measurements could be used instead of chemical phosphate determination. To evaluate rather small changes in phosphate transport and to eliminate the influence of tubular heterogeneity, the technique of crossed paired samples was applied. For this, control and test measurements were performed subsequently at the same tubule and in a second series the sequence was reversed, i.e. first the test and then the control measurement was performed. Furthermore, I will show you data from transport studies made by Evers et al. (3) with plasma membrane vesicles obtained from rat renal cortical slices by homogenization, and differential centrifugation in a calcium containing medium. Then I will mention data of Frömter et al. (4) on the intracellular electrical potential, when the phosphate and Na^+ concentration as well as the pH of the luminal perfusate was changed.

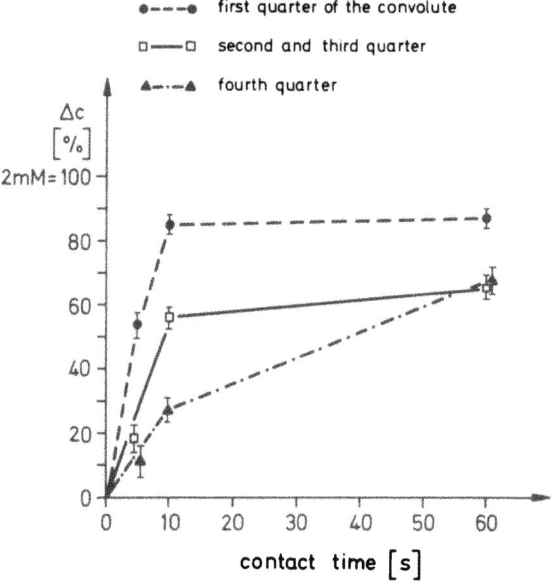

Figure 1. Phosphate transport as revealed by the transtubular P_i concentration differences (corrected for water fluxes) ± SE in the different segments of the proximal convolution at different contact times. Maximal possible Δc, i.e. the phosphate concentration in the capillary perfusate was 2 mM. The rats were chronically parathyroidectomized (Ullrich et al. 6).

Heterogeneity of the Proximal Convolution

In all local P_i transport studies we have to take into account the enormous heterogeneity of the proximal convolution as far as this transport system concerns (5,6). Figure 1 shows the increase of the transtubular concentration difference for phosphate which is caused by a decrease of the luminal concentration with time. The upper line is from the first quarter of the convolute, the line in the middle from the second and third quarter and the lower line from the last quarter. It can be seen that the reabsorption from the lumen is almost linear in the first 10 seconds and that the early part transports 4 times faster than in the late part.

Effect of PTH in Chronic and Acute Parathyroidectomized Rats

Figure 2 shows the effect of parathyroid hormone given intravenously to acute (>2 hr) and chronic (>2 days) parathyroidectomized rats. In acute PTX rats PTH reduces the P_i transport in the

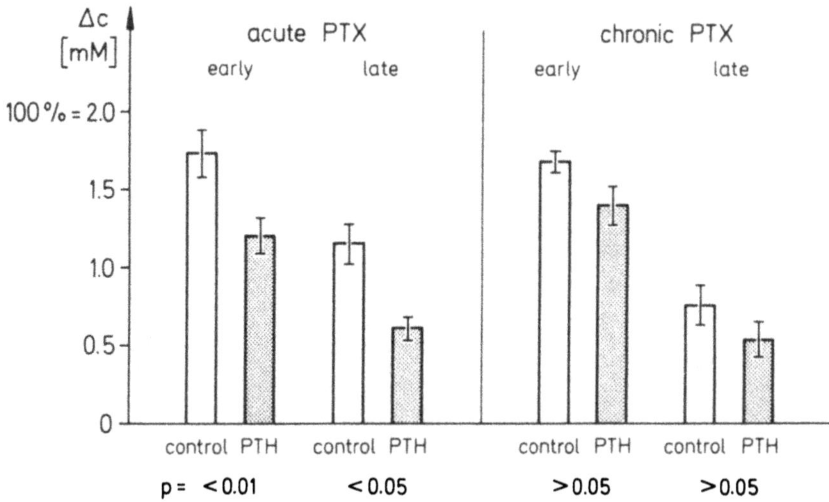

Figure 2. Effect of PTH on Δc (± SE) of phosphate on early and late proximal convolution of acute and chronic PTX rats. Contact time was 10 seconds (Ullrich et al. 6)

early and late proximal convolution by 30 and 40%. In the chronic PTX rats the changes are much smaller (about 20%). The same difference in the PTH response between acute and chronic PTX animals was also seen in free flow micropuncture in rats (7) and in dogs (8,9). Amiel et al. (10) suggested that the reduced plasma calcium level in chronic PTX rats compared with that of acute PTX animals would be at least partially responsible for this effect. It can, however, hardly be a direct effect of Ca^{++} on P_i transport, as the authors suppose, since the Ca^{++} concentration in our solutions was the same in all tests. Alternatively it might be that the different plasma Ca^{++} levels in the plasma of our experimental animals might have influenced the chain of events from PTH binding to inhibition of P_i transport. We were not able to test this hypothesis in the present experiments because PTH needs longer to act than the renal capillaries can be artificially perfused, so that we were forced to apply PTH to the whole animal, where it acted in the presence of either low or normal Ca^{++} levels. Cuche et al. (11) have indeed found in TPTX dogs that increasing the plasma calcium from the hypocalcemic level to the normal potentiates the phosphaturic effect of PTH. It is, however, also possible that other factors are responsible for the different response on PTH. Furthermore, it is not excluded that ectopic parathyroid tissue is already activated in the chronic parathyroidectomized rats.

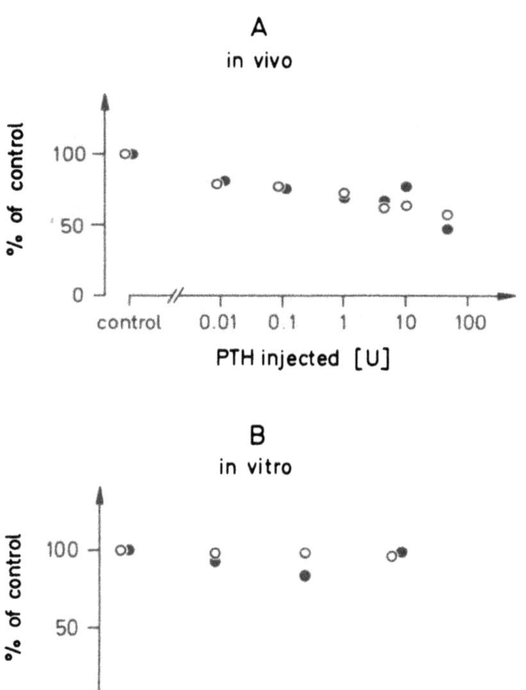

Figure 3. Effect of PTH on phosphate uptake by isolated brush border membrane vesicles, comparison of in vivo application (A) of PTH versus the effect of PTH on isolated membrane vesicles (in vitro B), shown in two characteristic experiments. Open circles represent phosphate uptake after 20 sec, closed dots uptake after one minute (Evers et al. 3).

At this place I want to show you data from Evers et al. (3) which indicate that the inhibition of the P_i transport, which is exerted by PTH, concerns the luminal transport step. As can be seen in Figure 3 the P_i transport into brush border vesicles is reduced up to 50%, when PTH was given 1 hr before sacrifice of normal animals, but not when it was added to the brush border vesicles directly.

Effect of Diet on Basal P_i Transport and PTH Effect

By using clearance techniques it was observed that the P_i content in the diet determines the P_i handling in the kidney and that this adaptation occurred also in PTX animals (12,13,14,15,16). We have now studied this adaptation in the proximal convolution (6). The Figure 4 shows the influence of the diet on phosphate reabsorption. This influence was so strong that in low P_i diet rats we had to reduce the exposure time to 5 sec, because during 10 sec exposure time the P_i transport seemed to reach already its steady state concentration. Thus, in the early and late proximal tubule the P_i reabsorption of rats on low P_i diet is approximately three times higher than with high P_i diet. If rats on high P_i diet are acutely parathyroidectomized their P_i transport rises in the early as well as in the late proximal convolution. But if PTH is given to rats on low P_i diet only the late parts of the convolution react. This finding might indicate that there are different secondary factors - as yet unknown - which modify the response of the tubular cell to PTH.

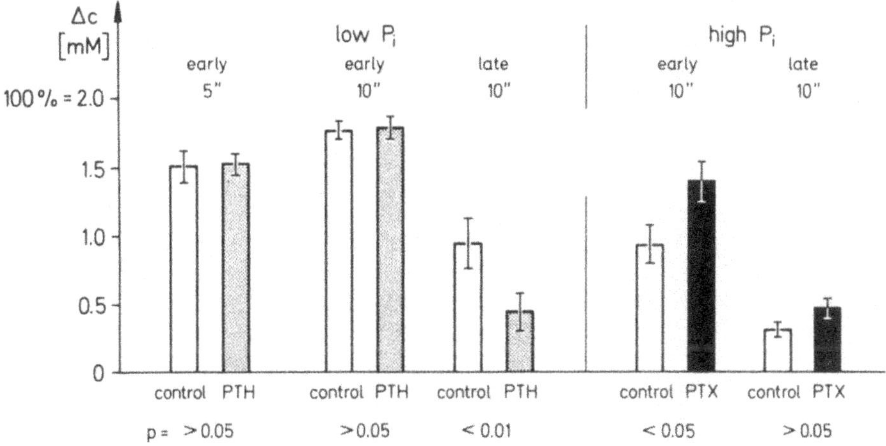

Figure 4. Effect of low (0.15%) and high (2%) phosphate diet on the phosphate transport (Δc ± SE) in the early and late proximal convolution of not parathyroidectomized rats. After the control period the rats on low P_i diet were infused with PTH, and the rats on high phosphate diet were acutely parathyroidectomized. Because the 10" values of rats on low P_i diet reached already the static head situation, the 5" values of this group have to be compared with the 10" values of the animals on high P_i diet (Ullrich et al. 6).

Na^+-P_i Cotransport in the Brush Border and its pH Dependence

In studies with brush border vesicles, which Kinne et al. (2) presented last year at the phosphate meeting in Heidelberg, it was shown that it is the electrochemical gradient for Na^+ ions which provides the driving force for P_i transport through the brush border membrane. With potassium in the incubation medium little difference in P_i uptake into the vesicles was seen, whether a gradient is present or not. With sodium, but in the absence of a gradient, the initial rate of uptake was 4 times higher than in the presence of potassium. This could be interpreted as Na^+ interacting with the phosphate transport system. But when a sodium gradient was present a typical overshoot of P_i uptake occurred. This is a clear sign that the Na^+ gradient provides the driving force for P_i transport. As shown in Figure 5, which is taken from Hoffmann et al. (18), the initial rate of phosphate increased in a characteristic way, when the Na^+ concentration in the incubation medium was increased. Furthermore, the transport was much higher when the incubation medium was alkaline, upper curve with pH of 8.0, than when it was more acid, medium curve with pH 7.4 or lower curve with pH 6.0. The fact that the curves are sigmoidal indicates that more than one sodium ion is accompanying one phosphate ion. A reciprocal plot 1/v against $1/Na^{+2}$ gave straight lines for all pH values. Thus, Hoffmann et al. (18) suggested that 2 sodium ions are transported in cotransport with one phosphate and that the alkaline form is preferentially transported under the conditions prevailing in the transport studies with vesicles. If both forms of the phosphate buffer, primary as well as secondary phosphate, are transported with 2 sodium ions, then the primary phosphate $H_2PO_4^- + 2Na^+$ should be positively charged and its transport should be electrogenic, while the secondary phosphate $HPO_4^{--} + 2Na^+$ ion should be electroneutral. This is indeed the case, as electrophysiological studies of Frömter et al. (4) revealed. If the tubular lumen is perfused with phosphate buffer plus sodium ions the tubular cells are depolarized, when the solution has an acid pH, but not when its pH is alkaline. Thus, the driving force for primary $H_2PO_4^-$ must be the electrochemical gradient for Na^+, but for secondary HPO_4^{--} it is only the chemical gradient for Na^+ ions. In the tubular cell in situ with the cell inside negativity of -70 mV the driving force for primary phosphate is therefore always greater than for secondary phosphate. Since, however, the pd in the experiments of Hoffmann et al. (18) with the brush border vesicles was not monitored, it is not known, whether the lower flux rates of primary phosphate are due to an increase of a vesicle inside more positive potential or to a lower permeability of the cell wall for that P_i buffer species. Clearly more work has to be done on that point. The data, however, show already the complex nature of pH changes on P_i transport (see 1).

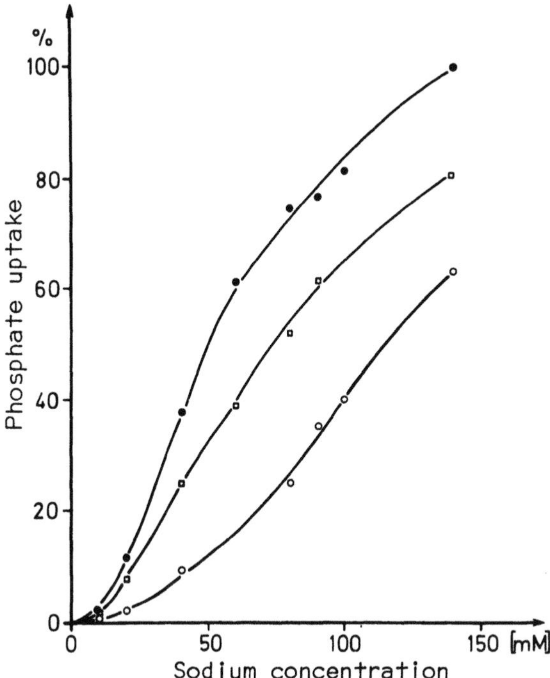

Figure 5. Phosphate uptake by isolated renal brush border vesicles. Influence of the Na^+ and H^+ ion concentration in the medium. Upper curve with pH 8.0, medium curve with pH 7.4 and lower curve with pH 6.0 (Hoffmann et al. 18).

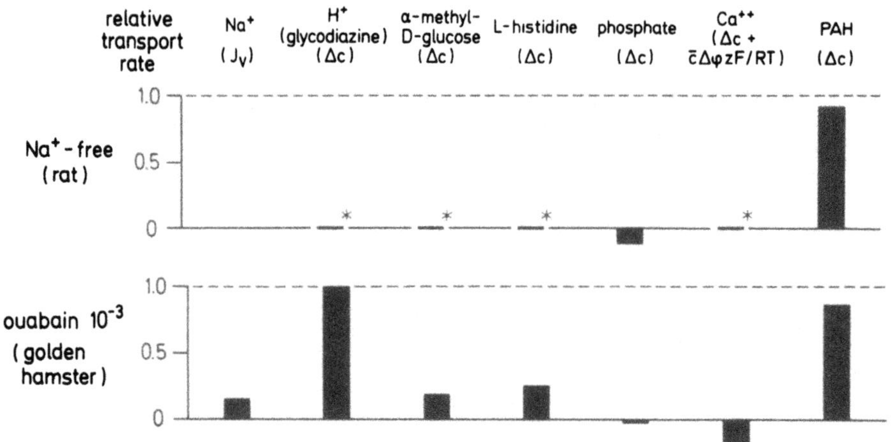

Figure 6. Effect of Na^+-free solutions and ouabain on the phosphate and other solute transport rates in the proximal convolution of the rat kidney. The values with asterisks are extrapolated. (Ullrich et al. 19, and from other papers).

Now I will show you some data gained with the method of doubly perfused tubules, which also document the role of Na^+ in P_i transport (19). When the transport experiments are performed with Na^+-free solutions, all Na^+-dependent transport processes vanish, except that of PAH (Figure 6). When in another set of experiments ouabain is given the same pattern is observed except for H^+ ions. Thus we can say, the active transport of phosphate, as well as that of Ca^{++}, amino acids, glucose is driven by the sodium gradient. The active transport of H^+ ions, however, is not driven by the Na^+ gradient, although it is apparently Na^+-dependent. (For the discussion of the latter phenomenon see Lit. 19).

Interrelationship of Proximal P_i Transport with Other Transport Processes

Pitts and Alexander (20) observed in 1944 that elevation of plasma glucose resulted in a depression of P_i reabsorption. Recently, de Rouffignac et al. (21) showed the same phenomenon by P_i tracer injection in the proximal tubule. The most probable explanation for the mutual interaction of P_i and glucose reabsorption is a competition for the common driving force, namely the electrochemical potential difference for Na^+ ions across the luminal cell membrane. This type of interaction was first revealed by Murer et al. (17) for mutual inhibition of glucose and amino acid transport in intestinal brush border vesicles.

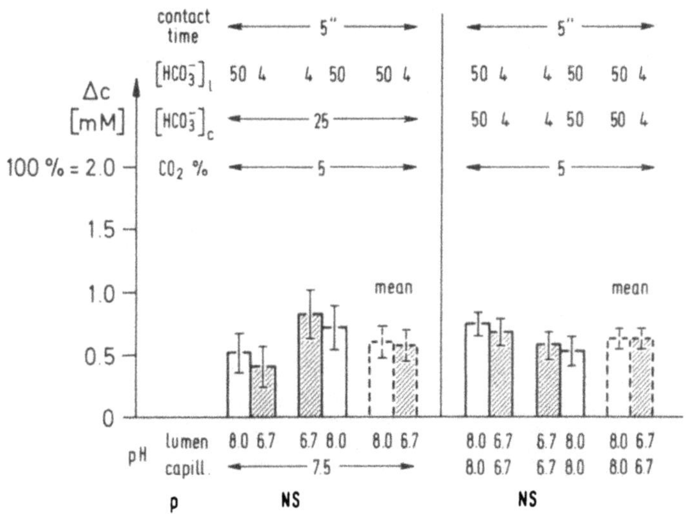

Figure 7. Lacking effect of pH changes in the perfusates on proximal phosphate reabsorption, as evaluated by the method of crossed paired samples (see introduction). The second samples on the same places show always a somewhat lower transtubular concentration difference. The reason for that is likely to be an increased backleak of the tubule for P_i (see Fig.9). The means contain all values with the same pH, independent of the sequence within the experiment. The reason that the absolute values in each paired group are different comes from the different proportion from the early and late proximal segment (Ullrich et al. 23).

More complicated interactions seem to exist between proximal P_i transport and proximal buffer reabsorption or H^+ secretion respectively. In an earlier paper (22) we have shown that tubular bicarbonate reabsorption - or H^+ secretion - rises linearly with the luminal bicarbonate concentration. If we, however, change the luminal or both, luminal and peritubular HCO_3^--concentrations from 4 to 50 mM and consequently the pH from 6.7 to 8.0, the transtubular P_i transport remains unchanged (23, Fig.7). Furthermore, when the HCO_3^- (or glycodiazine) buffer is completely omitted the P_i transport is reduced as is the transport of H^+ ions

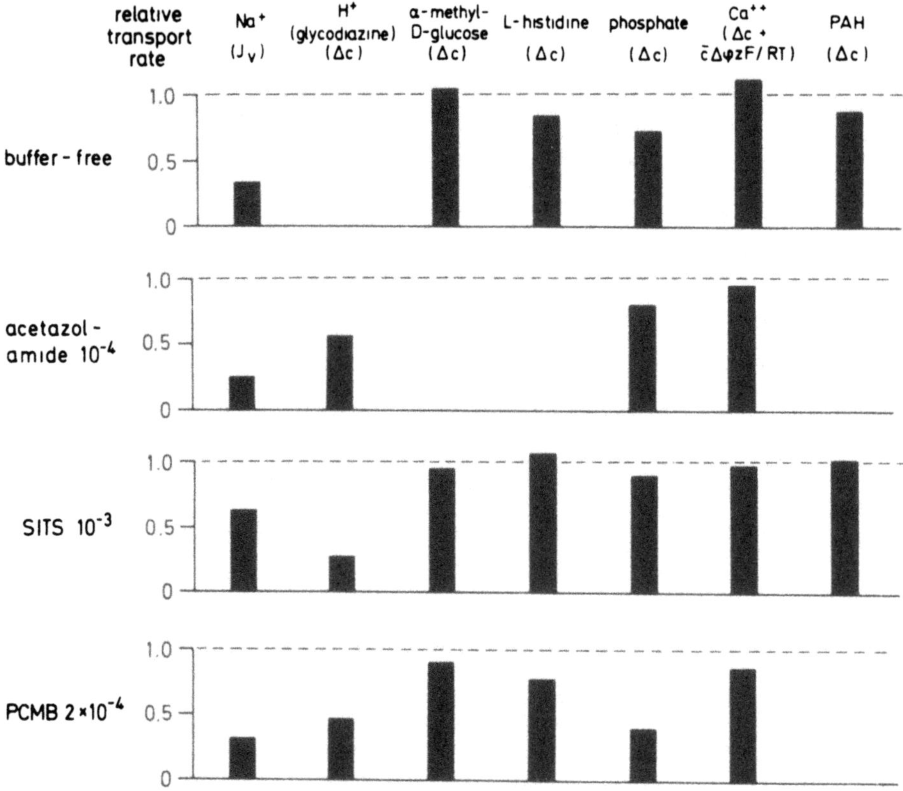

Figure 8. Pattern of the proximal transport rates, the P_i transport included, when the solutions contain no HCO_3^-- or glycodiazine buffer, when acetazolamide, SITS and pCMB is given (Ullrich et al. 19, and from other papers).

and that of Na^+ (Fig. 8). All other Na^+ coupled transport processes remain unchanged. A similar pattern of inhibition is seen when acetazolamide is given. The Na^+, H^+ and P_i transport is also reduced after pCMB. When the specific blocker of the chloride channel in the red cells, SITS, is given from the peritubular cell side the H^+ transport is primarily affected, the effect on Na^+ transport is smaller and that on P_i transport is almost missing (19). In all cases we do not know for certain what the single steps are, through which the P_i transport is inhibited. The possible ways can be seen from the summarizing Table.

Local Effect of Ca^{++} on P_i Absorption

The local effect of Ca^{++} ions on the P_i reabsorption was tested in chronic PTX rats (23). When the ionophore A23187 was added to the perfusate the P_i transport in the early as well as in the late part of the proximal convolution was not changed (Fig. 9), but when the solutions were changed from 1.5 mM to zero Ca^{++} about 20% inhibition of the net P_i transport was seen. This is, however, as we originally suspected, not due to an increased paracellular back flux of P_i . The influx of P_i from the peritubular cell side into the tubular lumen is not augmented but rather diminished, when Ca^{++} was omitted. Thus, we may conclude that Ca^{++} has a direct stimulatory effect on the P_i transport. I should mention that the effect of Ca^{++} on the paracellular P_i flux coincides nicely with that on the paracellular Cl^--flux, as was seen in electrical measurements made by Frömter (24).

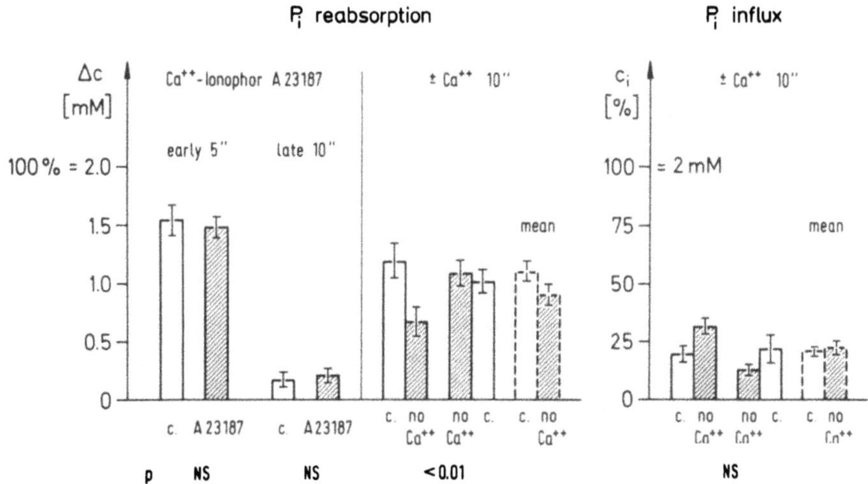

Figure 9. Effect of Ca^{++} on proximal P_i transport: the first two series show the effect of the Ca^{++} ionophore A23187 and of omission of calcium in the reabsorption of P_i. The last series shows the effect of omission of Ca^{++} on the P_i influx into the tubular lumen. In the latter case the luminal perfusate contained no Ca^{++} at time zero. In series 2 and 3 the method of crossed paired samples were applied. As in Fig. 7 the means contain all values with the same Ca^{++} concentration irrespective of the sequence within the experiment. Since all P_i influx studies are made on the late proximal tubule the differences between the groups seem to be significant. (Ullrich et al. 23).

TABLE

Factors which influence transtubular P_i transport

1. Influence on the transport machinery itself
   a. luminal:
      PTH, cAMP, diet.
      Not yet clarified: Heterogeneity, pH, Ca^{++}, pCMB.
   b. contraluminal:
      Not yet determined

2. Influence on the driving forces:
      Ouabain, omission of Na^+, other Na^+ driven substrates like glucose.
      Not yet clarified: pCMB.

3. Influence on the concentration of substrate
      ($HPO_4^{--}/H_2PO_4^-$ ratio): pH changes.

4. Combination of 2 and 3:
      Not yet clarified: Omission of HCO_3^- or similar buffer, acetazolamide

For summary I may refer to the Table where the factors, which influence the proximal P_i transport, are subdivided in those which 1. influence the transport machinery in the luminal and contraluminal cell membrane itself, included the shunt pathway, 2. change the driving forces and 3. change the concentration of the substrate, i.e. primary to secondary phosphate and vice versa. Since I have also included the not yet cleared points of attack of some substances the Table may serve as a check list for further experimental work.

REFERENCES

1. Knox, F.G., Greger, R.F., Lang, F.C., Marchand, G.R.: Renal handling of phosphate: Update: in Phosphate Metabolism. Eds. S.G. Massry and E. Ritz. Advances in Experimental Medicine and Biology, 81: 3-14, 1977. Plenum Press, New York

2. Kinne, R., Berner, W., Hoffmann, N., Murer, H.: Phosphate transport by isolated renal and intestinal plasma membranes. Update: in Phosphate Metabolism. Eds. S.G. Massry and E. Ritz. Advances in Experimental Medicine and Biology 81:265, 1977. Plenum Press New York.

3. Evers, C., Murer, H., Kinne, R.: Effect of parathyroid hormone on the transport properties of isolated renal brush border vesicles. J. Membr. Biol., in press

4. Frömter, E., Samarzija, I., Gessner, K.: Electrical analysis of Na^+-dependent cotransport systems in rat kidney proximal tubule. Proc. II. Europ. Coll. Renal Physiol. Balatonfüred 1977, Abstr. 28.

5. Baumann, K., de Rouffignac, C., Roinel, N., Rumrich, G., Ullrich, K.J.: Renal phosphate transport: Inhomogeneity of local transport rates and sodium dependence. Pflügers Arch. 356:287, 1975.

6. Ullrich, K.J., Rumrich, G., Klöss, S.: Phosphate transport in the proximal convolution of the rat kidney . I. Tubular heterogeneity, effect of parathyroid hormone in acute and chronic parathyroidectomized animals and effect of phosphate diet. Pflügers Arch., in press.

7. Kuntzinger, H., Amiel, C., Cailla, H., Delaage, M.: Effect of parathyroidectomy on renal tubular transport of cAMP and phosphate. Abstr. 26th Int. Congress Physiol. Paris 1977.

8. Knox, F.G., Lechene, C.P.: Effect of parathyroid hormone on distal phosphate reabsorption in the dog. Kidney Int. A 60, 1974.

9. Knox, F.G., Lechene, C.P.: Distal site of action of parathyroid hormone on phosphate reabsorption. Amer. J. Physiol. 229:1556, 1975.

10. Amiel., C., Kuntzinger, H., Couette, S., Coureau, C., Bergounioux, N.: Evidence for a parathyroid hormone-independent calcium modulation of phosphate transport along the nephron. J. clin. Invest. 57:256, 1976.

11. Cuche, J.L., Ott, C.E., Marchand, G.R., Diaz-Buxo, J.A., Knox, F.G.: Intrarenal calcium in phosphate handling. Amer. J. Physiol. 230:790, 1976.

12. McIntosh, G.H., Scott, D.: Renal regulation of phosphate excretion in the pig. Quartl. J. Exp. Physiol. 60:299, 1975.

13. Steele, T.H., DeLuca, H.F.: Influence of dietary phosphorus on renal phosphate reabsorption in the parathyroidectomized rat. J. clin Invest. 57:867, 1976.

14. Steele, T.H.: Renal resistance to parathyroid hormone during phosphorus deprivation. J. clin. Invest. 58:1461, 1976.

15. Tröhler, U., Bonjour, J.P., Fleisch, H.: Renal tubular adaptation to dietary phosphorus. Nature 261:145, 1976.

16. Tröhler, U., Bonjour, J.P., Fleisch, H.: Inorganic phosphate homeostasis: Renal adaptation to the dietary intake in intact and thyroparathyroidectomized rats. J. clin. Invest. 57:264, 1976.

17. Murer, H., Sigrist-Nelson, K., Hopfer, U.: Mechanism of sugar and amino acid interaction in intestinal transport. J. Biol. Chem. 250:7392, 1976.

18. Hoffmann, N., Thees, M., Kinne, R.: Phosphate transport by isolated renal brush border vesicles. Pflügers Arch. 362:147, 1976.

19. Ullrich, K.J., Rumrich, G., Klöss, S.: Coupling between proximal tubular transport processes: Studies with ouabain, SITS, and HCO_3^--free solutions. Pflügers Arch. 368:245, 1977.

20. Pitts, R.F., Alexander, R.S.: The renal reabsorptive mechanism for inorganic phosphate in normal and acidolic dogs. Amer. J. Physiol. 142:648, 1944.

21. De Rouffignac, C., Touvay, C., Poujeol, P., Corman, B.: Influence of glucose on renal reabsorption of phosphate in the rat. 27th Int. Congr. Physiol. Paris 1977, Abstr.

22. Ullrich, K.J., Radtke, H.W., Rumrich, G.: The role of bicarbonate and other buffers on isotonic fluid absorption in the proximal convolution of the rat kidney. Pflügers Arch. 330:149, 1971.

23. Ullrich, K.J., Rumrich, G., Klöss, S.: Phosphate transport in the proximal convolution of the rat kidney. II. Effect of pH, acetazolamide and calcium. Pflüger Arch., in preparation.

24. Frömter, E.: Passive transport properties of rat proximal tubule, in **Electrophysiology of the Nephron.** Satell. Symposium to the 27th Congr. of Physiol. Paris 1977.

RENAL TUBULAR TRANSPORT OF CALCIUM: UPDATE

Zalman S. Agus

University of Pennsylvania School of Medicine

Philadelphia, Pennsylvania, U.S.A.

Early studies of calcium transport emphasized the striking similarity between the renal handling of calcium and of sodium (1) and pioneering micropuncture studies suggested that calcium transport occurred throughout the nephron paralleling sodium (2,3). More recently, sophisticated studies by a number of investigators have allowed us to begin to dissect out various segments of the nephron in an attempt to define the site of action of the factors which regulate the urinary excretion of calcium. These studies have allowed the development of a concept of calcium transport which emphasizes the importance of the distal portions of the nephron in the determination of calcium excretion. In this review, I will discuss transport in the various segments of the nephron but because of time limitations, I will be able to emphasize only some of the recently studied important issues.

Micropuncture studies have now verified that about 60% of the total plasma calcium is ultrafiltered across the glomerulus (4,5). In the proximal tubule, about 55% of this filtered load is reabsorbed. The ratio of tubular fluid to ultrafiltrable calcium in a variety of studies is persistently greater than one (6). This value is consistent with a passive transport mechanism which would be dependent upon sodium and water reabsorption and many investigators have documented a parallelism in the proximal tubule (6). Recently, Ullrich et al (7) were able to evaluate directly the contribution of an active calcium transport mechanism in the proximal tubule of the rat (figure 1). Using stop flow microperfusion in combination with simultaneous perfusion of the peritubular capillaries, they arrived at an active transport rate of 3.4×10^{-13} mol/cm/second as shown by the solid bar. This represents approximately 20% of the total calcium reabsorptive rate as measured in-

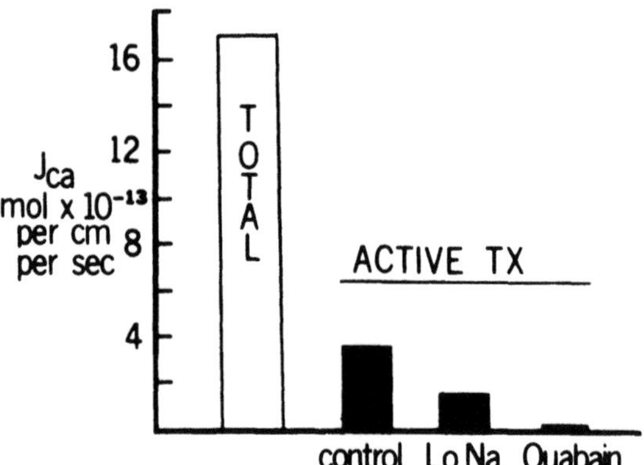

Figure 1. Calcium reabsorption (J Ca^{++}) in the proximal tubule of the rat. The open bar represents total net calcium reabsorption as measured by free flow micropuncture. Solid bars represent active calcium reabsorption measured during stop flow microperfusion with measurement of zero net flux transtubular concentration difference. Lo Na represents data obtained when sodium was removed from the perfusion solution. Data adapted from Ullrich et al (7).

dependently by free-flow micropuncture shown by the open bar. They also found that removal of sodium from the perfusion solution (labelled Lo Na in figure 1) or inhibition of sodium transport with ouabain virtually abolished the active component of calcium transport. They suggested therefore that the bulk of calcium transport in the proximal tubule is accounted for by passive forces and is sodium dependent. The smaller component of active transport seems also to be linked to sodium transport possibly via an ATPase system. The original parallelism noted between sodium and calcium handling by the kidney, therefore seems to be characteristic of the proximal tubule and with a few exceptions, multiple studies have been unable to demonstrate a dissociation between these ions at this site.

Some of the exceptions to this rule include calcium and sulfate infusion and possibly parathyroidectomy. The ratio of

TF/UF calcium has been observed to increase with infusion of calcium (8,9) and sulfate (10) and it seems likely that this is related to an increase in the fraction of calcium which is complexed in the glomerular filtrate and may not be available for reabsorption. Some studies have suggested that alterations in parathyroid hormone may selectively alter calcium reabsorption in this segment. Kuntziger and Amiel found a very high TF/UF calcium in acutely parathyroidectomized rats which fell with DBCAMP (11). Harris et al (12) found a fall in proximal TF/P calcium with PTH administration to acutely parathyroidectomized hamsters. The meaning of these observations is unclear and in our laboratory we have found no change in proximal TF/UF calcium in either the acutely parathyroidectomized dog (13) or rat (14). In any case, as we shall discuss shortly, current data suggest that the effect of PTH on urinary calcium excretion is due principally to an effect upon the terminal nephron.

As a general rule therefore, I think it is still reasonable to consider the proximal tubule as a site where under usual conditions, sodium and calcium transport are parallel and possibly linked.

Calcium transport in the pars recta has not been studied directly as yet. Studies by Jamison et al in the rat (15) and de Rouffignac et al in Psammomys (16) suggested that transport of sodium and calcium may not be parallel between the end of the convoluted proximal tubule and the ascending limb. Both groups of investigators found that the TF/UF calcium at the papillary tip was significantly lower than the TF/P Na in contrast to the proximal tubule where the reverse obtains. These data and the reversal of this pattern with furosemide suggest a major dissociation between calcium and sodium reabsorption in either the descending limb or the pars recta. More recently, calcium transport has been studied directly in the various segments of the loop with in vitro microperfusion. In the thin descending limb, Rocha et al (17) found a very low permeability coefficient to calcium from both bath to lumen and lumen to bath. When an osmotic gradient was imposed to simulate in vivo conditions of osmotic water extraction (figure 2), the rise in the volume marker, in this case iothalamate, was associated with an identical rise in the Ca^{45} ratio. Thus there was no significant efflux of calcium despite net water abstraction. Similarly in the thin ascending limb there was no evidence of net calcium transport.

In contrast however, the thick ascending limb was able to generate a calcium lumen to bath concentration gradient in the absence of water movement. The calculated <u>net</u> calcium reabsorption of approximately 10 peq/cm/min in this segment compares favorably with that which would be predicted from free flow micropuncture experiments. The observed flux ratio however was signi-

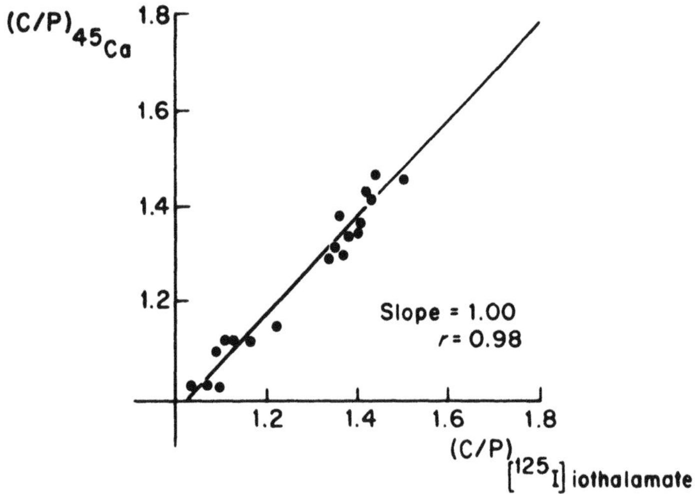

Figure 2. Correlation between fractional increase in calcium concentration to fractional increase in volume marker in the thin descending limb of Henle's loop during an imposed osmotic gradient. From Rocha et al (17).

ficantly greater than that predicted by the Ussing equation. The effects of the addition of ouabain are shown in figure 3. Addition of ouabain significantly reduced the potential difference by 67%. Despite this change and the associated inhibition of sodium and chloride transport calcium outflux only fell slightly by 21%. Taken together then these data suggest that the lumen positive PD is not the driving force for calcium reabsorption in this segment and that calcium transport across the TALH is by some mechanism other than simple diffusion. If these data are correct, and they need to be documented by further studies, then taken in conjunction with previous data including those of Jamison we could depict calcium transport up to the early distal tubule as follows.

Approximately 55% of the filtered load of calcium is reabsorbed in the proximal tubule. Within the pars recta, it is possible that another 10% is transported and this fraction seems to be inhibitable by furosemide. There is no transport in either the thin descending or ascending limb of the loop of Henle.

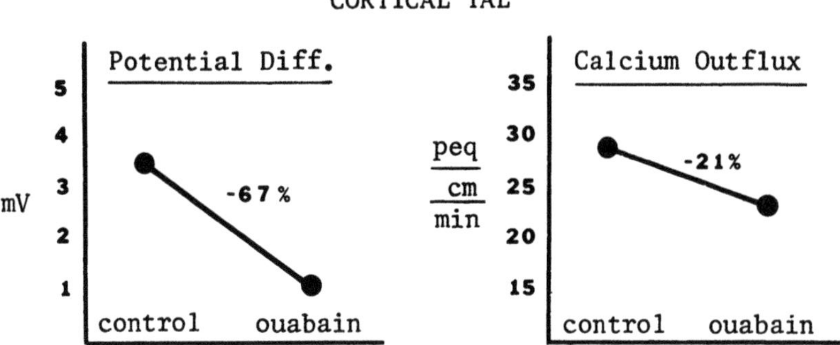

Figure 3. Effect of ouabain on potential difference and calcium outflux in the thick ascending limb of Henle's loop. Data adapted from Rocha et al(17).

Approximately 20% of the filtered load of calcium is reabsorbed in the thick ascending limb. The mechanism of transport is not clear but preliminary data suggest that it may be active transport independent of chloride transport. We presume that transport in this segment is also inhibited by furosemide based upon previous micropuncture studies but this has not been verified directly as yet.

The segment of the nephron beyond the loop of Henle although accounting for reabsorption of less than 10% of the filtered load seems to be the major site responsible for the regulation of urinary calcium excretion. In the distal tubule of the rat, Costanzo and Windhager have been able to demonstrate active calcium reabsorption (18). More recently, they have also been able to demonstrate an enhancement of both fractional and absolute calcium reabsorption along the length of the distal tubule with thiazide administration (19). These data differ from the effects of PTH and lend further support to the concept that thiazide has direct effects on calcium reabsorption independent of PTH. In an earlier study (21), we had shown that parathyroid hormone in the dog produced an inhibition of proximal tubular reabsorption of calcium as well as sodium and phosphate. As urinary calcium excretion fell despite the increased delivery from the proximal tubule, the data suggested that the hypocalciuric effect of PTH was beyond the proximal tubule in some segment of the distal nephron. The more terminal portions of the nephron, i.e. the late distal tubule and collecting duct however, seem to be the site of final modulation of urinary calcium excretion. Recent studies evaluating the effects of metabolic acidosis, parathyroid hormone and chronic phosphate depletion have in common the fact that while changes may be observed within distal tubule samples, virtually all studies indicate major effects beyond the late distal tubule. Examples of these types of studies are data we have obtained in the rat attempting to localize the site of the increased calcium excretion observed with saline loading and thyroparathyroidectomy (14).

Saline loading in intact rats produced a natriuresis of 3.3% and a calciuria of 1.8% compared to 0.14% sodium excretion and 0.2% calcium excretion in non-diuretic controls. Superimposition of thyroparathyroidectomy had no further effect upon sodium excretion but markedly increased calcium excretion to 5.5%. Figure 4 demonstrates the fraction of the filtered load of sodium and of calcium remaining in the late distal tubule in the non-diuretic and saline loaded intact rats. Despite differences in delivery out of the proximal tubule, as shown by the thin lines, there was no difference between the two groups in the amount of sodium or calcium remaining in the late distal tubule. The increased sodium and calcium excretion with saline loading therefore must have been due to inhibition of transport in the terminal nephron. In figure 5, we have depicted the fraction of the load delivered to the terminal nephron which was reabsorbed there. Saline loading significantly reduced reabsorption of both sodium and calcium in this segment. Superimposition of thyroparathyroidectomy upon saline loading had no effect upon sodium transport in this segment but calcium transport was virtually abolished. We therefore concluded that the terminal nephron is the major site of action of parathyroid hormone and further is the most important site in the final regulation of urinary calcium excretion.

Sutton et al in the dog (20) and Harris et al in the hamster (12) have also presented similar data and there seems to be general agreement that a major action of parathyroid hormone is enhancement of calcium reabsorption in the terminal segments of the nephron. These data of course assume nephron homogeneity and more direct studies of these segments are necessary before we can be sure. There is a great deal of evidence that the proximal and phosphaturic effects of PTH are mediated by generation of CAMP, but the evidence that this was also true for enhancement of calcium reabsorption was less definite. Thus neither Kuntziger in the rat (11) nor we in the dog (21) were able to demonstrate a fall in urinary calcium excretion with cyclic AMP or DBCAMP infusion. Recently however Burnatowska et al presented data demonstrating a marked reduction in fractional calcium excretion with

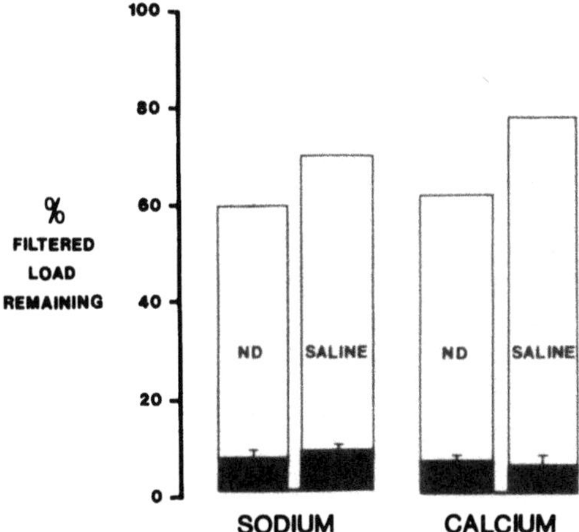

Figure 4. Fraction of the filtered load of sodium and of calcium remaining in the late distal tubule in non-diuretic and saline loaded intact rats. Delivery out of the proximal tubule is indicated by thin lines. From Agus et al (14).

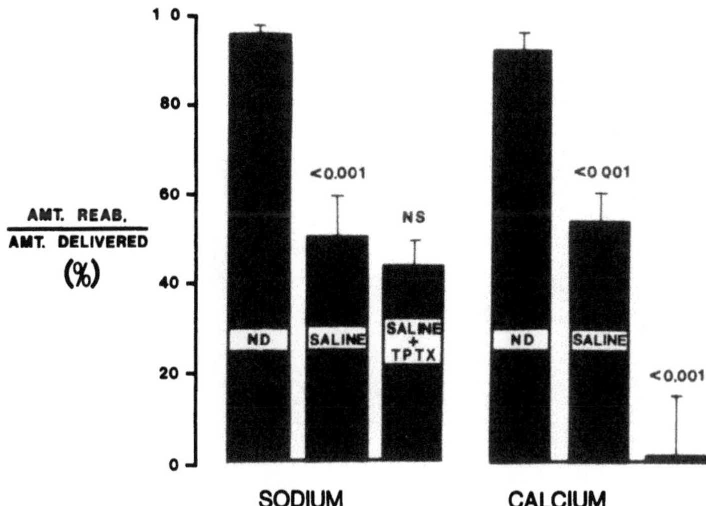

Figure 5. Fraction of the load of sodium and calcium delivered to the terminal nephron which is reabsorbed there in non-diuretic (ND), saline loaded, and thyroparathyroidectomized saline loaded rats. From Agus et al (14).

CAMP and DBCAMP infusion in the acutely TPTX hamster (22). These data and previously published data by Chabardes (23) are consistent with mediation of the hypocalciuric effects of PTH in the terminal nephron by CAMP.

The hypercalciuria of chronic phosphate depletion has been the subject of intense study and more data will be presented at this meeting. The two questions that have been evaluated are first the site of altered calcium transport and secondly, the role of PTH suppression. In the dog, we have demonstrated inhibition of proximal tubular reabsorption of sodium and calcium with phosphate depletion (13), as shown in figure 6. Acute infusion of phosphate (figure 7), in thyroparathyroidectomized dogs, markedly reduced calcium excretion to normal levels but the proximal tubular defect was unchanged. These data suggest that although calcium reabsorption may be inhibited in the proximal and distal portion of the nephron, it is the distal nephron which is responsible for the hypercalciuria. Quamme et al (24) also found impaired calcium reabsorption in both proximal and distal segments of the nephron in the dog and suggested that a major effect of phosphate infusion was to enhance calcium reabsorption beyond the distal puncture site, presumably the terminal nephron.

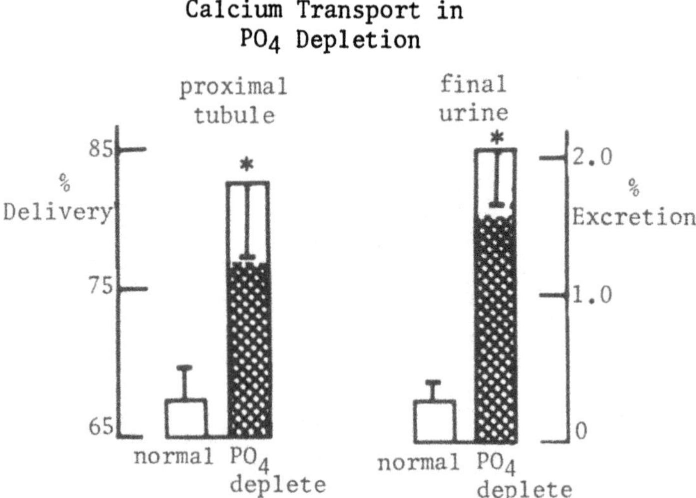

Figure 6. Effect of chronic phosphate depletion on calcium delivery from the proximal tubule and calcium excretion in the final urine. From Goldfarb et al (13).

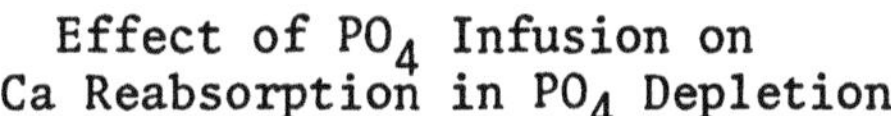

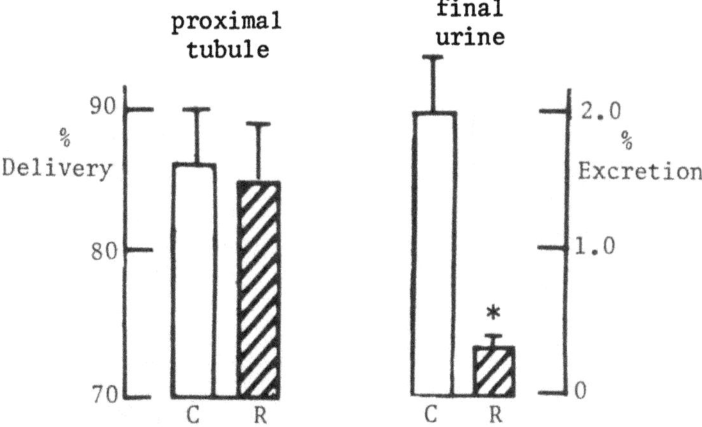

Figure 7. Effect of phosphate infusion on calcium delivery from the proximal tubule and calcium excretion in the final urine. C = control collections in phosphate depleted dogs prior to phosphate infusion. R = recollection after phosphate infusion. From Goldfarb et al (13).

The second question, i.e. the role of PTH, is more difficult to answer. It is clear that phosphate administration to TPTX PO_4 depleted dogs will correct the hypercalciuria. PO_4 administration alone however is an anticalciuric maneuver and its effects in phosphate depletion may therefore be non-specific. Possibly more to the point is the fact that three groups of investigators - ourselves (13), Quamme et al (24) and Coburn and Massry (25) have been unable to completely correct the hypercalciuria of the phosphate depleted dog with acute intravenous PTH administration. We have also evaluated the effect of subacute intraperitoneal PTH administration in phosphate depleted rats (26). Administration of PTE 3-10 units IP q8h for 24 hours, a dose which will raise the serum calcium by 0.2 mEq/L, significantly lowered calcium excretion in the TPTX PO_4 depleted animals to levels comparable to those obtained in intact PO_4 depleted animals receiving only the vehicle. Both groups however remained significantly calciuric when compared to normal controls. Thus, while not conclusive, I believe the data indicate that at least part of the defect in terminal nephron calcium transport in phosphate depletion is not explained by PTH suppression.

Figure 8 represents a summary of the current data concerning tubular calcium transport. As some of the data is preliminary and some unconfirmed this figure should be considered as a tentative proposal. The proximal tubule where 50-60% of the filtered load is reabsorbed continues to be a site where there is a strong link between sodium and calcium transport, with few exceptions, principally increased complex formation such as with sulfate or in hypercalcemia.

There is now indirect, and I emphasize indirect, data to suggest that up to 10% of the filtered load of calcium may be transported in the pars recta and that possibly there is a sodium-calcium dissociation at this site.

The first data from isolated tubule perfusion suggests virtually no calcium transport in the descending limb or thin ascending limb of the loop of Henle. Active calcium transport possibly distinct from chloride transport occurs in the thick ascending limb of the cortex where approximately 20% of the filtered load is reabsorbed. There is adenylate cyclase activity in this segment (23) and some data suggests that PTH may enhance calcium transport in this segment although this is not the major site of action of PTH on calcium transport.

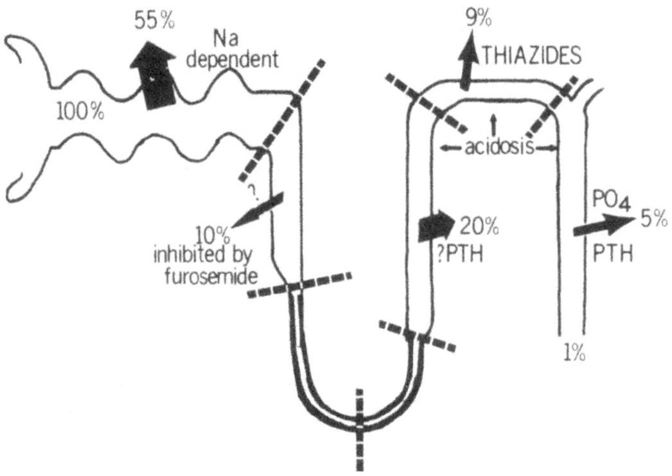

Figure 8. Segmental calcium reabsorption. See text.

Active calcium transport seems to take place in the distal tubule as well with reabsorption of up to 10% of the filtered load. Thiazides are able to dissociate sodium and calcium transport with inhibition of sodium and enhancement of calcium reabsorption.

The terminal nephron, that is the late distal tubule and the collecting system while responsible for reabsorption of only 5-6% of the filtered calcium load, seems to be the major site for the final regulation of urinary calcium excretion. Current data suggests that these segments are the major site of action of parathyroid hormone, and are responsible for the alterations in calcium excretion observed with metabolic acidosis and chronic phosphate depletion.

In studies by Sutton (27,28), the source of the calciuria in chronic metabolic acidosis appears to be within the distal nephron. Correction with intravenous sodium bicarbonate was associated with increased reabsorption beyond the distal puncture site. Thus although there are influences in the early portions of the nephron, similar to phosphate depletion, it appears that the terminal nephron is the important regulator of urinary calcium excretion in chronic metabolic acidosis.

It is unfortunate that a major site of regulation of calcium excretion is inaccessible to micropuncture and consequently, the bulk of this data is dependent upon observed differences between late distal tubule and final urine. Hopefully, in the next several years, we will see more direct data from perfusion of isolated collecting tubules.

Finally, the other aspect of calcium transport that we have not yet begun to unravel is the nature of the mechanism of transport and the manner in which these various factors alter net calcium reabsorption. Hopefully, with the advent of isolated tubular perfusion and electron probe microanalysis applied to intracellular events we will be able to evaluate some of these problems directly.

Acknowledgements

I should like to thank Dr. Martin Goldberg and the following colleagues who performed the experiments from our laboratory summarized in this paper. Drs. Stanley Goldfarb, Peter J.S. Chiu, Morris Grabie, Kai Lau, Randy Westby and Ms. Dorothy Senesky. This work was supported by research grants HL-00340 and AM-19478 and a Research Career Development Award, 1-K04-AM00258 from the National Institutes of Health.

REFERENCES

1. Walser, M. Calcium clearance as a function of sodium clearance in the dog. Am. J. Physiol. 200: 1099, 1961.
2. Lassiter, W.E., Gottschalk, C.W., and Mylle, M.: Micropuncture study of renal tubular reabsorption of calcium in normal rodents. Am. J. Physiol. 204: 771, 1963.
3. Duarte, C.G. and Watson, J.F.: Calcium reabsorption in proximal tubule of the dog nephron. Am. J. Physiol. 212: 355, 1967.
4. Harris, C.A., Baer, P.G., Chirito, E., and Dirks, J.H.: Composition of mammalian glomerular filtrate. Am. J. Physiol. 227: 972, 1974.
5. LeGrimellec, C., Poujeol, P., and de Rouffignac, C.: ^{3}H-Inulin and electrolyte concentrations in Bowman's capsule in rat kidney. Pflug. Arch. 354: 117, 1975.
6. Goldberg, M., Agus, Z.S., and Goldfarb, S.: Renal handling of phosphate, calcium and magnesium. IN: The Kidney, ed. Rector, F.E. and Brenner, B.M., 1976.
7. Ullrich, K.J., Rumrich, G., and Kloss, S.: Acute Ca^{2+} reabsorption in the proximal tubule of the rat kidney. Pflug. Arch. 364: 223, 1976.
8. Edwards, B.R., Sutton, R.A.L., and Dirks, J.H.: Effect of calcium infusion on renal tubular reabsorption in the dog. Am. J. Physiol. 227: 13, 1974.
9. LeGrimellec, C., Roinel, N., and Morel, F.: Simultaneous Mg, Ca, P, K and Cl analysis in rat tubular fluid. III. During acute Ca plasma loading. Pflug. Arch. 346: 171, 1974.
10. Lechene, C., Abraham, E., and Warner, R.: Effect of sulfate loading on ionic distribution along the rat nephron. Clin. Res. 23: 432A, 1975.
11. Kuntziger, H., Amiel, D., Roinel, N., and Morel, F.: Effects of parathyroidectomy and cyclic AMP on renal transport of phosphate, calcium and magnesium. Am. J. Physiol. 227: 905, 1974.
12. Harris, C.A., Burnatowska, M., Sutton, R.A.L., and Dirks, J.H.: Evidence for parathyroid hormone (PTH) enhancement of calcium and magnesium reabsorption in the terminal nephron segment of the hamster. Clin. Res. 24: 401A, 1976.
13. Goldfarb, S., Westby, G.R., Goldberg, M., and Agus, Z.S.: Renal tubular effects of chronic phosphate depletion. J. Clin. Invest. 59: 770, 1977.
14. Agus, Z.S., Chiu, P., and Goldberg, M.: Regulation of urinary calcium excretion in the rat. Am. J. Physiol., 1977, in press.
15. Jamison, R.L., Frey, N.R., and Lacy, F.B.: Calcium reabsorption in the thin loop of Henle. Am. J. Physiol. 227: 745, 1974.
16. De Rouffignac, C., Morel, F., Moss, N., and Roinel, N.: Micropuncture study of water and electrolyte movements along the loop of Henle in Psammomys with special reference to magnesium, calcium and phosphorus. Pflug. Arch. 334: 309, 1973.
17. Rocha, A.S., Magaldi, J.B., and Kokko, J.P.: Calcium and phosphate transport in isolated segments of rabbit Henle's loop. J. Clin. Invest. 59: 975, 1977.

18. Costanzo, L.S. and Windhager, E.E.: Characteristics of calcium transport in the distal convoluted tubule. Abstracts of 9th Annual Meeting of the Am. Soc. of Nephrology, p. 3, 1976.
19. Costanzo, L.S. and Windhager, E.E.: Distal reabsorption of calcium: effect of load and chlorothiazide (CTZ). Fed. Proc. 35: 466, 1976.
20. Sutton, R.A.L., Wong, N.L.M., and Dirks, J.H.: Effects of parathyroid hormone on sodium and calcium transport in the dog nephron. Clin. Sci. & Mol. Med. 51: 345, 1976.
21. Agus, Z.S., Gardner, L.B., Beck, L.H., and Goldberg, M.: Effects of parathyroid hormone on renal tubular reabsorption of calcium, sodium and phosphate. Am. J. Physiol. 224: 1143, 1973.
22. Burnatowska, M.A., Harris, C.A., Sutton, R.A.L., and Dirks, J.H.: Effects of PTH and CAMP on renal handling of calcium, magnesium and phosphate in the hamster. Abstracts of 9th Annual Meeting of the Am. Soc. of Nephrology, p. 2, 1976.
23. Chabardes, D., Imbert, M., Cligne, A., Montegut, M., and Morel, F.: PTH sensitive adenyl cyclase activity in different segments of the rabbit nephron. Pflug. Arch. 354:229, 1975.
24. Quamme, G.A., O'Callaghan, T.O., Wong, N.L.M., Sutton, R.A.L., and Dirks, J.H.: Hypercalciuria in the phosphate-depleted dog. A micropuncture study. Abstracts of the 9th Annual Meeting of the Am. Soc. of Nephrology, p. 6, 1976.
25. Coburn, J.W. and Massry, S.G.: Changes in serum and urinary calcium during phosphate depletion: studies on mechanisms. J. Clin. Invest. 49:1073, 1970.
26. Grabie, M., Goldfarb, S., Lau, K., Agus, Z.S. and Goldberg, M.: Enhancement of the hypercalciuria of phosphate depletion by parathyroidectomy. Clin. Res. 25:432A, 1977.
27. Sutton, R.A.L., Wong, N.L.M., and Dirks, J.H.: The hypercalciuria of metabolic acidosis - a specific impairment of distal calcium reabsorption. Clin. Res. 23:434A, 1975.
28. Sutton, R.A.L., Wong, N.L.M., and Dirks, J.H.: Renal tubular Na and Ca reabsorption: dissociation of maneuvers which increase bicarbonate excretion. Clin. Res. 24:413A, 1976.

RENAL HANDLING OF MAGNESIUM

J.H. Dirks and G.A. Quamme

Department of Medicine, University of British Columbia,

Vancouver, B.C., Canada

ABSTRACT

Renal handling of magnesium is principally a filtration reabsorption process with a capacity to maximally conserve and reject magnesium when appropriate. Micropuncture studies in the dog, hamster and Psammomys, aided by ultramicroanalysis of tubular fluid with the electron microprobe, have recently added much to our knowledge of renal magnesium physiology. At the glomerulus, 70-80% of total plasma magnesium is freely filterable. Magnesium concentration rises above its ultrafilterable value along the proximal tubule, though there is a wide dispersion of concentration ratios. Mean end proximal tubule fluid to ultrafilterable (TF/UF) magnesium, reaches a mean of 1.5 in the dog and 1.65 in the rat when TF/P inulin values average 2.0 and 2.4, and is probably due to available proximal tubule in these two species. Net proximal magnesium reabsorption constitutes 25% of the filtered load and can be reduced by saline and magnesium infusion. Unlike other solutes including calcium, magnesium is poorly coupled to sodium in the proximal tubule which is poorly permeable to magnesium. The precise mechanisms of proximal magnesium transport remain undefined. In the descending limb, magnesium rises 3-5 fold above ultrafilterable concentration due to water removal in the renal medulla. There is evidence that during acute magnesium infusion, entry of magnesium into the lumen may occur prior to the hairpin bend. The ascending limb avidly reabsorbs some 60-70% of the filtered magnesium and mean distal TF/UF concentrations approximate 0.6. Ascending limb magnesium transport may be active or possibly passive accompanying active chloride removal. Furthermore, magnesium transport in this segment may be progressively reduced by acute magnesium infusion, non-reabsorbable anions and furosemide. Relatively little magnesium reabsorption occurs in the distal convoluted tubule and collecting duct under normal circumstances with about 10% of the filtered magnesium being excreted. However, there is some clearance and micropuncture evidence that suggests magnesium addition in the terminal segments during acute magnesium infusion. Data in the hamster which is highly sensitive to the action of parathyroid hormone (PTH) suggests that PTH increases magnesium as well as calcium reabsorption in the ascending limb, and beyond the distal tubule puncture site. This effect is mimicked by cyclic AMP infusion. Other factors that affect magnesium handling deserve detailed study by a variety of micropuncture approaches. The exact homeostatic mechanisms which regulate renal tubular magnesium reabsorption require further identification.

The kidney plays an important role in magnesium homeostasis. The regulatory mechanisms of magnesium handling by the kidney largely remains unknown. Normally 5-20% of the filtered load is excreted in the urine. This may drop to near unmeasurable levels in dietary magnesium deficit and rise to high levels in dietary magnesium surfeit or magnesium infusion. Some of the factors that alter magnesium reabsorption are listed in Table 1.

TABLE I

Factors Known to Alter Magnesium Reabsorption

Increase	Decrease
Magnesium deficiency	Magnesium excess
Parathyroid hormone	Hypercalcemia
Cyclic AMP	Mineralocorticoids
	Alcohol
	Osmotic diuretics
	Diuretics (Ethacrynic acid, Furosemide)
	Extracellular volume expansion

Micropuncture studies have indicated that diffusible plasma magnesium is filtered at the glomerulus and excreted in the urine after reabsorption of its major fraction at various sites along the nephron (1,2). Direct micropuncture of the long loops of Henle demonstrate the ascending limb is the major site of reclamation of filtered magnesium (3,4). We will attempt to review some of the evidence for these conclusions and speculate on some of the mechanisms which may be involved in transcellular transport of magnesium. This subject is covered in more detail elsewhere (5).

Glomerulus

Plasma magnesium is filtered at the glomerular membrane to the extent of 70-80% as measured by in vitro techniques and by direct micropuncture of surface glomeruli in the Munich-Wistar strain of rat (6,7).

Proximal Tubule

Micropuncture of late proximal tubules in rat, Psammomys, hamster and dog have consistently demonstrated magnesium concentration of the late tubular fluid to exceed that obtained from the early puncture site, Table 2 (3,4,8-10). Thus the tubular fluid to ultrafilterable (TF/UF) magnesium ratio rises along the proximal tubule but to a lesser extent than that of inulin. This is in contrast to the other major cations, the TF/P ratios of which remain close to unity as water is abstracted. Figure 1 illustrates these ratios along the length of the proximal nephron; although there is much scatter in the reported values, the TF/UF magnesium in most instances is less than the TF/P inulin indicating some net magnesium reabsorption in the proximal tubule (Table 2).

TABLE 2

Proximal Tubule Fluid to Ultrafiltrate Inulin and Magnesium Ratios

		TF/P_{In}	TF/UF_{Mg}
Morel et al (8)	rat	-	1.81
Brunette et al (9)	dog	1.50 ±0.04	1.05 ±0.03
Le Grimellec et al (10)	rat	2.13 ±0.04	1.67 ±0.05
Brunette et al (4)	rat	2.36 ±0.10	1.65 ±0.09
De Rouffignac et al (3)	Psammomys	2.10 ±0.37	1.52 ±0.44
Quamme et al (11)	dog	2.11 ±0.06	1.50 ±0.06

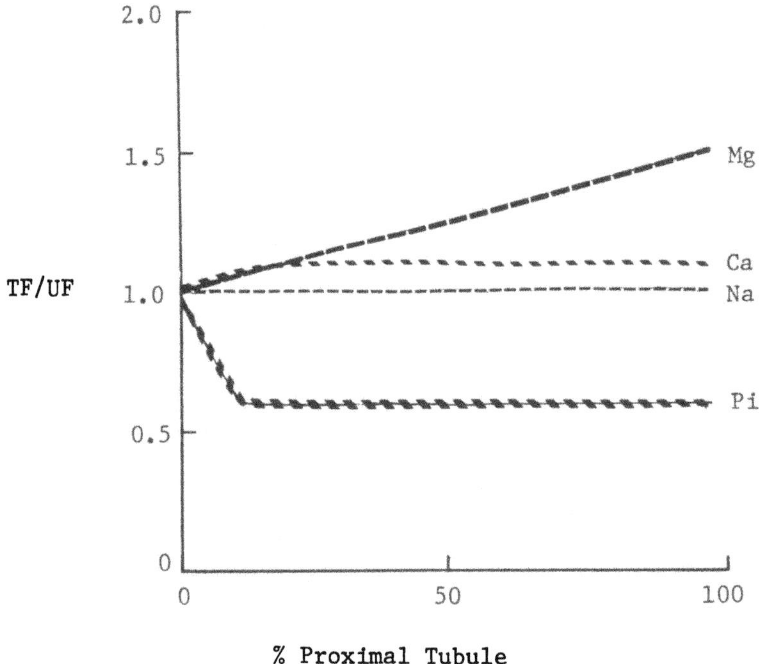

Figure 1. Tubular fluid to ultrafilterable magnesium, calcium, sodium and phosphate as a function of proximal length.

Evidence suggests the proximal tubular epithelium to be relatively impermeable to magnesium ions. Brunette and Aras in the rat, demonstrated that the excretory pattern of radioactive ^{28}Mg, when injected into the proximal tubule, was the same as that of inulin suggesting poor permeability of the tubular epithelium to magnesium (12). In addition microinjection studies with ^{28}Mg failed to show any passage of the isotope from the superficial capillary to the tubular lumen. Recent studies from our laboratory confirm these conclusions. In vivo perfusion of individual nephrons with magnesium-free solutions results in no measurable influx of magnesium into the lumen. Obviously, the permeability of the tubular epithelium is of great importance in determining the efficiency of net transport during continuous perfusion of the tubule. The differential permeability of magnesium to sodium and water have been used to explain the phenomenon of increasing magnesium concentration along the proximal tubule.

Loop of Henle

Tubular fluid obtained from the early distal tubule contains magnesium at a lesser concentration than does the glomerular filtrate. Table 3 reviews reported values for the distal tubule in hydropenia, magnesium infusion, as well as several experimental manoeuvres. The normal TF/UF magnesium ratios ranged from 0.50 to 0.80 in all animal species studied to date. This fact, taken with the inulin ratio for these animals demonstrates the loop of Henle is the major nephron segment reclaiming a significant portion of the filtered load. These data are derived from superficial nephrons which are accessible to micropuncture and do not include the long-loop nephrons which may contribute more to the final urinary magnesium than their small number would lead one to expect. Data available from the desert rat (Psammomys obsesus) by direct micropuncture of Henle's loops demonstrates a TF/UF magnesium of 5.08, less than the TF/P inulin ratio at the hairpin turn (3). Thus magnesium is concentrated by water removal down the descending limb and avidly reabsorbed in the ascending limb, probably the thick portion of Henle's loop. In this study de Rouffignac and colleagues observed a good correlation of tubular fluid electrolytes and osmolarity rather than with inulin concentration, suggesting medullary recycling of electrolytes including magnesium. Brunette et al also reported a TF/UF magnesium of 3.24 at the hairpin turn of the papillary loop of rats corresponding to TF/P inulin ratio of 4.54 (4). They then investigated the long loops in the papilla under conditions of acute magnesium loading. TF/UF magnesium was observed to exceed that for inulin (4.25 and 3.32 respectively) indicating net addition of magnesium to the lumen between the late proximal tubule and bend of the loop of Henle (18). In both of these conditions magnesium was extensively reabsorbed in the ascending limb of the loop. Thus the permeability of the ascending limb to magnesium appears to be quite different from that of the proximal tubule where magnesium is relatively impermeable.

Terminal Nephron

The terminal segments of the nephron, i.e., distal convoluted tubule and collecting duct appear to have very little additional effect on the reabsorptive pattern for magnesium in normal conditions. The fractions of filtered magnesium remaining at the various sites along the nephron are summarized in Figure 2. Reabsorption in these segments, as calculated from superficial nephrons accessible to micropuncture and the final urine,has been demonstrated in these segments following a number of experimental manoeuvres including acute plasma phosphate loading and following parathyroid hormone infusion (15, 12). Magnesium secretion has also been suggested following acute $MgSO_4$ loading with furosemide (15) (Table 3).

TABLE 3

Tubular Fluid to Ultrafilterable Inulin and Magnesium Ratios obtained from the Distal Tubule in Control, Hydropenia and following a Number of Experimental Conditions.

	TF/P_{In}	TF/UF_{Mg}
Morel et al (8)		
rat - control		0.79
Wen et al (13)		
dog - ECF expansion	4.20 ±0.34	0.55 ±0.07
- $MgSO_4$	3.19 ±0.32	1.89 ±0.13
- $MgSO_4$ + Furosemide	2.59 ±0.25	1.79 ±0.16
- $MgCl_2$	2.75 ±0.15	1.84 ±0.09
Le Grimellec et al (7)		
rat - normal	4.79 ±0.17	0.70 ±0.04
Le Grimellec et al (14)		
rat - control	4.43 ±0.21	0.65 ±0.07
- $MgCl_2$ loading	3.71 ±0.18	1.30 ±0.09
Le Grimellec et al (15)		
rat - control	4.72 ±0.25	0.92 ±0.06
- Pi loading	3.69 ±0.26	0.92 ±0.11
Le Grimellec et al (16)		
rat - control	4.67 ±0.28	0.54 ±0.06
Ca^{++} loading	4.96 ±0.46	1.13 ±0.11
Kuntziger et al (17)		
rat - TPTX	7.10 ±0.63	0.58 ±0.01
- cAMP infusion	5.45 ±0.32	1.02 ±0.14
Brunette et al (4)		
rat - hydropenic	5.55 ±0.27	0.80 ±0.06
Brunette et al (18)		
rat - $MgCl_2$ loading	6.87 ±0.50	3.92 ±0.27
de Rouffignac et al (3)		
Psammomys - saline	4.29 ±1.43	0.69 ±0.28
Quamme et al (11)		
dog - hydropenic	5.50 ±0.26	0.60 ±0.07

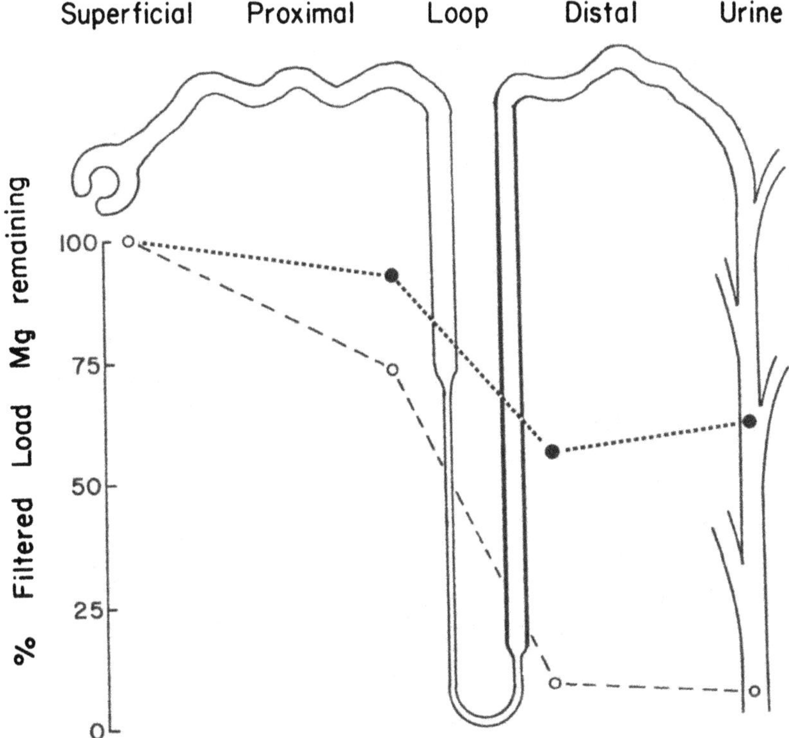

Figure 2. Fractions of ultrafilterable magnesium remaining along the nephron in normal, hydropenic conditions (0-----0) and following acute $MgCl_2$ loading (●......●).

Magnesium Infusion

A number of factors have been shown to affect urinary magnesium excretion (Tables 1 and 3). The most studied by micropuncture techniques is that of elevation of plasma magnesium by acute administration of magnesium salts ($MgCl_2$ and $MgSO_4$). These studies reported that proximal TF/P inulin ratio was significantly reduced after infusion of magnesium resulting in a marked increase in magnesium and water delivery to the loop. Distal TF/UF magnesium ratios rose significantly with a marked increase in distal fractional rejection(Table 3, Figure 2). This is reflected as a massive hypermagnesiuria in the final urine attaining excretions in excess of 60% of the filtered load. A number of studies have reported a maximal tubular reabsorptive capacity (Tm) for magnesium (1, 14, 19). As the plasma magnesium was acutely elevated 2-3 fold, a Tm was reached in the dog (19). Micropuncture studies in the rat suggests this occurs in the ascending limb of Henle (14). This tubular reabsorption maximum appears to be increased by parathyroid hormone (PTH) and reduced by the elevation of serum calcium (14).

Magnesium Deficiency

In states of magnesium deprivation the kidney is extremely effective in reclaiming filtered magnesium despite falling plasma levels. The mechanisms involved are not known nor has this syndrome been studied by micropuncture techniques.

Interrelationship of Magnesium to Sodium and Calcium

Magnesium excretion has been demonstrated to follow closely that of sodium and calcium. Manoeuvres which have been shown to increase sodium excretion such as extracellular volume expansion, renal vasodilation, increased glomerular filtration rate or increased perfusion pressure are associated with proportional increases in urinary magnesium excretion (1, 2). Micropuncture studies indicate that proximal magnesium transport is reduced after saline infusion to the same extent as is sodium reabsorption (9). It has further been demonstrated that the infusion of magnesium salts with the attendant hypermagnesemia causes an increase in the urinary excretion of calcium whilst hypercalciuria is associated with an increase in the excretion of magnesium (19,20). This has led some authors to suggest a common reabsorptive mechanism for these two divalent cations (1,2). However, sodium reabsorption is inhibited by both these manoeuvres, hence it is not clear whether it is a direct mechanism or secondary to depressed sodium movement. One could postulate either the cations moving via a common carrier which would require receptors common to both or independent transport systems associated only by the need for active sodium and/or chloride transport.

Hormonal Effects

The physiological importance of parathyroid hormone in the renal homeostasis of magnesium is uncertain. Initial observations suggested that excess PTH may result in increased urinary excretion of magnesium (22,23). This observation is mitigated by the fact that hypercalcemia was present and may inhibit tubular reabsorption of magnesium. More recent studies have concluded that parathyroid hormone decreases fractional magnesium excretion (19). These latter observations are compatible with our recent micropuncture studies with thyroparathyroidectomized (TPTX) hamsters, in which acute administration of PTH significantly decreased the fractional excretion of magnesium. This action of PTH appears to take place in the distal segments of the nephron including the ascending limb, the major site of magnesium reabsorption. However, the acute administration of cyclic AMP, the proposed mediator of PTH action, failed to lower magnesium excretion in TPTX rats (17). This may well be due to the acute effect of PTH or cyclic AMP in reducing proximal reabsorption of sodium and magnesium thus increasing distal delivery.

The relation between aldosterone secretion and magnesium homeostasis is well recognized (24,25). Chronic administration of mineralocorticoids cause increased urinary excretion of magnesium and this is reversed with spironolactone administration or adrenal insufficiency (2). The site of this renal action is unclear but likely reflects volume expansion with associated increased proximal delivery of sodium, calcium and magnesium to the distal sites where mineralocorticoids may enhance sodium reabsorption without affecting calcium and magnesium transport. A number of hormones including thyroid hormone, growth hormone and vitamin D have been shown to increase magnesium excretion. The detailed mechanisms for these actions have not been delineated and may be extrarenal in origin. In addition, many of these circumstances involve a concomitant natriuresis and may reflect associated transport changes with magnesium.

Metabolic Factors and Diuretics

Alcohol, whether administered chronically or acutely, has been shown to increase urinary magnesium excretion. Administration of alcohol results in hypermagnesuria and hypercalciuria without natriuresis or changes in glomerular filtration rate and renal blood flow. This has also been observed following ingestion of glucose or other rapidly metabolizable substances (26). It is not known whether this is a direct effect on renal transport or secondary to increases in production of metabolic intermediates which may either form non-reabsorbable magnesium complexes, change intraluminal pH or inhibit reabsorption by other means. No micropuncture studies are yet available to discern the site of these metabolic effects.

Acute administration of diuretic agents (furosemide and ethacrynic acid) increases fractional urinary excretion of magnesium proportional to the increased sodium excretion (27, 28). The major site of electrolyte inhibition by diuretics is the ascending limb of the loop of Henle. The effect of these agents on magnesium reabsorption at this site has not been investigated by micropuncture in the hydropenic state. However, the effect of furosemide was tested subsequent to $MgSO_4$ loading in dogs and appeared to have little or no effect on magnesium transport per se, while sodium reabsorption was greatly inhibited (13). The effect of thiazide diuretics on magnesium excretion appears to be variable. Only small increases in magnesium clearance have been observed following administration of chlorothiazide (3). The action of these diuretics on magnesium reabsorption needs to be investigated by micropuncture techniques.

Speculation on Cellular Aspects of Magnesium Reabsorption

Models to explain the mechanisms by which cellular magnesium is regulated have been proposed by a number of investigators (29-34). Many of these models are speculative and much of the evidence is based on that obtained for cells other than kidney. Figure 3 illustrates a hypothetical cell of the thick ascending limb of Henle's loop. Magnesium must transfer through at least three membrane barriers, the luminal membrane, the invaginated basilar membrane associated with an abundance of mitochondria and finally the capillary endothelium. Any attempt to describe the control and the regulation of magnesium must take into account first the concentration of ionized magnesium in the cytosol and secondly the generally well recognized cellular events in which it is involved; including ribosome stability and the functioning of intracellular enzymes. Thus intracellular concentrations must be regulated within limits compatible with these activities. Intracellular concentration of magnesium has been reported to range from 2-20 mM in a number of different cells and is much higher than reported for calcium, important to this however, is the free magnesium ion concentration. The exact ionized fraction is not known but it is presumed that a fraction of the total quantity is bound and unavailable for the transport pool. Appreciating the maximum values, entry of magnesium across the luminal membrane would be against a concentration gradient. The luminal concentration being approximately 1.5 mEq/L and 0.5 mEq/L in proximal and distal tubules respectively. This entry step, however, would be down an electrical potential gradient of some 60-70 mV in both these segments. At the basilar membrane magnesium is shuttled down a concentration gradient to the pericapillary space and against a high electrical gradient. A number of mechanisms have been associated with this membrane with regard to transcellular effluxes. They include an active independent pump perhaps related to magnesium activated ATPase activity which is generally recognized to exist at this site. In addition, an ATP independent magnesium efflux has been postulated which reflects magnesium extrusion in exchange for external sodium; a mechanism similar to that proposed for calcium (31, 35). Moreover. the thick ascending limb of Henle's loop has been demonstrated to actively transport chloride from the lumen to the peritubular side and it has been postulated the major cations follow passively. This may also apply to magnesium.

The role of intracellular organelles and compartments of differing activities are unknown. Mitochondria have been reported to take magnesium in exchange for hydrogen ion and is deposited as a phosphate complex (36). Borle and colleagues propose mitochondria control intracellular calcium concentrations and may regulate transcellular transport (32). Terepka and associates assign a crucial role to the external plasma membrane of calcium transporting

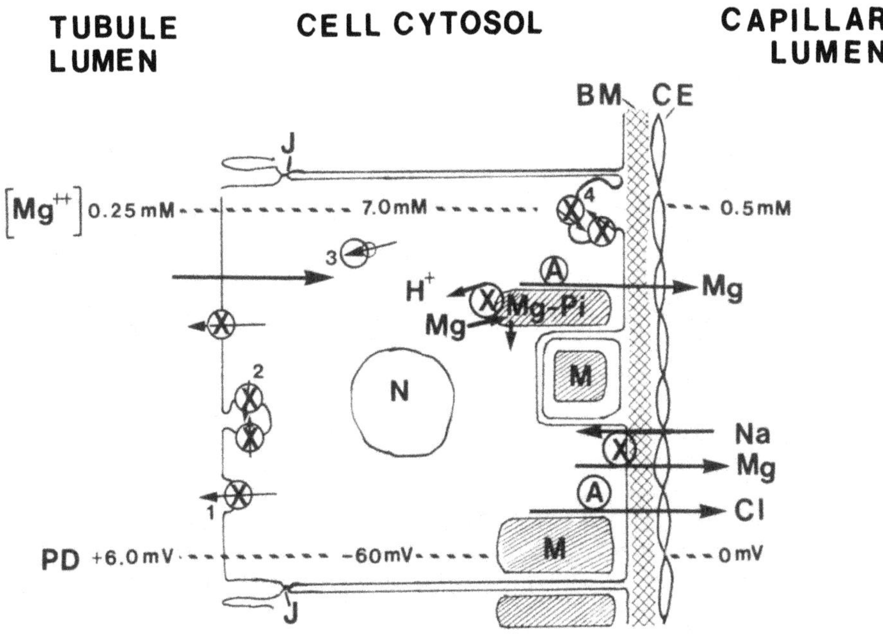

Figure 3. Schematic depiction of a cell model of thick ascending limb of Henle's loop for transcellular transport of magnesium. The abbreviations are: J= tight junction; N = nucleus; M = mitochondrium; BM = basement membrane; CE = capillary endothelium.

cells (35). They postulate outwardly directed membrane calcium pumps which invaginate forming endocytotic vesicles which move to the basal membrane and release their calcium load by exocytosis. A number of factors require explanation, such as the mechanisms for cation binding selectivity, energy input, sodium dependency, polarization of membrane function and hormonal regulatory mechanisms. Whether this form of packaging can be applied to transport of magnesium remains speculative.

SUMMARY

In summary, magnesium reabsorption occurs throughout the proximal and distal segments of the nephron. The proximal tubule is less permeable to magnesium than calcium and sodium with most of the filtered load being reclaimed in the ascending loop of Henle. In contrast to calcium and sodium a tubular reabsorptive maximum has been demonstrated for magnesium and under certain circumstances secretion has been demonstrated in the terminal nephron segments. Although many factors are known to affect magnesium reabsorption the mechanism of the renal homeostasis remains to be determined.

REFERENCES

1. Massry, S.G. and Coburn, J.W. The hormonal and nonhormonal control of renal excretion of calcium and magnesium. Nephron 10: 66, 1973.
2. Walser, M. Divalent Cations: Physiochemical state in glomerular filtrate and urine and renal excretion. In Orloff J. and Berliner, R.W. (editors): Handbook of Physiology: Renal Physiology. Williams and Wilkins Co., Baltimore, 1973.
3. De Rouffignac, C., Morel, F., Moss, N., and Roinel, N. Micropuncture study of water and electrolyte movements along the loop of Henle in Psammomys with special references to magnesium, calcium and phosphorus. Pflugers Arch. 344: 309, 1973.
4. Brunette, M.G., Vigneault, N. and Carriere, S. Micropuncture study of magnesium transport along the nephron in young rat. Amer. J. Physiol. 227: 891, 1974.
5. Sutton, R.A.L., Quamme, G.A., Dirks, J.H. Transport of calcium, magnesium and inorganic phosphate in the kidney. In Transport Across Biological Membranes. Editors G. Giebisch, D.C. Tosteson and H.H. Ussing (in preparation).
6. Brunette, M.G. and Crochet, M.D. Fluoremetric method for the determination of magnesium in renal tubule fluid. Anal. Biochem. 65: 79, 1975.
7. LeGrimellec, C., Poujeol, P. and De Rouffignac, C. H^3-Inulin and electrolyte concentrations in Bowman's capsule in rat kidney. Comparison with artificial ultrafiltration. Pflugers Arch. 354: 117, 1975.

8. Morel, F., Roinel, N., LeGrimellec, C. Electron probe analysis of tubular fluid composition. Nephron 6: 350, 1969.
9. Brunette, M.G., Wen, S.F. and Dirks, J.H. Micropuncture study of magnesium reabsorption in the proximal tubule of the dog. Amer. J. Physiol. 216: 1510, 1969.
10. LeGrimellec, C., Roinel, N. and Morel, F. Simultaneous Mg, Ca, P, K, Na and Cl analysis in rat tubular fluid. II. During acute Mg plasma loading. Pflugers Arch. 340: 197, 1973.
11. Quamme, G.A., Roinel, M., Wong, N.L.M., de Rouffignac, C., Morel, F., and Dirks, J.H. A micropuncture study of magnesium reabsorption in the dog kidney. 2nd Int. Congress on Magnesium, Montreal, Quebec, 1976.
12. Brunette, M. and Aras, M. A microinjection study of nephron permeability to calcium and magnesium. Amer. J. Physiol. 221: 1442, 1971.
13. Wen, S.F., Evanson, R.L. and Dirks, J.H. Micropuncture study of renal magnesium transport in proximal and distal tubule of the dog. Amer. J. Physiol. 219: 570, 1970.
14. LeGrimellec, C., Roinel, N., and Morel, F. Simultaneous Mg, Ca, P, K, Na and Cl analysis in rat tubular fluid. II. During acute Mg plasma loading. Pflugers Arch. 340: 197, 1973.
15. LeGrimellec, C., Roinel, N., Morel, F. Simultaneous Mg, Ca, P, K, and Cl analysis in rat tubule fluid. IV. During acute phosphate plasma loading. Pflugers Arch. 346: 189, 1974.
16. LeGrimellec, C., Roinel, N. and Morel, F. Simultaneous Mg, Ca, P, K, Na, and Cl analysis in rat tubular fluid. III. During acute Ca plasma loading. Pflugers Arch. 346: 171, 1974.
17. Kuntziger, H., Amiel, C., Roinel, N., and Morel, F. Effects of parathyroidectomy and cyclic AMP on renal transport of phosphate, calcium and magnesium. Amer. J. Physiol. 227: 905, 1974.
18. Brunette, M.G., Vigneault, N. and Carrier, S. Micropuncture study of renal magnesium transport in magnesium in magnesium-loaded rats. Amer. J. Physiol. 229: 1695, 1975.
19. Massry, S.G., Coburn, J.W. and Kleeman, C.R. Renal handling of magnesium in the dog. Amer. J. Physiol. 216: 1460, 1969.
20. Coburn, J.W., Massry, S.G. and Kleeman, C.R. The effect of calcium infusion on renal handling of magnesium with normal and reduced glomerular filtration rate. Nephron 7: 131, 1970.
21. Massry, S.G., Ahumada, J.J., Coburn, J.W. and Kleeman, C.R. Effect of $MgCl_2$ infusion on urinary Ca and Na during reduction in their filtered loads. Amer. J. Physiol. 219: 881, 1970.
22. Heaton, F.W. The parathyroid glands and magnesium metabolism in the rat. Clin. Sci. 28: 543, 1955.
23. Barnes, B.A., Krane, S.M. and Cope, O. Magnesium studies in relation to hyperparathyroidism. J. Clin. Endocr. and Metab. 17: 1407, 1957.
24. Hanna, S. and MacIntyre, I. Influence of aldosterone on metabolism of magnesium. Lancet 2: 348, 1960.

25. Horton, R. and Biglieri, E.G. Effect of aldosterone on the metabolism of magnesium. J. Clin. Endocr. & Metab. 22: 1187, 1962.
26. Lindeman, R.D., Adler, S., Yungst, M.J., and Beard, E.S. Influence of various nutrients on urinary divalent cation excretion. J. Lab. Clin. Med. 70: 236, 1967.
27. Duarte, C.G. Effects of ethacrynic acid and furosemide on urinary calcium. phosphate and magnesium. Metabolism 17: 867, 1968.
28. Eknoyan, G., Suki, W.N. and Martinez-Maldonado, M. Effect of diuretics on urinary excretion of phosphate, calcium, and magnesium in thyroparathyroidectomized dogs. J. Lab. Clin. Med. 76: 257, 1970.
29. Spencer, T. and Bygrove, F.L. The role of mitochondria in modifying the cellular ionic environment. Bioenergetics 4: 347, 1973.
30. Sordahl, L.A. Effects of magnesium, rubidium red and antibiotic ionophone A23187 on initial rates of calcium uptake and release by heart mitochondria. Arch. Biochem. Biophys. 167: 104, 1974.
31. Carapali, E. and Crompton, M. Calcium ions and mitochondria p. 89, Symposium of the Society for Experimental Biology. Calcium in Biological Systems. Editor Duncan, C.J., Cambridge University Press, 1976.
32. Baker, P.F. The regulation of intracellular calcium. p. 67 Editor Duncan, C.J. Cambridge University Press, 1976.
33. Borle, A.B. and Anderson, J.H. A cybernetic view of cell calcium metabolism. p. 141. Editor Duncan, C.J. Cambridge University Press, 1976.
34. Baker, P.F. and Crawford, A.C. Mobility and transport of magnesium in squid giant axons. J. Physiol. (Lond.) 227: 855, 1972.
35. Terepika, A.R., Coleman, J.R., Armbrecht, H.J., and Gunter, T.E. Transcellular transport of calcium. p. 117, Editor Duncan, C.J. Cambridge University Press, 1976.
36. Allison, A.C. and Davies, P. Mechanism of endocytosis and exocytosis. Symp. Soc. Exp. Biol., 28: 419, 1974.
37. Bronk, J.R. and Leese, H.J. Accumulation of amino acids and glucose by the mammalian small intestine. Symp. Soc. Exp. Biol. 28: 283, 1974.
38. Brierley, G., Murer, E., Bachmann, E., and Green, D.E. Studies on ion transport. II. The accumulation of inorganic phosphate and magnesium ions by heart mitochondria. J. Biol. Chem. 238: 3482, 1963.
39. Schatzmann, H.J. Active calcium transport and Ca^{++} activated ATPase in human red cells. Curr. Topics Membrane Transports 6: 125, 1975.
40. Blaustein, M.P. The interrelationship between sodium and calcium fluxes across cell membranes. Rev. Physiol. Biochem. Exp. Pharmacol. 70: 33, 1974.

AN EVALUATION OF POSSIBLE SITES OF PHOSPHATE SECRETION IN THE RAT NEPHRON.

Franklyn G. Knox, John Haas, and Theresa Berndt

Nephrology Research Laboratory, Departments of Physiology & Biophysics and Medicine, Mayo Clinic & Mayo Foundation, Rochester, Minnesota U.S.A.

Although net secretion of phosphate has been demonstrated in non-mammalian species, the secretion of phosphate in mammals has been difficult to demonstrate using clearance methods (1). In these studies, plasma phosphate was elevated by infusion of phosphate and the clearance of phosphate was compared to the clearance of a glomerular marker (usually inulin). The results were equivocal with some investigators reporting net secretion, while others did not. In recent studies by Boudry et al (2), phosphate clearances were greater than inulin clearances in conscious rats when plasma Pi concentration was corrected for ultrafilterability. Likewise, in studies by Troehler et al (3), rats fed a high phosphate diet for 10 days and then infused acutely with phosphate, had a FE_p% of 97% without correction for plasma ultrafilterability. Since it is highly unlikely that unidirectional outflux of phosphate (reabsorption) was abolished completely in these studies, this data has been taken as evidence for a secretory component of net phosphate transport if not net secretion per se.

In microperfusion studies by Murayama, Morel and LeGrimellec, proximal tubules were perfused with low phosphate solutions and phosphate backflux evaluated (4). The backflux was 17% of the net flux and due to the scatter of the data this value was not significantly different from zero. In more recent studies by Boudry et al (2) in phosphate and PTH loaded rats, both backflux and net secretion of phosphate were reported for the proximal tubule. However, no marker for contamination of microperfusate was included in these studies. In similar studies by Greger et al (5), a marker for contaminated samples was included and phosphate trnasport in the proximal tubule was found to be essentially a unidirectional reabsorptive process without a significant backflux or secretory component. The luminal phosphate concentration at the site of collection was close to zero and might be explained either by the absence of phosphate backflux or by a balance between a small secretory flux relative to a predominant reabsorptive flux. In a recent stationary split droplet study in intact rats, significant phosphate influx into phosphate free droplets was observed (6). However, this was attributed to emptying of the cellular pool rather than transcellular backflux. In split droplet studies only about 0.5 nl of the perfusion fluid is exposed to the cellular pool, whereas in microperfusion studies, the cellular pool is exposed to about 60 nl. In isolated perfused tubules of the rabbit net phosphate transport in the proximal tubule was shown to be essentially a unidirectional process (7). Lumen to bath flux was 6.60 $\pm$ 1.4 pmol/mm·min whereas bath to lumen flux was only 0.45 $\pm$ 0.08 pmol/mm·min. Thus, although a small backflux of phosphate in the proximal tubule may be demonstrable, it is probably negligible in regard to regulation of net phosphate reabsorption (8).

Boudry et al have reported net entry of phosphate along the terminal part of the nephron in phosphate loaded rats as determined from the fractional delivery of phosphate in superficial distal tubules and urine (2). They interpreted this as evidence for net secretion of phosphate based on the assumption that the superficial nephrons are representative of the entire nephron population.

We re-evaluated and extended these studies as follows: first, during phosphate loading, differences in phosphate delivery between superficial distal tubules and urine were evaluated utilizing internal controls to detect pitfalls in micropuncture and microanalytic methodologies (9). Accordingly, contamination of micropuncture samples with collecting duct fluid was evaluated by measuring single nephron glomerular filtration rates and tubule fluid to plasma potassium concentration ratios. The same microanalytic methods and standard solutions were used for both phosphate and inulin measurements in tubule fluid and urine. Second, additional studies were performed to determine if greater phosphate delivery by deep nephrons contributed to this addition of phosphate in the collecting system.

In the first group of 8 anesthetized Munich-Wistar rats, following an infusion of phosphate and parathyroid hormone (PTH), fractional delivery of phosphate (FD_p%) from superficial distal tubules was 56 $\pm$ 6%, significantly less, ($p < .01$), than the amount appearing in the urine, 67 $\pm$ 6%. In a second group of 6 rats we determined whether this difference could be accounted for by a higher FD_p% in the deep nephrons. Free flow micropuncture collections were taken from deep nephrons (ascending limb of the loop of Henle in the papilla) superficial nephrons, (distal tubules in the cortex), and urine (duct of Bellini). The FD_p% in deep nephrons was 78 ± 10%, significantly greater than superficial nephrons, 51 ± 6% ($p < .005$), and urine 72 ± 10% ($p < .05$).

Thus we found that the fraction of filtered phosphate excretion in the urine was significantly greater than that delivered from the superficial distal tubule of phosphate loaded rats. (Figure 1).
These data are in good agreement with those of Boudry et al (2). This difference in phosphate delivery between superficial nephrons and urine raises the question whether this finding is due to net phosphate secretion in the collecting system or heterogeneity of nephron function with phosphate delivery in deep nephrons greater than that in superficial nephrons. Boudry et al ascribed this difference to net secretion of phosphate with the assumptions that the micropunctured nephrons are representative of cortical nephrons and that there is a clearly defined percentage distribution of nephrons. If superficial nephrons represent 55% of the filtered phosphate, they calculated that phosphate reabsorption would have to be completely abolished along the entire length of deep nephrons to account for the results on the basis of nephron

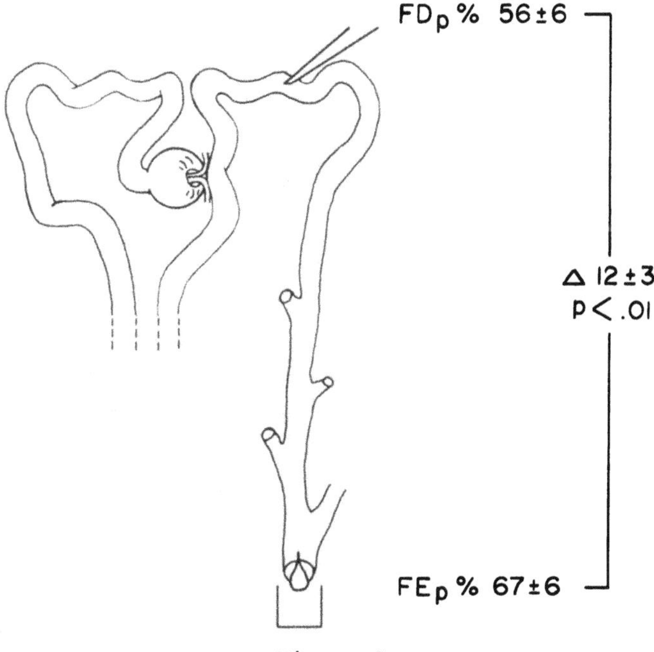

Figure 1

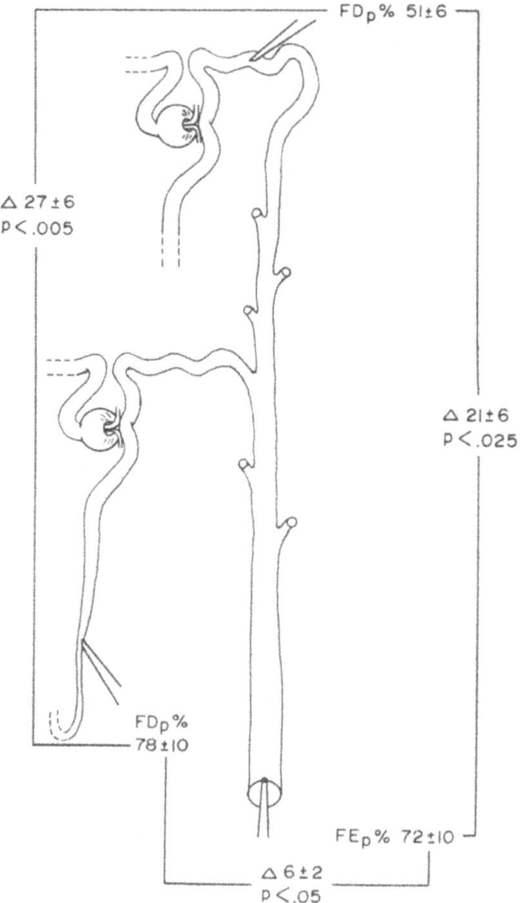

Figure 2. Heterogeneity of phosphate transport.

heterogeneity. In our experiments, a greater fraction of the filtered load of phosphate was delivered to the urine from the deep nephrons than from the superficial nephrons (Figure 2). This large difference in fractional delivery of phosphate was not due to contamination of deep nephron samples with collecting duct fluid as verified by comparisons of potassium concentrations and filtration rates. Previous studies from our laboratory (10,11) and isolated microperfusion studies (12) indicate that the difference in phosphate delivery between superficial and deep nephrons is probably not due to reabsorption of phosphate by the ascending limb of Henle's loop. If the phosphate transport characteristics of the deep nephrons represent a larger fraction of the total nephron population than the superficial, the addition of phosphate to the urine could be accounted for by nephron heterogeneity.

However, since the precise distribution of deep and superficial nephrons in regard to phosphate transport is unknown, a secretory component cannot be ruled out from these results. We conclude that the addition of phosphate to the collecting system is due, at least in part, to greater phosphate delivery from deep nephrons in phosphate loaded rats. Thus although secretion of phosphate cannot be ruled out by studies to date, the presence and site of phosphate secretion remains to be definitively demonstrated.

REFERENCES

1. Knox, F.G., Schneider, E.G., Willis, L.R., Strandhoy, J.W., and Ott, C.E.: Site and control of phosphate reabsorption by the kidney. Kidney Int. 3:347-353, 1973.
2. Boudry, J.F., Troehler, U., Toubai, M., Fleisch, H., and Bonjour, J.P.: Secretion of inorganic phosphate in the rat nephron. Clin. Sci. Mol. Med. 48:475-489, 1975.
3. Troehler, U., Bonjour, J.P., and Fleisch, H.: Inorganic phosphate homeostasis. Renal adaptation to the dietary intake in intact and thyroparathyroidectomized rats. J. Clin. Invest. 57:264-273, 1976.
4. Murayama, Y., Morel, F., and LeGrimellec, C.: Phosphate, calcium and magnesium transfers in proximal tubules and loops of Henle, as measured by single nephron microperfusion experiments in the rat. Pflugers Archiv. 333:1-16, 1972.
5. Greger, R.F., Lang, F.C., Knox, F.G., and Lechene, C.P.: Absence of significant secretory flux of phosphate in the proximal convoluted tubule. Am. J. Physiol. 232:F235-238, 1977.
6. Shirley, D.G., Poujeol, P., and LeGrimellec, C.: Phosphate, calcium and magnesium fluxes into the lumen of the rat proximal convoluted tubule. Pflugers Archiv. 362:247-254, 1976.
7. Dennis, V.W., Woodhall, P.B., and Robinson, R.R.: Characteristics of phosphate transport in isolated proximal tubule. Am. J. Physiol. 231:979-983, 1976.
8. Schneider, E.G., and McLane, L.A.: Evidence for a peritubular-to luminal flux of phosphate in the dog kidney. Am. J. Physiol. 1:159-166, 1977.
9. Knox, F.G., Haas, J.A., Berndt, T., Marchand, G.R., Youngberg, S.P.: Phosphate transport in superficial and deep nephrons in phosphate loaded rats. Am. J. Physiol., in press, 1977.
10. Lang, F.C., Greger, R.F., Marchand, G.R., and Knox, F.G.: Stationary microperfusion study of phosphate reabsorption in proximal and distal nephron segments. Pflugers Archiv., in press, 1977.
11. Haas, J.A., Larson, M., Marchand, G.R., Lang, F., Greger, R., and Knox, F.G.: Phosphaturic effect of furosemide, role of PTH and carbonic anhydrase. Am. J. Physiol. 1:F105-110, 1977.
12. Rocha, A.S., and Magaldi, J.B.: Calcium and phosphate transport in isolated segments of Henle's loop. J. Clin. Invest. 59:975-984, 1977.

ATTEMPTS TO DEMONSTRATE PHOSPHATE SECRETION IN THE RAT

E. J. Weinman, S. Sansom and W. N. Suki

VA Hospital and Baylor College of Medicine

Houston, Texas 77211 USA

The renal tubular secretion of phosphate from peritubular capillary blood into the tubular lumen has been conclusively demonstrated in some non-mammalian kidneys, yet the presence of such a pathway in the mammalian kidney is still in question (1-9). It is generally agreed that, in the mammalian kidney, the reabsorption of phosphate filtered at the glomerulus is the predominant transport process. Recent studies in man, dog and rat, however, have reopened the question of the existence of a phosphate secretory mechanism (7-9). The current investigations were designed to re-examine this question, utilizing a modification of the precession technique.

METHODS

Male Sprague-Dawley rats were anesthetized with Nembutal (50-60 mg/kg body wt) and the left kidney prepared for micropuncture. The left ureter was catheterized with a length of PE-50 tubing equal to that of the ureter and bladder catheter draining the right kidney. Ten nanoliters of an isotonic saline solution containing tracer quantities of ^{32}P phosphate and ^{3}H inulin were microinjected into the peritubular capillaries of the left kidney, following which urine was serially collected in 20-sec aliquots from both left and right kidneys. For each capillary microinjection the ratio of ^{32}P phosphate to ^{3}H inulin in the urine is divided by the ^{32}P to ^{3}H ratio in the microinjection solution. This term is designated as the "Ratio of Counts" and is calculated for each microinjection at the arrival time of inulin in the urine and at peak inulin excretion. The presence of more phosphate, that is, a higher Ratio of Counts in the urine from the left kidney as compared to that of the right kidney at the urinary arrival time of inulin, is taken as an index of phosphate entry from peritubular blood into the lumen.

To consider the differences in isotope recoveries between the left and right kidneys as a measure of phosphate secretion requires that there was no distortion of the anatomic relationship between the peritubular capillaries and the renal tubular cells as a consequence of puncturing the capillary and that there were no significant functional differences between the two kidneys.

Preliminary studies indicated that the results were not due to technical artifacts of the micropuncture techniques. The equality of renal function between the two kidneys was ascertained by the following observations:

First, the urine flow rate of the left kidney was 90% or more of that of the right kidney; second, the lack of differences in the urinary arrival time of inulin or the urine inulin concentrations at peak inulin excretion; third, the equality of the urine-to-perfusion solution Ratio of Counts in both kidneys following the intravenous infusion of the isotopes; and fourth, in all groups of animals listed on Table 1, the Ratio of Counts at peak inulin excretion in both kidneys was equal.

Thus, given the absence of technical artifacts and the equality of phosphate handling between the two kidneys, the differences in the Ratio of Counts at the arrival time of inulin between the experimental left and contralateral right kidney may be utilized as an index of phosphate secretion.

TABLE 1

$^{32}P/^{3}H$ Urine/Perfusion Solution Ratio of Counts at Peak Inulin Excretion

	Experimental (L) Kidney	Contralateral (R) Kidney	*P*
Control (n=17)	0.15±0.01	0.16±0.01	N.S.
Parathyroid Hormone (n=17)	0.23±0.02	0.21±0.02	N.S.
Phosphate (n=15)	0.70±0.03	0.70±0.03	N.S.
Bicarbonate (n=17)	0.24±0.03	0.25±0.02	N.S.
Acetazolamide (n=15)	0.21±0.015	0.22±0.01	N.S.
Cyanide in Solution (n=14)	0.17±0.02	0.15±0.02	N.S.
Cyanide Systemic (n=10)	0.16±0.02	0.14±0.01	N.S.

Values represent mean ± S.E.M.; n = number of intracapillary microinjections. *P* values compare values of left and right kidneys of the same group of animals.

RESULTS AND DISCUSSION (TABLE 2)

Control animals received an infusion of 5% mannitol in isotonic saline at a rate of 12 ml/hr to insure high urine flow rates. The Ratio of Counts in the left kidney at the arrival time of inulin averaged 0.24±0.02, a value significantly higher than that of the right kidney, which averaged 0.18±0.01. The additional infusion of parathyroid hormone at a rate of 15 units/kg body wt/hr inhibited phosphate reabsorption as indicated by the higher Ratio of Counts in the right kidney as compared to those obtained in control animals. The Ratio of Counts in the left micropunctured kidney was 0.39±0.03, and was significantly higher than that of the right kidney. In animals receiving parathyroid hormone, the Ratio of Counts in the left kidney was 77% higher than that of the right kidney compared to a 33% difference in control animals. This suggests that parathyroid hormone enhanced the entry of phosphate from peritubular blood into the tubular fluid and that the phosphaturia following parathyroid hormone administration may be the consequence of both an inhibition of reabsorption and an increase in secretion.

Since the results in control animals and in animals receiving parathyroid hormone indicated the entry of phosphate into the tubular lumen, several additional experimental maneuvers known to alter phosphate excretion were performed. The intravenous infusion of phosphate at a rate of 18 μmole of phosphate per min increased the Ratio of Counts at the urinary arrival time of inulin from both kidneys. The differences between the left and right

TABLE 2

$^{32}P/^{3}H$ Urine/Perfusion Solution Ratio of Counts at Arrival Time of Inulin

	Experimental (L) Kidney	Contralateral (R) Kidney	*P*
Control (n=17)	0.24±0.02	0.18±0.01	<0.01
Parathyroid Hormone (n=17)	0.39±0.03	0.22±0.02	<0.01
Phosphate (n=15)	0.76±0.03	0.71±0.04	N.S.
Bicarbonate (n=17)	0.30±0.03	0.27±0.02	N.S.
Acetazolamide (n=15)	0.29±0.02	0.29±0.015	N.S.
Cyanide in Solution (n=14)	0.31±0.05	0.16±0.02	<0.01
Cyanide Systemic (n=10)	0.34±0.06	0.17±0.02	<0.01

Values represent mean ± S.E.M.; n = number of intracapillary microinjections. *P* values compare values of left and right kidneys of the same group of animals.

kidneys, observed in control animals, however, was obliterated by phosphate loading. This finding may indicate either that phosphate infusion saturated an active secretory process or that the apparent inhibition of secretion was the consequence of a decrease in the specific activity of the radioactive phosphate. To distinguish between these possibilities, the effects of the metabolic inhibitor cyanide were examined. Cyanide was added to the microinjection solution (5×10^{-3} M) or infused systemically (7.6 μmole/kg/hr). Whether added to the microperfusion solution or administered systemically, cyanide did not obliterate the evidence for phosphate secretion, that is, the Ratio of Counts in the left kidney was significantly higher than that of the right kidney. The percent difference between the left and right kidneys in animals receiving cyanide was actually higher than that observed in control animals. The preliminary conclusion to be drawn from these results is that phosphate secretion is not an active process but, rather, appears to represent a passive back-leak. Moreover, this passive back-leak is increased by cyanide.

Re-examining for a moment the effects of phosphate loading which abolished the evidence for phosphate secretion, the results of the cyanide studies suggest that this result was not due to saturation of an active transport system. The apparent inhibition of phosphate secretion in phosphate-loaded animals may be the result of the dilution of the radioactive phosphate into a larger unlabeled phosphate pool in the kidney, thereby reducing the possibility of detecting secretion of the radioactive phosphate by the methods employed.

We next examined the effects of bicarbonate infusion (5% mannitol in isotonic sodium bicarbonate infused at a rate of 12 ml/hr) and the effects of acetazolamide (25 mg/kg body wt/hr, administered intravenously). Both the infusion of bicarbonate and the infusion of acetazolamide are known to increase phosphate excretion, and these findings are confirmed in the current studies (10). Of interest, however, both maneuvers decreased the differences in the Ratio of Counts between the two kidneys, thus obliterating the evidence for phosphate secretion. While both bicarbonate and acetazolamide alkalinize the urine, their systemic effects are quite different and the common denominator between them with respect to phosphate handling by the kidney is not known. In other preliminary studies, the infusion of hydrochloric acid also abolished the evidence for phosphate secretion. It would appear, then, that systemic, intracellular and/or intratubular pH may affect phosphate secretion but, at the present time, the mechanism is unknown and requires additional study (11).

Evidence for the renal tubular secretion of phosphate has been demonstrated in a variety of non-mammalian species but, to date, the question of the presence of a phosphate secretory mechanism in the mammalian kidney has not been resolved (2-4,12). Although stopped-flow and precession studies in the dog have advanced suggestive evidence for phosphate secretion, these studies could not always be confirmed, and have been criticized on methodologic grounds (11,13-19). In 1962, following a series of negative experimental maneuvers to demonstrate phosphate secretion in the dog, Handler concluded that evidence for phosphate secretion in the mammalian kidney is yet to be demonstrated (5). In other studies performed under specific experimental conditions, a fractional excretion of phosphate of over 100% has been observed occasionally (20; Suki, unpublished observations). When such results are corrected for protein binding and the Donnan's equilibrium, however, the fractional excretion is not sufficiently greater than 100% to be unequivocal. The question of phosphate secretion in the mammalian kidney was reopened by the observations of Glorieux and Scriver in patients with vitamin D-resistant rickets in whom the fractional excretion of phosphate exceeded 100% (9). In a series of micropuncture studies by Boudry and co-workers in rats receiving exogenous infusions of parathyroid hormone and phosphate, $TF/P_{phosphate/inulin}$ ratios in the proximal convoluted tubule of over one were reported, and indirect evidence for phosphate secretion in the collecting ducts was also suggested (7). Schneider et al. performed an interesting series of studies, using techniques analagous to those of the present study, and advanced evidence that phosphate secretion does occur in the dog (8). On the other hand, Greger, Lang, Knox and Lechene microperfused segments of the rat proximal tubule and were unable to demonstrate phosphate entry into the tubule (6). Their study, however, does not exclude the possibility that the secreted phosphate was back-reabsorbed or the possibility that the phosphate secretory site is located in nephron segments other than the proximal convoluted tubule. The results of the current investigations do present evidence for phosphate secretion in the rat, probably by a non-energy requiring mechanism. It is not possible at the present time, however, to assess the physiologic importance of this mechanism in the overall renal handling of phosphate.

ACKNOWLEDGMENTS

The authors gratefully acknowledge the technical assistance of Deborah Steplock and the secretarial assistance of Polly Dunham. This work was supported in part by a Clinical Investigatorship award from the Veterans Administration (to Dr. Weinman) and by a grant from the National Aeronautics and Space Administration, NAS 9-14715 (to Dr. Suki).

REFERENCES

1. Levinsky, N.G., and Davidson, D.G.: Renal action of parathyroid extract in the chicken. Am. J. Physiol. 191:530, 1957.

2. Marshall, E.J. Jr., and Graffin, A.L.: Excretion of inorganic phosphate by the aglomerular kidney. Proc. Soc. Exp. Biol. Med. 31:44, 1933.

3. Walker, A.M., and Hudson, C.C.: The role of the tubule in the excretion of inorganic phosphate by the amphibian kidney. Am. J. Physiol. 118:167, 1937.

4. Wolback, R.A.: Phlorizin and renal phosphate secretion in the spiny dogfish *Squalus acanthias*. Am. J. Physiol. 219:886, 1970.

5. Handler, J.S.: A study of renal phosphate excretion in the dog. Am. J. Physiol. 202:787, 1962.

6. Greger, R.F., Lang, F.C., Knox, F.G., and Lechene, C.P.: Absence of significant secretory flux of phosphate in the proximal convoluted tubule. Am. J. Physiol. 232:F235, 1977.

7. Boudry, J.-F., Troehler, U., Touabi, M., Fleisch, H., and Bonjour, J.-P.: Secretion of inorganic phosphate in the rat nephron. Clin. Sci. Molec. Med. 38:375, 1975.

8. Schneider, E.G., and McLane, L.A.: Evidence for a peritubular to luminal flux of phosphate in the dog kidney. Am. J. Physiol. 232:159, 1977.

9. Glorieux, F., and Scriver, C.R.: Loss of a parathyroid hormone-sensitive component of phosphate transport in x-linked phosphatemia. Science 175:997, 1972.

10. Fulop, M., and Brazeau, P.: The phosphaturic effect of sodium bicarbonate and acetazolamide in dogs. J. Clin. Invest. 47: 983, 1968.

11. Carrasquer, G., and Brodsky, W.A.: Elimination of transient secretion of phosphate by alkalinization of plasma in dogs. Am. J. Physiol. 201:499, 1961.

12. Clark, N.B., and Dantzler, W.H.: Renal tubular transport of calcium and phosphate in snakes. Role of parathyroid hormone. Am. J. Physiol. 223:1455, 1972.

13. Davis, B.B., Kedes, L.H., and Field, J.B.: Demonstration of distal tubular flux of phosphorus using modified stop-flow analysis. Metabolism 15:482, 1966.

14. Foulkes, E.C.: The precession clearance of phosphate in the dog and the action of parathyroid hormone. (Abstract) Fed. Proc. 26:376, 1967.

15. Lambert, P.P., Vanderveiken, F., deKoster, J.P., Kahn, R.J., and Myttenaere, M.: Study of phosphate excretion by the stopped-flow technique. Effects of parathyroid hormone. Nephron 1:103, 1964.

16. Mudge, G.H., Berndt, W.O., and Valtin, H.: Tubular transport of urea, glucose, phosphate, uric acid, sulfate and thiosulfate. *In* Orloff, J. and Berliner, R.W., eds., Handbook of Physiology, Section 8: Renal Physiology. Washington, D.C., American Physiological Society, pp. 587-652, 1973.

17. Orloff, J.: Pitfalls in the use of stop-flow for the localization of diuretic action with special reference to Na reabsorption. Ann. N.Y. Acad. Sci. 139:344, 1966.

18. Samiy, A.H., Hirsch, P.F., and Ramsay, A.G.: Localization of phosphaturic effect of parathyroid hormone in the nephron of the dog. Am. J. Physiol. 208:73, 1965.

19. Zins, G.R., and Weiner, I.M.: Bidirectional urate transport limited to the proximal tubule in dogs. Am. J. Physiol. 215: 411, 1968.

20. Pitts, R.F.: The excretion of urine in the dog. Am. J. Physiol. 106:1, 1933.

PHOSPHATE AND GLUCOSE TRANSPORT IN THE PROXIMAL CONVOLUTED TUBULE:

MUTUAL DEPENDENCY ON SODIUM

Vincent W. Dennis and Peter C. Brazy

Division of Nephrology, Duke University Medical Center

Durham, North Carolina 27710

The possibility that diverse solutes such as glucose and amino acids may influence phosphate transport in the proximal renal tubule (1) has provided a basis for various theories regarding the mechanism of phosphate absorption. Such theories may include a polyfunctional carrier, a common, limited energy source or shared driving forces. Thus, as with other epithelia (2), absorptive processes in the proximal convoluted tubule may share a common element such as coupling to sodium transport. In this regard, the present studies were designed to examine the relationship between glucose and phosphate absorption in isolated proximal convoluted tubules from the rabbit kidney and to document that sodium transport is necessary for the renal absorption of both these solutes.

METHODS

Individual proximal convoluted segments from the rabbit kidney were perfused in vitro with an artificial fluid resembling glomerular ultrafiltrate but of variable composition. Normal rabbit serum was used as the bath. Radioisotopic techniques were used to measure the lumen-to-bath fluxes of phosphate (J-Phos; pmol/mm·min) and glucose (J-Gluc) during perfusion with normal physiological fluids as well as during perfusion with fluids wherein glucose was selectively replaced with sodium chloride.

RESULTS

In paired studies (n=12 tubules), J-Phos decreased from 9.34 ± 1.48 to 6.28 ± 1.20 pmol/mm·min ($P < 0.01$) when glucose was added to the perfusate. Phlorizin 10^{-5}M in the lumen reduced the lumen-

Table 1: Effect of ouabain on glucose and phosphate absorption by isolated proximal convoluted tubules.

Ouabain (M)	J-Gluc (pmol/mm·min)	J-Phos (pmol/mm·min)
0	87.5 ± 6.4	5.87 ± 0.80
10^{-5}	24.5 ± 3.3	0.50 ± 0.10

to-bath flux of glucose from 80 ± 5 to 11 ± 2 pmol/mm·min ($P < 0.001$) and under similar conditions increased J-Phos from 6.94 ± 1.89 to 9.06 ± 2.01 pmol/mm·min ($P < 0.02$). Phlorizin had no effect on J-Phos when glucose was absent from the perfusate. As shown in Table 1, ouabain 10^{-5}M in the bath reduced the lumen to bath fluxes of both phosphate and glucose to values approaching their bath-to-lumen fluxes (3, 4).

DISCUSSION

These data indicate that in this system intraluminal glucose interacts directly with phosphate absorption. This interaction is related to the transport of glucose rather than merely its presence or absence from the lumen. Moreover, to the extent that ouabain represents a specific inhibitor of active sodium transport, the observation that the net transport of both phosphate and glucose are essentially eliminated by ouabain suggests that mutual dependency on sodium transport may represent the functional site where glucose and phosphate transport interact.

REFERENCES

1. Pitts, R. F., and Alexander, R. F.: The renal reabsorption mechanism for inorganic phosphate in normal and acidotic dogs. Am. J. Physiol. 142:648, 1944.

2. Schultz, S. G. and Curran, P. F.: Coupled transport of sodium and organic solutes. Physiol. Rev. 50:637, 1970.

3. Dennis, V. W., Woodhall, P. B., and Robinson, R. R.: Characteristics of phosphate transport in isolated proximal tubule. Am. J. Physiol. 231:979, 1976.

4. Tune, B. M. and Burg, M. B.: Glucose transport by proximal renal tubules. Am. J. Physiol. 221:580, 1971.

FACTORS INVOLVED IN THE ALTERED PHOSPHATE REABSORPTION DURING PHOSPHATE LOADING IN THYROPARATHYROIDECTOMIZED RATS*

F. Lang, H. Oberleithner, R. Greger, and P. Deetjen

Physiologisches Institut, Universität Innsbruck

Fritz-Pregl-Str. 3, A - 6020 Innsbruck, Austria

Several investigators (3,4,5,9) observed a decline of renal phosphate reabsorption after prolonged intravenous infusion of phosphate. Similarily high phosphate diets are known to produce phosphaturia and phosphate depletion enhances renal phosphate reabsorption (11,12). The decline of renal phosphate reabsorption during acute or chronic phosphate loading was demonstrated in both, intact and thyroparathyroidectomized (TPTX) rats. Irrespective of the potentially different mechanisms involved in acute and chronic phosphate loading, the kidney appears to be capable to adjust phosphate reabsorption to phosphate input even in the absence of parathyroid hormone.

Alterations induced by phosphate loading

In order to test, whether the decline of renal phosphate reabsorption is mediated by alterations in acid base balance or plasma electrolyte concentrations, clearance studies were performed in TPTX rats. The animals were initially infused with 0.2 ml/min kg BW saline. After a control period of 1 h the infusate was replaced by 0.2 ml/min kg BW phosphate 100 mmol/l made isotonic with sodium chloride and adjusted to pH 7.4. Analytical and experimental procedures will be described in detail elsewhere (10). All data presented in this paper are given ± SEM.

Fig. 1 summarizes the results of this series: GFR remained virtually constant. Since plasma phosphate concentration increased from 2.5 to 5.3 mmol/l, filtered load exceeded the maximal tubular

*Footnote: This study was supported by "Legerlotz Stiftung" and by "Deutsche Forschungsgemeinschaft".

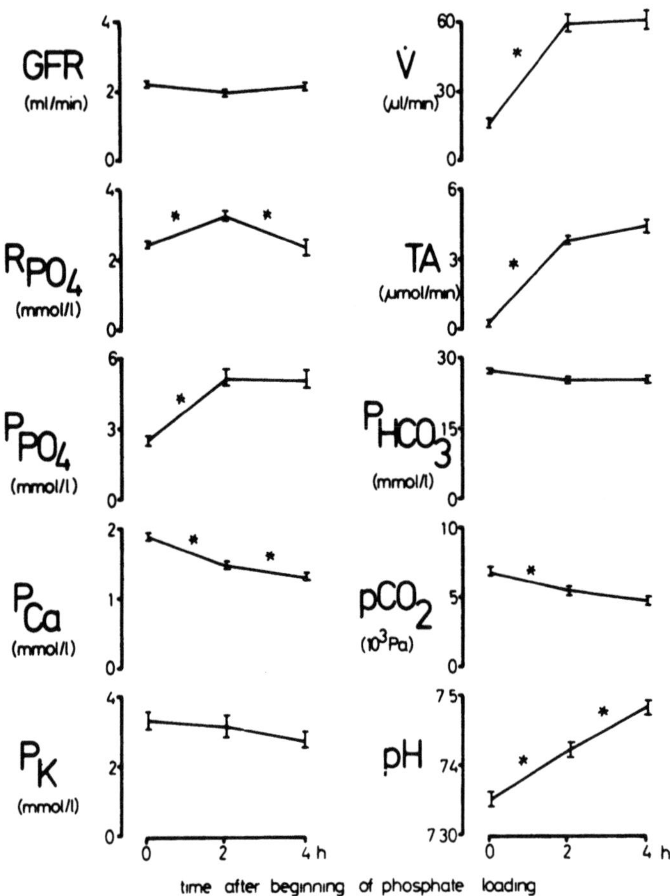

Fig.1: Variables during phosphate loading
*Indicates significant change ($p < 0.05$) between two subsequent periods. Abbreviations used: GFR = glomerular filtration rate, $\dot{V}$ = urinary flow rate, R_{PO_4} = phosphate reabsorption per unit GFR, P_{PO_4}, P_{Ca}, P_K and P_{HCO_3} = plasma concentrations of phosphate, calcium, potassium and bicarbonate, TA = titratable acid, pCO_2 = plasma CO_2 pressure (in Pascale), pH = plasma pH.

transport rate for phosphate, which appeared to be 3.3 mmol/l GFR after 2 h. Despite the fact that plasma phosphate remained virtually constant within the next two hours, phosphate reabsorption declined significantly to 2.4 mmol/l. Urinary titratable acid increased in parallel to the phosphate excretion, since urinary pH remained low (control: 5.6 ± 0.1, 2h: 5.9 ± 0.2, 4h: 6.3 ± 0.1). Thus, excreted phosphate served as a proton acceptor and allowed excessive excretion of hydrogen ions. Furthermore, phosphaturia led to osmotic diuresis with an increase of urinary flow rate from 16 to 60 μl/min. The increase in urinary flow rate was not a consequence of volume expansion, which was avoided in this study (see above). The increased excretion of titratable acid partially explains the development of alkalosis. Plasma pH increased from 7.35 to 7.48. Interestingly, alkalosis even followed the infusion of acid phosphate solutions (pH 5.8). If the enhanced excretion of titratable acid were the only cause for the development of alkalosis, plasma bicarbonate should increase. However, bicarbonate did not significantly change during phosphate loading. Instead, pCO_2 decreased significantly from 6.6 to 4.4 kilopascale. The reason for the respiratory alkalosis is most likely the drop in plasma calcium (from 1.9 to 1.3 mmol/l). Increased calcium in the cerebrospinal fluid is known to suppress ventilation (8). Plasma potassium decreased from 3.4 to 2.8 mmol/l, however, the decrease was not statistically significant.

The role of acid base balance for the decline in phosphate reabsorption

During phosphate loading, the decline of phosphate reabsorption was significantly correlated with the increase of plasma pH ($p<0.01$) and bicarbonate ($p<0.05$). However, renal phosphate reabsorption and pH were correlated with the duration of phosphate loading and hence the correlation might have been factitious. Therefore, in an additional series of experiments, attempts were made to reverse the alkalosis during continued infusion of phosphate. To this end, the animals were offered 5 % CO_2 and 95 % O_2 for respiration, 2 hours after the beginning of phosphate loading. In addition, neutral phosphate was replaced by acid phosphate (pH 5.8) in the infusate. In fact, plasma pH increased from 7.39 ± 0.01 to 7.50 ± 0.02 within the first two hours and declined thereafter to 7.38 ± 0.04. At the same time, however, phosphate reabsorption continued to decline (from 3.95 ± 0.3 to 3.6 ± 0.6 and 2.6 ± 0.3 mmol/l GFR). Bicarbonate remained constant during the procedure. From this series we conclude that the decline of phosphate reabsorption is not a result of the alkalosis induced by phosphate loading. This does not rule out that alkalosis contributes to the decline of phosphate reabsorption. However, the influence of alkalosis on phosphate reabsorption is still a matter of debate (7). In any case other - more important - factors must be operative during phosphate loading.

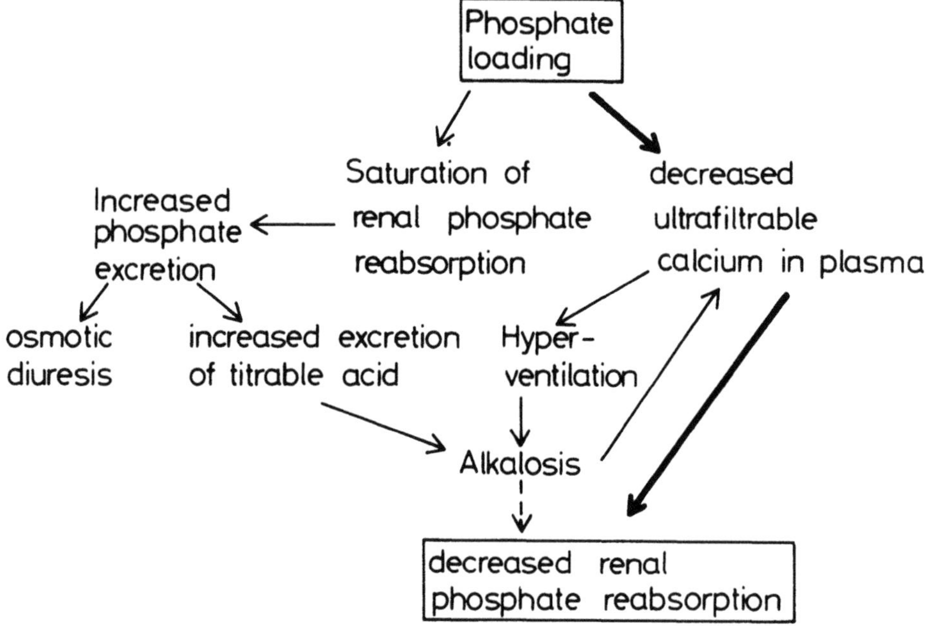

Fig. 2: Alterations induced by phosphate loading

The role of plasma calcium for the decline in phosphate reabsorption

Since plasma calcium decreased in parallel to the decline of phosphate reabsorption, it appeared reasonable to assume that calcium might mediate the alteration in phosphate transport. Furthermore, calcium has been shown to increase phosphate reabsorption (1,6), although this effect was not invariably demonstrated (2). On the other hand, the correlation of plasma calcium and phosphate reabsorption could again reflect a coincidence of time course. Therefore, calcium (2 μmol/min during 1/2 hour followed by 0.7 μmol/min) was infused 4 hours after the beginning of phosphate load. As exspected, plasma calcium declined during phosphate load (1h: 1.55 ± 0.1 mmol/l; 2.5h: 1.41 ± 0.1 mmol/l; 4h: 1.23 ± 0.1 mmol/l) and increased after calcium infusion (1.5h: 1.66 ± 0.2 mmol/l, 2,5h: 1.82 ± 0.1 mmol/l) despite continued phosphate infusion. Renal phosphate reabsorption declined as usually within the first four hours (1h: 2.8 ± 0.4 mmol/l GFR; 2.5h: 2.6 ± 0.3 mmol/l GFR; 4h: 2.1 ± 0.3) but increased after calcium infusion despite continued phosphate load (1.5h: 2.8 ±

0.4 mmol/l GFR; 2.5h: 3.2 ± 0.5 mmol/l GFR). Thus, elevation of calcium to control levels completely reversed the decline of phosphate reabsorption.

In another series of experiments, ^{33}Phosphate and ^{3}H-inulin containing saline solution was microinfused into single proximal tubules, and urine collected serially. The continuous microinfusion period was 60 min and 1 μmol calcium was added to the kidney surface after 30 min. Addition of calcium was followed by a significant reduction of phosphate recovery over inulin (ΔR = 14 ± 4%). We therefore conclude that calcium has a direct effect on the kidney.

Fig. 2 summarizes the effects observed in this study under phosphate loading. In respect to the decline of phosphate reabsorption, calcium appears to be the crucial parameter.

References

1. Amiel, C., Kuntziger, H., Couette, S., Coureau, C., Bergounioux: Evidence for a Parathyroid Hormone-Independent Calcium Modulation of Phosphate Transport along the Nephron. J.Clin.Invest. 57, 256-263 (1976)
2. Cuche, J.L., Ott, C.E., Marchand, G.R., Knox, F.G.: Lack of Effect of Hypocalcemia on Renal Phosphate Handling. J.Lab. Clin.Med.88, No. 2, 271-275 (1976)
3. Engle, J.E., Steele, T.H.: Renal phosphate reabsorption in the rat: Effect of inhibitors. Kidney Intern. 8, 98-104 (1975)
4. Frick, A.: Reabsorption of Inorganic Phosphate in the Rat Kidney. Pflügers Arch. 304, 351-364 (1968)
5. Le Grimellec, C., Roinel, N., Morel, F.: Simultaneous Mg, Ca, P, K, Na and Cl Analysis in Rat Tubular Fluid. Pflügers Arch. 346, 171-188 (1974)
6. Le Grimellec, C., Roinel, N., Morel, F.: Simultaneous Mg, Ca, P, K and Cl Analysis in Rat Tubular Fluid. Pflügers Arch. 346, 189-204 (1974)
7. Knox, F.G., Greger, R., Lang, F., Marchand, G.R.: Renal Handling of Phosphate: Update. Plenum Press, N.Y. (in press)
8. Koepchen, H.P.: Atmungsregulation in: Physiologie des Menschen (Gauer,O.H., Kramer,K., Jung,R., ed.) Volume 6, Urban & Schwarzenberg, Munich 1972
9. Lang, F., Greger, R., Marchand, G., Knox, F.G.: Saturation kinetics of phosphate reabsorption in rats. 2nd Intern. Workshop on Phosphate. Plenum Press, New York.
10. Oberleithner, H., Greger, R., Lang, F.: Role of calcium in the decline of phosphate reabsorption during phosphate loading in TPTX animals. In preparation.
11. Steele, T.H., De Luca, H.F.: Influence of Dietary Phosphorus

on Renal Phosphate Reabsorption in the Parathyroidectomized Rat. J. Clin. Invest. 57, 867-874 (1976)

12. Troehler, U., Bonjour, J.P. and Fleisch, H.: Inorganic phosphate homeostasis. Renal adaptation to the dietary intake in intact and thyroparathyroidectomized rats. J.Clin.Invest. 57: 264-273 (1976)

EFFECT OF VOLUME EXPANSION ON PHOSPHATE TRANSPORT IN UREMIC DOGS

Sung-Feng Wen, James W. Boynar, Jr. and Robert W. Stoll

Department of Medicine, University of Wisconsin Center for Health Sciences, Madison, Wisconsin 53706, U.S.A.

Functional adaptation for renal phosphate transport in chronic renal failure has generally been considered to be mainly the result of secondary hyperparathyroidism (1, 2). On the other hand, it has also been reported that uremic animals can maintain phosphate homeostasis in the absence of parathyroid glands (3). Our present clearance and micropuncture studies were designed to re-evaluate the role of parathyroid hormone (PTH) in phosphate adaptation of uremic remnant kidney dogs.

METHODS

Unilateral remnant kidney model was induced in 25 dogs by ligation of 2/3 - 5/6 branches of left renal artery and this was followed by contralateral nephrectomy 3-8 weeks later. Another week was allowed before the micropuncture experiments were carried out. All animals were studied before and after extracellular volume expansion (VE) to 10% of body weight. Of the 13 dogs which had thyroparathyroidectomy (TPTX) 1-3 days before the experiments, 6 had fractional excretion (FE) of phosphate less than 16% (RK-I + TPTX) and 7 had FE phosphate greater than 19% (RK - II + TPTX). The other 12 dogs with intact parathyroids were divided into 6 dogs with plasma creatinine lower than 3.5 mg/100 ml (RK-I) and 6 dogs with that higher than 3.5 mg/100 ml (RK-II). Tubule fluid (TF) phosphate was analyzed by a colorimetric method (4, 5) and inulin by a fluorometric technique (6).

RESULTS AND DISCUSSION

Clearance and micropuncture data are summarized in the table.

Exptl Groups		GFR ml/min	UF_{PO4} mmol/L	FE_{PO4} %	SNGFR nl/min	$\left(\frac{TF}{P}\right)_{IN}$	$\left(\frac{TF}{UF}\right)_{PO4}$	RF_{PO4} %
NML	H	33.4	2.25	5.2	67	1.71	0.72	42
	VE	34.9	2.08	27.8**	70	1.27**	0.81**	64 **
NML +TPTX	H	32.3	2.12	3.7	67	1.63	0.63	39
	VE	35.8	1.99	11.8**	73	1.31	0.80**	60 **
RK-I	H	11.4	2.06	39.4	102	1.44	0.95	65
	VE	13.2	1.79**	55.9*	111	1.24**	0.94	77*
RK-I +TPTX	H	13.4	1.78	7.0	97	1.48	0.96	65
	VE	15.4	1.64*	40.0**	98	1.21**	0.97	81**
RK-II	H	8.7	2.33	48.2	114	1.39	1.04	74
	VE	9.8**	2.08	57.1**	125	1.23*	1.05	83*
RK-II +TPTX	H	8.1	1.97	32.7	96	1.53	1.05	70
	VE	9.3*	1.71**	51.4**	101	1.32**	1.06	81*

All data are mean values of the micropunctured kidney.
GFR = Glomerular filtration rate; UF = Plasma ultrafiltrate;
SN = Single nephron; RF = Remaining fraction in proximal tubule;
NML = Normal dogs; RK = Remnant kidney; H = Hydropenia; *P<0.05;
**P<0.01

High FE phosphate in the remnant kidney dogs with intact parathyroids indicates phosphate adaptation. With moderate renal failure, phosphate adaptation is primarily due to secondary hyperparathyroidism since TPTX reduced FE phosphate to normal. However, the phosphaturic response to volume expansion in these TPTX remnant kidney dogs was exaggerated, suggesting that extracellular volume may contribute to phosphate adaptation in the absence of PTH. When more severe renal failure was induced, FE phosphate remained high even with TPTX, indicating that factors other than PTH could be responsible for phosphate adaptation in advanced chronic renal failure. High proximal TF/UF phosphate ratios in all remnant kidney groups indicate that phosphate adaptation in the proximal tubule is independent of PTH or the severity of the renal disease. However, the final adaptation along the nephron as expressed by FE phosphate is determined by alteration in phosphate transport distal to the late proximal tubule sites. It is concluded that both PTH and non-PTH factors are important in functional adaptation for phosphate transport in chronic renal failure.

REFERENCES

1. Slatopolsky E, Gradowska L, Kashemsant C, Keltner R, Manley C and Bricker NS: The control of phosphate excretion in uremia. J Clin Invest 45: 672, 1966.
2. Slatopolsky E, Robson AM, Elkan I and Bricker NS: Control of phosphate excretion in uremic man. J Clin Invest 47: 1865, 1968.
3. Swenson RS, Weisinger JR, Ruggeri JL and Reaven GM: Evidence that parathyroid hormone is not required for phosphate homeostasis in renal failure. Metabolism 24: 199, 1975.
4. Chen, Jr. PS, Toribara TY and Warner H: Microdetermination of phosphorus. Anal Chem 28: 1756, 1956.
5. Wen SF: Micropuncture studies of phosphate transport in the proximal tubule of the dog. The relationship to sodium reabsorption. J Clin Invest 53: 143, 1974.
6. Vurek GG and Pegram SE: Fluorometric method for determination of nanogram quantities of inulin. Anal Biochem 16: 409, 1966.

MICROPUNCTURE STUDY OF PHOSPHORUS TRANSPORT IN GENETIC HYPO-PHOSPHATEMIC MICE

M.G. BRUNETTE, S.D. GIASSON, N. VIGNEAULT, S. CARRIERE

MAISONNEUVE-ROSEMONT HOSPITAL-UNIVERSITY OF MONTREAL

5415 l'ASSOMPTION BLVD. MONTREAL P.Q. H1T 2M4, CANADA

Altough hypophosphatemic vitamin D-resistant rickets was first described by Albright and coll. in 1937 (1) the pathogenesis of this disease is still unknown. Two opposing hypothesis exist regarding the primary defect responsible for the constant hypophosphatemia. The first suggests a faulty intestinal absorption of calcium with secondary hyperparathyroidism, whereas the second places the initial responsibility on a defect of renal transport of phosphorus. The measurement of serum immunoreactive PTH has been found normal or low by Rook and coll (9), and by Arnaud (2), slightly increased by Lewy (7), and definitely increased by Reitz (8). Since the hyperparathyroidism is not a constant finding and when present, it seems not pronounced enough to explain the biological trait of the disease the hypothesis of a primary renal defect seems more probable.

Until recently, the exclusive incidence of the vitamin D-resistant rickets in humans has greatly reduced the possibilities of investigation. The recent discovery by Eicher and collaborators (5) of a mutant strain of mice presenting all the characteristics of the human disease provides an opportunity to obtain new information.

The present paper describes a micropuncture study of phosphorus transport in the proximal tubule of these mice which were kindly supplied by Dr. Eicher and Dr. Scriver.

METHODS

13 control and 6 hypophosphatemic (Hyp) male mice were anesthetized with inactin, 120 mg/K intraperitoneal. Catheters were placed in the carotid artery and jugular vein for blood sampling and intravenous perfusion. Urine was collected through a bladder catheter. The left kidney was prepared for micropuncture through an abdominal incision, and the proximal convoluted tubule punctured through the capsule. Inulin (In) and inorganic phosphorus (Pi) clearance were performed every second hour during the time of micropuncture.

The intratubular phosphorus concentration was determined by a new procedure, recently developed in our laboratory. This technique is based on the reaction between phosphate converted to hexadimolybdatophosphate, with thiamine and Borax, resulting in a highly fluorescent thiochrome. The micro adaptation of this reaction permits the measurement of Pi in 3 nl samples of tubular fluid (TF) (4). The tubular fluid inulin was measured using the fluorometric method of Vurek and Pegram (11).

RESULTS

The clearance data are presented in table 1. The plasma concentration of Pi is 85.10 ± 2.27 mg/L and 48.43 ± 3.29 mg/L in normal and Hyp mice respectively. The GFR is also significantly lower in Hyp than in control mice, despite the fact that the weight of both groups was comparable. The Pi concentration in urine is lower in Hyp mice than in their controls, but since the urinary volume (UV) is relatively high in the first group, the phosphaturia is similar in the two series of animals. However, due to the different plasma concentration of Pi (P Pi), the fractional excretion (FE Pi) is largely increased in Hyp compared to the corresponding value in normal (N) mice.

Table 2 summarizes the micropuncture data obtained in N and Hyp mice. The mean TF Pi is not significantly different in the two series of animals. However, because of the low P Pi in Hyp mice, the TF/P Pi and the fractions of filtered Pi which are unreabsorbed (% E Pi) are significantly higher in the latter group than in the control, indicating a relative defect of Pi transport at this level.

Conclusions concerning distal reabsorption are hazardous since no distal micropunctures have been performed. However, in normal mice approximately 24 % of the filtered Pi remains at the end of the proximal tubule (TF/P In > 2) the corresponding FE Pi in urine is 15.81 %. If comparison between these two values is acceptable, it can be assumed that about 10 % of the filtered load is reabsorbed in the distal segments of the nephron. In Hyp mice, the % E Pi

Table I. Clearance data

TYPE OF MICE	P Pi mg/L	U Pi ug/ul	V ul/min	UV Pi ug/min	GFR ul/min	FE Pi %
CONTROL n=21 (13 mice)	85.10 ± 2.27	4.30 ± 0.53	0.41 ± 0.05	1.79 ± 0.31	132.71 ± 12.90	15.81 ± 1.90
Hyp. n= 14 (6 mice)	48.43 ± 3.29	1.74 ± 0.20	0.68 ± 0.14	1.12 ± 0.22	90.64 ± 14.88	35.34 ± 5.26
Significance	P<0.0005	P<0.05	P<0.025	NS	P<0.025	P<0.0005

Table II. Micropuncture data

TYPE OF MICE	TF Pi mg/L	TF/P Pi	TF/P In	% E Pi
CONTROL n=21 (13 mice)	62.00 ± 3.48	0.73 ± 0.04	1.64 ± 0.10	49.10 ± 4.59
Hyp. n=14 (6 mice)	57.57 ± 7.10	1.19 ± 0.12	1.52 ± 0.13	78.68 ± 7.39
Significance	NS	P<0.0005	NS	P<0.0025

does not vary significantly along the proximal tubule. However, all of the values whose mean is 78.68 % are far above the corresponding FE (35.34 %) suggesting a relatively greater distal fractional Pi reabsorption than in normal mice. But since the filtered load is lower in Hyp mice than in the N mice, it is probable that the absolute quantities of Pi reabsorbed in the distal parts of the nephron are similar in the two series of animals.

DISCUSSION

The phosphaturia in Hyp mice and N mice are comparable. The lack of Pi retention in the hypophosphatemic animals suggests an abnormal renal leak of this electrolyte. The present study shows a Pi transport defect in the proximal tubule. A primary defect at this level could involve the luminal membrane carrier, the metabolism of cyclic AMP system, the number of the basolateral membrane receptors, the basolateral membrane permeability of Pi efflux or the intracellular metabolism of inorganic vs organic phosphorus. Normal Pi transport through the apical membrane of the proximal tubule depends on the Pi gradient (6), the TF pH (6), the Na (3, 6) and glucose transport (10).

According to our data, the TF Pi concentration is normal in Hyp mice and since the intracellular pool of Pi is also normal (5) the defect does not result from an increased intra luminal-intra cellular gradient of Pi concentration. TF pH, Na, and glucose have not been measured. Clearance studies however did not detect any abnormal glucosuria (5) and in our study the mean TF/P In does not significantly differ between the two series of animals, suggesting that water and therefore Na proximal transport is not modified.

An intrinsic defect of cyclic AMP metabolism or an abnormal response of cyclic AMP to PTH or calcitonin, resulting in an overactivity of this system might be responsible for the relative hyperphosphaturia and should be investigated in these mice. The intracellular calcium concentration is an important regulating factor of adenyl cyclase activity and may be modified by the phosphorus depletion.

Finally, a Pi transport defect can also be secondary to an extra renal effect such as a hypersecretion of PTH or calcitonin. Normal PTH levels have been found in these mice (5) but no data concerning the serum calcitonin are available.

In conclusion, the finding of a proximal tubular defect of Pi transport in hypophosphatemic vitamin D-resistant rickets does not solve the problem of the pathogenesis, but has resulted in the evolution of a more precise hypothesis for further investigation.

REFERENCES

1. ALBRIGHT, F., BUTLER, A.M., and BLOOMBERG, E.
Rickets resistant to vitamin D therapy.
Amer. J. dis. child. 54: 529-547, 1937.

2. ARNAUD, C., GLORIEUX, F., and SCRIVER, C.
Serum parathyroid hormone in X-linked hypophosphatemia.
Science 173: 845-847, 1971.

3. BAUMANN, K., ROUFFIGNAC, C., de, ROINEL, N., RUMRICH, G. and ULLRICH, K.J.
Renal phosphate transport: inhomogeneity of local proximal.
Pflügers Arch 356: 287-297, 1975.

4. BRUNETTE, M.G., VIGNEAULT, N., and DANAN, G.
A new fluorometric method for the determination of picomoles of inorganic phosphorus. Application to the renal tubular fluid.
Analytical Biochemistry. In Press.

5. EICHER, E.M., SOUTHARD, J.L., SCRIVER, C.R., and GLORIEUX,F.
Hypophosphatemia: mouse model for human familial hypophosphatemic vitamin D-resistant rickets.
Proc. Natl. Acad. Sci. U.S.A. 73: 4667-4671, 1976.

6. HOFFMANN, N., THEES, M., and KINNE, R.
Phosphate transport by isolated renal brush border vesicles.
Pflügers Arch. 362: 147-156, 1976.

7. LEWY, J.E., CABANE, C., REPETTO, H.A., CANTERBURRY, J.M., and REISS, E.
Serum parathyroid hormone in hypophosphatemic vitamin D-resistant rickets.
J. Pediat. 81: 294-300, 1972.

8. REITZ, R.E., and WEINSTEIN, R.L.
Parathyroid hormone secretion in familial vitamin D-resistant rickets.
New England J. med. 289: 941-945, 1973.

9. ROOF, B.S., PIEL, C.F., and GORDAN, G.S.
Nature of defect responsible for familial vitamin D-resistant rickets based on parathormone assay.
Clin. Res. 20: 624, 1972.

10. ROUFFIGNAC, C. de, TOUVAY, C., POUJEOL, P., and CORMAN, B. Influence of glucose on renal reabsorption of phosphate in the rat.
XXVII International congress of physiology-Paris-1977.

11. VUREK, G.G., and PEGRAM, S.E.
Fluorometric method for the determination of nanograms quantities of inulin.
Anal. Biochem. 16: 409-414, 1966.

REGULATION OF THE TUBULAR TRANSPORT OF PHOSPHATE IN THE RAT: ROLE OF PARATHYROID HORMONE AND 1,25-DIHYDROXY-VITAMIN D_3

J.-P. Bonjour, C. Preston, U. Troehler, and H. Fleisch
Department of Pathophysiology, University of Berne, Murtenstrasse 35, 3010 Berne, Switzerland

In the growing rat, the kidney responds to variation in the supply (1,2) and probably also to the demand (3) of the organism for inoganic phosphate (Pi) by changing its tubular capacity to transport Pi. The adaptive response in reducing the net tubular reabsorption of Pi by animals fed a high Pi diet can be observed in both intact (1) and thyroparathyroidectomized (TPTX) rats (1,2). However, after thyroparathyroidectomy the capability of the renal tubule to adapt to a high Pi intake is reduced (4). The disappearance of the direct influence by parathyroid hormone (PTH) on the tubular Pi transport may explain this phenomenon. However, removal of the parathyroid glands leads to a reduced production of 1,25-dihydroxyvitamin D_3 (1,25-$(OH)_2D_3$) (5), a metabolite which influences markedly Pi homeostasis (6,7). Therefore the question arises whether or not the diminished production of 1,25-$(OH)_2D_3$ in TPTX rats contributes to the reduced tubular response due to a high Pi supply. To investigate this problem, the influence of 1,25-$(OH)_2D_3$ on the renal handling of Pi was studied in TPTX rats which were fed a high (1.2 g %) or low (0.2 g %) phosphorus diet. As reported in detail elsewhere (8) 1,25-$(OH)_2D_3$ was administered chronically at the dose of 13 pmol twice daily during the 7 days preceding the clearance study. This dose was selected because it normalized without overcorrecting the low intestinal Ca (9) and P (10) absorption in TPTX rats.

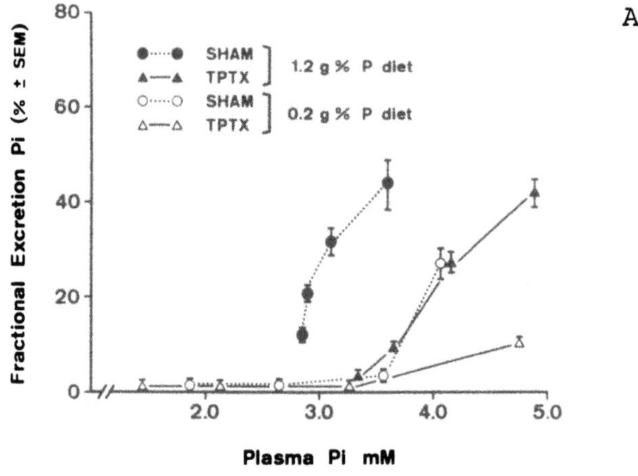

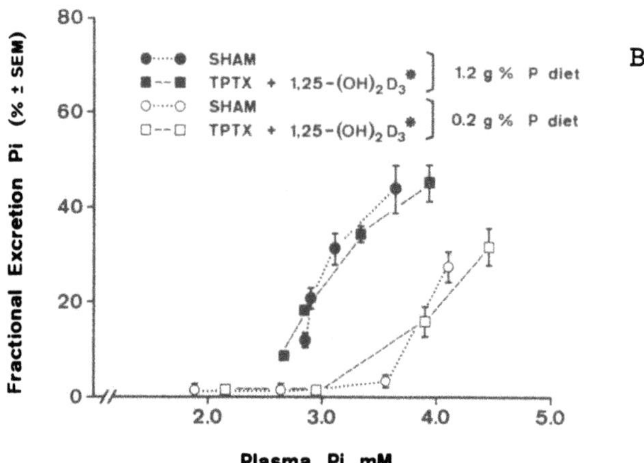

Figure 1: Fractional excretion of Pi determined under acute i.v. sodium chloride and stepwise-increasing sodium phosphate infusion in A: sham-operated (SHAM) and thyroparathyroidectomized (TPTX); in B: SHAM and TPTX treated with 1,25-$(OH)_2D_3$. All rats were pair-fed low or high Pi diet. * 2 x 13 pmol/day i.p. for 7 days (adapted from reference 8).

The dramatic effect of 1,25-$(OH)_2D_3$ on the renal handling of Pi when chronically administered to TPTX rats is illustrated on Figure 1. Indeed the marked impact of TPTX on the renal handling of Pi (Figure 1A) is completely corrected by 1,25-$(OH)_2D_3$ (Figure 1B). On both low and high Pi diets TPTX rats supplemented with 1,25-$(OH)_2D_3$ appear to have the same renal handling of Pi as sham-operated counterparts (Figure 1B). Note that in TPTX rats fed low Pi diet, 1,25-$(OH)_2D_3$ does not alter the ability of the kidney to excrete a urine which appears virtually free of Pi up to a plasma Pi concentration of 3.0 - 3.5 mM (Figure 1B). Our results show that 1,25-$(OH)_2D_3$ given in physiological amounts to TPTX rats restore the ability of the tubular Pi transport system to adjust to conspicuous variations in the Pi intake. This observation indicates that PTH is not essential for the tubular Pi adaptation.

The mechanism by which 1,25-$(OH)_2D_3$ enhances the tubular capacity to excrete Pi does not seem to include the adenylcyclase system (8). In TPTX rats fed high Pi diet the normalization of the renal handling of Pi induced by 1,25-$(OH)_2D_3$ was not associated with a correction of urinary cAMP excretion (8). The effect of 1,25-$(OH)_2D_3$ on the renal handling of Pi in TPTX rats was not associated with a change in the overall tubular capacity to transport calcium (11) or urinary pH (8). The effect of 1,25-$(OH)_2D_3$ was also maintained under marked extracellular volume expansion and conspicuous increase in the fractional excretion of Pi (8). Thus the chronic administration of 1,25-$(OH)_2D_3$ appears to affect quite selectively the tubular Pi transport system.

Among several other vitamin D metabolites tested, including 25-$(OH)D_3$, 24R,25-$(OH)_2D_3$, 1,24R,25-$(OH)_3D_3$ and 1,24S,25-$(OH)_3D_3$, the 1,25-$(OH)_2D_3$ derivative was most potent in increasing the tubular capacity to excrete Pi by TPTX rats (12). This selective and potent influence of 1,25-$(OH)_2D_3$ on the tubular Pi transport strongly suggests that this effect is of physiological significance.

The results of the experiments presented above strongly suggest that PTH by its acute and direct effect on the tubular Pi transport system is not the most important regulator of Pi excretion. Indeed as shown on Figure 1B the mechanism of Pi adaptation can fully operate in the absence of this hormone. Furthermore other experiments indicate that the adaptation mechanism is also capable of controlling the tubular phosphaturic response to PTH. Indeed, as previously reported by Harter et al. (13), the prior dietary intake of Pi can alter markedly the tubular phosphaturic response to PTH. This observation has been recently confirmed in two laboratories (3,14). Our experiments show that this influence of the dietary supply of Pi is, at least in part, independent of the filtered load of Pi (Figure 2). In addition our experiments show that in TPTX rats fed a low Pi diet, blockage of bone mineralization by the diphosphonate disodium ethane-1-hydroxy-1,1-diphosphonate (EHDP) is not only associated with an increased capacity to excrete Pi (3) but also with a phosphaturic response to PTH similar to that observed in the animals receiving a high Pi diet. This result suggests that not only the supply but also the demand in Pi of the organism could markedly alter the acute phosphaturic response to PTH.

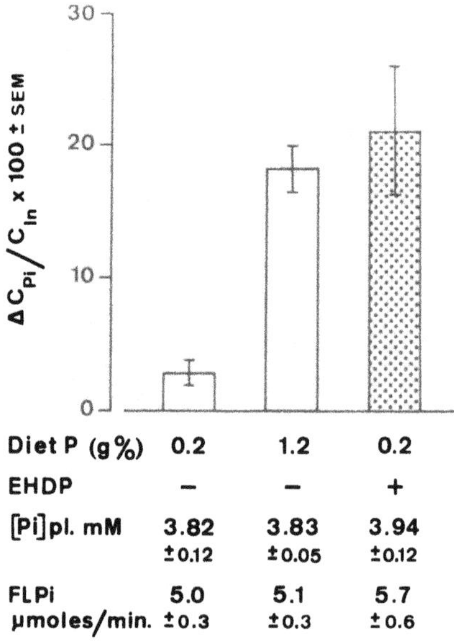

Figure 2: Phosphaturic response to parathyroid hormone in TPTX rats. The increase (Δ) in the fractional excretion of Pi [clearance (C) Pi/Inulin (In)] was determined at similar plasma Pi concentration ([Pi]Pl.) and filtered load of Pi (FLPi) in TPTX rats fed low or high Pi diet. Acute infusions of sodium phosphate were used to match the filtered load of Pi. One group of TPTX rats, fed low Pi diet, received EHDP during the 7 days preceding the renal study. The diphosphonate was given at a dose (10 mg P/kg s.c. per day) which blocks bone mineralization (15,16). All values are means ± SEM.

In summary, the reduced capability of the tubular Pi transport to adapt to a high Pi diet in TPTX rats can be normalized by physiological doses of $1,25\text{-}(OH)_2D_3$. This suggests that the chronic consequence of a lack of PTH could be due,at least in part, to the reduced production of $1,25\text{-}(OH)_2D_3$. The mechanism of Pi adaptation appears to be the most important regulator of Pi excretion in the growing rats, since it can markedly alter the acute phosphaturic response to parathyroid hormone.

Acknowledgements

We acknowledge Miss J. Bornand and Mrs. G. Kunz for their excellent technical assistance, Mrs.C. Stieger for drawing the figures and Mrs. B. Gyger for preparing the manuscript. This work was supported by the Swiss National Science Foundation (3.725.76), by F. Hoffmann-La Roche & Co., Basle, Switzerland, and by the Procter and Gamble Company, Cincinnati, Ohio, USA.

References

1. Troehler, U., Bonjour, J.-P., and Fleisch, H.: Inorganic phosphate homeostasis. Renal adaptation to the dietary intake in intact and thyroparathyroidectomized rats. J.Clin.Invest. 57: 264, 1976.

2. Steele, T.H., and DeLuca, H.F.: Influence of dietary phosphorus on renal phosphate reabsorption in the parathyroidectomized rats. J.Clin.Invest. 57: 867, 1976.

3. Bonjour, J.-P., Troehler, U., Mühlbauer, R., Preston, C., and Fleisch, H.: Is there a bone-kidney link in the homeostasis of inorganic phosphate (Pi)? In: Phosphate Metabolism. Plenum Press, New York, 319, 1977.

4. Troehler, U., Bonjour, J.-P., and Fleisch, H.: Renal tubular adaptation to dietary phosphorus. Nature 261: 145, 1976.

5. Garabedian, M., Holick, M.F., DeLuca, H.F., and Boyle, I.T.: Control of 25-hydroxycholecalciferol metabolism by parathyroid gland. Proc.Nat.Acad.Sci 69: 1673, 1972.

6. DeLuca, H.F., and Schnoes, H.K.: Metabolism and mechanism of action of vitamin D. Ann.Rev.Biochem. 45: 631, 1976.

7. Garabedian, M., Pezant, E., Miravet, L., Fellot, C., and Balsan, S.: 1,25-dihydroxycholecalciferol effect on serum phosphorus homeostasis in rats. Endocrinology 98: 794, 1976.

8. Bonjour, J.-P., Preston, C., and Fleisch, H.: Effect of 1,25-dihydroxyvitamin D_3 on the renal handling of Pi in thyroparathyroidectomized rats. J.Clin.Invest., in press.

9. Rizzoli, R., Fleisch, H., and Bonjour, J.-P.: Effect of thyroparathyroidectomy on calcium metabolism in rats: Role of 1,25-dihydroxyvitamin D_3. Amer.J. Physiol., in press.

10. Rizzoli, R., Fleisch, H., and Bonjour, J.-P.: Role of 1,25-dihydroxyvitamin D_3 on intestinal phosphate absorption in rats with a normal vitamin D supply. J. Clin.Invest., in press.

11. Hugi, K., Fleisch, H., and Bonjour, J.-P.: Renal handling of calcium in rats: Influence of parathyroid hormone (PTH) and 1,25-dihydroxyvitamin D_3 (1,25-$(OH)_2D_3$). Kidney Int. 12: 75, 1977.

12. Bonjour, J.-P., Preston, C., Rizzoli, R., and Fleisch, H.: Vitamin D metabolites and phosphate transport. In: Proceedings of the 6th Parathyroid Conference, Vancouver, June 12-17, 1977, in press.

13. Harter, H.R., Mercado, A., Rutherford, E., Rodriguez, H., Slatopolsky, E., and Klahr, S.: Effect of phosphate depletion and parathyroid hormone on renal glucose reabsorption. Amer.J.Physiol. 227: 1422, 1974.

14. Steele, T.H.: Renal resistance to parathyroid hormone during phosphorus deprivation. J.Clin.Invest. 58: 1461, 1976.

15. Gasser, A.B., Morgan, D.B., Fleisch, H.A., and Richelle, L.J.: The influence of two diphosphonates on calcium metabolism in the rat. Clin.Sci. 43: 31, 1972.

16. Schenk, R., Merz, W.A., Mühlbauer, R.C., Russell, R.G.G., and Fleisch, H.: Effect of ethane-1-hydroxy-1,1-diphosphonate (EHDP) and dichloromethylene diphosphonate (Cl_2MDP) on the calcification and resorption of cartilage and bone in the tibial epiphysis and metaphysis of rats. Calc.Tiss.Res. 11: 196, 1973.

IMPORTANCE OF 25-HYDROXYLATION TO THE RENAL TUBULAR ACTIONS OF VITAMIN D METABOLITES

Jules B. Puschett and John Szramowski

Allegheny General Hospital and University of Pittsburgh Medical School, Pittsburgh, Pennsylvania
320 E. North Avenue, Pittsburgh, Pennsylvania 15212

Experimental observations from my own laboratory as well as data from other workers have documented an acute effect of vitamin D and certain of its metabolites on renal tubular electrolyte transport (1-5). Both in the dog and the rat, the infusion of the biologically active derivative of vitamin D_3, 25-hydroxycholecalciferol (25 HCC) and 1,25-dihydroxycholecalciferol (1,25 DHCC) has been demonstrated to produce an acute enhancement of phosphate (1-5), calcium and sodium (4,5) reabsorption. Recently, a series of additional metabolites and analogues has been discovered (6). Their subsequent characterization and synthesis have provided us with the opportunity to study the structural requirements of these vitamin D_3 derivatives with regard to their ability to alter renal tubular transport. The protocol utilized for these studies was identical to that originally described (1).

Studies were performed in dogs with chronic, stable hypoparathyroidism. Thyroparathyroidectomy had been performed at least 48 hours and usually 72 hours to 1 week prior to the experiments. Thyroid hormone was replaced. Animals were accepted for study only if glandular ablation resulted in a fall in serum calcium concentration of at least 30% from pre-operative values. Because baseline phosphate excretion is quite low in the TPTX dog, potentially obscuring any further decline in its excretion induced by the metabolites, phosphaturia was first produced by the administration of vasopressin and modest volume expansion. When steady-state saline-vasopressin diuresis had been established, either one of the vitamin D_3 derivatives or the vehicle alone was administered. No effort was made to vitamin D-deplete the animals. Only those dogs with stable levels of glomerular filtration rate and effective renal plasma flow were accepted for data analysis. Calcium was added to the infusion solution in amounts calculated to keep its ultrafilterable serum concentration constant throughout the study. In figure 1 are shown the data for glomerular filtration rate, effective renal plasma flow and percentage phosphate excretion obtained when 25-100 units (approximately .625-2.5 μg) of 25 HCC or 1,25 DHCC was infused. Sustained volume expansion plus the continued infusion of vasopressin resulted in a mild increase in phosphate excretion from control to experimental phases of the investigations performed in animals which were given only the vehicle. Contrarily, a sharp reduction in phosphate excretion resulted from the infusion of both 25 HCC and 1,25 DHCC which was not related to alterations in renal hemodynamics, as evidenced by the lack of any consistent variation in either GFR or effective renal plasma flow (figure 1). Likewise, there was no alteration in filtration fraction. As was the case for phosphate excretion, sustained volume expansion and continued vasopressin administration resulted in a mild ever-increasing calciuria (figure 2). However, the infusion of both 25 HCC and 1,25 DHCC acutely reduced calcium excretion, as was the case with respect to phosphate. Furthermore, these changes were paralleled by the effect of both metabolites on sodium excretion, which did not change in the control dogs, but fell consistently after the infusion of each of the metabolites (figure 2). Additionally, the changes were not the result of any alterations in serum ultrafilterable calcium concentration (SUF_{Ca})(1,2).

An analogue of vitamin D_3 which is capable of enhancing intestinal calcium transport and has proven effective in the therapy of uremic bone disease and hypoparathyroidism is 1,α-hydroxycholecalciferol (1,α HCC). Presumably, its activity is related to its conversion to the 1,25-dihydroxylated metabolite (7). The trihydroxylated dervative, 1,24,25-trihydroxycholecalciferol (1,24,25 THCC) is a metabolic product of 1,25 DHCC and possibly also of 24,25 DHCC. Whether it has biological activity or is merely a degradation product is not presently known (6). Employment of 1,α HCC provided us with the opportunity to evaluate the importance of 25-hydroxylation to the renal tubular action of the vitamin D metabolites. Study of 1,24,25 THCC enabled us to determine whether it was effective in altering renal tubular transport and to evaluate the possibility that it was the tissue active form of the vitamin in the kidney (2).

In figure 3 are presented data from a study in which 25 units of 1,α HCC was infused. There occurred an abrupt reduction in percentage phosphate excretion without an effect on the excretion of calcium or sodium. No consistent variation in either GFR or C_{PAH} was noted. A similar situation was obtained when 1,24,25 THCC was administered (figure 4). Again, enhancement of phosphate reabsorption was unaccompanied by an alteration in sodium or calcium transport such as that observed with 25 HCC and 1,25 DHCC (cf. figures

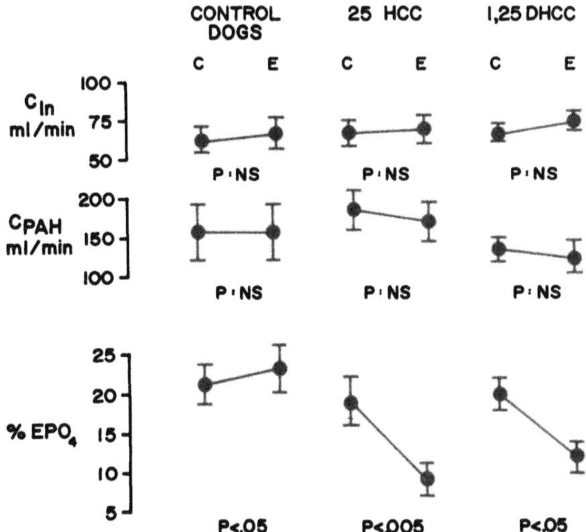

Figure 1. Mean values(±SE) during control (C) and experimental (E) phases of studies in which either 25-hydroxycholecalciferol (25 HCC), 1,25-dihydroxycholecalciferol (1,25 DHCC) or the vehicle alone (control dogs) was administered to chronically thyroparathyroidectomized dogs. There were no changes in glomerular filtration rate (C_{In}) or effective renal plasma flow (C_{PAH}) in any of the experimental groups. The percentage of filtered phosphate excreted (%EPO_4) fell after both metabolites but rose slightly in the control dogs. Data from (1,2).

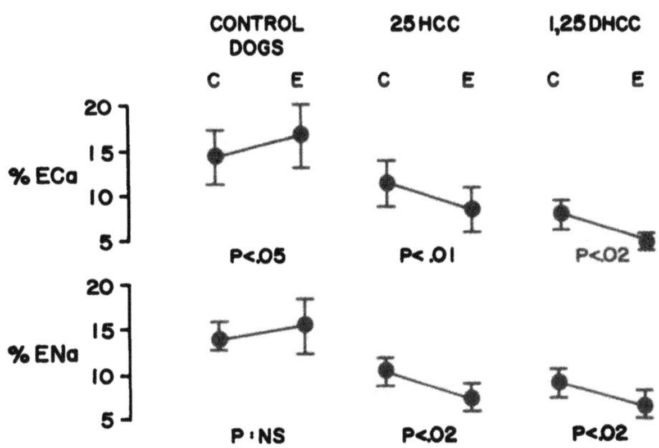

Figure 2. The action of 25 HCC and 1,25 DHCC on the percentage of filtered calcium (%ECa) and sodium (%ENa) excreted compared to observations in control animals. Data from (1,2).

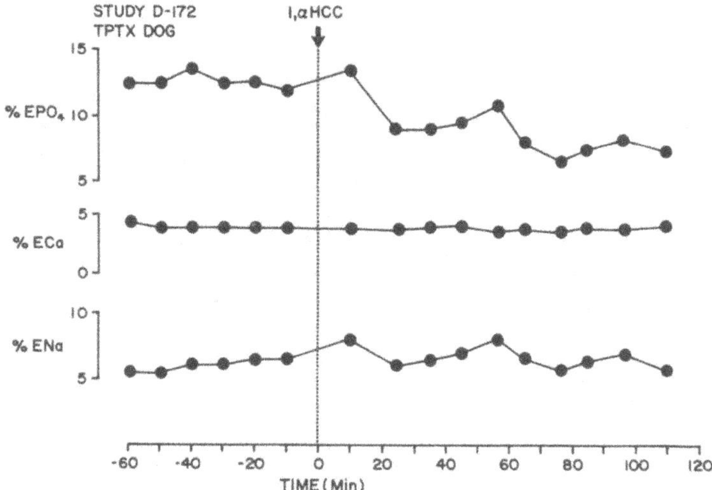

Figure 3. Effects of 1,α-hydroxycholecalciferol (1,αHCC) on the percentage of filtered phosphate (%EPO4), calcium (%ECa) and sodium (%ENa) excreted in a representative study. The metabolite was administered at the arrow.

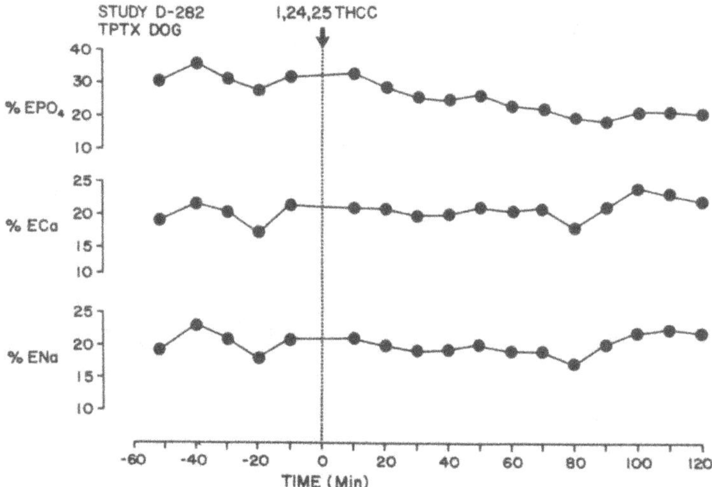

Figure 4. The effects of 1,24,25-trihydroxycholecalciferol (1,24,25 THCC) on the percentage excretion rates of phosphate (%EPO$_4$), calcium (%ECa) and sodium (%ENa). The metabolite was given at the arrow.

1 and 2). The phosphate excretion changes obtained with 1,α HCC and 1,24,25 THCC likewise could not be attributed to variation in SUF_{Ca}, which did not change.

The data can be explained on either or both of two bases: first, 1,α HCC and 1,24,25 THCC may act at different sites within the nephron than those acted upon by 25 HCC or 1,25 DHCC. Second, it may be that in order for a metabolite of vitamin D_3 to alter calcium and sodium transport, it must not only have a hydroxyl group in the 25-position, but that grouping must also be sterically unhindered. The data thus far available do not elucidate which of these mechanisms (or others) is responsible for the experimental observations presented. Further studies will be required to resolve these questions, some of which are currently underway.

REFERENCES

1. Puschett, J.B., Moranz, J. and Kurnick, W.S.: Evidence for a direct action of cholecalciferol and 25-hydroxycholecalciferol on the renal transport of phosphate, sodium and calcium. J. Clin. Invest. 51:373,1972.

2. Puschett, J.B., Fernandez, P.C., Boyle, I.T., Gray, R.W., Omdahl, J.L. and DeLuca, H.F.: The acute renal tubular effects of 1,25-dihydroxycholecalciferol. Proc. Soc. Exp. Biol. Med. 141:379, 1972.

3. Puschett, J.B., Beck, W.S.,Jr., Jelonek, A. and Fernandez, P.C.: Study of the renal tubular interactions of thyrocalcitonin, cyclic adenosine 3',5'-monophosphate, 25-hydroxycholecalciferol, and calcium ion. J. Clin. Invest. 53:756, 1974.

4. Puschett, J.B., Beck, W.S., Jr. and Jelonek, A.: Parathyroid hormone and 25-hydroxy vitamin D : synergistic and antagonistic effects on renal phosphate transport. Science. 190:473, 1975.

5. Popovtzer, M.M., Robinette, J.B., DeLuca, H.F. and Holick, M.F.: The acute effect of 25-hydroxycholecalciferol on renal handling of phosphorous. Evidence for a parathyroid hormone-dependent mechanism. J. Clin. Invest. 53:913, 1974.

6. DeLuca, H.F.: Vitamin D endocrinology. Ann. Int. Med. 85:367, 1976.

7. DeLuca, H.F.: Metabolism of vitamin D: current status. Am. J. Clin. Nutr. 29:1258, 1976.

HAS VITAMIN D A DIRECT RENAL EFFECT ON THE TUBULAR REABSORPTION OF PHOSPHATE?

A study in parathyroidectomized (PTX) and non-PTX man

S. Madsen and K. Ølgaard

Medical Dept. P, Division of Nephrology,

Rigshospitalet, 2loo Copenhagen Ø, Denmark

The parathyroid hormone has a key role in the regulation of the renal handling of phosphate (1, 2, 3), but it has become increasingly evident that other factors are, or may be, involved in this important homeostatic mechanism. These factors are primarily the pH, the extracellular volume, the circadian rhythm, dietary phosphate, steroids, diuretics, ionized calcium, calcitonin, and vitamin D.

The parathyroid hormone (PTH) exhibits a direct renal phosphaturic effect, and most observations support the hypothesis, that this effect is mediated via stimulation of the renal adenyl cyclase. The importance of the parathyroid hormone was stressed in our previous investigation (4, 5), where a significant inverse correlation was demonstrated between the serum concentration of immunoreactive parathyroid hormone (i-PTH) and the renal handling of phosphate, while the latter did not correlate with either the extracellular volume, standard bicarbonate or serum calcium.

The renal effect of vitamin D is more controversial and it remains to be clarified whether biologically active vitamin D exhibits a direct stimulating effect on the tubular reabsorption of phosphate in man. Conflicting data have been obtained from investigations on experimental animals concerning the effect of vitamin D on the renal handling of phosphate. A direct, as well as lack of a direct renal effect of vitamin D on the tubular reabsorption of phosphate in the dog and the rat has been reported (6). Large species differences seem to exist in this field and investigations on experimental

animals may not allow conclusions concerning the effect of vitamin D on the human kidney.
1-alpha-hydroxycholecalciferol (1α-OH-D_3), a crystalline vitamin D analog, which is converted in the liver (7) to the genuine active vitamin D (1.25$(OH)_2$-D_3), has recently become available (8). The present study was undertaken _in man_ to elucidate the effect of 1α-OH-D_3 treatment on the renal handling of phosphate and on the parathyroid function.
The maximal tubular reabsorption of phosphate (TmP) is highly correlated to the glomerular filtration rate (GFR) (9), and therefore to reduce the contribution of GFR to the variation of TmP, the latter must be expressed in relation to GFR. This TmP/GFR index, which was used in the present investigation, appears to be the most consistent index of renal phosphate handling (1o).

MATERIAL

The material consists of 1) patients with functioning parathyroid glands (_non-PTX_ patients) and 2) totally parathyroidectomized patients (_PTX_ patients).

Non-PTX patients

These patients were fundamentally the same as in our previous report (4, 5), except that 5 patients had to be omitted (2 had initiated hemodialysis, 1 received intensive steroid treatment, 1 was hypercalcemic and 1 died after a cerebral hemorrhage). The material therefore consisted of 1o patients (5 females, 5 males) aged 22-58 years (mean 38) with creatinine clearances of 4-65 ml/min (mean 39.6). Six patients (3 females, 3 males) aged 22-58 years (mean 36) had well functioning kidney allografts with creatinine clearances of 43-65 ml/min (mean 59.1). The average time of the present investigation after the kidney transplantation was 18 months (range 6-6o). The transplanted patients received a daily prednisone dosage of 7.5-25 mg (mean 15.o) which was unaltered throughout the study. None of these patients showed clinical or biochemical signs of rejection during the study. Four patients (2 females, 2 males) aged 23-5o years (mean 4o) had varying degrees of chronic renal insufficiency with creatinine clearances of 4-2o ml/min (mean 1o.4). The nephrological disease in 2 patients was chronic interstitial nephropathy, in 1 patient chronic glomerulonephritis and in 1 polycystic kidney disease. No patient received dialysis treatment; 5

patients received diuretic treatment, which was withdrawn 24 hours prior to the study.

PTX patients

Five totally parathyroidectomized patients, 4 females and 1 male, with a mean age of 48 years (range 3o-55) were studied. Two patients (nos. 11 and 12) had well functioning kidney allografts with stable creatinine clearances of 85 and 6o ml/min, 38 and 81 months after grafting. At the time of the present study patient no 11 received 7.5 mg of prednisone and loo mg of azathioprine/day, while patient no 12 had been without prednisone treatment for 15 months, but still received azathioprine loo mg/day. Patient no 11 was totally parathyroidectomized 14 months after grafting (24 months prior to the present investigation) due to persisting hyperparathyroidism. Patient no 12 was totally parathyroidectomized during hemodialysis treatment 5 months before grafting (86 months prior to the present investigation).
Three female patients (nos. 13, 14 and 15) with stable creatinine clearances of about 6o ml/min had been thyroidectomized 14, 6 and 23 years prior to the present investigation. During surgery they were accidentally parathyroidectomized, and developed typical hypocalcemic tetany postoperatively.
In all 5 patients, continued calciferol treatment was necessary to prevent development of symptomatic hypocalcemia, and they were therefore considered to be totally parathyroidectomized. Apart from calciferol, which was given to all 5 patients, and the immunosuppressive treatment given to patient no 11 and 12, they received no other medication at the time of the present study.

METHODS

The serum concentration of i-PTH (11) and the maximal tubular reabsorption of phosphate (TmP) was estimated in the <u>non-PTX</u> patients in two 12o-min periods during an i.v. infusion of phosphate as described elsewhere (4, 5) and the glomerular filtration rate (GFR) was measured by the single injection technique of ^{51}Cr-EDTA (12), whereupon the TmP/GFR index was calculated (9). Determination of the TmP/GFR index has in our hands been found to be reproducible with a coefficient of variation of 14% by duplicate measurements in 25 individuals (13). The lo <u>non-PTX</u> patients were then treated with 1α-OH-D_3 (Leo Pharmaceutical Products, Copenhagen) for 8o days and the i-PTH and TmP/GFR index reestimated.

Four of the PTX patients (nos. 11-14) were normocalcemic on calciferol treatment. Calciferol was withdrawn and subsequently the patients were carefully followed by clinical observation as well as by weekly determination of ionized calcium in whole blood (b-Ca^{++}) (14). They were all moderately hypocalcemic 14-72 days (mean 3o) later, with b-Ca^{++} between o.73 and o.91 mmol/l (normal range 1.o2-1.18) but without manifest tetany.

Patient no 15 was hypocalcemic due to deficient control. Also in this patient calciferol was withdrawn and at the time of the present study her b-Ca^{++} was o.81 mmol/l. During hypocalcemia the TmP/GFR index was determined in these 5 PTX patients during an i.v. phosphate infusion (4, 5). The patients then received 1α-OH-D_3 in a dose varying between 1 and 4 μg/day and stable normocalcemia was thereby reestablished in the course of 14-27 days (mean 17.8). During normocalcemia exactly the same investigations were carried out as during hypocalcemia.

Studies in the rat suggest that in the absence of circulating PTH, the tubular phosphate transport system may operate at its maximal reabsorptive capacity in the sense that no further increase can take place by any stimulation, including vitamin D. We therefore investigated whether thyrotoxic patients exhibit TmP/GFR values in excess of those obtained in parathyroidectomized patients. The TmP/GFR index was measured in two thyrotoxic patients, one female and one male, 62 and 68 years of age, with creatinine clearances of 85 and 1oo ml/min, respectively.

Finally it was investigated whether the decrease in TmP induced by hyperglycemia could be counteracted by treatment with 1α-OH-D_3. In one parathyroidectomized patient (no 13) TmP/GFR was determined in one 12o-min period with normoglycemia and in one period with hyperglycemia before as well as after administration of 1α-OH-D_3. Hyperglycemia was induced by i.v. injection of 5o ml 5o% glucose at time zero and at time 6o min during the second 12o-min period.

RESULTS

Non-PTX patients

The values for TmP/GFR index, i-PTH and serum calcium as determined in the 1o patients before and after 8o

Table I
TmP/GFR, i-PTH and serum calcium in lo non-parathyroidectomized patients before (B) and after (A) treatment with 1α-OH-D_3.

PATIENT NO.	TMP/GFR (μMOL/ML)		I-PTH (NG/ML)		SERUM CALCIUM (MMOL/L)	
	B	A	B	A	B	A
1	0.85	0.92	2.1	2.0	2.60	2.62
2	0.77	0.84	1.9	2.2	2.39	2.44
3	0.72	0.80	2.4	2.3	2.68	2.54
4	0.69	0.77	2.8	1.2	2.41	2.64
5	0.58	0.65	3.3	2.3	2.48	2.72
6	0.42	0.71	3.0	1.9	2.49	2.51
7	0.38	0.58	4.3	3.2	2.67	2.65
8	0.35	0.39	3.5	3.0	2.08	2.47
9	0.11	0.32	9.5	6.3	2.38	2.54
10	0.03	0.26	13.0	4.1	2.27	2.41
MEAN CHANGE (%)	26.5% ↑		37.0% ↓		4.5% ↑	

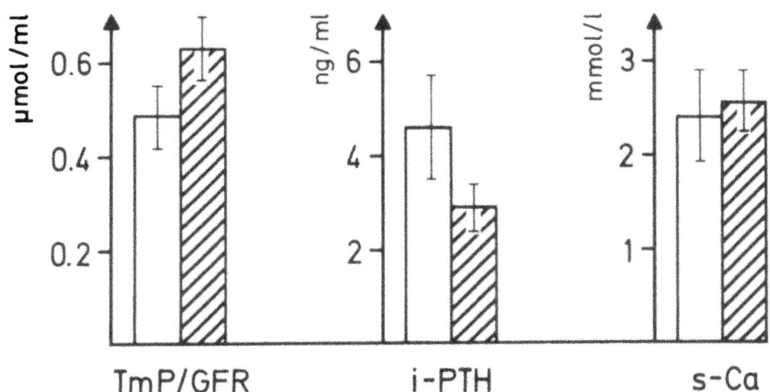

Fig. 1
TmP/GFR, i-PTH and serum calcium (mean ± SEM) in lo non-parathyroidectomized patients before (□) and after (▨) 8o days of treatment with 1α-OH-D_3.

days of treatment with 1α-OH-D_3 are given in Table I. The TmP/GFR values varied over a wide range (o.o3-o.85 µmol/ml) prior to the treatment and a significant ($p < o.ol$) increase (mean 26.5%) was seen after the treatment. The i-PTH values varied similary over a wide range (1.9-13.o ng/ml) and decreased (mean 37.o%) significantly ($p < o.ol$) after the treatment (Fig. 1). Serum calcium increased by 4.5% ($p < o.o5$), while the extracellular volume and standard bicarbonate remained unchanged.

Before the administration of 1α-OH-D_3 a significant inverse correlation ($r = -o.87$; $p < o.ool$) was found between the TmP/GFR index and i-PTH, while the extracellular volume and the serum concentrations of standard bicarbonate and calcium did not correlate to the index. After 8o days of treatment with 1α-OH-D_3 an inverse significant correlation ($r = -o.79$; $p < o.ol$) persisted between the same two parameters. The slopes and intercepts of these two regression lines did not differ

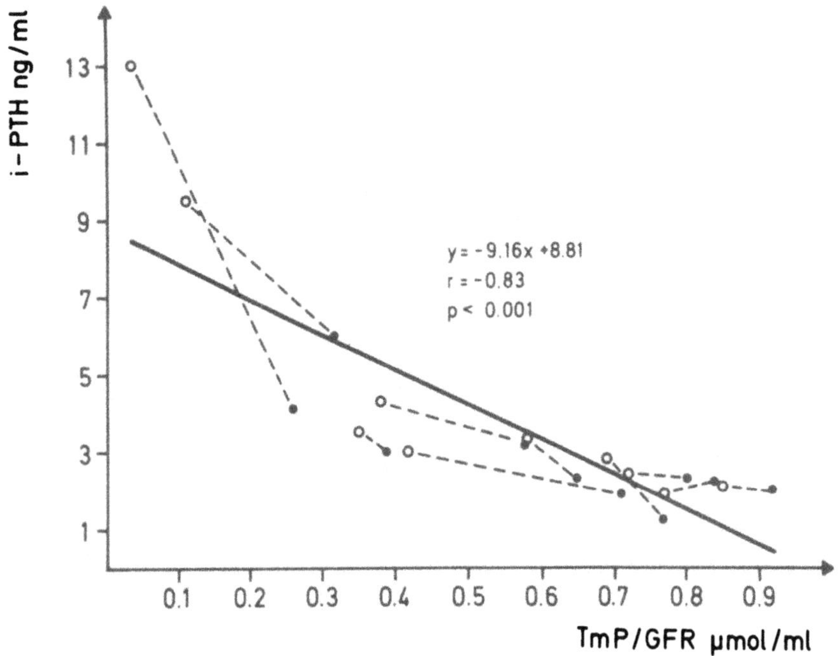

Fig. 2
Correlation between TmP/GFR and i-PTH in lo non-parathyroidectomized patients before (o) and after (●) 8o days of treatment with 1α-OH-D_3. --- = individual course of each patient.

Table II
TmP/GFR, i-PTH and ionized calcium in whole blood (b-Ca^{++}) in 5 parathyroidectomized, vitamin D deficient patients before (B) and after (A) treatment with 1α-OH-D_3.

PATIENT NO.	TMP/GFR (µMOL/L)		I-PTH (NG/ML)		B-CA^{++} (MMOL/L)	
	B	A	B	A	B	A
11	1.54	1.32	1.8	1.8	0.83	1.02
12	1.37	1.18	1.8	1.8	0.74	0.98
13	1.06	1.02	1.6	1.6	0.81	1.07
14	0.99	0.99	1.6	1.5	0.91	1.09
15	0.92	0.79	1.7	1.8	0.73	1.01
MEAN CHANGE (%)	17.2% ↓		0%		28.8% ↑	

significantly. Consequently a significant inverse correlation (r = -o.83; p < o.ool) could be demonstrated between the TmP/GFR index and i-PTH in the lo patients, whether or not they received 1α-OH-D_3. This regression line is reproduced in Fig. 2, which also shows the individual course of each patient. Finally, the variations in extracellular volume, standard bicarbonate and serum calcium during the study did not correlate to the changes in the TmP/GFR index.

PTX patients

Table II shows the values of b-Ca^{++}, TmP/GFR and i-PTH before and after treatment with 1α-OH-D_3. The patients were hypocalcemic before treatment, due to withdrawal of calciferol (patient no 11-14) or due to deficient control of calciferol dosage (patient no 15). The mean b-Ca^{++} during hypocalcemia was o.8o mmol/l (range o.73-o.91).
Stable normocalcemia was established following 14-27 (mean 17.8) days of treatment with 1α-OH-D_3, and b-Ca^{++} increased by o.23 mmol/l (range o.18-o.28). The mean

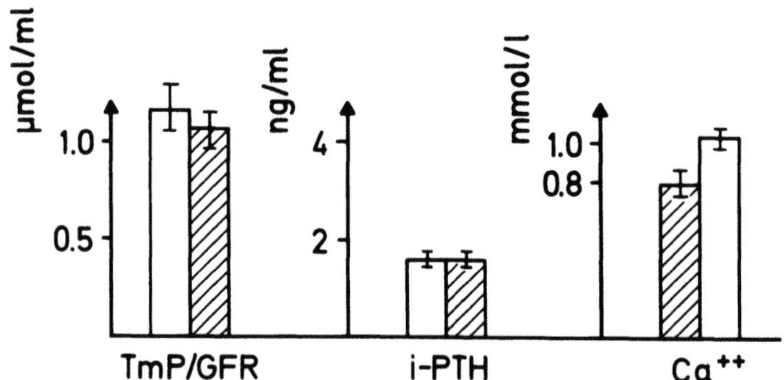

Fig. 3
TmP/GFR, i-PTH and Ca^{++} (mean $\pm$ SEM) in 5 parathyroidectomized patients before (▭) and after (▨) treatment with 1α-OH-D_3.

b-Ca^{++} during normocalcemia was 1.o3 mmol/l (range o.98-1.o9).
Serum i-PTH was unchanged at low values (mean 1.7 ng/ml) before as well as after treatment with 1α-OH-D_3.
The TmP/GFR remained unchanged in one patient (no 14), while a small but insignificant ($p > o.o5$) decrease was observed in 4 patients (nos. 11, 12, 13 and 15) after treatment with 1α-OH-D_3 (Fig. 3). The mean decrease in TmP/GFR was only o.12 µmol/ml and was uncorrelated ($p > o.o5$) to the increase in b-Ca^{++}.
Standard bicarbonate was identical before (mean 23.2 mmol/l, range 21.7-24.5) and after (mean 24.1 mmol/l, range 21.4-25.5) treatment with 1α-OH-D_3. The extracellular volume likewise remained unchanged before (mean 12.2 l, range lo.7-13.8) and after (mean 11.5 l, range 9.5-13.6) treatment.

Hyperthyroid patients

The TmP/GFR was 1.54 and 1.56 µmol/ml, respectively, in the two hyperthyroid patients and thus 45.8% and 47.5% higher than the mean of all values in the hypoparathyroid patients. The i-PTH values of these 2 patients were within the normal range (1.7 and 1.8 ng/ml, respectively).

Table III
TmP/GFR in a parathyroidectomized patient (no 13) during normo- (N) and hyperglycemia (H), before (B) and after (A) treatment with 1α-OH-D_3.

	Plasma glucose mmol/l		Diuresis ml/120 min		b-Ca mmol/l	TmP/GFR µmol/ml		i-PTH ng/ml
	N	H	N	H		N	H	
B	5.8	19.0x)	650	235	0.81	1.06	0.62	1.6
A	4.7	17.1x)	320	235	1.07	1.02	0.73	1.6

TmP/GFR during normo-and hyperglycemia

In one patient (no 13) TmP/GFR was measured during normoglycemia and during hyperglycemia, before as well as after treatment with 1α-OH-D_3. It appears, from Table III, that hyperglycemia resulted in a considerable depression (41.5%) of TmP/GFR and that treatment with 1α-OH-D_3 did not counteract this depression.

DISCUSSION

The influence of vitamin D on the renal handling of phosphate has been a matter of controversy (5). The availability of the biologically active 1α,25(OH)$_2$$D_3$ or the more convenient 1α-OH-D_3 has recently made it possible to study the renal effects of these compounds.

In the present investigation, long-term administration of 1α-OH-D_3 to non-PTX patients increased the TmP/GFR index and serum calcium significantly and resulted in a significant decline in i-PTH. Furthermore, the linear correlation as previously found (4, 5), persisted between TmP/GFR and i-PTH after the treatment with 1α-OH-D_3, while serum calcium, standard bicarbonate and the extra-

cellular volume remained uncorrelated to the TmP/GFR index. This suggests that the 1α-OH-D_3 induced changes in the renal handling of phosphate may be explained by the parallel suppression of PTH (15).
However, it does not rule out the possibility, that vitamin D beside the effect (directly and/or via increase in Ca^{++}) on the parathyroid glands exerts a direct action on the renal tubular transport of phosphate. We therefore investigated PTX patients with the aim of examining the effect of 1α-OH-D_3 on TmP/GFR under conditions, where concomitant suppression of PTH could be excluded. The TmP/GFR ratios of the parathyroidectomized patients were higher than in patients with preserved parathyroid glands. This finding is in good agreement with the previously demonstrated (4, 5) inverse correlation between TmP/GFR and i-PTH. Furthermore, in no case did the TmP/GFR ratio increase after treatment with 1α-OH-D_3. Thus, as shown in Fig. 2 and Fig. 3 the hypoparathyroid patients responded in a manner which differed distinctly from patients with intact parathyroid glands (13). In fact, a small, but insignificant decrease in the ratio was observed in 4 of the 5 hypoparathyroid patients.
By itself this finding does not prove that 1α-OH-D_3 is without stimulating effect on tubular phosphate reabsorption. The TmP/GFR in parathyroidectomized man may be maximal in the sense that no further increase is possible by any stimulus, including biologically active vitamin D. In agreement with Bijvoet (9) we have, however, found that thyrotoxic patients may exhibit TmP/GFR ratios considerably in excess of the ratios in hypoparathyroid patients, indicating that TmP/GFR is not maximal in hypoparathyroid man. Further, the results shown in Table III demonstrate that 1α-OH-D_3 does not counteract the depression of TmP/GFR, which can be induced by hyperglycemia. Based on all the presented evidence the present investigation suggests that biologically active vitamin D does not directly stimulate tubular phosphate reabsorption in man, and that the previously demonstrated antiphosphaturic effect of 1α-OH-D_3 is mediated largely, if not exclusively, via a concomitant suppression of PTH.
This conclusion is in accordance with the results of several investigations on normal and parathyroidectomized rats (6), most recently confirmed by Popovtzer et al (16), who reported that 25-hydroxycholecalciferol reduced urinary phosphate excretion only in normal, but not in parathyroidectomized rats.
Our findings on human beings, as well as the above mentioned findings on rats, are, however, at variance with the studies of Puschett et al (17), who found that active

vitamin D increases tubular phosphate reabsorption in volume expanded parathyroidectomized dogs. Species differences, as well as differences in experimental design, may account for this discrepancy.
Further work is necessary to finally settle the problem regarding the effect of vitamin D on the renal handling of phosphate. Apart from micropuncture studies, further information may be obtained from investigations on patients under conditions, where the effect of vitamin D, PTH and calcium can be dissociated.

SUMMARY

The effect of 1-alpha-hydroxycholecalciferol (1α-OH-D_3) on the renal handling of phosphate and the immunoreactive parathyroid hormone in serum (i-PTH) has been studied in 1o patients with a wide range of glomerular filtration rate (GFR), maximal tubular reabsorption of phosphate (TmP) and i-PTH. The patients were treated with 2 µg 1α-OH-D_3 per day for approximately 8o days. Before and after this period of treatment, the TmP, i-PTH, ^{51}Cr EDTA clearance, extracellular volume, standard bicarbonate, and serum calcium were measured in each patient. The TmP/GFR ratio was used as an index of the renal handling of phosphate.
The index increased significantly (mean 26.5%, $p < o.o1$) during the treatment, while i-PTH decreased significantly (mean 37.o%, $p < o.o1$). A significant inverse correlation was demonstrated between the TmP/GFR index and i-PTH both before ($r = -o.87$; $p < o.oo1$) and after ($r = -o.79$; $p < o.o1$) the administration of 1α-OH-D_3, while none of the other factors investigated were correlated to the index.
This may suggest that the stimulating effect of biologically active vitamin D on the tubular reabsorption of phosphate is mediated via the parallel suppression of PTH, but does not exclude that biologically active vitamin D exerts a direct effect on the human renal tubule. Therefore, the effect of 1α-OH-D_3 was studied in 5 totally parathyroidectomized patients, in whom concomitant suppression of PTH would not occur. Estimation of TmP/GFR was performed 1) when the patients were vitamin D depleted and hypocalcemic, and 2) after 14-27 days of treatment with 1α-OH-D_3 to obtain stable normocalcemia. In patients with absent parathyroid function, no increasing effect of 1α-OH-D_3 on TmP/GFR could be demonstrated. It is therefore concluded 1) that 1α-OH-D_3 exhibits no antiphosphaturic effect in the absence of PTH and 2) that the previously demonstrated antiphosphaturic

effect of 1α-OH-D_3 in man is mediated via a concomitant suppression of PTH.

REFERENCES

1. Agus, Z.S., Gardner, L.B., Beck, L.H., and Goldberg, M.: Effects of parathyroid hormone on renal tubular reabsorption of calcium, sodium, and phosphate. Am. J. Physiol. 224: 1143, 1973.

2. Falls, W.F., Carter, N.W., Rector, F.C., and Seldin, D.W.: The mechanism of impaired phosphate reabsorption in chronic renal disease. Clin. Res. 14: 74, 1966.

3. Slatopolsky, E., Robson, A.M., Elkan, I., and Bricker, N.S.: Control of phosphate excretion in uremic man. J. Clin. Invest. 47: 1865, 1968.

4. Madsen, S., Ølgaard, K., and Ladefoged, J.: Renal handling of phosphate in relation to serum parathyroid hormone levels. Acta Med. Scand. 2oo: 7, 1976.

5. Madsen, S., Ølgaard, K., and Ladefoged, J.: The maximal tubular reabsorption of phosphate in relation to serum parathyroid hormone. In: Phosphate Metabolism. ed. Massry, S.G. and Ritz, E. Plenum Press. New York and London, 1977, p. 141.

6. Bonjour, J.P., and Fleisch, H.: The effect of vitamin D and its metabolites on the renal handling of phosphate. In: Vitamin D, Biochemical, Chemical and Clinical Aspects Related to Calcium Metabolism. ed. Norman, A.W. et al. Walter de Gruyter. Berlin. New York, 1977, p. 419.

7. Zerwekh, J.E., Brumbaugh, P.F., Haussler, D.H., Cork, D.J., and Haussler, M.R.: 1α-hydroxyvitamin D_3. An analog of vitamin D which apparently acts by metabolism to 1α,25-dihydroxy vitamin D_3. Biochemistry 13: 4o97, 1974.

8. Holick, M.F., Semmler, E.J., Schnoes, H.K., and DeLuca, H.F.: 1α-hydroxy derivative of vitamin D_3. A highly potent analog of 1α,25-dihydroxy vitamin D_3. Science 18o: 19o, 1973.

9. Bijvoet, O.L.M.: Relation of plasma phosphate concentration to renal tubular reabsorption of phosphate. Clin. Sci. 37: 23, 1969.

1o. Stamp, T.C.B., and Stacey, T.E.: Evaluation of theoretical renal phosphorus Threshold as an index of renal phosphorus handling. Clin. Sci. 39: 5o5, 197o.

11. Almqvist, S., Hjern, B., and Wästhed, B.: The diagnostic value of a radioimmunoassay for parathyroid hormone in human serum. Acta Endocrinol. 78: 493, 1975.

12. Nosslin, B.: Determination of clearance and distribution volume with the single injection technique. Acta Med. Scand. suppl. 442: 97, 1965.

13. Madsen, S., Ølgaard, K., and Thaysen, J. Hess: The effect of 1-α-hydroxycholecalciferol on the renal handling of phosphate in parathyroidectomized man. Acta Med. Scand. In press 1977.

14. Madsen, S., and Ølgaard, K.: Evaluation of a new automatic calcium ion analyzer. Clin. Chem. 23: 69o, 1977.

15. Madsen, S., Ølgaard, K., and Ladefoged, J.: 1-alpha-hydroxycholecalciferol-induced changes in the renal handling of phosphate and the serum parathyroid hormone level. Acta Med. Scand. 2oo: 351, 1976.

16. Popovtzer, M.M., Robinette, J.B., DeLuca, H.F., and Holick, M.F.: The acute effect of 25-hydroxycholecalciferol on renal handling of phosphorus. J. Clin. Invest. 53: 913, 1974.

17. Puschett, J.B., Moranz, J., and Kurnick, W.S.: Evidence for a direct action of cholecalciferol and 25-hydroxycholecalciferol on the renal transport of phosphate, sodium and calcium. J. Clin. Invest. 51: 373, 1972.

OUTFLUX OF ^{45}CALCIUM ALONG THE RAT NEPHRON*

R. Greger, F. Lang, H. Oberleithner, and P. Deetjen

Physiologisches Institut, Universität Innsbruck

Fritz-Pregl-Str. 3, A - 6020 Innsbruck , Austria

From previous micropuncture data (1,4-6,9-15,17,19) it was postulated that calcium is reabsorbed in the proximal tubule and in addition in the distal tubule and/or collecting duct. This was concluded by comparing the amount of calcium present at the distal puncture site and that in final urine. Although this discrepancy between distal and urinary calcium load as detected by free flow micropuncture and clearance techniques might reflect distal reabsorption of calcium, it is no direct prove for that. A similar result might be obtained if there was nephron heterogeneity in regard to calcium reabsorption with the implication that deeper nephrons reabsorb calcium more avidly than superficial ones.

The microinfusion technique easily can distinguish between these two explanations. Using this technique a saline solution containing tracer concentrations of $^{45}CaCl_2$ and ^3H inulin was microinfused continuously for several minutes at a flow rate of 2 nl/min into the free flowing tubule fluid of nephron segments of different location. Ipsilateral and contralateral urine were collected continuously and fractional recovery of calcium was calculated.

The results obtained in three groups of rats (intact, acutely thyroparathyroidectomized = TPTX, and acutely TPTX substituted with PTH) indicated (7) that the vast majority of the amount of ^{45}Ca infused into proximal nephron segments is reabsorbed, both in the presence and absence of PTH. This is in good

*Footnote: This study was supported by "Legerlotz Stiftung".

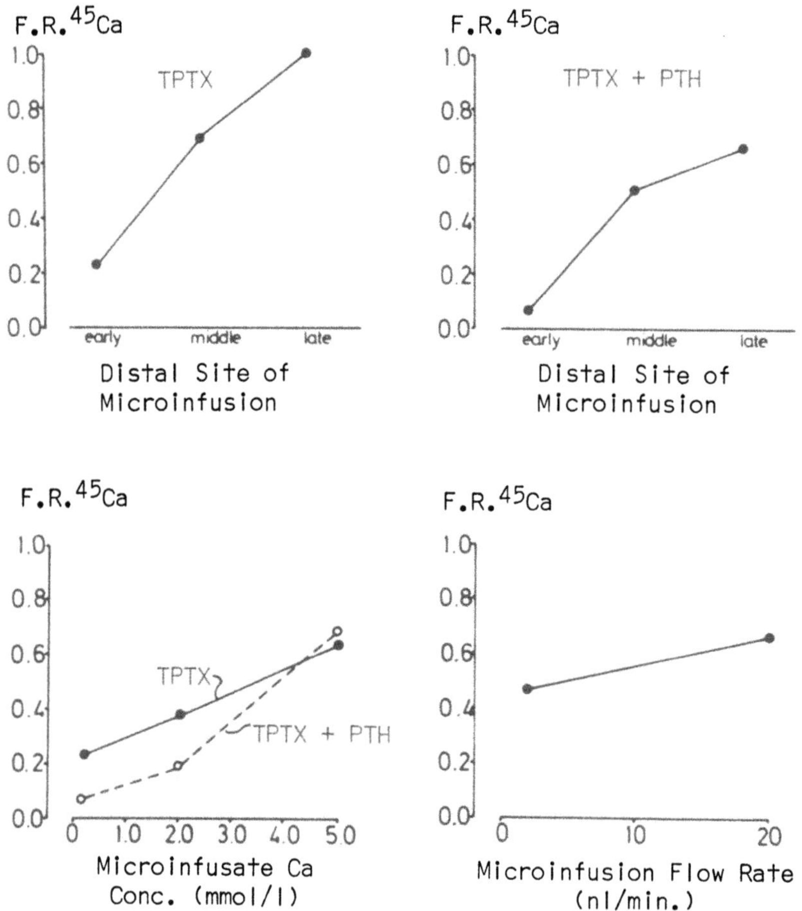

Fig.1: Determinants of fractional urinary recovery of ^{45}Ca (F.R.^{45}Ca) after distal microinfusion. Left upper panel: F.R.^{45}Ca in correlation to the distal site of microinfusion for TPTX rats. Right upper panel: The same graph for TPTX rats substituted with PTH. PTH lowers F.R. ^{45}Ca for corresponding distal nephron sites. Left lower panel: Correlation of F.R.^{45}Ca to the calcium concentration in the microinfusate. Closed circles and the solid function correspond to TPTX rats, open circles and the dashed line to TPTX rats substituted with PTH. Right lower panel: Dependence of F.R.^{45}Ca on the microinfusion flow rate.

agreement to previous reports (1,2,4-6,8-15,17,19). Since the proximal tubule (2,13,16,18) and the loop of Henle (13) are permeable to calcium, the measured ^{45}Ca outflux is an overestimate of the net reabsorption of calcium.

After distal microinfusion (Fig. 1) fractional urinary recovery of ^{45}Ca was variable and depended on: 1) the site of distal microinfusion, 2) the presence or absence of PTH, 3) the calcium concentration in the microinfusate, and 4) the microinfusion flow rate. Ad 1): Urinary ^{45}Ca recovery was almost complete if microinfusions were carried out into the very last loops of the distal convolution. Recovery was incomplete for the microinfusions into early distal tubules. Ad 2): For comparable distal segments the intact and the PTH substituted animals showed lower recoveries of ^{45}Ca than the TPTX animals. Furthermore, with a time delay of some 30 min synthetic PTH (10 IU prime, 17 IU/h) decreased the recovery of ^{45}Ca in early distal tubules of TPTX rats. In these experiments microinfusions were performed for at least one hour in the same distal tubule such as to allow direct comparison of ^{45}Ca recoveries in the absence and presence of PTH. Ad 3) and 4): Both, increases in microinfusate calcium concentration (0.17-5.0 mmol/l) and increases in microinfusion flow rate (2-20 nl/min) resulted in highly significant increases in fractional urinary recovery of ^{45}Ca.

The data obtained for the distal tubule indicate: 1) Calcium is reabsorbed along the distal convoluted tubule. Since at this site no significant back leakage of calcium occurs (3) the measured tracer outflux represents net reabsorption. 2) The collecting duct system seems not to contribute significantly to the distal reabsorption since fractional urinary recovery is essentially complete if tracers are microinfused at a late distal site. Furthermore, the increase in fractional urinary recovery of ^{45}Ca after microinfusion at increased flow rate or with increased calcium concentration suggests that calcium reabsorption takes place in the distal convolution and not in the collecting duct system since there - after convergence of several distal tubules to form one collecting duct - the experimental manoeuvers are probably of little effect. 3) Distal calcium reabsorption is enhanced in the presence and diminished in the absence of PTH.

References:

1. Agus, Z.S., Gardner, L.B., Beck, L.H., Goldberg, M.: Effects of parathyroid hormone on renal tubular reabsorption of calcium, sodium, and phosphate. Am.J.Physiol. 224, 1143-1148 (1973).
2. Brunette, M., Aras, M.: A microinjection study of nephron permeability to calcium and magnesium. Am.J.Physiol. 221,1442-1448 (1971).
3. Constanzo,L.S., Windhager, E.E.: Characteristics of calcium transport in the distal convoluted tubule. Kidney Int.10,489 (1976)

4. Duarte, C.G., Watson, J.F.: Calcium reabsorption in proximal tubule of the dog nephron: Am.J.Physiol. 212, 1355-1360 (1967)
5. Edwards, B.R., Sutton, R.A.L., Dirks, J.H.: Effect of calcium infusion on renal tubular reabsorption in the dog. Am.J.Physiol. 227, 13-18 (1974)
6. Frick, A., Rumrich, G., Ullrich, K.J., Lassiter, W.E.: Microperfusion study of calcium transport in the proximal tubule of the rat kidney. Pflügers Arch. 286, 109-117 (1965)
7. Greger, R., Lang, F. and Oberleithner, H.: Distal site of calcium reabsorption in the rat kidney. Pflügers Arch. submitted.
8. Jamison, R.L., Frey, N.R., Lacy, F.B.: Calcium reabsorption in the thin loop of Henle. Am.J.Physiol. 227, 745-751 (1974)
9. Kövér, G.: Effect of hypercalcaemia on tubular calcium and phosphate transport. Acta Physiol. Acad. Sci, Hung. 45, 95-107 (1974)
10. Kuntzinger, H., Amiel, C., Roinel, N., Morel, F.: Effects of parathyroidectomy and cyclic AMP on renal transport of phosphate, calcium, and magnesium. Am.J.Physiol. 227, 905-911 (1974)
11. Lassiter, W.E., Gottschalk, C.W., Mylle, M.: Micropuncture study of renal tubular reabsorption of calcium in normal rodents. Am.J.Physiol. 204, 771-775 (1963)
12. Le Grimellec, C., Roinel, N., Morel, F.: Simultaneous Mg, Ca, P, K, Na and Cl analysis in rat tubular fluid. III during acute Ca plasma loading. Pflügers Arch. 346, 171-188 (1974)
13. Murayama, Y., Morel, F., Le Grimellec, C.: Phosphate, calcium, and magnesium transfers in proximal tubules and loops of Henle, as measured by single nephron microperfusion experiments in the rat. Pflügers Arch. 333, 1-16 (1972)
14. Quamme, G.A., Wong, N.L.M., Sutton, R.A.L., Dirks, J.H.: Interrelationships of chlorothiazide and parathyroid hormone: a micropuncture study. Am.J.Physiol. 229, 200-205 (1975)
15. Schneider, E.G., Strandhoy, J.W., Willis, J.R., Knox, F.G.: Relationship between proximal sodium reabsorption and excretion of calcium, magnesium and phosphate. Kidney Int. 4, 369-376 (1973)
16. Shirley, D.G., Poujeol, P., Le Grimellec, C.: Phosphate, calcium and magnesium fluxes into lumen of the rat proximal convoluted tubule. Pflügers Arch. 362, 247-254 (1976)
17. Sutton, R.A.L., Wong, N.L.M., Dirks, J.H.: Effects of parathyroid hormone on sodium and calcium transport in the dog nephron. Clin. Sci. Mol. Med. 51,345-351 (1976)
18. Ullrich, K.J., Capasso, G., Rumrich, G., Klöss, S.: Effect of parathyroid hormone on the active Ca^{++}-reabsorption in the proximal convolution of the rat kidney. Pflügers Arch. 359, R 118 (1975)
19. Ullrich, K., Rumrich, G., Klöss, S.: Acitve Ca^{2+}-reabsorption in the proximal tubule of the rat kidney. Dependence on sodium and buffer transport. Pflügers Arch. 364, 223-228 (1976)

Intestinal Transport of Phosphate

INTESTINAL INORGANIC PHOSPHATE TRANSPORT

Marlin W. Walling

VA Wadsworth Hospital Center and Schools of Dentistry

and Medicine, Univ. of Calif., Los Angeles, California

Evidence indicating that the intestinal absorption of phosphate occurs, at least in part by regulated processes, has been available since the 1930's when balance studies showed that vitamin D increased both calcium and phosphate absorption (1-3). However, it was not until the extensive studies of Harrison and Harrison in the early 1960's that it became clear that vitamin D directly effected inorganic phosphate (Pi) absorption by mammalian small intestine (4). The transport-mediated changes in Pi concentration between the outer and inner compartments of everted gut sacs reported by the Harrisons are much larger than the changes that could result solely from effects of the transmural potential difference (PD) which is about 5 mV, so that these results (4) clearly indicate active Pi absorption. Nevertheless, in several studies in which bidirectional Pi fluxes were analyzed in relationship to the PD by means of the Ussing flux ratio test (5), the observed ratios were not different from those predicted as the result of the electrical gradients (6,7). This apparent discrepancy in results can most likely be explained by an increasing body of data which indicate that the activity of intestinal Pi absorptive processes tends to reflect the needs of the animal for this molecule. Effects of metabolic phosphate requirements were clearly indicated by studies of Carlsson when he observed that diets adequate in calcium but deficient in phosphorus elicited an increase in intestinal calcium absorption in the rat (8). Subsequent work by Tanaka and DeLuca demonstrated that phosphorus depletion increased the conversion of ^{3}H-25 hydroxyvitamin D_3 (25-OH-D_3) to ^{3}H-1α,25 dihydroxyvitamin D_3 (1,25$(OH)_2D_3$) indicating that either blood or tissue phosphate levels directly or indirectly influence the activity of renal 25-OH-D_3-1α-hydroxylase (9). This observation has been confirmed by several investigators. In light of these interrelationships between Pi and vitamin D metabolism, it is not surprising that most of the pathophysiological states in which Caniggia and Gennari observed Pi malabsorption in man are conditions in which alterations in vitamin D metabolism are quite possible, e.g., cirrhosis, chronic uremia, myxedema, diabetes, hypoparathyroidism, chronic glucocorticoid therapy and even post-menopausal osteoporosis (10).

The movement of phosphate across the intestinal epithelium almost certainly occurs by two distinct routes, cellularly mediated active transport and diffusion between cells through the paracellular "shunt" pathway. These paracellular channels are about twice as permeable to monovalent cations as to monovalent anions (11) and it is unclear what the anticipated partial conductance of a polyatomic anion such as phosphate might be. However, we must assume that any net diffusion of Pi ions across the epithelium will probably occur by this route. This is because the diffusional entry of Pi into the cells will be greatly retarded by the highly electronegative cell interior (at least -50 mV (12)), which, combined with the data suggesting that intracellular diffusible Pi levels may be rather high (about 5 mM (13)), makes it quite unlikely that extracellular Pi activities large enough to drive net diffusional entry will be reached under physiologic conditions. However, before the effects of electrochemical gradients on the equilibrium distributions of Pi across cell membranes can be estimated, the valence as well as the concentration (activity) must be known and since the pK_2 for phosphoric acid is 7.2, Pi will be nearly equally distributed between the mono- and divalent species at a physiological pH of 7.4. Thus, the diffusional gradients for these two species will be quite different because a valence of 2 rather than 1 will double the value of an exponential term rather than having only a simple proportional effect.

The problems of charge and electrochemical gradients can be overcome for studies of Pi influx into the cell by the use of resealed membrane vesicles as has been reported by Berner et al. (14). For the transepithelial transport of Pi, these problems in analysis of the data can be eliminated if experiments are conducted in the absence of electrochemical gradients. This is because at steady-state, diffusional fluxes will be equal in both directions and will cancel themselves out, requiring any significant net flux which is observed to be the result of some type of active transport process. This latter approach is employed in the present studies in which the Ussing-technique (15) is used to eliminate electrical gradients by passing a nulling or short-circuit current (SCC) and chemical and hydrostatic gradients are avoided by using equal volumes of identical buffer on both sides of the intestine.

RESULTS AND DISCUSSION

For a detailed description of the modified Ussing Technique we have employed the reader is referred to prior publications (16-18). The buffer used in the studies that follow was a pH 7.4 Krebs-Ringer solution with HCO_3-buffering (16), which contained 1.25 mM Ca, 2.4 mM Pi and 11 mM D-glucose unless indicated otherwise. The serosal muscle coat was removed by blunt microdissection, a procedure that has been shown to greatly enhance the oxidative metabolism of the intestine in vitro (19). This procedure not only improves the in vitro viability of the epithelium, but for Pi in particular, it decreases the time required for ^{32}P-Pi to reach a steady-state flux rate. Finally, this maneuver also enhances the access of compounds added to the serosal incubation medium to the basal lateral plasma membranes of the epithelial cells. The results of a three hour experiment conducted with jejunum obtained from vitamin D-deficient rats (8-10 wks) that had been received 270 ng doses of $1,25(OH)_2D_3$, 72, 48 and 24 hrs before study are shown in Figure 1. In these experiments, the concentration of Pi was 0.5 mM and the mucosal buffer contained 20 mM D-mannitol while the serosal solution contained 20 mM D-glucose.

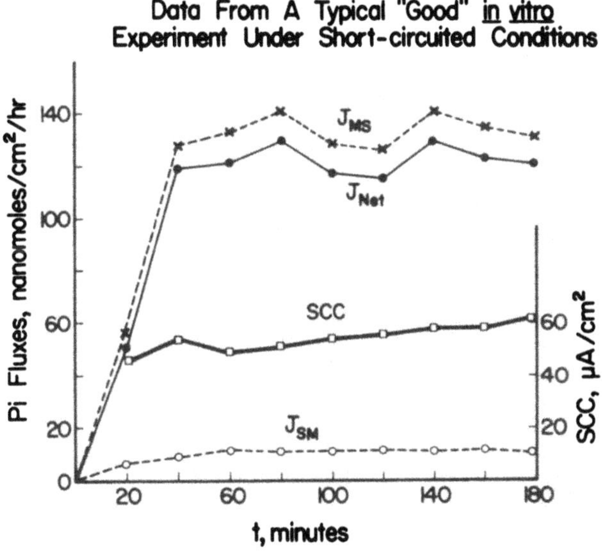

Figure 1. Pi transport across jejunum from $1,25(OH)_2D_3$-treated rats in which there was adequate conductance matching for the entire 3 hrs.

Conductance matched within 25% on the tissues for both Jms and Jsm throughout the experiment. The absence of mucosal glucose accounts for the relatively low SCC, which nevertheless was stable over the 3 hr period (Fig. 1). Both Pi Jms and Jsm reached steady-state rates in terms of the tracer measurements of fluxes by about 60 min and remained constant over the subsequent 2 hr period (Fig. 1) as did net Pi absorption, which in the absence of electrochemical gradients represents active transport. In most studies in which we wish to only compare the steady-state rates across intestine as a function of varing conditions (age, vitamin D-deficiency, repletion with vitamin D metabolites, etc.) studies were generally conducted for only 2 hrs.

Table 1

ACTIVE TRANSPORT OF CALCIUM AND PHOSPHATE ACROSS NORMAL ADULT RAT INTESTINE

Fluxes in nanomoles. cm^{-2}. hr^{-1} ± 1 SEM

$J_{Net} = J_{MS} - J_{SM}$

Tissue	N	J_{Net} Calcium	J_{Net} Phosphate
Duodenum	8	- 26.2 ± 3.6	- 18.5 ± 2.4
Jejunum	9	- 18.0 ± 1.9	- 16.4 ± 2.2
Ileum	7	- 17.6 ± 3.2	- 23.0 ± 2.5
Colon	4	1.6 ± 3.2	0.6 ± 0.6

[Ca] = 1.25 mM, [Pi] = 2.4 mM

When normal adult rats are fed a diet containing adequate levels of Ca and phosphorus (e.g., Purina Lab Chow) active intestinal absorption of these elements is not observed, and in fact, as shown in Table 1, there appears to be active secretion by the entire small bowel. Whether or not this secretion represents a significant excretory route is unclear, however, the data suggest that in a non-growing animal, an adequate amount of both Ca and Pi can be absorbed by passive diffusion and/or solvent drag. When dietary Ca is restricted in these adult animals, active absorption of this element is stimulated in response to increased metabolic needs (15,20,21) (most probably by increased conversion of 25-OH-D to $1,25(OH)_2D$) and, although it has only been tested in growing (22) and not in adult animals, dietary phosphorus restriction would presumably have a similar effect on absorption.

Effects of Vitamin D-metabolites on Pi Absorption

The availability of chemically synthesized vitamin D-metabolites and analogs has greatly facilitated the study of the effects of these molecules on intestinal function. In the rat, $1,25(OH)_2$-D_3 is by far the most potent form of the prohormone in the stimulation of active Pi as well as Ca absorption (23) and therefore, was used to study the Pi transport response of different segments of small intestine. The results in Table 2 show that even after 6-8 weeks of vitamin D-depletion, active absorption of Ca is still observed in the duodenum while active Pi absorption persists in the jejunum, otherwise the vitamin D-deficient intestine appears to function in a manner similar to adult small bowel. The persistance of these active absorptive processes may reflect incomplete vitamin D-deficiency or may indicate effects of the stress of growth through unelucidated mechanisms. The response of the small intestine to a single, pharmacological dose of $1,25(OH)_2D_3$ (975 pmoles), together with the approximate time at which a maximal stimulation was observed, also appear in Table 2. While changes in both active calcium and Pi absorption are observed in all three segments, the duodenum was most responsive to $1,25(OH)_2D_3$ in terms of increased calcium absorption, jejunum exhibited the greatest Pi response and ileum appeared to undergo a slower, but nearly equal stimulation of both Ca and Pi absorption. This general result has been confirmed in more extensive studies reported elsewhere (23), in which the same segmental response pattern was also observed after repeated doses of $1,25(OH)_2D_3$ or $24R,25(OH)_2D_3$. In these studies conducted with rats that had been vitamin D-deficient for 8-10 wks, $24R,25(OH)_2D_3$ was about 50% less potent than equimolar doses of $1,25(OH)_2D_3$ in stimulating the active absorption of Ca and Pi. In a prior study of duodenal transport, we had observed similar effects of single 1.3 nmoles doses of $1,25(OH)_2D_3$, $1,24R,25(OH)_3D_3$ and 13 nmoles of $24R,25(OH)_2D_3$ in intact rats and while the response to the two former compounds was relatively unaffected by nephrectomy, this extremely large dose of $24R,25(OH)_2D_3$ was apparently entirely inactive in the absence of renal tissue (24).

Table 2

ACTIVE TRANSPORT OF CALCIUM AND PHOSPHATE ACROSS VITAMIN D-DEFICIENT RAT INTESTINE ± 1α,25-$(OH)_2$ VITAMIN D_3

Vitamin D-deficient

Tissue	N	J_{Net} Calcium	J_{Net} Phosphate
Duodenum	10	+ 18.6 ± 4.3	- 18.3 ± 1.8
Jejunum	7	- 11.0 ± 1.5	+ 28.1 ± 7.3
Ileum	7	- 25.1 ± 5.1	- 44.8 ± 6.0

+ 975 pmoles 1α,25-$(OH)_2D_3$

Tissue	N	J_{Net} Calcium	J_{Net} Phosphate	Time
Duodenum	9	+ 117.9 ± 6.1	+ 15.0 ± 3.6	24 hr
Jejunum	6	+ 5.0 ± 1.5	+ 80.4 ± 11.1	24 hr
Ileum	6	+ 0.3 ± 2.1	- 12.8 ± 2.0	96 hr

Fluxes in nanomoles. cm^{-2}. hr^{-1} ± 1 SEM

[Ca] = 1.25 mM, [Pi] = 2.4 mM

This indicates that in the rat, the stimulation of active Pi as well as Ca absorption compounds in the vitamin D series requires the presence of a hydroxyl group in the 1α position (or its steric equivalent).

Mode of Action of Vitamin D on Intestinal Absorption

There are several possible means by which intestinal absorption may be increased. First of all, increased net movement from the lumen to the blood can occur by simple diffusion, but only if there are favorable electrochemical gradients. The second means of change is via alterations in active transport processes. This may involve increases in active absorption as well as decreases in active secretion and may also be combined with alterations in diffusional permeability. Before the mode of action of vitamin D on the intestine can be fully understood, information is needed on: 1) the portion of Pi and Ca flux that occurs via the paracellular "shunt" pathway and 2) whether or not the vitamin D status of the animal alters the permeability of this route. Since direct evidence is lacking on both the preceeding points, the best indication of the diffusional permeability of the epithelium which is available in existing data are measurements of electrical conductance. This is because the partial conductances of monovalent ions through the shunt pathway account for more than 80% of the total tissue conductance (11) so that this parameter primarly reflects shunt permeability. In a very large number of experiments conducted with the Ussing technique, no significant change in conductance has been consistently noted in rat intestine as a function of vitamin D-status (23). In fact, in the few groups in which there have been apparent differences, conductance was decreased by $1,25(OH)_2D_3$ treatment. It should be pointed out, however, that these studies were not designed to carefully evaluate conductance changes and differences in "edge damage" and effective absorptive area could obscure moderate alterations.

In rat intestine, not only is conductance apparently unaltered by vitamin D-status but the flux of both Pi and Ca in the blood to lumen or serosal to mucosal direction (Jsm) is unchanged as well (16,21,23,24). Since the results in Tables 1 and 2 show that there is active secretion of Pi and Ca in the absence of electrochemical gradients (also see reference 23), part of Jsm must certainly occur through cells rather than between them. While the relative distribution might change, the sum of these two processes that comprise Jsm is unaltered by vitamin D. This of course requires that changes in net absorption must occur via variations in the movement from lumen to blood or mucosal to serosal flux (Jms) and this appears to definitely be the case (16,21,23,24). Thus, it appears to be safe to conclude that in the rat, the <u>major</u> effects of hormonally active forms of vitamin D on both Ca and Pi absorption occur through increases in cellularly-mediated active transport processes which are expressed in Jms.

The fact that the Pi absorptive process is regulated means that the net movement of this ion across the gut epithelium may appear as net secretion, net absorption or no net flux, depending on the metabolic status of the animal. This almost certainly explains the conflicting conclusions of earlier studies with regard to the energetic requirements of the process (4,6,7). It also is interesting to consider the case in which the observation of no net flux may be the result of equal but opposite active transport processes rather than indicating the absence of active transport. This situation exists because there appear to be graded responses of the active absorptive system (23) with zero net flux necessarily occurring in the transition from secretion to absorption.

Effects of PTH and Cyclic 3', 5' Adenosine Monophosphate (cAMP) on Jejunal Pi Transport

Because of the tremendous alterations in renal tubular Pi reabsorption that occur in response to PTH and the similarities between many renal and intestinal epithelial transport processes, a direct effect of PTH on gut Pi absorption is a reasonable possibility. However, if we assume that PTH effects intestinal epithelium by the same mechanism as it acts on renal cells, then it should activate adenylate cyclase and increase cellular levels of cAMP. When both of these parameters were examined by Kimberg and his co-workers, no effect of PTH on intestinal adenylate cyclase (25) or mucosal cAMP levels (Brasitus, Walling and Kimberg, unpublished observations) was detected. In 1973, the author undertook a large series of experiments in Dr. Kimberg's laboratory on the direct effects of PTH and salmon calcitonin (SCT) on intestinal transport function when the hormones were added to solutions bathing the serosal surface of the gut in the Ussing apparatus. While 10 μg/ml of SCT did cause a small but consistent stimulation of intestinal SCC and active Cl secretion (26) (generally is an indication of an elevation of cAMP), the same high dose of PTH had no apparent effect. Lower doses of both SCT and PTH were without effect. Interestingly, in spite of the cAMP-like effect of SCT, we were unable to detect an elevation of cellular cAMP in response to this hormone (26). The preceeding experiments were conducted using intestine from normal adult rats in which there is little active absorption of Ca and Pi and usually active secretion of these molecules is observed (e.g., see Table 1). Therefore, it is possible that this experimental model might have accounted for the lack of hormonal effects on Ca and Pi transport (PTH had no effect, while SCT increased bidirectional Ca fluxes with no change in Jnet (26)). Recently, evidence for PTH and SCT sensitive adenylate cyclase in rat gut was pursued further by looking for effects in tissues taken from growing animals. In the first series of experiments we homogenized scraped epithelia, centrifuged this material at 2000 x g for 20 min and assayed adenylate cyclase activity in the resulting pellet (27). Studies were conducted using rats that had been raised from weaning on a non-rachitogenic, vitamin D-deficient diet and then subsequently were injected with 1:1 propanediol-ethanol solvent or 975 pmoles of $1,25(OH)_2D_3$ 48 and 24 hrs before study. In the vitamin D-deficient animals (n = 8) basal adenylate cyclase activity was 11.1 pmoles cAMP/mg prot/min ± 1.1 SEM; +PTH, 10^{-7}M = 12.3 ± 1.5; +SCT, $2(10)^{-7}$M = 12.4 ± 1.3; and +NaF, 10^{-2}M = 76.8 ± 8.0. In the $1,25(OH)_2D_3$ treated animals (n = 8) basal activity = 23.0 ± 2.2; +PTH = 21.3 ± 2.5; +SCT = 23.5 ± 2.0, (+ vasoactive intestinal peptide, $2(10)^{-6}$M = 40.3 ± 2.1; and +NaF, 10^{-2}M = 86.9 ± 8.5. Clearly, there was a VIP effect and no PTH or SCT effect in either group (biological activity of the hormones was confirmed in other cell types (27)). Just as clearly, $1,25(OH)_2D_3$-treatment caused a doubling of basal adenylate cyclase activity ($P<0.001$) while F-stimulated activity was unchanged. This change in basal adenylate cyclase activity confirms our earlier report of a $1,25(OH)_2D_3$-mediated elevation of duodenal cAMP and adenylate cyclase levels (28). The nature of this steroid hormone effect on the activity of an enzyme generally regulated by polypeptide hormones is at best, unclear. However, our initial studies do not indicate a direct interaction of the hormone with adenylate cyclase receptors. Data obtained in partially purified BL membranes prepared from duodenal epithelial cells in which the $1,25(OH)_2D_3$ was added using ethanol as a vehicle, showed a marked effect on the ethanol alone with no further change due to $1,25(OH)_2D_3$ (adenylate cyclase activities as pmoles cAMP/mg prot/min were: basal = 6.5; basal +ethanol = 11.5; $1,25(OH)_2D_3$ 10^{-6}M = 11.9; 10^{-7}M = 12.8; 10^{-8}M = 12.0; 10^{-9}M = 11.6; 10^{-10}M = 12.5; 10^{-11}M = 11.6; prostaglandin E_1 $(10)^{-6}$M = 16.0; and 10mM NaF = 104.4). The effects of PTH were also studied in this partially purified BL membrane preparation over a range of concentrations from 10^{-6} to 10^{-11}M and again no effects were observed while vasoactive intestinal peptide produced marked stimulation of the enzyme (basal activity = 8.4; + VIP = 23.7). Thus, preparations which respond to a known polypeptide hormone stimulator, are unaffected by PTH.

If we assume that PTH would effect the intestine in the same manner as it does the renal proximal tubule, then it should inhibit Pi absorption. Therefore, it would be more probable that an effect would be observed on intestine with a high level of active Pi absorption. Because we were unable to obtain any evidence of a direct PTH-stimulation of adenylate cyclase activity in intestinal epithelium of duodenum, jejunum or ileum of normal growing or adult rats as well as vitamin D-deficient or $1,25(OH)_2D_3$-stimulated animals, the alternative was to elevate cellular cAMP by addition of exogenous nucleotide. Because of its greater membrane permeability, dibutyryl cAMP (DbcAMP) was used. Because jejunum exhibits the greatest Pi absorptive stimulation following $1,25(OH)_2D_3$-treatment (23), this segment was used from animals treated as described in the results shown in Figure 1. To be sure that Pi absorption was not at a maximal rate, a Pi concentration below our observed Km values (29) and similar to the Km reported by Berner et al. (14) was used, i.e., 0.24mM. Mucosal glucose was replaced by mannitol to maximize the number of Na molecules available for Pi transport and to eliminate the possibility of Pi and glucose competing for a finite quantity of Na-gradient for coupled entry into the cells. Studies were carried out by mounting four adjacent pieces of jejunum (with the muscle coats removed) with two pieces used for Jms and two for Jsm. After control periods of 80 to 100 min, the best pairing of Jms and Jsm was done using conductance matching and 1mM DbcAMP was then achieved in the serosal compartments of one Jms-Jsm pair by dissolving crystalline material directly in the buffer. Within 2 min, SCC began to rise and was maximally elevated 15-20 min. When DbcAMP was added after a 80 min control period, it was often difficult to be sure of the initial steady-state flux rate, but no makred change in Pi transport was noted. Because good viability was observed for 3 hrs (Fig. 1), 18 experiments were carried out in which a 2 hr baseline was obtained and then DbcAMP was added to one Jms-Jsm pair. The data from the seven studies in which conductance matching stayed within acceptable limits (30% (18)) are shown in Table 3.

Table 3

Effects of 1mM DbcAMP on Active Jejunal Pi Absorption

	ΔNet Absorption Nanomoles/cm^2/hr		ΔShort Circuit-Current $\mu A/cm^2$	
	Control	+DbcAMP	Control	+DbcAMP
	- 3.1	+ 5.5	+ 8	+155
	- 2.0	+16.6	+18	+108
	- 6.6	+ 8.6	0	+ 87
	-13.5	- 1.9	0	+116
	-24.1	-17.8	+ 3	+ 76
	+ 0.4	-11.9	+ 8	+ 87
	- 3.2	- 0.4	+17	+110
Mean =	- 7.4±3.2SE	-0.2±4.5	+ 8±2	+105±10
% Change =	-7%	-0.1%	+16.4%	+212%

Differences are between steady-state values for the first 2 hrs vs. the rates for the 3rd hr with or without DbcAMP.

The SCC was increased 212% by DbcAMP while only a slight, 16%, increase was noted in controls (Table 3). In spite of this clear indication of marked changes in jejunal transport function (the SCC increase is primarily the result of active Cl secretion), the active absorption of Pi was not altered by treatment (Table 3).

Thus neither PTH nor its "second messenger" in the kidney markedly alter gut Pi absorption, at least under the conditions that we employed. Therefore, it appears that the major hormonal regulation of intestinal Pi absorption is mediated by 1,25$(OH)_2D_3$, with PTH effects occurring via stimulation of synthesis of this hormone rather than a direct action. However, data of Borle et al. indicate PTH effects on intestinal cell metabolism (30), so that effects other than on adenylate cyclase should be considered.

The Role of Ca in Pi Transport

The function of Ca ions in Pi absorption is unclear. Harrison and Harrison found that removal of Ca abolished concentrative Pi transport by everted gut sacs (4) and a similar observation was made by Chen et al. in rat duodenum but not in the jejunum (31). However, there have been several other reports in which the presence or absence of Ca had little or no effect on Pi transport (13,32-34) or even increased it (35). We found that the presence of Ca in the serosal but not the mucosal bathing media was necessary for the general "transport" viability of rat gut in vitro, and that 1,25-$(OH)_2D_3$-stimulated active Pi absorption occurred with no mucosal Ca (except possibly in the unstirred layer on the BB surface (23). The lack of a Ca-requirement for Pi to cross the brush border (BB) membrane is indicated by the results of Berner et al. in which Pi influx into vesicles was unaltered by Ca (14). However, the results of Neville and Holdsworth (35) show a marked effect of luminal Ca on mucosal Pi metabolism so that events subsequent to BB Pi influx may be altered by this ion.

Carrier-Mediation of Pi Transport

The observation of Pi active transport processes implies the existence of molecules that facilitate the movement of Pi across intestinal cells. Since the thermodynamic requirements of Pi transport indicate the need for energy coupling at the BB membrane (14, 29), it is not surprising that carrier-kinetics have been observed across the surface. In their extensive studies of rat BB membrane Pi kinetics, Berner et al. reported an apparent Km for Na-dependent Pi influx of 1.1 $(10)^{-4}$M and observed competitive inhibition by arsenate (14). We have found a higher Km for Pi influx into intact jejunal epithelia in vitro (about 3mM) but have not corrected our values for Na-independent Pi cellular influx or paracellular Pi movement (29). Data obtained for 10-40 min Pi uptake across the BB membrane indicate processes with Km's of 10^{-4} and 10^{-6}M for human duodenum (36) and 2 $(10)^{-4}$M for chick jejunum (37). However, ^{32}P-Pi crosses the entire intestinal wall in less than 10 min (our unpublished data and ref. 37) so that 10 min or longer uptake periods reflect several processes rather than just BB influx. In addition, it appears that in contrast to the kidney, where dibasic Pi appears to be most readily reabsorbed (38,39), monobasic Pi is preferentially absorbed by the gut (14,29). If this is the case, then Km values should be calculated using the concentration of $H_2PO_4^-$ rather than total Pi to give a more accurate indication of the "true" affinity of the transport site.

Finally, the most likely candidate for a molecule that is involved in Pi transport is alkaline phosphatase. However, evidence on this point is currently circumstantial, at best (33,40).

Na-Dependence of Pi Transport

Experiments by McHardy and Parsons in vivo (41) and Harrison and Harrison in vitro (42) both indicated that Pi absorption by rat small bowel increased proportionally with increasing concentrations of Na in the medium. Taylor later made a similar observation in chick ileum (34). These data clearly indicate a Na-stimulatory effect on intestinal Pi absorption, but reflect changes via at least two processes. One process is cellularly-mediated Pi transport and the other is paracellular diffusion which will be altered because the electrical gradient across the epithelium is directly related to the concentration of Na. This can be seen in the results in Table 4 in which the PD (calculated from SCC/G) increased from about -0.3 mV to +4.8 mV as the [Na] was raised from 25 to 144mM. Thus, under

Table 4

Effects of Na Concentration on $1,25\text{-}(OH)_2D_3$-Stimulated

Jejunal Pi Absorption and Electrical Parameters

[Na] mM		Jms[a]	Jsm	Jnet	SCC[b]	G[c]
25	5	55.8± 8.8	37.0± 1.3	18.8±5.6	-4.7±1.5	18.3±1.1
90	5	116.6±15.9	51.6±12.1	65.0±7.4	87.7±7.4	27.8±3.0
144	7	167.1±16.2	65.6±13.3	101.6±9.4	142.1±6.3	29.9±2.1

[a] Fluxes in nmoles/cm^2/hr; all numbers ± SEM

[b] μA/cm^2/hr

[c] mmmhos/cm^2

open-circuited conditions such as exist in vivo or with everted gut sacs, the electrical gradient actually changes from one that should slightly retard net Pi diffusion toward the blood or serosal surface to a gradient favoring diffusional absorption as the [Na] increases. The changes in Pi fluxes that occurred in response to alterations in [Na] with the PD nulled by a SCC appear in Table 4. The rats used were vitamin D-deficient for 8-10 wks after weaning and then received 1.3 nmole doses of $1,25(OH)_2D_3$, 48 and 24 hrs before sacrifice so that the effects of Na concentration on vitamin D-stimulated cells could be studied. Interestingly, both Pi Jms and Jsm increased in proportion to the larger levels of Na. This is consistent with Na effecting Pi fluxes across both the basal lateral (BL) and brush border (BB) plasma membranes, with the BB effect having been well documented by Berner et al. (14). Analysis of Pi fluxes relative to the approximate electrochemical gradients across both BL and BB membranes of intestinal cells indicates that Pi entry across both surfaces must be the result of active transport while exit is consistent with a distribution that could be produced by diffusion alone (29). As is the case for amino acids and hexoses, the coupling of Pi fluxes to the Na gradient into the intestinal cell may provide the energy for Pi transport as well as providing for electroneutral entry, particularly since it appears that 1 Na is transported with 1 H_2PO_4 (14). Once inside, the electronegativity of this compartment would provide the gradient for net Pi diffusion out of the cell (a similar model for intestinal Pi absorption has been proposed by Kinne's group, based on data obtained from membrane vesicles (14)). Thus, active Pi absorption and active Pi secretion could represent manifestations of the same Na-dependent process. Secretion would be observed when: a) there are more sites for coupled Na-Pi entry on the BL membrane than on the BB membrane and b) the permeability of the BB membrane to Pi is greater than that of the BL membrane. Active absorption would exist when: a) there are more sites for coupled Na-Pi in the BB membrane than in the BL membrane and b) the permeability of the BB membrane to Pi is lower than the BL membrane. Thus $1,25(OH)_2D_3$, for example, could increase active Pi absorption by producing a decrease in the passive permeability of the BB membrane or an increase in the permeability of the BL membrane to Pi together with somehow elevating the number of BB membrane Na-Pi transport sites. While the permeability changes have not been studied, $1,25(OH)_2D_3$ does increase BB membrane Pi influx in the presence of a high Na concentration (29) and the stimulation of BB Pi uptake is blocked by cyclohexamide (37), suggesting that such a transport site is indeed synthesized in response to the hormone.

Acknowledgments

Thanks are due P. Holliday, C. Schaefer and E. Tallos for expert assistance and Dr. J.W. Coburn for encouragement and facilities. Supported by VA Medical Research Funds and USPHS Grant AM-14750. Vitamin D metabolites were furnished by Hoffman-La Roche, Nutley, N.J. courtesy of Dr. A. W. Norman.

References

1. Harris, J.L., and Innes, J.R.M.: The mode of action of vitamin D. Studies on hypervitaminosis D. The influence of the calcium phosphate intake. Biochem. J. 25:367, 1931.

2. Nicolaysen, R.: Studies upon the mode of action of vitamin D. II. The influence of vitamin D on the faecal output of endogenous calcium and phosphorus in the rat. Biochem. J. 31:107, 1937.

3. Nicolaysen, R.: Studies upon the mode of action of vitamin D. III. The influence of vitamin D on absorption of calcium and phosphorus. Biochem. J. 31:122, 1937.

4. Harrison, H.E., and Harrison, H.C.: Intestinal transport of phosphate: action of vitamin D, calcium, and potassium. Am. J. Physiol. 201:1007, 1961.

5. Ussing, H.H.: The distinction by means of tracers between active transport and diffusion. The transfer of iodide across the isolated frog skin. Acta Physiol. Scand. 19:43, 1949.

6. Asano, T.: Transport of calcium and inorganic phosphate across the intestinal wall of the rat. Seitai no Kagaku 11:55, 1960.

7. Noble, H.M., and Matty, A.J.: The effect of thyroxine on the movement of calcium and inorganic phosphate through the small intestine of the rat. J. Endocr. 37:111, 1967.

8. Carlsson, A.: The effect of vitamin D on the absorption of inorganic phosphate. Acta Physiol. Scand. 31:301, 1954.

9. Tanaka, Y., and DeLuca, H.F.: The control of 25-hydroxyvitamin D metabolism by inorganic phosphorus. Arch. Biochem. Biophys. 154:566, 1973.

10. Caniggia, A., and Gennari, C.: Absorption du phosphate radioactif chez l'homme et sa regulation. In Symposium Internatinal sur Phosphate et Metabolisme Phosphocalcique. Sandoz Edition's, Paris, 1970, pp. 209-235.

11. Frizzell, R.A., and Schultz, S.G.: Ionic conductances of extracellular shunt pathway in rabbit ileum. J. Gen. Physiol. 59: 318, 1972.

12. Okada, Y., Sato, T., and Inouye, A.: Effects of potassium ions and sodium ions on membrane potential of epithelial cells in rat duodenum. Biochim. Biophys. Acta 413:104, 1975.

13. Kowarski, S., and Schachter, D.: Effects of vitamin D on phosphate transport and incorporation into mucosal constituents of rat intestinal mucosa. J. Biol. Chem. 244:211, 1969.

14. Berner, W., Kinne, R., and Murer, H.: Phosphate transport into brush border membrane vesicles isolated from rat small intestine. Biochem. J. 160:467, 1976.

15. Ussing, H.H., and Zerahn, K.: Active transport of sodium as the source of electric current in the short-circuited isolated frog skin. Acta Physiol. Scand. 23:110, 1951.

16. Walling, M.W., and Rothman, S.S.: Phosphate-independent, carrier-mediated active transport of calcium by rat intestine. Am. J. Physiol. 217:1144, 1969.

17. Walling, M.W., and Kimberg, D.V.: Active secretion of calcium by adult rat ileum and jejunum in vitro. Am. J. Physiol. 225: 415, 1973.

18. Walling, M.W., and Kimberg, D.V.: Effects of 1α,25-dihydroxyvitamin D_3 and _Solanum glaucophyllum_ on intestinal calcium and phosphate transport and on plasma Ca, Mg, and P levels in the rat. Endocrinology 97:1567, 1975.

19. Frizzell, R.A., Marksheid-Kaspi, L., and Schultz, S.G.: Oxidative metabolism of rabbit ileal mucosa. Am. J. Physiol. 226: 1142, 1974.

20. Kimberg, D.V., Schachter, D., and Schenker, H.: Active transport of calcium by intestine: effects of dietary calcium. Am. J. Physiol. 200:1256, 1961.

21. Walling, M.W., and Kimberg, D.V.: Calcium absorption or secretion by rat ileum in vitro: effects of dietary calcium intake. Am. J. Physiol. 226:1124, 1974.

22. Walling, M.W., Brautbar, N., and Coburn, J.W.: Jejunal phosphate active transport: effects of phosphorus depletion and vitamin D. Federation Proc. 36:1097, 1977.

23. Walling, M.W.: Intestinal Ca and phosphate transport: differential responses to vitamin D_3 metabolites. Am. J. Physiol. _In Press_.

24. Walling, M.W., Hartenbower, D.L., Coburn, J.W., and Norman, A.W.: Effects of 1α,25-, 24R,25-, and 1α,24R,25-hydroxylated metabolites of vitamin D_3 on calcium and phosphate absorption by duodenum from intact and nephrectomized rats. Arch. Biochem. Biophys. 182:251, 1977.

25. Kimberg, D.V., Field, M., Johnson, J., Henderson, A., and Gershon, E.: Stimulation of intestinal mucosal adenyl cyclase by Cholera enterotoxin and prostaglandins. J. Clin. Invest. 50:1218, 1971.

26. Walling, M.W., Brasitus, T.A., and Kimberg, D.V.: Effects of calcitonin and substance P on the transport of Ca, Na and Cl across rat ileum in vitro. Gastroenterology 73:89, 1977.

27. Minkin, C., Blackman, L., Newbrey, J., Pokress, Posek, R., and Walling, M.: Effects of parathyroid hormone and calcitonin on adenylate cyclase in murine mononuclear phagocytes. Biochem. Biophys. Res. Commun. 76:875, 1977.

28. Walling, M.W., Brasitus, T.A., and Kimberg, D.V.: Elevation of cyclic AMP levels and adenylate cyclase activity in duodenal mucosa from vitamin D-deficient rats by 1α,25-dihydroxycholecalciferol. Endocr. Res. Commun. 3:83, 1976.

29. Walling, M.W.: Effects of 1α,25-dihydroxy-vitamin D_3 on active intestinal inorganic phosphate absorption. In Vitamin D: Biochemical Chemical and Clinical Aspects Related to Calcium Metabolism. Ed. Norman, A.W., Schaefer, K., Coburn, J.W., DeLuca, H.F., Fraser, D., Grigoleit, and von Herrath, D.: Walter de Gruyter, Berlin, N.Y., 1977, pp 321-330.

30. Borle, A.B., Keutmann, H.T., and Neuman, W.F.: Role of parathyroid hormone in phosphate transport across rat duodenum. Am. J. Physiol. 204:705, 1963.

31. Chen, T.C., Castillo, L., Korycka-Dahl, M., and DeLuca, H.F.: Role of vitamin D metabolites in phosphate transport of rat intestine. J. Nutr. 104:1056, 1974.

32. Helbock, H.J., Forte, J.G., Saltman, P.: The mechanism of calcium transport by rat intestine. Biochim. Biophys. Acta 126:81, 1966.

33. Wasserman, R.H., and Taylor, A.N.: Intestinal absorption of phosphate in the chick: effect of vitamin D_3 and other parameters. J. Nutr. 103:586, 1973.

34. Taylor, A.N.: In vitro phosphate transport in chick ileum: effect of cholecalciferol, calcium, sodium and metabolic inhibitors. J. Nutr. 104:489, 1974.

35. Neville, E., and Holdworth, E.S.: Phosphorus metabolism during transport of calcium. Biochim. Biophys. Acta 163:362, 1968.

36. Short, E.M., Binder, H.J., and Rosenberg, L.E.: Familial hypophosphatemic rickets: defective transport of inorganic phosphate by intestinal mucosa. Science 179:700, 1973.

37. Peterlik, M., and Wasserman, R.H.: Effect of vitamin D_3 and 1,25-dihydroxy-vitamin D_3 on intestinal transport of phosphate. In Phosphate Metabolism, Ed. Massry, S.G., and Ritz, E. Plenum Press, N.Y. and Lond. 1977, pp. 323-332.

38. Baumann, K., de Rouffignac, C., Roinel, N., Rumrich, G., and Ullrich, K.J.: Renal phosphate transport: Unhomogeneity of local proximal rates and sodium dependence. Pflugers Arch. 356:287, 1975.

39. Hoffman, N., Thees, M., and Kinne, R.: Phosphate transport by isolated renal brush border vesicles. Pflugers Arch. 362: 147, 1976.

40. Moog, F., and Glazier, H.S.: Phosphate absorption and alkaline phosphatase activity in the small intestine of the adult mouse and of the chick embryo and hatched chick. Comp. Biochem. Physiol. 42A:321, 1972.

41. McHardy, G.J.R., and Parsons, D.S.: The absorption of inorganic phosphate from the small intestine of the rat. Quart. J. Exp. Physiol. 41:398, 1956.

42. Harrison, H.E., and Harrison, H.C.: Sodium, potassium, and intestinal transport of glucose, L-tyrosine, phosphate and calcium. Am. J. Physiol. 205:107, 1963.

VITAMIN D-DEPENDENT PHOSPHATE TRANSPORT BY CHICK INTESTINE: INHIBITION BY LOW Na^+ AND N-ETHYLMALEIMIDE

Meinrad Peterlik

Department of General and Experimental Pathology,

University of Vienna, Austria

In vitamin D-deficient chicks the duodenum displays a high capacity of phosphate (P_i) transfer from lumen to blood side, while jejunum and ileum show only low rates of transepithelial P_i transport. Vitamin D_3 stimulates intestinal phosphate absorption in all parts of the chick small intestine: The increment in P_i absorption due to vitamin D_3 is relatively small in the duodenum and also in the ileum. However, in the jejunum the vitamin increases the rate of P_i transfer to a level comparable to that displayed by the duodenum. In the jejunum, entry of P_i from the lumen is by a carrier-mediated energy-dependent transport mechanism presumably located at the brush border. Vitamin D_3 enhances the maximal velocity of this process two- to threefold. This effect is probably due to the action of the active metabolite, 1,25-dihydroxy-vitamin D_3. The exact mechanism by which the latter stimulates P_i influx is not known at present. However, a protein synthetic step seems to be necessary for enhancement of P_i absorption by the hormonally acting sterol (1, 2, 3).

Evidence is now accumulating that vitamin D affects intestinal phosphate transport apart from its effect on the calcium absorptive process: In everted chick ileum (4) and jejunum (unpublished results), phosphate transport proceeds unaffected by the lack of calcium in the incubation solution. In addition, the effect of vitamin D on P_i entry across the mucosal surface in chick jejunum could be separated from vitamin D-dependent induction of calcium-binding protein (2). The latter parallels vitamin D-dependent calcium transfer across various epithelia in almost any instance (5). Further evidence for separate calcium and phosphate pathways and for their independent effectuation by vitamin D was obtained during characterization of intestinal P_i transport systems. The present study describes two conditions which selectively inhibit vitamin D-dependent phosphate transport in everted chick jejunum and in cultured embryonic chick duodenum while not affecting the respective calcium movements. Thus, regulation of intestinal phosphate absorption by vitamin D should be considered as a different facet of vitamin D action on the cellular level.

EXPERIMENTAL

One day-old White Leghorn cockerels were raised on a rachitogenic (vitamin D-deficient) diet for 4 weeks in a windowless room under constant lighting. Diet composition was exactly as described by Corradino and Wasserman (6), except that soy bean protein was substituted by vitamin D-free casein. The animals were fasted 18 hr before the experiment.

4 cm long everted gut sacs were prepared from the jejunum of either vitamin D-deficient (-D) or vitamin D-repleted (+D) chicks. The latter received 1000 I.U. vitamin D_3 in 0.2 ml propylene glycol by intramuscular injection 48 hr before use.

The buffer used for incubation and filling of the everted gut sacs was Krebs-Henseleit bicarbonate buffer continously gassed with a O_2/CO_2 (95/5 %) mixture. Phosphate concentration in the serosal solution (0.4 ml per gut sac) and in the mucosal (bathing) solution was adjusted to 4.0 mM and 1.2 mM, respectively. Calcium concentration was 0.6 mM on both sides of the gut. Radiotracers (0.5 µCi/ml Ca-45 and 0.2 µCi/ml P-32) were added to the mucosal buffer only. In some experiments, sodium in the mucosal and serosal incubation solutions was isosmotically replaced by choline. NaCl was substituted by choline chloride, and $NaHCO_3$ by choline hydrogencarbonate. Isotonicity was checked with an osmometer (Knauer, Germany). The everted gut sacs were incubated for 20 min in 5.0 ml buffer at 32° C in a metabolic shaker (120 oscillations/min).

P_i was determined with the Fiske and Subbarow method (7). Calcium was measured by atomic absorption spectrophotometry (8). P-32 and Ca-45 were determined by liquid scintillation counting using a double-channel method. Sample preparation was done by routine methods.

Embryonic chick duodena were cultured using the technique described by Corradino (9). Briefly, duodena from 20 day-old embryos were slit open and placed mucosa side up on a grid in a Petri dish. McCoy's 5A (modified) medium was added so that the guts were barely in contact with the medium. The duodena were cultured for 48 hr either in the absence (-D) or presence of 26 μM vitamin D_3 (+D). The covered dish was kept at 37° C in an incubator gassed with a 95/5 % air/CO_2 mixture.

For determination of phosphate and calcium accumulation, the cultured duodena were incubated at 37° C for 30 min in 3.0 ml of Krebs-Henseleit bicarbonate buffer. A "low sodium" buffer was prepared by isotonic replacement of NaCl by mannitol. Both buffers contained 1.2 mM P_i and 0.25 mM Ca. Concentration of radiotracers was the same as given above.

Phosphate and calcium movements were calculated according to Kowarski and Schachter (10).

RESULTS AND DISCUSSION

The following conditions were found most suitable for the assessment of basal and vitamin D-dependent phosphate and calcium movements in everted chick jejunum. At 1.2 mM P_i in the mucosal solution, the P_i transport system is certainly saturated (K_m = 0.2 mM) (2, 3). There is no change in mucosal flux rates within an incubation period of 30 min. An initial serosal P_i concentration of 4.0 mM counteracts passive vitamin D-independent out-of-tissue movement of phosphate into the serosal compartment and, consequently, P_i net transfer across the serosal border is zero. These "standard conditions", therefore, allow measurement of P_i movements across the mucosal border without interference by net changes across the contralateral surface (3). The rate of transmural transfer of P_i, however, increases non-linearly with time (Fig. 1). The vitamin D effect on P_i absorption from the lumen is not apparent in the over-all transport before 20 min. After that time, increase in serosal P_i concentration is caused by the increasingly higher extent of mucosa-to-serosa phosphate transport (not shown).

At 0.6 mM Ca, there is no net change of Ca across both surfaces of the everted gut. The vitamin D effect on the Ca absorptive process can be evaluated by measuring the rate of Ca exchange across the mucosal border (by determination of tissue uptake of Ca-45). In addition transepithelial transport of Ca proceeds linearly with time and, in contrast to P_i transport, provides a sensitive measure of the vitamin D effect on calcium absorption (Fig. 1).

Effect of Extracellular Na^+ on P_i and Ca Fluxes

A sodium-sensitive step can be implicated in P_i translocation across the small intestine (4, 12). The results shown in Fig. 2 indicate that sodium-dependency of the absorptive process resides in sensitivity towards Na^+ of the P_i entry step from the lumen into the epithelial cell layer. This pathway is also primarily affected by vitamin D. In both the +D and -D group, substitution of mucosal Na^+ by choline enhances net secretion

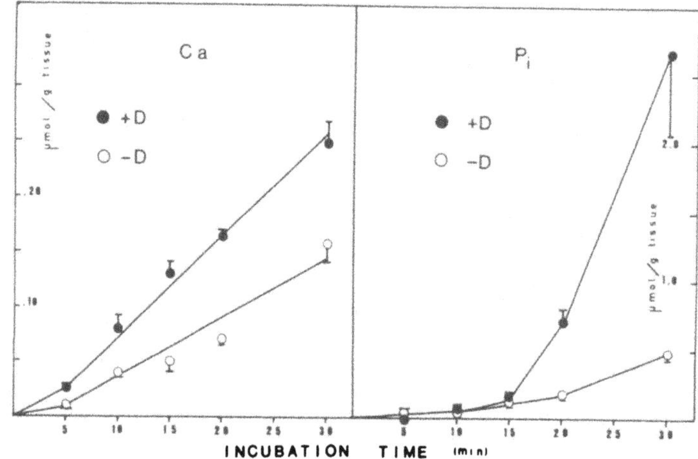

Figure 1: Effect of vitamin D on mucosa-to-serosa transport of P_i and Ca. Data are expressed as means $\pm$ S.E.M. from 12 to 33 everted gut sacs. Ca transport in the +D group is significantly different from -D (at least at $P<0.025$ level) at any point of time. Phosphate transfer in +D differs from -D only at 20 and 30 min ($P<0.001$).

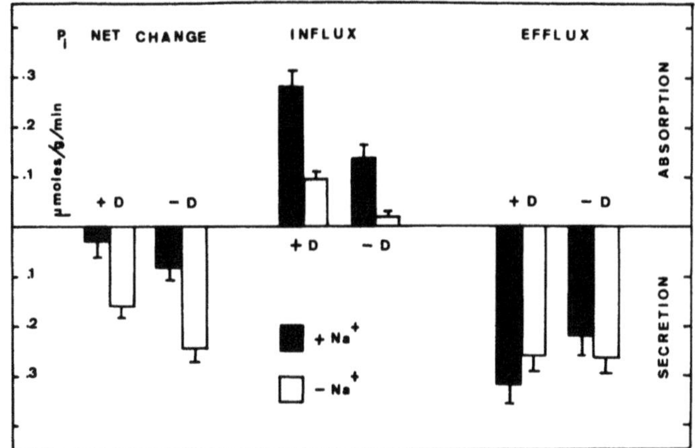

Figure 2: Influence of extracellular Na^+ on phosphate movements across mucosal border in chick jejunum. Data are given as means $\pm$ S.E.M. from 6 to 12 determinations. Net change and influx in $+D/+Na^+$ and $-D/+Na^+$ groups differed significantly ($P<0.001$) from $+D/-Na^+$ and $-D/-Na^+$ groups, respectively. Pertinent +D and -D groups also differed at the $P<0.001$ level.

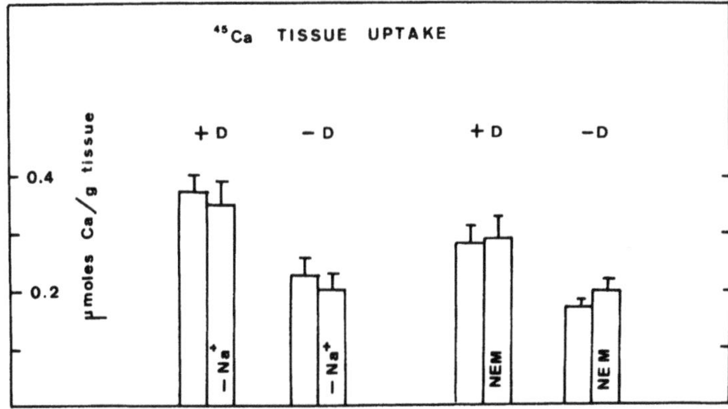

Figure 3: Uptake of Ca from mucosal solution in Na^+-free state ($-Na^+$) and in presence of 0.5 mM N-ethylmaleimide (NEM). Neither treatment had any influence on Ca movement into tissue. Values are means $\pm$ S.E.M. from 6 everted gut sacs.

of P_i into the lumen. This results from the reduced rate of P_i influx in the sodium-free state while no change in efflux from the tissue is apparent.

Ca influx determined under steady-state conditions displays no dependence on mucosal Na^+ either in vitamin D-repleted or -deficient chicks (Fig. 3). These findings were substantiated by measurement of mucosa-to-serosa Ca fluxes. Any reduction of Ca uptake from the luminal side would result in a depressed rate of over-all translocation of Ca across the gut wall. However, substitution of Na^+ by choline on both sides of the gut had no influence whatsoever on the transfer of Ca from the lumen to the serosal side (Fig. 4).

Another example for a differential effect of low extracellular sodium on phosphate and calcium transport is observed in embryonic chick duodenum. Maintained in organ culture, this tissue is sensitive to vitamin D (9). Presence of vitamin D_3 in the culture medium enhances tissue accumulation of Ca and P_i (9, 12). Apparently, vitamin D action involves enhancement of a saturable, energy dependent step in the uptake process of phosphate (12). Incubation in "low sodium" buffer considerably reduces the capacity of both +D and -D duodena to accumulate P_i and diminishes the difference between the +D and -D group. Calcium uptake, on the other hand, in-

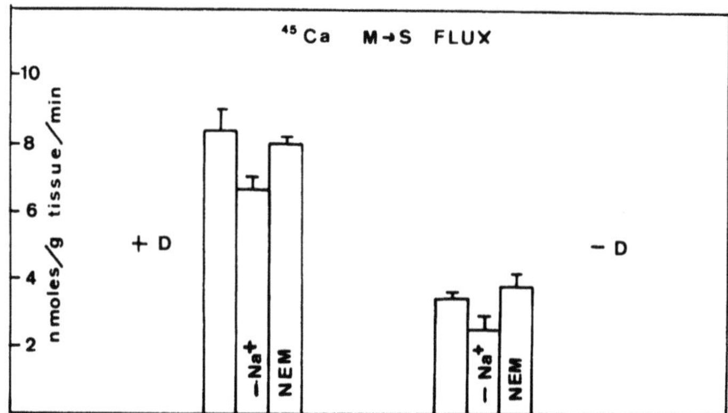

Figure 4: Mucosa-to-serosa (M-S) flux of Ca in Na^+-free state and in presence of 0.5 mM N-ethylmaleimide (NEM). Data are means ± S.E.M. from 6 to 12 determinations.

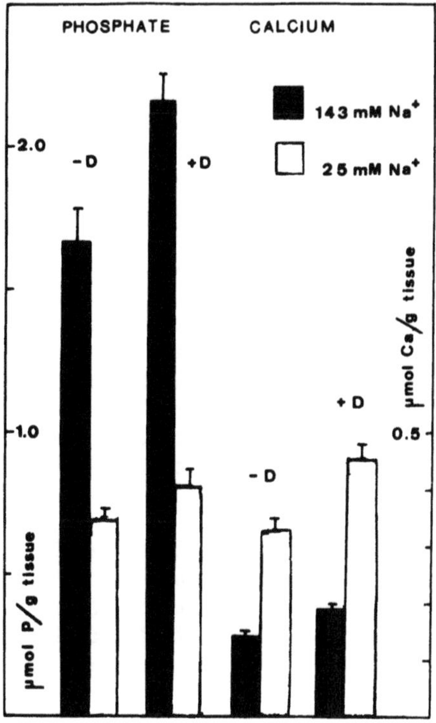

Figure 5: Effect of low sodium concentration on phosphate and calcium transport in embryonic chick duodenum. Guts were cultured in absence (-D) or presence (+D) of 26 µM vitamin D_3. Results are expressed as mean ± S.E.M. Statistically significant differences at least at $P<0.025$ level were found between "normal" and "low Na^+" groups, and between pertinent +D and -D groups.

creases more than twofold under identical conditions. In addition, the effect of vitamin D on Ca accumulation is even more evident at 25 mM Na^+ than at normal Na^+ concentrations (Fig. 5).

Inhibition of Phosphate Absorption by N-Ethylmaleimide

Phosphate transport across the inner mitochondrial membrane can be inhibited by SH-blocking reagents, e. g. N-ethylmaleimide (NEM) (13). Since P_i transfer across the luminal pole of the intestinal epithelial cell is also carrier mediated (1, 2, 3), it was of interest to know whether SH-groups are essential for the function of this "phosphate pump". When everted gut sacs are incubated in the presence of 0.5 mM NEM in the mucosal solution, there is net secretion of P_i into the luminal solution in both the +D and -D group (Fig. 6). Measurement of radiotracer fluxes clearly shows that NEM does not render the plasma membrane more permeable for outward movement of P_i but rather inhibited uphill movement of phosphate in the opposite direction.

Findings on Ca transfer during blocking of SH-groups on the mucosal surface also speak against unspecific alteration of membrane permeability by NEM. Inward movement of Ca as well as total transfer of Ca across the gut wall - in contrast to phosphate movements in the same direction - are obviously not affected by 0.5 mM NEM (Fig. 3 and 4).

It should be noted that 0.5 mM NEM does not abolish any vitamin D increment of P_i influx (Fig. 6). Even when 1.5 mM NEM is included in the mucosal bathing solution, P_i influx in the +D group is not further reduced and the difference due to vitamin D repletion still persists (results not shown). This finding bears on the question

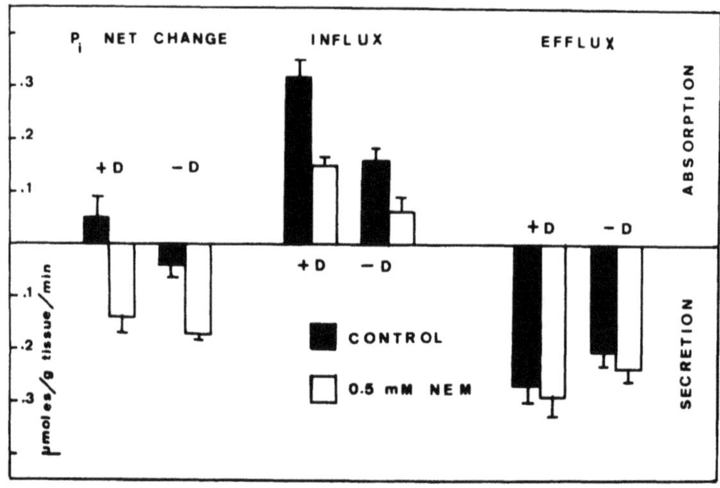

Figure 6: Inhibition of phosphate absorption by N-ethylmaleimide (NEM). Differences in net change and influx are significant at P<0.001 level (means ± S.E.M. from 12 to 14 gut sacs).

whether vitamin D induces a P_i transport system different from that existing in vitamin D-deficient chicks. If the action of the vitamin on P_i transport would involve activation of a pre-existing transport system or synthesis of identical carrier complexes, one would expect reduction of the P_i entry rate to identical levels in the +D and -D state. However, persistence of a vitamin D increment even at the highest NEM concentration used points at a part of the vitamin D-induced P_i transport system being insensitive to NEM.

Furthermore, a similar phenomenon can be observed when phosphate absorption is depressed by lack of extracellular sodium. Again, there is a significant difference in P_i influx between +D and -D everted gut sacs in the sodium-free state (Fig. 2). This suggests that primarily the rate of basal (vitamin D-independent) P_i uptake is affected by low extracellular Na^+. Further evidence for this assumption is obtained from the experiments with embryonic chick duodenum. This tissue displays a high rate of basal (-D) P_i accumulation which is only moderately stimualted by vitamin D_3 (Fig. 5). Consequently, phosphate accumulation is considerably depressed by low Na^+ in the incubation medium and only a slight effect of vitamin D on P_i absorption can be detected.

Although these findings do not represent conclusive evidence they, however, suggest that vitamin D induces a phosphate transport mechanism which differs from the transport system already existing in the -D state by its (partial) insensitivity to extracellular Na^+ and to SH-blocking reagents. On the other hand, the latter conditions do allow to distinguish between cellular pathways of phosphate and calcium transfer. Inhibition of P_i transport by NEM and low Na^+ while not affecting or even stimulating the Ca transport system (as in the case of embryonic chick duodenum) obviously excludes the possibility of coupled phosphate and calcium transfer across the intestine and fosters the idea of independent vitamin D action on both absorptive mechanisms.

ACKNOWLEDGEMENTS

These investigations were supported by Grant No. 3031 from the Fonds zur Förderung der wissenschaftlichen Forschung in Österreich. The expert technical assistance of Mrs. Heidi Duffek and Mr. Peter Wyskowsky is thankfully acknowledged.

REFERENCES

1. Peterlik, M., and Wasserman, R.H.: Basic features of the vitamin D-dependent phosphate transport by chick jejunum in vitro. Fed. Proc. 34:887, 1975

2. Peterlik, M., and Wasserman, R.H.: Control of intestinal phosphate absorption by vitamin D. Isr. J. Med. Sci 12: 1492, 1976

3. Peterlik, M., and Wasserman, R.H.: Effect of vitamin D_3 and 1,25-dihydroxyvitamin D_3 on intestinal transport of phosphate. In: Phosphate Metabolism (ed. by Massry, S.G., and Ritz, E.), p. 323, Plenum Press, New York 1977

4. Taylor, A.N.: In Vitro Phosphate Transport in Chick Ileum: Effect of Cholecalciferol, Sodium and Metabolic Inhibitors. J. Nutr. 104:489, 1974

5. Wasserman, R.H., and Corradino, R.A.: Vitamin D, Calcium and Protein Synthesis. In: Vitamins and Hormones 31:43, Academic Press, New York 1973

6. Corradino, R.A., and Wasserman, R.H.: Strontium Inhibition of Vitamin D_3-Induced Calcium-Binding Protein (CaBP) and Calcium Absorption in Chick Intestine. Proc. Soc. Exp. Biol. Med. 133:960, 1970

7. Fiske, C.H., and SubbaRow, Y.: The colorimetric determination of phosphorus. J. Biol. Chem. 66:375, 1925

8. Paschen, K., and Fuchs, C.: A new micro-method for Na, K, Ca and Mg determinations in a single serum dilution by atomic-absorption spectrophotometry. Clin. Chim. Acta 35:401, 1971

9. Corradino R.A.: Embryonic chick intestine in organ culture. A unique system for the study of the intestinal calcium absorptive mechanism. J. Cell. Biol. 58:64, 1973

10. Kowarski, S., and Schachter,DD.: Effects of Vitamin D on Phosphate Transport and Incorporation into Mucosal Constituents of Rat Intestinal Mucosa. J. Biol. Chem. 244:211, 1969

11. Kinne, R., Berner, W., Hoffmann, N., and Murer, H.: Phosphate Transport by Isolated Renal and Intestinal Plasma Membranes. In: Phosphate Metabolism (ed. by Massry, S.G., and Ritz, E.), p. 265, Plenum Press, New York 1977

12. Peterlik, M.: Effects of Vitamin D_3 on Phosphate Transport by Embryonic Chick Duodenum. Abstr. 6th Int. Conf. Endocrinology, London, July 1977

3. Coty, W.A., and Pedersen, P.L.: Phosphate Transport in Rat Liver Mitochondria. Kinetics, Inhibitor Sensitivity, Energy Requirements, and Labelled Components. Mol. Cell. Biochem. 9:109, 1975

THE INTESTINAL PHOSPHATE TRANSPORT UNDER CONDITION OF EXPERIMENTAL HYPERCALCEMIA

R.S.Lorenc, L.Poniatowski, T.K.Gray

Dpt. of Biochemistry, Medical Center of Postgraduate Education, Warsaw, Poland; CRU University of North Carolina, Chapel Hill N.C., USA.

The progress in knowledge about Vitamin D metabolism and mechanisms of its action in the last ten years has brought us to the formulation of several questions about hormonal factors involved in phosphate transport mechanisms, phosphate homeostasis and phosphate homeostasis hormonal regulation. Beside broadly described phosphaturic effect of parathyroid hormone also active metabolite of Vitamin D_3, 1,25 $(OH)_2D_3$, in serum phosphate homeostasis recently has been suggested as an important factor /1/.
In this report we have attempted to evaluate the role of Vitamin D and synthetic analogue of 1,25 $(OH)_2D_3$, metabolized to 1,25$(OH)_2D_3$ /2/, 1α- OH D_3 on serum phosphate homeostasis and on *in vivo* and *in vitro* intestinal phosphate transport values.

Experimental Procedures

The data which are presented herein were obtained employing the *in vitro* gut sac technique of Schachter et al. /3/ modified with respect to phosphate transport by Harrison et al. /4/. The *in vivo* perfusion system employed was described in detail by Szecówka et al. /5/. Intestinal gut sacs were prepared from 10 cm segments of duodenum or jejunum. In the *in vivo* studies, solutions containing 2 mM phosphate buffer along with a poorly

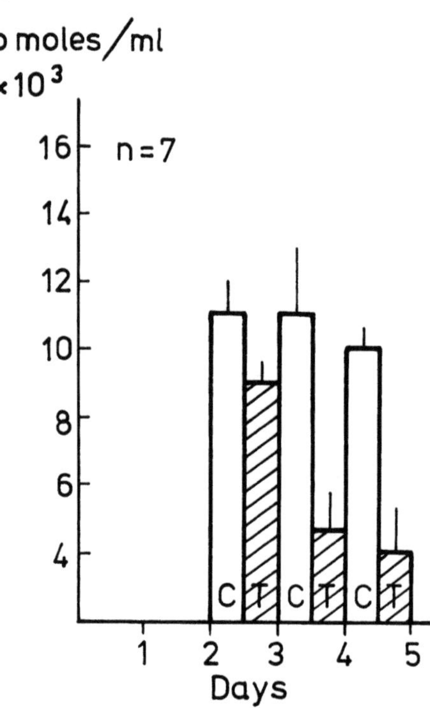

Figure 1. The pattern of cAMP concentration in the urine of the rats treated with 260 nmoles of Vitamin D_3 per day (T) and control (C) groups. Vertical lines: standard deviation. All data statistically significant between groups in student t test.

absorbed polyethylene glycol marker were infused into an cannulated 30 cm duodeno-jejunal segment of the small intestine. Intestinal effluents and blood were analyzed for total calcium /6/ and inorganic phosphorus /7/. The values for each animal in the experimental group were pooled and expressed as the mean value in nmoles/cm/h $\pm$ standard error. Polyethylene glycol was determined by the method of Malawer et al. /8/. The significance were analyzed in Student's t test. All animals were Wistar albino rats from our own inbreeding colony fed the normal standard diet. The weight of the animals was 110-140 g. Vitamin D_3 was obtained from Serva, 1α- OH D_3 was a generous gift obtained from Leo Pharmaceutical, Dennmark.

The Experimental Model

The groups of animals were treated orally for six days with 650 nmoles of Vitamin D_3 or with 520 pmoles of 1α- OH D_3 in i.p. injections for four days. Control groups were dosed with corresponding amounts of vehicle. The estimation of cAMP

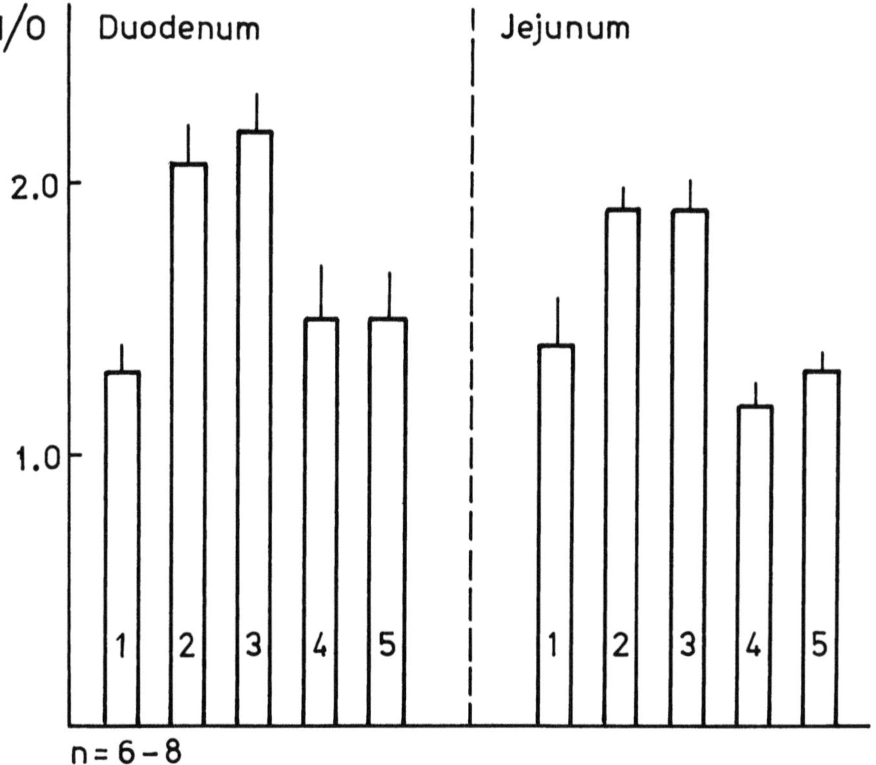

Figure 2. Intestinal phosphate transport in duodenum and jejunum measured in vitro by means of the everted gut sac method /4/. The experiment was performed on the sixth day of vitamin D_3 treatment (650 nmoles per day) or on the fourth day of 1α - OH D_3 treatment (520 pmoles per day). 1. Control group; 2. Vitamin D_3 treated animals; 3. 1α - OH D_3 treated animals; 4. TPTX animals; 5. TPTX animals treated for six days with vitamin D_3. Vertical lines: standard error. Groups 2,3, significantly different in student's t test from 1,4,5.

concentration /9/ in the urine of Vitamin D dosed animals shows a significant decrease of cAMP level in comparison with the control group (Figure 1). In addition to the increased serum calcium level this observation creates some additional argument for the supression of PTH secretion in the condition of experimental hypercalcemia.

TABLE 1. Serum Phosphate and Calcium Responses to 260 nmoles Vitamin D_3 per day over six days, of rats on standard diet.

Surgical treatment	Vitamin D_3 administration	Serum Phosphate	Serum Calcium
Sham	-	7.42 $\pm$ 0.3 /8/	9.19 $\pm$ 0.2 /8/
Sham	+	7.63 $\pm$ 0.2 /8/	11.62 $\pm$ 0.3 /8/ x
TPTX	-	13.66 $\pm$ 0.6 /15/	4.92 $\pm$ 0.3 /15/
TPTX	+	8.04 $\pm$ 0.4 /15/X	9.68 $\pm$ 0.4 /15/ x

The animals were treated orally with Vitamin D_3 dissolved in propylene glycol or corresponding amounts of vehicle. TPTX - the animals were thyroparathyroidectomized one day before the start of the experiment. The number in parenthesis represents the number of animals in the group. The data are expressed as the mean $\pm$ standard deviation. X means significance in Student's t test.

TABLE 2. Serum Phosphate and Calcium Responses to 520 pmoles of 1α - OH D_3 per day, of rats on standard diet.

Surgical treatment	Duration of treatment	1α - OH D_3 administration	Serum Phosphate	Serum Calcium
Sham	2 days	-	7.39 $\pm$ 0.3 /10/	9.23 $\pm$ 0.2 /10/
Sham	2 days	+	9.12 $\pm$ 0.2 /10/ X	10.72 $\pm$ 0.1 /10/X
Sham	4 days	-	7.32 $\pm$ 0.3 /10/	9.36 $\pm$ 0.2 /10/
Sham	4 days	+	8.52 $\pm$ 0.2 /10/ X	10.62 $\pm$ 0.2 /10/X
TPTX	4 days	-	12.20 $\pm$ 0.4 /15/	5.55 $\pm$ 0.4 /15/
TPTX	4 days	+	13.38 $\pm$ 0.4 /15/ X	7.68 $\pm$ 0.3 /15/X

The animals were injected i.p. with 1α - OH D_3 or vehicle. The number in parenthesis represents the number of rats in each group. The data are expressed as the mean $\pm$ standard deviation. X means significance between groups in Student's t test.

The Effect of Vitamin D_3 or 1α - OH D_3 on Serum Calcium and Phosphate Level in Normal - Vitamin D Supplemented and Thyroparathyroidectomized (TPTX) Animals

The results in Table I and Table II show the response of treated animals to supraphysiological doses of Vitamin D_3 and physiological doses of 1α - OH D_3. In all cases Vitamin D_3 or 1α - OH D_3 supplementation caused the increase in serum calcium. A marked difference was visualized between Vitamin D_3 and 1α - OH D_3 when serum phosphate level was analyzed. Contrary to Vitamin D_3 that didn't effect the serum phosphate level in intact animals and decreased to normal the serum phosphate level in TPTX 1α - OH D_3 treatment caused the increase in serum phosphate in all groups. It can be pointed out that this data are in some contradiction to the observation of Garabedian et al. /1/ who have ascribed the regulatory phosphate mechanism to $1,25(OH)_2D_3$.

The Effect of the Sustained Vitamin D_3 or 1α - OH D_3 Treatment on Intestinal Phosphate Transport in vitro

Both in duodenal and the jejunal segments of the small intestine the long-term treatment of the intact animals under study caused an increase in the intestinal phosphate transport values. We interpreted this data as a direct effect of $1,25\ (OH)_2D_3$ that can be metabolized from Vitamin D_3 or 1α - OH D_3 and stored in the intestinal tissue in the analyzed experimental model. The additional argument for this interpretation is connected with the observation that Vitamin D_3 does not cause any increase in intestinal phosphate transport in TPTX animals who because of absence of PTH are devoid of the possibility of the synthesis of the $1,25\ (OH)_2D_3$ /10/.

The Effect of Vitamin D_3 or 1α - OH D_3 on Phosphate Transport in vivo

As shown in Figure 3, the dosing of intact and TPTX animals with 1α - OH D_3 is followed by the increase of the intestinal phosphate absorption values. In the case of Vitamin D_3 treated animals a much more complicated pattern of intestinal phosphate absorption data has been observed. In intact animals the in vivo intestinal phosphate transport was not changed, which is

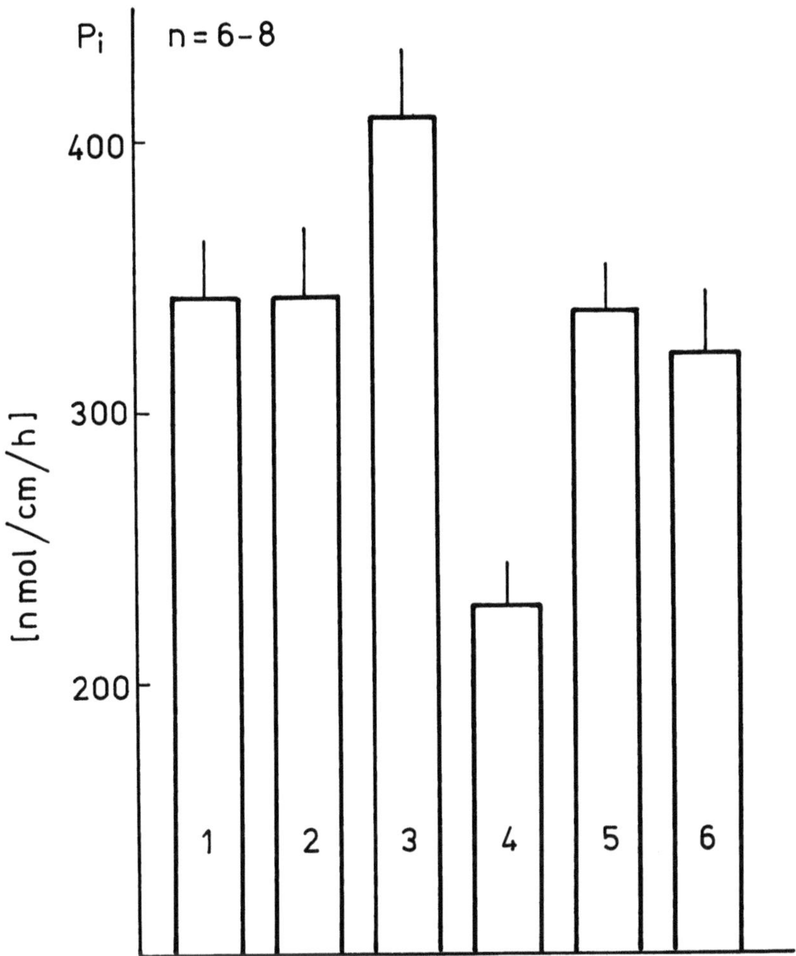

Figure 3. Phosphate transport in the duodeno-jejunal segment of the small intestine measured in the cannulated segment of intestine by means of the in vivo perfusion in the condition as described in Fig. 2. Group 6: includes data obtained from the group of TPTX animals treated during four days with 520 pmoles of 1α - OH D_3 per day. Vertical lines represents standard error. Group 3 different in student t test from 1 and 2 and group 4 from 1,2,3,5 and 6.

contrary to in vitro studies. The observed phenomenon corresponded with lack of change in serum phosphate over the whole Vitamin D treatment. We are going to correlate the increase of intestinal phosphate absorption in the case of Vitamin D-dosed TPTX animals with the decrease of phosphate gradient connected with hypophosphatemic action of Vitamin D in this group of animals.

Summary

The analysis of the serum calcium and phosphate level changes in intact Vitamin D - dosed animals showed the increasing serum calcium values without any concomitant change in serum phosphate concentration. The observed discrepancy of intestinal phosphate transport in vitro and in vivo studies together with the effect of Vitamin D towards normalizing serum phosphate level in TPTX Vitamin D - dosed animals suggest the presence of Vitamin D as some phosphate regulatory factor. The participation of the possible role of 25 OH D_3 in the observed phenomenon is under current investigations. In PTH supressed hypercalcemic conditions we did not reproduce, with the usage of 1α - OH D_3, the regulatory effect of 1,25 $(OH)_2D_3$ described by Garabedian et al. /1/.

Acknowledgments

Thanks are due to Mrs. I. Dargiel-Targońska, Miss M.E. Williams and Mrs. D. Pool for expert technical assistance. Supported in part by Wroclaw Politechnic's I,22,02,04, PAN II, 1,1,10 and by NIH, AM17835/TKG/.

References

1. Garabedian, M., Pezant, E., Miravet, L., Fellot, C., and Balsan, S. 1976: 1,25-Dihydroxycholecalciferol Effect on Serum Phosphorus Homeostasis in Rats, Endocrinology, 98, 794.

2. Fukushima, M., Suzuki, Y., Tohira, Y., Matsunaga, I., Ochi, K., Nagano, H., Nishii, Y., Suda, T., 1975: Metabolism of 1α-Hydroxyvitamin D_3 to 1,25-Dihydroxyvitamin D_3 in Perfused Rat Liver. Biochem. Biophys. Res. Comm. 66, 632.

3. Schachter, D., Rosen, S., 1959: Active transport of ^{45}Ca by the small intestine and its dependence on Vitamin D. Am. J. Physiol. 196, 357.

4. Harrison, H.E., Harrison, H.C., 1961: Intestinal transport of phosphate: action of Vitamin D, calcium and potassium. Am. J. Physiol. 201, 1007.

5. Szecówka, J., Poniatowski, L., Lorenc, R., 1977: The Intestinal Calcium and Phosphate Transport under Conditions of Experimental Hypercalcemia, Acta Physiol. Pol., 28, 127.

6. Kocacs, K., Tarnowsky, S., 1964: Microdetermination of calcium. J. Clin. Path., 13, 160.

7. Chen, P.S., Toribary, T.Y., 1956: Microdetermination of phosphorus. Anal. Chem., 28, 1756.

8. Malawer, S.J., Powell, D.W., 1967: An Improved turbidometric analysis of PEG in estimating intestinal water volume. Gastroenterology, 53, 250.

9. Steiner, A.L., 1973: Radioimmunoassay for the Cyclic Nucleotides, Pharmacol. Rev., 25, 73.

10. Garabedian, M., Holick, M.F., DeLuca, H.F., Boyle, I.T., 1972: Control of 25 - Hydroxycholecalciferol Metabolism by Parathyroid Glands, Proc. Nat. Acad. Sci. USA, 69, 1673.

Metabolism of Phosphate and Other Minerals in Disease States

URINARY PHOSPHATE AND CYCLIC AMP IN PSEUDOHYPOPARATHYROIDISM

Saulo Klahr and Eduardo Slatopolsky

Washington University School of Medicine, Department of Medicine, Renal Division, 4550 Scott Avenue, St. Louis, Missouri 63110 U.S.A.

In a 1942 article in Endocrinology, Albright, Burnett, Smith, and Parson (1) described a syndrome characterized by hypocalcemia and hyperphosphatemia, in the absence of renal insufficiency, in which there was little or no restoration of serum calcium and phosphorus values to normal after administration of parathyroid extract. Albright et al termed this syndrome, which resembled hypoparathyroidism, pseudohypoparathyroidism and postulated that its pathophysiology was due to resistance of the kidney and the skeleton to the action of parathyroid hormone. Albright et al, in their first report, were struck by the physical appearance of the patients with this syndrome. They were of short stature, had round faces and short necks, short phalanges, metacarpal and metatarsal bones, exostosis, and ectopic calcium deposits. It was shown subsequently that some patients with certain of these physical characteristics had a normal response to the action of parathyroid hormone and have normal serum calcium and phosphorus, so called pseudo-pseudohypoparathyroidism (2,3). In addition, patients with hypocalcemia and renal resistance to the phosphaturic action of parathyroid hormone but without the somatic characteristics of classic pseudohypoparathyroidism have also been described (3).

The observation that the mechanism of the action of parathyroid hormone is apparently mediated through activation of adenylate cyclase both in kidney and bone (4,5) and the finding by Chase, Melson, and Aurbach (6) that the urinary excretion of cyclic adenosine-3',5'-monophosphate (cyclic AMP) did not increase after administration of parathyroid hormone to patients with pseudohypoparathyroidism (PHP) gave support to the hypothesis that the metabolic defect in this disorder could be caused by a lack of, or defective forms of, PTH sensitive receptors or adenylate cyclase in bone and kidney (6). The observations of Bell et al (7) that dibutyryl cyclic AMP administration increased the serum calcium, lowered the serum phosphorus and increased urinary phosphorus excretion in patients with PHP are compatible with this postulate. However, several recent observations raise some doubts as to the validity of the above hypothesis to explain both the renal and bone resistance to the action of PTH. For example, certain patients with PHP develop skeletal changes of osteitis fibrosa similar to those seen in primary hyperparathyroidism (8-12). In addition, it has been shown that administration of vitamin D or its metabolites restores to normal the calcemic response of patients with PHP (13,14). Furthermore, removal of the parathyroid glands in a patient with PHP resulted in more marked hypocalcemia, suggesting previous responsiveness of the skeleton to the circulating levels of PTH (3). This evidence would suggest that the skeletal resistance is only partial or that the hypocalcemia of PHP is due to mechanisms other than skeletal resistance. Postulated mechanisms to explain this hypocalcemia include decreased calcium absorption from the intestine (8) and a renal calcium leak (15). But these 2 disorders alone may not explain the hypocalcemia.

The long-held concept that the renal resistance to the action of parathyroid hormone is due to a defective adenyl cyclase system has been challenged by two basic observations. In a patient with the somatic characteristics of PHP who died, studies of the renal adenyl cyclase system in vitro revealed normal activation of the enzyme by PTH and fluoride (16). In addition, a small number of patients with hypocalcemia and elevated levels of circulating PTH in whom the kidney responds to PTH administration with an increase in the urinary excretion of cyclic AMP but no phosphaturia have been recently described (17, 18; Brickman, unpublished observations). This syndrome has been termed pseudohypoparathyroidism Type II, and it can be distinguished from "classic" or pseudohypoparathyroidism Type I, by the increased urinary excretion of cyclic AMP in response to PTH. However, the rise in phosphate excretion, as in PHP Type I, is also absent (see Table I). Decreased urinary phosphate excretion in response to PTH has been demonstrated by us (19) and others (20) in phosphate depleted animals. As shown in Table II phosphate depleted dogs had a substantial rise in urinary cyclic AMP, although somewhat less than normal animals, but no increase in phosphate excretion in response to PTH administration. A blunted phosphaturic response to PTH has been described also in conditions in which single nephron GFR is decreased and proximal tubular reabsorption is increased (renal artery stenosis, unilateral ureteral ligation) (21).

TABLE I

Effect of parathyroid extract on the urinary excretion of sodium, bicarbonate, phosphate and cyclic AMP in a patient with pseudohypoparathyroidism Type II

Ccr ml/min	$U_{c-AMP}V$ pmoles/min	FE_{PO_4} %	$U_{Na}V$ µEq/min	FE_{Na} %	$U_{HCO_3}V$ µEq/min
94	2,164	6.6	29.3	0.2	3.2
85	2,714	6.0	21.8	0.2	2.8
100	2,278	6.0	25.4	0.2	3.5
Parathyroid extract (250 USP U) i.v. over 5 minutes.					
113	50,226	9.0	675.8	4.4	72.5
103	10,186	9.0	413.5	2.9	68.3
106	5,848	9.0	234.8	1.6	52.1

Abbreviations: Ccr, creatinine clearance; $U_{c-AMP}V$, urinary cyclic AMP excretion; FE_{PO_4}, fractional phosphate excretion; $U_{Na}V$, urinary sodium excretion; FE_{Na}, fractional sodium excretion; $U_{HCO_3}V$, urinary bicarbonate excretion.

TABLE II

Urinary excretion of cyclic AMP and PO_4 in normal and phosphate depleted dogs

	NORMAL		PO_4 DEPLETED	
	Basal	PTH	Basal	PTH
c-AMP (pmole/min)	952 ± 40	3,162 ± 75	387 ± 22	1,208 ± 168
$U_{PO_4}V$ (µg/min)	21 ± 3	529 ± 179	15.4 ± 0.2	15.6 ± 0.6

For abbreviations see Table I.

Since the phosphaturic response to PTH is absent or markedly blunted in PHP, it is of interest to analyze the effect of PTH administration on the urinary excretion of other solutes in this syndrome. Parathyroid hormone has been shown to decrease the reabsorption of fluid, sodium, bicarbonate, phosphate, and calcium in the proximal tubule (22). PTH administration in addition to being phosphaturic increases urinary sodium and bicarbonate excretion. Moses et al (15) demonstrated increased urinary sodium and bicarbonate excretion in response to PTH administration, similar to that seen in normal individuals, in 3 of 5 patients with PHP that they studied (see Figure 1). These results suggest that the decreased reabsorption of sodium, bicarbonate and water by the proximal tubule in response to PTH occurs by mechanisms independent of cyclic AMP generation or that only small increases in cyclic AMP are needed to depress the reabsorption of fluid and electrolytes by the kidney. In this respect the recent observations of Sinha et al (23) are of interest. These investigators examined the effects of acetazolamide administration (a carbonic anhydrase inhibitor) on phosphate excretion in 8 patients with PHP. In these 8 patients administration of parathyroid extract, as expected, produced no increase in urinary cyclic AMP and increased phosphate clearance very little or not at all. Acatazolamide significantly increased mean phosphate clearance in all patients without changing urinary cyclic AMP excretion (Figure 2). The diuretic, administered for 4 days at doses of 250-275 mg daily, was shown to increase mean serum calcium in each one of the patients with PHP and to lower the mean serum phosphate when it was abnormally elevated in all of them. Urinary calcium excretion was not consistently altered. These results indicate that patients with PHP are capable of responding to acetazolamide with a modest phosphaturia which is not cyclic AMP mediated. These results indicate that phosphate reabsorption in pseudohypoparathyroidism Type I can be blocked by agents that inhibit phosphate reabsorption through mechanisms which are independent of cyclic AMP generation. It is of interest that in the case of PHP Type II reported by Rodriguez et al (18) the intravenous administration of acetazolamide did not increase phosphate excretion (see Table III). This observation, coupled with the fact that there is increased excretion of cyclic AMP after the administration of PTH, suggests that in PHP Type II the defect in phosphate excretion is located beyond the generation of cyclic AMP presumably involving the transport of phosphate per se. Consequently, agents that block phosphate reabsorption, by mechanisms independent of cyclic AMP generation, may not increase urinary phosphate excretion in PHP Type II. In this respect the recent observations by Knox and his co-workers (24) on the effects of PTH and acetazolamide on phosphate excretion in the hamster are of interest. They found that administration of PTH did not increase phosphate excretion in the hamster, although it decreased the excretion of calcium and increased the urinary excretion of cyclic AMP. In this respect this animal model resembles PHP Type II. This lack of a phosphaturic response to PTH was not reversed by administration of 25(OH)vitamin D_3 or infusions of calcium or phosphate. These latter data are somewhat different from those observed in our patient with PHP Type II in whom calcium administration restored

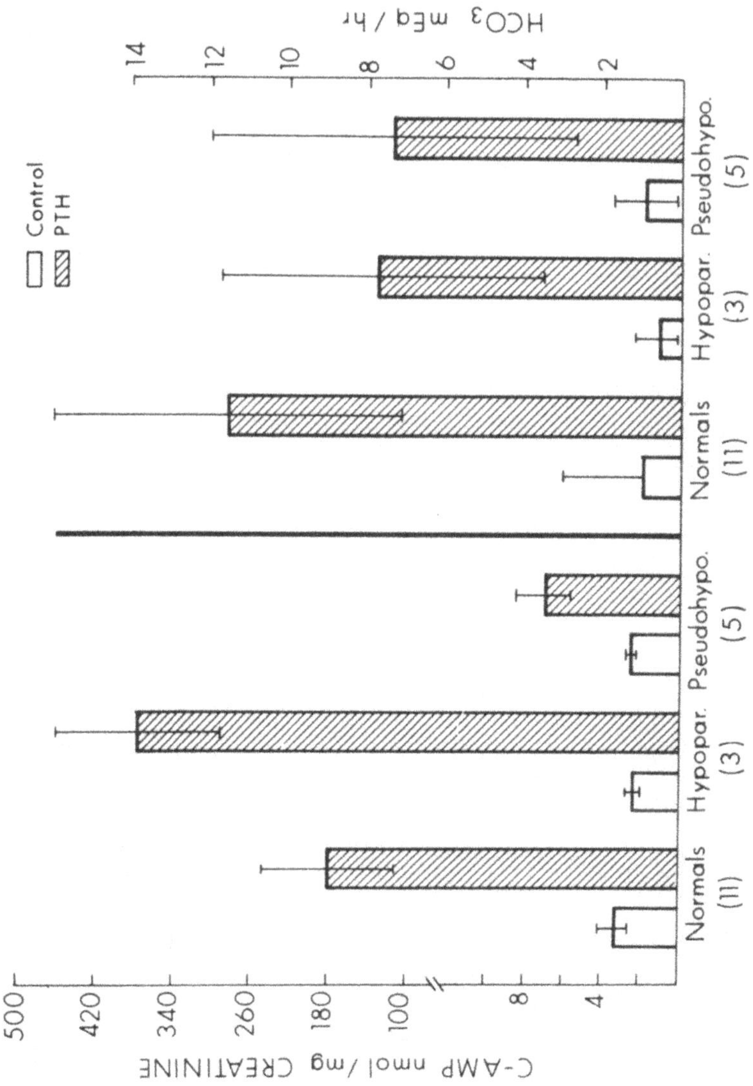

FIG. 1: Effects of PTH administration on urinary c-AMP and bicarbonate excretion in normals and patients with hypo or pseudohypoparathyroidism (from Moses et al., Am. J. Med. 61:184, 1976)

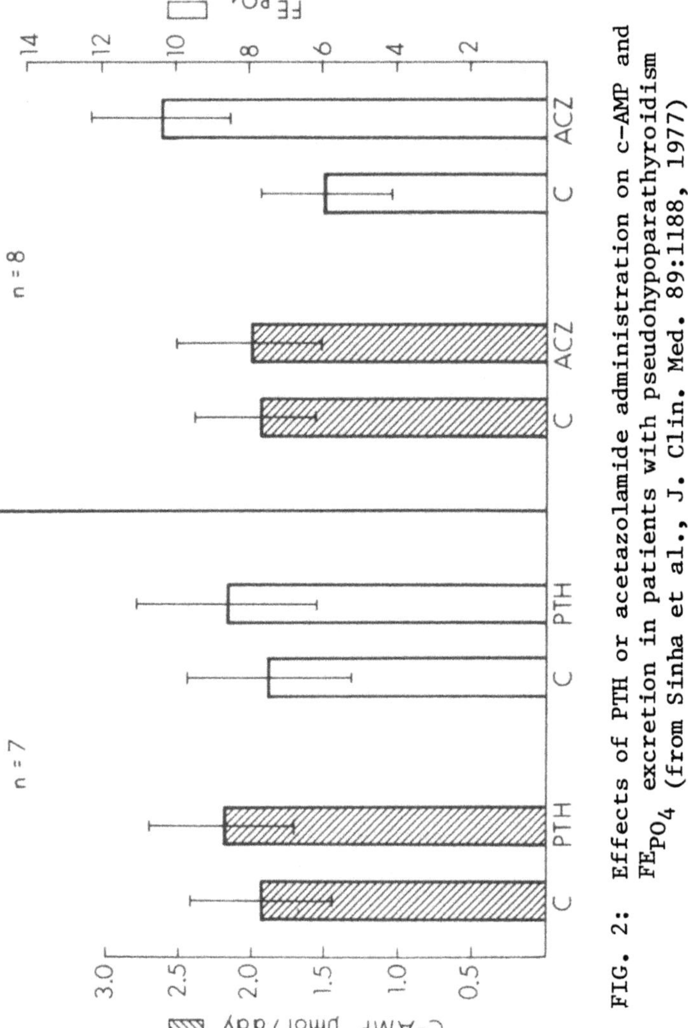

FIG. 2: Effects of PTH or acetazolamide administration on c-AMP and FE_{PO_4} excretion in patients with pseudohypoparathyroidism (from Sinha et al., J. Clin. Med. 89:1188, 1977)

TABLE III

Effect of acetazolamide on the urinary excretion of sodium, bicarbonate, phosphate, and cyclic AMP in a patient with pseudohypoparathyroidism Type II

Ccr ml/min	$U_{Na}V$ µEq/min	FE_{Na} %	$U_{HCO_3}V$ µEq/min	$U_{PO_4}V$ µg/min	FE_{PO_4} %	c-AMP pmoles/min
104	44.9	0.3	12.5	140	3.2	1869
102	47.6	0.3	14.5	110	2.5	1916
104	42.0	0.29	12.6	80	2.2	1730
Acetazolamide 10 mg/kg I.V. followed by infusion delivering 10 mg/kg/hr.						
103	530.3	3.5	497.1	70	2.2	1680
93	506.0	3.8	581.1	50	1.7	1606
95	508.6	3.8	688.7	90	3.7	1588
91	386	3.1	993.0	40	1.5	1426

Abbreviations as in Table I.

the phosphaturic response to PTH towards normal. Calcitonin, another phosphaturic hormone also failed to increase phosphate excretion in the hamster though it markedly increased the urinary excretion of cyclic AMP. Pre-treatment of the hamsters with ammonium chloride, which resulted in a decrease in plasma and urinary pH, resulted in demonstrable increases in the excretion of phosphate, as well as cyclic AMP in response to PTH and calcitonin. Acetazolamide had no phosphaturic effect in ammonium chloride loaded hamsters and it decreased cyclic AMP and calcium excretion. Alkalinization of the urine by acetazolamide did not prevent the phosphaturic effect of parathyroid hormone in ammonium chloride loaded hamsters, but it blocked the increase in urinary cyclic AMP excretion. These data suggested that systemic or intracellular pH, but not intraluminal pH, play an important role in the phosphaturic response to PTH in the hamster.

Treatment of patients with PHP with vitamin D restores the phosphaturic response to PTH, despite no increase in the urinary excretion of cyclic AMP. Albright and his co-workers (1) had already shown in 1942 that administration of large doses of dihydrotachysterol (AT-10) resulted in a decrease in serum phosphorus and an increase in serum calcium in a patient with PHP. Subsequently, Suh et al (13) studied the response to bovine parathyroid extract in an 11½ year old girl with PHP before and during treatment with large doses of vitamin D_2. Prior to vitamin D_2 therapy there was a slight but subnormal calcemic response and no phosphaturic response to large doses of parathyroid extract. Response to the same dose of parathyroid extract was tested again while the patient was receiving sufficient vitamin D_2 (100,000 IU/day) to restore serum calcium, serum phosphate, and the renal handling of phosphate to normal ranges. The serum calcium rose promptly from 10 to 14.4 mg/100 ml in response to intramuscular parathyroid extract injection and there were marked increases in urinary phosphate excretion rate and phosphate clearance and a decrease in the tubular reabsorption of phosphate. These data suggested, therefore, that large doses of vitamin D_2 improved the responsiveness of this patient with PHP to parathyroid extract. By contrast, Birkenhager et al (25) reported a 14 year old girl with PHP who after one year of treatment with dihydrotachysterol showed a somewhat greater but not normal phosphaturic response to parathyroid extract but no change in cyclic AMP excretion after parathyroid extract. Stögmann and Fischer (14) also showed in a 15 year old girl with PHP that, following normalization of the serum calcium concentration with vitamin D, serum immunoreactive PTH and phosphate concentrations returned to their normal range, and phosphaturia could be clearly stimulated and hypercalcemia induced by parathyroid extract. On the other hand, the urinary cyclic AMP excretion could not be stimulated, suggesting that in this case there appears to be no relationship between the urinary excretion of cyclic AMP and the phosphaturic effect of parathyroid extract.

Vitamin D_3 must undergo two enzymatic hydroxylations before it can function at the target cells. The first metabolic step in conversion of vitamin D_3 to $25(OH)D_3$ is in the liver. Under appropriate conditions, $25(OH)D_3$ then undergoes hydroxylation in the kidney to $1,25(OH)_2$ vitamin D_3, the principal metabolically active form of the vitamin (26). Factors that trigger the conversion of $25(OH)D_3$ to $1,25(OH)_2D_3$ include hypocalcemia, parathyroid hormone and hypophosphatemia (27-30). The fact that parathyroid hormone deficiency (or refractoriness) and hyperphosphatemia are features of hypoparathyroidism and pseudohypoparathyroidism led Kooh et al (31) to postulate that the conversion of $25(OH)D_3$ to $1,25(OH)_2D_3$ might be impaired in these diseases. They compared the therapeutic requirements of $25(OH)D_3$ and $1,25(OH)_2D_3$ in 2 children with hypoparathyroidism and one child with PHP. In both conditions minute amounts of $1,25(OH)_2D_3$ (.04 to .08 ug/kg B.W./day) quickly corrected hypocalcemia and increased intestinal calcium absorption. On the other hand, the effective dose of $25(OH)D_3$ to maintain normocalcemia was 3 to 4 ug/kg B.W./day in the two conditions. Thus, the dosage ratio of $25(OH)D_3$ to $1,25(OH)_2D_3$ approximated 100 to 1. These findings suggested an impaired conversion of $25(OH)D_3$ and $1,25(OH)_2D_3$ to $1,25(OH)_2D_3$ in both HP and PHP. Drezner et al (32) studied 4 patients with PHP and measured the plasma levels of both $25(OH)D_3$ and $1,25(OH)_2D_3$. Measurements indicated that in these 4 patients the levels of $25(OH)D_3$ were within normal limits. On the other hand, the levels of $1,25(OH)_2D_3$ were decreased in the 3 patients in whom the measurement was made. These patients on bone biopsy showed morphologic evidence of increased osteoclastic activity and osteomalacia. Drezner et al (32) proposed that in PHP there is a deficiency of $1,25(OH)_2D_3$ possibly resulting from a genetic renal lesion. Further evidence for a defect in the formation of $1,25(OH)_2D_3$ in PHP has been presented by Sinha, DeLuca and Bell (33). These investigators tested the effects of $1,25(OH)_2D_3$ 1 ug/day for 12 days on serum calcium and phosphorus, balances of calcium and phosphorus and serum parathyroid hormone in 3 patients with well-documented PHP. Serum $25(OH)D_3$ was also determined. Before treatment fecal calcium was increased, serum calcium was abnormally low and serum parathyroid hormone and serum $25(OH)D_3$ were abnormally increased. With $1,25(OH)_2D_3$, fecal calcium decreased, serum and urinary calcium increased, and serum parathyroid hormone decreased to or towards the normal range. After treatment this sequence of events was reversed. These findings support the hypothesis that diminished intestinal absorption of calcium, hypocalcemia and secondary hyperparathyroidism in PHP

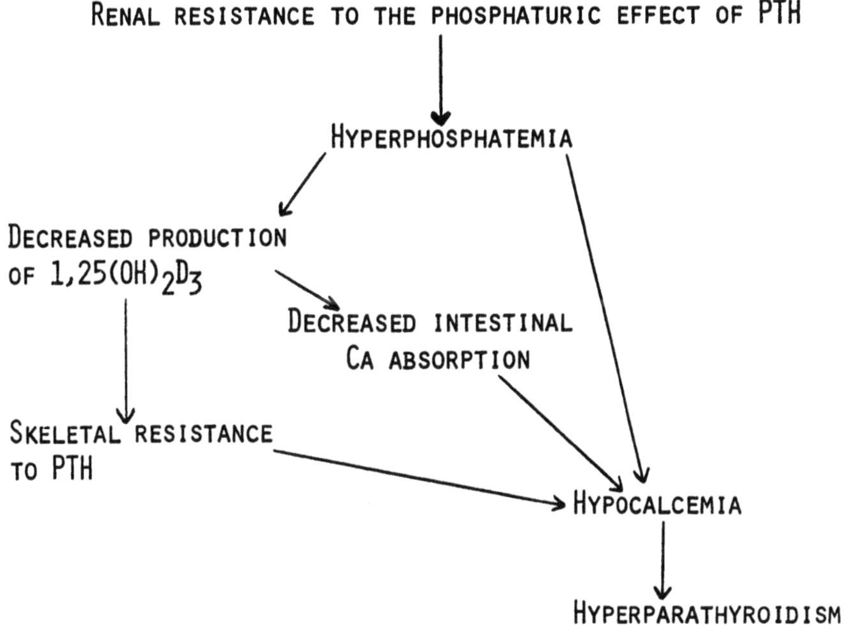

FIG. 3: Pathogenesis of metabolic abnormalities in PHP.

resulted from a defect in the formation of $1,25(OH)_2D_3$, in the kidney and that this compound is a new and useful specific means for treatment of the abnormal calcium metabolism in this disorder. Brickman et al (34) have tested the phosphaturic response to 150 U of parathyroid extract in 9 patients with PHP before and during treatment with 2 ug of $1,25(OH)_2D_3$ for 5-10 days. In these 9 patients, there was a significantly greater phosphaturic response to PTH during treatment with $1,25(OH)_2D_3$ than before; however, the response in urinary cyclic AMP excretion was unaffected. In 2 patients with PHP, correction of hypocalcemia by $CaCl_2$ infusion for 36-48 hours did not affect the response to parathyroid extract. These data demonstrate that administration of $1,25(OH)_2D_3$ restores a PTH dependent phosphaturic response in PHP. This occurred without a change in urinary cyclic AMP excretion, suggesting the participation of a non-adenyl cyclase dependent, PTH-mediated transport in PHP patients treated with $1,25(OH)_2D_3$.

Figure 3 presents the possible pathogenesis of the metabolic abnormalities seen in PHP. It is postulated that the renal resistance to the phosphaturic effect of PTH in patients with PHP may be accompanied by "resistance" in the conversion of $25(OH)D_3$ to $1,25(OH)_2D_3$. Decreased plasma levels of $1,25(OH)_2D_3$ will lead to skeletal resistance to the action of PTH and decreased intestinal calcium absorption. These two mechanisms coupled with hyperphosphatemia will lead to hypocalcemia which in turn will result in hyperparathyroidism.

ACKNOWLEDGMENTS

The original work reported in this manuscript was supported by U.S.P.H.S. NIAMDD grant AM-09976.

We would also like to thank Mrs. Patricia Verplancke for her assistance in the preparation of this manuscript.

REFERENCES

1. Albright, F., Burnett, C.H., Smith, P.H., and Parson, W.: Pseudohypoparathyroidism--an example of the "Seabright-Bantam Syndrome". Endocrinology 30:922, 1942.

2. Albright, F., Forbes, A.P., and Henneman, P.H.: Pseudo-pseudohypoparathyroidism. Trans. Assn. Amer. Phys. 65:337, 1952.

3. Potts, John J., Jr.: Pseudohypoparathyroidism, in The Metabolic Basis of Inherited Disease edited by J.B. Stanbury, J.B. Wyngaarden and D.S. Gredrickson, p. 1305, McGraw-Hill, New York, 1970.

4. Chase, R., Fedak, S.A. and Aurbach, G.D.: Activation of skeletal adenyl cyclase by parathyroid hormone in vitro. Endocrinology 84:761, 1969.

5. Chase, L.R. and Aurbach, G.D.: Parathyroid function and the renal excretion of 3',5'-adenylic acid. Proc. Nat. Acad. Sci. USA 58:518, 1967.

6. Chase, L.R., Melson, G.L., and Aurbach, G.D.: Pseudohypoparathyroidism -- Defective excretion of 3',5'-AMP in response to parathyroid hormone. J. Clin. Invest. 48:1832, 1969.

7. Bell, N.H., Avery, A., Sinha, T., Clark, C., Allen, D., and Johnston, C., Jr.: Effects of dibutyryl cyclic adenosine-3', 5'-monophosphate and parathyroid extract on calcium and phosphorus metabolism in hypoparathyroidism and pseudohypoparathyroidism. J. Clin. Invest. 51:816, 1972.

8. Bell, N.H., Gerard, E.S. and Bartter, F.C.: Pseudohypoparathyroidism with osteitis fibrosa cystica and impaired absorption of calcium. J. Clin. Endocrinol. 23:759, 1963.

9. Kolb, F.O., and Steinbach, H.L.: Pseudohypoparathyroidism with secondary hyperparathyroidism and osteitis fibrosa. J. Clin. Endocrinol. 22:59, 1962.

10. Zampa, G.A. and Zucchelli, P.C.: Pseudohypoparathyroidism and bone demineralization: Case report and metabolic studies. J. Clin. Endocrinol. 25:1616, 1965.

11. Allen, E.H., Millard, F.J.C., and Nassim, J.R.: Hypoparathyroidism. Arch. Dis. Child. 43: 295, 1968.

12. Singleton, E.B. and Teng, C.T.: Pseudohypoparathyroidism with bone changes simulating hyperparathyroidism (report of a case). Radiology 78:388, 1962.

13. Suh, S.M., Fraser, D., Kooh, S.W.: Pseudohypoparathyroidism responsiveness to parathyroid extract induced by vitamin D therapy. J. Clin. Endocrinol. Metab. 30:609, 1970.

14. Stögmann, W., Fischer, J.A.: Pseudohypoparathyroidism: Disappearance of the resistance to parathyroid extract during treatment with vitamin D. Am. J. Med. 59:140, 1975.

15. Moses, A.M., Breslau, N., and Coulson, R.: Renal responses to PTH in patients with hormone-resistant (pseudo) hypoparathyroidism. Am. J. Med. 61:184, 1976.

16. Marcus, R., Wilber, J.F., and Aurbach, G.D.: Parathyroid hormone-sensitive adenyl cyclase from the renal cortex of a patient with pseudo-hypoparathyroidism. J. Clin. Endocrinol. 33: 537, 1971.

17. Drezner, M., Neelon, F.A., Lebovitz, H.E.: Pseudohypoparathyroidism type II: a possible defect in the reception of the cyclic AMP signal. N. Engl. J. Med. 289:1056, 1973.

18. Rodriguez, H.J., Villarreal, H., Jr., Klahr, S., Slatopolsky, E.: Pseudohypoparathyroidism type II: Restoration of normal renal responsiveness to parathyroid hormone by calcium administration. J. Clin. Endocrinol. Metab. 39:693, 1974.

19. Harter, H., Mercado, A., Rutherford, E., Rodriguez, H.J., Slatopolsky, E., and Klahr, S.: Effect of phosphate depletion and parathyroid hormone on renal glucose reabsorption. Am. J. Physiol. 227:1422, 1974.

20. Steele, T.H.: Renal resistance to parathyroid hormone during phosphorus deprivation. J. Clin. Invest. 58:1461, 1976.

21. Purkerson, M.L., Rolf, D.B., Chase, L.R., Slatopolsky, E., and Klahr, S.: Tubular reabsorption of phosphate after release of complete ureteral obstruction in the rat. Kidney Internat. 5:326, 1974.

22. Goldberg, M., Agus, Z.S., and Goldfarb, S.: Renal handling of calcium and phosphate in: 2nd Rev. of Physiol. Kidney and Urinary Tract Physiology, Vol. II, Ed. by K. Thurman, University Park Press, Baltimore, 1976.

23. Sinha, T.K., Allen, D.O., Queener, S.F., and Bell, N.H.: Effects of acetazolamide on the renal excretion of phosphate in hypoparathyroidism and pseudohypoparathyroidism. J. Lab. Clin. Med. 89:1188, 1977.

24. Knox, F.G., Preiss, J., Kim, J.K. and Dousa, T.P.: Mechanism of resistance to the phosphaturic effect of the parathyroid hormone in the hamster. J. Clin. Invest. 59:675, 1977.

25. Birkenhager, J.C., Seldenrath, H.J., Hackeng, W.H.L., Schellekens, A.P.M., van der Veer, A.L.J. and Roelfsema, F. Calcium and phosphorus metabolism, parathyroid hormone, calcitonin and bone histology in pseudohypoparathyroidism. Europ. J. Clin. Invest. 3:27, 1973.

26. DeLuca, H.F.: Vitamin D: The vitamin and the hormone. Fed. Proc. 33:2211, 1974.

27. Garabedian, M., Holick, M.F., DeLuca, H.F., et al.: Control of 25-hydroxycholecalciferol metabolism by parathyroid glands. Proc. Natl. Acad. Sci. USA 69:1673, 1972.

28. Rasmussen, H., Wong, M., Bikle, D., et al: Hormonal control of the renal conversion of 25-hydroxycholecalciferol to 1,25-dihydroxycholecalciferol. J. Clin. Invest. 51:2502, 1972.

29. Fraser, D.R., Kodicek, E.: Regulation of 25-hydroxycholecalciferol-I-hydroxylase activity in kidney by parathyroid hormone. Nature 241:163, 1973.

30. Tanaka, Y., DeLuca, H.F.: The control of 25-hydroxyvitamin D metabolism by inorganic phosphorus. Arch. Biochem. Biophys. 154:566, 1973.

31. Kooh, S.W., Fraser, D., DeLuca, H.F., Holick, M.F., Belsey, R.E., Clark, M.B., and Murray, T.M.: Treatment of hypoparathyroidism and pseudohypoparathyroidism with metabolites of vitamin D: Evidence for impaired conversion of 25-hydroxyvitamin D to 1-α-25-dihydroxyvitamin D. New Engl. J. Med. 293:840, 1975.

32. Drezner, M.K., Neelon, F.A., Haussler, M., McPherson, H.T., and Lebovitz, H.E.: 1,25-dihydroxycholecalciferol deficiency: The probable cause of hypocalcemia and metabolic bone disease in pseudohypoparathyroidism. J. Clin. Endocrinol. Metab. 42:621, 1976.

33. Sinha, T.K., DeLuca, H. and Bell, N.H.: Evidence for a defect in the formation of 1-α-25-dihydroxyvitamin D in pseudohypoparathyroidism. Metabolism 26:731, 1977.

34. Brickman, A.S., Norman, A.W., and Coburn, J.W.: Restoration of PTH-dependent phosphaturia by 1,25(OH)$_2$ vitamin D$_3$ in pseudohypoparathyroidism I. Kidney Internat. 10:488, 1976.

ROLE OF PHOSPHATE AND PYROPHOSPHATE IN SOFT TISSUE CALCIFICATION

Allen C. Alfrey and Lloyd S. Ibels

Denver V.A. Hospital and Univ. of Colo. Medical Center

Denver, Colorado 80220

Extraskeletal calcification is a common complication of chronic renal failure. With the advent of chronic hemodialysis this complication has been seen with increasing frequency and it is now apparent that it is a significant cause of morbidity and mortality in this patient population (1-3). Studies in our laboratory have been directed at characterizing the crystalline features and inorganic constituents of these deposits, defining their pathogenesis and determining the clinical consequences of extraskeletal calcification.

Abnormal Pyrophosphate Metabolism in Uremia

It has largely been assumed that at the body pH the only solid form of calcium-phosphate that can exist is apatite (4). However, using x-ray diffractive techniques it was subsequently shown that in uremic patients calcium-phosphate deposits exist in at least two different crystalline forms (5,6). The deposits which form in arteries and about joints give apatitic diffraction patterns; whereas, those deposits occurring in the heart, lung and skeletal muscles consistently have amorphous x-ray diffraction patterns. This would suggest that in these latter deposits that an inhibitor or stabilizer is present which prevents their transformation to apatite. Upon analysis two crystal inhibitors, pyrophosphate and magnesium, were found to be present in increased amounts in visceral calcification as compared to apatitic arterial and periarticular deposits (7). In fact approximately 30% of the phosphorus in these former deposits is present as pyrophosphate (Table I).

Further confirmation for the presence of pyrophosphate in visceral calcium-phosphate deposits was obtained by infrared analysis which showed P-O bondings (7).

TABLE I

Visceral Calcification	Ca	Mg	PO_4	P_2O_7
	← mg/gram dry tissue →			
Mean	47.2	4.91	26.6	11.0
SD	39.2	3.86	19.2	11.8
Arterial & Periarticular				
Mean	244	4.80	111	1.83
SD	68	0.94	4	1.49
Control				
Mean	0.60	0.57	2.5	0.80
SD	0.20	0.07	0.4	0.40

Additional evidence has been presented to suggest a generalized disturbance in pyrophosphate metabolism in uremic patients. Russell et al (8) found elevated plasma pyrophosphate levels and David et al (9) increased serum pyrophosphate levels in a number of uremic patients. In addition bone pyrophosphate levels have been found to be elevated in some uremic patients. Elevated bone pyrophosphate levels appear to be more common in patients with visceral calcium-phosphate deposits which are high in pyrophosphate than in bone obtained from uremic patients who are free of this complication (10). (Table II).

TABLE II

	Bone	Lung	
	P_2O_7	Ca	P_2O_7
Uremic	← mg/gram dry tissue →		
Group I			
Mean	0.41	1.64	1.06
SD	0.15	0.60	0.44
Group II			
Mean	2.23	21.2	4.32
SD	1.68	18.4	1.89
Normal			
Mean	0.396	0.60	0.80
SD	.088	0.20	0.40

In an attempt to determine how pyrophosphate is deposited in bone and soft tissues a number of studies have been performed. First, it has been shown that the in vitro uptake of pyrophosphate and diphosphonates by uremic visceral calcium-phosphate deposits was markedly decreased (10) whereas uremic bone having high bone pyrophosphate adsorbed as much pyrophosphate as control bone or synthetic apatite (11). These studies show that at least in bone, pyrophosphate is not primarily surface limited. Secondly, bone and visceral calcification was subjected to treatment with inorganic pyrophosphatase. The pyrophosphate present in both of these tissues was found to be resistant to hydrolysis with pyrophosphatase. This would be consistent with the pyrophosphate being deposited in the transphosphorylated form (12) or else present as the magnesium salt (13) since these compounds are resistant to hydrolysis with pyrophosphatase and increased magnesium is commonly present in tissues which contain large amounts of pyrophosphate. In an attempt to determine if magnesium pyrophosphate was present in visceral calcification selective chelation studies were performed using EDTA and EGTA. Since EGTA does not chelate magnesium but does chelate calcium it was felt that if pyrophosphate existed as an insoluble magnesium salt it should remain in this state following EGTA chelation. However, as can be seen in Table III, magnesium was as readily solubilized as calcium with EGTA chelation.

TABLE III

	Specimen 1			Specimen 2			Synthetic Mg P_2O_7
	Ca	Mg	P_2O_7	Ca	Mg	P_2O_7	Mg
	← mg/100 ml →						
Water	2	0.6	0.3	0.90	0.38	0.18	8.8
EDTA	76	8.4	12.7	138	12	16.5	812.6
EGTA	66	7.4	9.5	91	8	9.3	64.8

These studies make it unlikely that pyrophosphate exists as the magnesium salt. It would thus appear that magnesium and pyrophosphate are either entrapped within the crystal structure or an integral part of the crystal unit since magnesium and pyrophosphate are released during disruption of the crystal's integrity by calcium chelation. This would further suggest that magnesium and pyrophosphate may be deposited by separate and unrelated mechanisms in the bone and soft tissue of uremic patients.

Formation and Resolution of Extraskeletal Calcification

In order to study the pathogenesis and physiological importance of extraskeletal calcification three animal models have been developed. These consist of an acute uremic model (ureteral ligation) (ARF), reversed acute uremic model (removal of ureteral ligatures) (RAU) and chronic renal failure model (1 7/8 nephrectomies)(CU). During two days of acute uremia tissue calcium levels rapidly rise in the aorta, kidney, lung and heart. In spite of reinstitution of normal renal function by releasing the ureteral ligatures the extraskeletal calcium-phosphate deposits persist and calcification in the aortas actually appears to intensify. In the chronically uremic animal visceral calcification also occurs to an equal or greater severity than found in the acute uremic model (Table IV).

In the acute uremic model the deposits can be totally prevented either by prior parathyroidectomy or preventing the hyperphosphotemia by previous phosphate depletion.

TABLE IV

	Heart	Kidney	Lung	Aorta
	← mmol/kg dry weight →			
ARF	19 ± 6	30 ± 18	28 ± 31	172 ± 197
RAU	16 ± 14	69 ± 88	66 ± 83	887 ± 747
CU	43 ± 48	251 ± 241	183 ± 218	500 ± 758
Control	8 ± 4	10 ± 3	15 ± 3	24 ± 15

Similarly in the chronic renal failure model phosphate depletion prevents calcification in all viscera. One reason calcification does not occur is that renal failure does not develop in the phosphate depleted animals. The plasma creatinine at time of study was 1.0 ± .1 mg/100 ml in the phosphate depleted group as compared to 3.2 ± 0.4 mg/100 ml in the non-phosphate depleted group. It is suggested that renal failure occurred in the remnant kidney of the non-phosphate depleted animals as a result of renal calcification which incites a fibrotic and inflammatory response in this organ. Phosphate depletion prevented calcification of the remnant kidney in the depleted group and renal function did not deteriorate.

This is further supported by data in figure 1. It can be appreciated that in heart and lung calcium content does not increase until the terminal phases of renal failure when phosphate is also elevated. In contrast, the calcium content of the kidney begins to significantly rise prior to the development of severe uremia and precedes the rise in other organs. These studies further suggest that hyperphosphotemia plays an important role in the pathogenesis of lung, heart and aorta (not shown) calcification but other mechanisms may be responsible for renal calcification.

CONCLUSION

The following scheme of extraskeletal calcification is suggested. As a consequence of progressive loss of renal function serum phosphorus increases. The rise in serum phosphorus is associated with a small fall in serum calcium which in turn stimulates release of parathyroid hormone. In addition the rise in phosphorus may also accelerate pyrophosphate production. It would appear from the data presented that pulmonary, myocardial and possibly

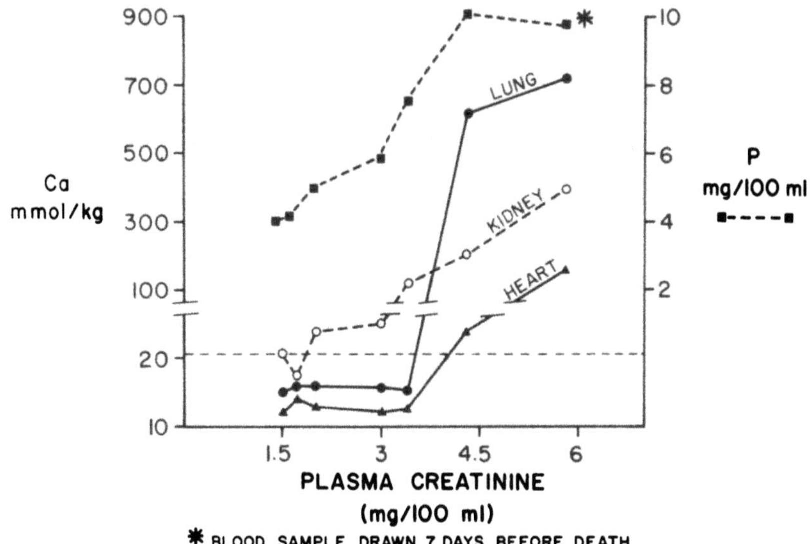

Figure 1
Effect of uremia on calcium content of heart, kidney and lung.

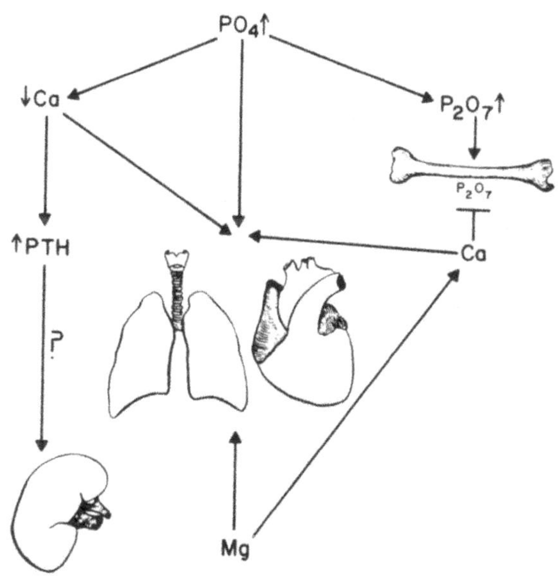

Figure 2
Pathogenesis of extraskeletal calcification.

aortic calcification are largely if not entirely a result of the rise in phosphorus to a critical level where the solubility product of Ca-P is exceeded and precipitation occurs. The fact that parathyroidectomy prevents calcification in the acute uremic model does not exclude the above mechanism in that the product was also lower as a result of hypocalcemia. This same criticism would apply to Bernstein et al (14) work which showed parathyroidectomy was effective in preventing calcification in chronically uremic rats.

Renal calcification may be a result of different pathogenic mechanisms in that it tends to occur earlier in uremia at a time when other organs do not calcify. It is possible that parathyroid hormone as has been shown in regards to brain calcium in uremia (15) is involved in this phenomena.

Pyrophosphate could have a contributory effect on extraskeletal calcification. It would prevent calcium uptake by bone and encourage its deposition in other organs. Furthermore, it would tend to stabilize soft tissue deposits and alter their crystalline features.

REFERENCES

1. Parfitt, A.M.: Soft tissue calcification in uremia. Arch. Intern. Med. 124:544, 1969.

2. Terman, D., Alfrey, A.C., Hammond, W.S., Donnedlinger, T., Ogden, D.A. and Holmes, J.H.: Cardiac calcification in uremia. Am. J. Med. 50:744, 1971.

3. Conger, J.D., Hammond, W.S., Contiguglia, S.R. and Alfrey, A. C.: Clinical correlates of metastatic pulmonary calcification in chronic renal failure. Ann. Intern. Med. 83:330, 1975.

4. Neuman, W.F. and Neuman, M.W.: The chemical dynamics of bone mineral. Univ. of Chicago press, Chicago, Ill., 1958, p. 35.

5. Contiguglia, S.R., Alfrey, A.C., Miller, N., Runnells, D. and LeGeros, R.Z.: Nature of soft tissue calcification in uremia. Kidney Int. 4:229, 1973.

6. LeGeros, R.Z., Contiguglia, S.R. and Alfrey, A.C.: Evidence for two types of calcium-phosphate deposits in uremia. Calcif. Tissue Res. 13:173, 1973.

7. Alfrey, A.C., Solomons, C.C., Ciricillo, J. and Miller, N.L.: Extraosseous calcification: Evidence for abnormal pyrophosphate metabolism in uremia. J. Clin. Invest. 57:693, 1976.

8. Russell, G., Bisaz, S. and Fleisch, H.: Pyrophosphate and diphosphonates in calcium metabolism and their possible role in renal failure. Arch. Intern. Med. 124:571, 1969.

9. David, S.D., Sakai, S., Granda, J., Cheigh, J.S., Riggio, R. R., Stenzel, K.H. and Rubin, A.L.: Role of pyrophosphate in renal osteodystrophy. Trans. Amer. Soc. Artif. Internal Organs 19:440, 1973.

10. Conger, J.D. and Alfrey, A.C.: Letter to the Editor. Ann. Intern. Med. 84:2240225, 1976.

11. Alfrey, A.C. and Solomons, C.C.: Bone pyrophosphate in uremia and its association with extraosseous calcification. J. Clin. Invest. 57:700, 1976.

12. Krane, S.M. and Glimcher, M.J.: Transphosphorylation from nucleoside di- and triphosphates by apatite crystals. J. Biol. Chem. 237:2991, 1962.

13. Cathla, G. and Brunel, C.: L'Activite pyrophosphatasique de la phosphatase alcaline du cerveau. Biochim. Biophys. Acta 315:73, 1973.

14. Bernstein, D.S., Pletka, P., Hattner, R.S., Hampers, C.L. and Merrill, J.P.: Effect of total parathyroidectomy and uremia on the chemical composition of bone, skin and aorta in the rat. Isr. J. Med. Sci. 7:513, 1971.

15. Arieff, A.I. and Massry, S.G.: Calcium metabolism of brain in acute renal failure. Effects of uremia, hemodialysis and parathyroid hormone. J. C.in. Invest. 53:387, 1974.

VISCERAL CALCIFICATION AND THE CaXP PRODUCT

Velentzas, C., Meindok, H., Oreopoulos, D.G.,
Meema, H.E., Rabinovich, S., Jones, M., Sutton, D.,
Rapoport, A., and deVeber, G.A.

Toronto Western Hospital, 399 Bathurst Street,
Toronto, Canada. M5T 2S8

Soft-tissue calcification (metastatic calcification) frequently complicates diseases characterized by hypercalcemia or hyperphosphatemia. Calcification of the arteries or the periarticular tissues can be demonstrated easily by radiological means (1) but calcification of viscera, such as lungs or stomach cannot; even if, on histological examination, it is extensive. For this reason we stand in urgent need of a method for the antemortem diagnosis of visceral calcification because it would improve our efforts to prevent or treat this complication. Recently several workers (2-6) have reported that the visceral uptake of bone-seeking radionuclides during the course of a bone scan indicates calcification, and have demonstrated the presence of calcium crystals in these tissues on histological examination. Using this technique, the incidence of visceral calcification was studied retrospectively in 40 patients - 22 with chronic renal failure, nine with hypercalcemia secondary to malignancy and nine with primary hyperparathyroidism. We also examined the role of the concentration of serum calcium (Ca), phosphorus (P), and the CaXP product on such calcification. This paper describes our findings.

MATERIAL, METHODS AND RESULTS

These 40 patients included 22 with chronic renal failure on dialysis, nine with malignant disease and hypercalcemia, and nine with primary hyperparathyroidism. Visceral uptake of bone seeking radionuclides in the course of bone scan was first observed in patients with chronic renal failure and patients with hypercalcemia and malignancy. Following this observation we studied the bone scan of 22 renal failure patients on dialysis (12 men and 10 women) and nine patients with hypercalcemia secondary to malignancy (5 men and 4 women). Since most of the patients with chronic renal failure have a degree of primary hyperparathyroidism, and in order to elucidate the role of hyperparathyroidism per se in the development of visceral calcification, we also reviewed the bone scans of nine patients with primary hyperparathyroidism (5 men and 4 women).

Bone scintigraphy was performed 2½ hours after the injection of 99^{m}Tc methylene **diphosphonate** or 3½ hours after the injection of 99^{m}Tc polyphosphate **(10mCi/m^{2}** body surface). We consider that uptake in lungs or stomach was abnormal when such uptake was equal to or greater than that by the ribs.

Increased lung uptake, indicating calcification, was observed in 11 patients with chronic renal failure (50%) and four of those with malignancy and hypercalcemia (44%). In the latter group two had malignant lymphoma, one had plasma-cell leukemia and one had multiple myeloma. In addition to the lung uptake, three of the renal failure patients and two of those with malignancy and hypercalcemia showed radionuclide uptake by the stomach. No evidence of visceral radionuclide uptake was obtained in the remaining 11 renal failure patients, in the five patients with malignancy and hypercalcemia or in any of the patients with primary hyperparathyroidism.

Table 1 shows the average serum Ca, P and CaXP product obtained in each patient during the three-month period preceding the bone scan or throughout their period of hospitalization (if shorter than three months) and the maximum CaXP product. This table also shows normal values obtained from 90 volunteers.

Examination of the data indicates that elevation of serum calcium alone could not explain the visceral uptake. Similarly, the changes in serum P and the average CaXP product were not consistent with the hypothesis that elevation of these factors alone is responsible for the production of visceral calcification. Thus, although in each group both P and CaXP were higher in patients with visceral uptake than in those without, no consistent pattern emerged when renal failure patients with visceral uptake were compared with those in the malignant group who had no uptake. Actually, those renal failure patients without uptake had higher mean values than "malignant" patients with uptake. However, the maximum CaXP product was consistently higher in those with visceral uptake than in those without.

Figure 1 compares the maximum CaXP product in these 40 patients with that of the controls. It is obvious that, with few

TABLE 1

Mean Of The Average Serum Ca, P, CaXP Values And The Mean Of The Maximum CaXP Products Observed Before The Scan

Groups	N Pts	Ca	P	CaXP	Maximum CaXP	Comparisons of Maximum CaXP	
CRF with visceral uptake	11	9.7±0.9	6.9±2.4	68.3±20.6	84.3±23.7	1 vs 2	$p < 0.001$
CRF without visceral uptake	11	8.6±0.8	5.9±0.8	51.8±10.5	59.2±14.0	2 vs 6	$p < 0.001$
Malignancy with visceral uptake	4	11.3±2.5	4.2±1.4	50.5±21.7	72.2± 6.4	3 vs 4	$p < 0.005$
Malignancy without visceral uptake	5	13.5±0.9	2.9±0.6	36.4± 6.8	49.3± 6.7	4 vs 6	$p < 0.001$
Primary hyperparathyroidism	9	11.4±2.1	2.5±0.6	30.4± 7.1	35.0± 8.0	5 vs 6	N.S.
Normal	90	9.5±0.4	3.5±0.5	33.9± 5.4			

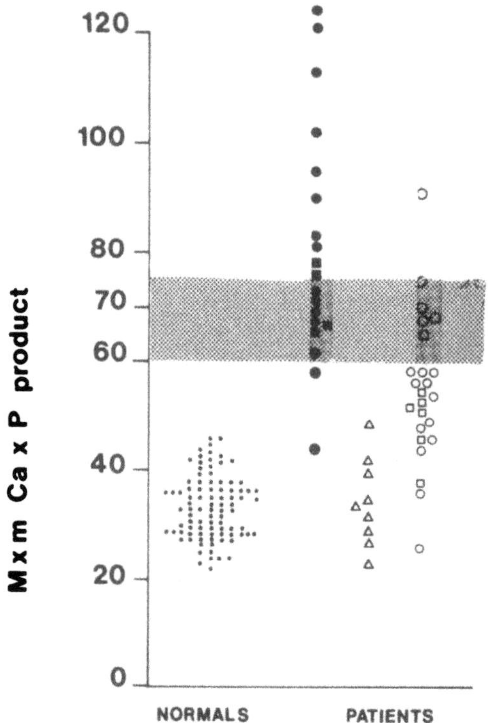

Figure 1.-The maximum CaXP product observed in each of the patients during the three-month period prior to the scan.

exceptions, bone-seeking radionuclides are not deposited in the viscera when the CaXP product remains below 60 but occurs almost always when the CaXP product is above 75. In the zone between 60 and 75, calcification will or will not occur, depending on such contributing factors as pH and the presence or absence of inhibitors of calcification.

DISCUSSION

Visceral uptake of bone-seeking radionuclides has been described during the course of bone scan in 12 patients (2-8). Autopsy was performed in six of these and in two of our patients with malignancy and hypercalcemia. In seven of these eight patients, with visceral radionuclide uptake, subsequent histological examination demonstrated calcium crystals in the corresponding organs. This evidence supports the view that visceral uptake of bone-seeking radionuclides provides a reliable indication of visceral calcification. Our histological observations showed that the site of calcification in the lung was in the perialveolar space.

The frequency of lung calcification among our renal failure patients (50%) (based on radionuclide uptake) and among those with hypercalcemia and malignancy (44%) is similar to that reported earlier, based on histological examination (9,10).

The results of this study indicate that the serum CaXP product is a critical factor in the development of visceral calcification although the precise level of CaXP product above which precipitation of calcium phosphate salts may occur (saturation level) is still controversial (9,12). Our data support an earlier estimate (11) that a CaXP product of 60 reflects the point of saturation calcium phosphate in serum above which spontaneous precipitation may occur. Thus, 13 of our 15 patients (77%) who had visceral calcification had a CaXP product above 60, and 21 of the 25 patients (74%) who had a CaXP product less than 60 had no visceral calcification. Changes in blood pH or in the concentration of inhibitors of calcification probably explain the appearance of visceral calcification in patients whose CaXP product was less than 60 and the absence of calcification in those whose product was higher than 60 (10,12). The absence of visceral calcification among our patients with primary hyperparathyroidism suggests that increased levels of parathyroid hormone do not induce this complication unless they are accompanied by a high CaXP product. In the only reported instance of primary hyperparathyroidism associated with visceral calcification (13) the CaXP product was higher than 75.

We have concluded that visceral calcification is a frequent complication of renal failure or hypercalcemia secondary to malignancy, but is rare among patients with primary hyperparathyroidism. The single most important factor in the development of this complication is an increase in the CaXP product above 60.

SUMMARY

The authors studied the presence of visceral calcification as evidenced by the visceral uptake of bone-seeking radionuclides during the course of a bone scan among 22 patients with terminal renal failure maintained on dialysis, nine patients with hypercalcemia secondary to malignancy, and nine patients with primary hyperparathyroidism. Uptake by the lungs or stomach was observed in 11 renal failure patients (50%) and in four of those with malignancy and hypercalcemia (44%). None of the patients with primary hyperparathyroidism had evidence of visceral calcification. The serum CaXP product was significantly higher among those with visceral calcification than those without. The results of this study indicate that a CaXP product of 60 represents the saturation product of calcium phosphate in serum above which spontaneous precipitation of this salt may occur in such viscera as stomach and lungs.

REFERENCES

1. Meema, H.E., Oreopoulos, D.G., and deVeber, G.A.: Arterial calcifications in severe chronic renal disease and their relationship to dialysis treatment, renal transplant and parathyroidectomy. Radiology 21:315, 1976.

2. Holmes, R.: Detection of diffuse metastatic pulmonary calcification with radiostrontium. J. Nucl. Med. 11:327, 1970.

3. Chaudhuri, T.K., Chaudhuri, T.K., Muilenburg, M.I., and Christie, J.H.: Abnormal deposition of radiostrontium in lungs. Chest 61:190, 1972.

4. Grames, G.M., Sanser, D.D., Jansen, C., Soderblom, R.E., Hodgkin, J.E., and Stilson, M.S.: Radionuclide detection of diffuse interstitial pulmonary calcification. J.A.M.A. 230:992, 1974.

5. Richards, G.A.: Metastatic calcification detected through scanning with ^{99m}Tc polyphosphate. J. Nucl. Med. 46:188, 1974.

6. McLaughlin, A.F.: Uptake of ^{99m}Tc bone scanning agent by lungs with metastatic calcification. J. Nucl. Med. 16:322, 1975.

7. Schlangen, J.T., and Pauwels, E,K.J.: Die Diagnostik der Calcinosis pulmonis durch Szintigraphische Untersuchungen. Fortschr. Geb. Roentgenstr. Nuklearmed. 124:119, 1976.

8. Devacaanthan, K., Tap, A.V., Changes, Z., and Stein, R.M.: Pulmonary calcification in chronic renal failure: use of diphosphonate scintiscan as a diagnostic pool. Clin. Nephrol. 6:488, 1976.

9. Conger, J.D., Hammon W.S., and Alfrey, A.C.: Pulmonary calcification in chronic dialysis patients. Ann. Intern. Med. 83:330, 1975.

10. Mulligan, R.M.: Metastatic calcification. Arch. Pathol. 43:117, 1947.

11. Hebert, L.A., Lemann, J., Jr., Peterson, J.R., and Lennon, E.J.: Studies of the mechanism by which phosphate infusion lowers serum calcium concentration. J. Clin. Invest. 45: 1886, 1966.

12. Oreopoulos, D.G., Pitel, S., Husdan, H., deVeber, G.A., and Rapoport, A.: Contrasting effects of hemodialysis and peritoneal dialysis on the inhibition of in vitro calcification by uremic serum. Can. Med. Assoc. J. 110:43, 1974.

13. Schully, R.E., Galdabini, J.J., and McNeely, B.U.: Weekly clinicopathological exercises. N. Engl. J. Med. 295:433, 1976.

ORTHOPHOSPHATE AND OTHER PHOSPHATE COMPOUNDS IN RELATION TO STONE FORMATION

H. Fleisch

Department of Pathophysiology, University of Berne, Murtenstrasse 35, 3010 Berne, Switzerland

Introduction

It has been reported repeatedly that the ingestion of orthophosphate leads to a decrease in the formation of urinary calcium stones in man (1,2,3,4). The suggestion has therefore been made that stone formers may be treated by the administration of phosphate salts. Although some authors could not find such an effect (5), and even though a clearcut double-blind trial is still lacking, the bulk of evidence seems to suggest that such a beneficial effect is real. Now the question arises by what mechanism does this effect take place.

The current knowledge about mechanisms of urinary stone formation is centered around three basic concepts: a) the relationship between the solubility of the solid phase formed and the concentration of the forming substances in urine, b) the role played by activators of crystallization and aggregation, and c) the role played by inhibitors of these two processes.

Saturation of Urine

It is presently generally accepted that urine, even in normal people, is ordinarily supersaturated with respect to calcium oxalate (6), the three main calcium phosphate salts octocalcium phosphate (6), hydroxyapatite (6)

and brushite (7), as well as sodium and ammonium urate (8). With respect to magnesium ammonium phosphate, supersaturation occurs only once urine becomes alkaline due to infections (6). Thus the physicochemical conditions are fulfiled for the formation of crystals to occur.

One possible way of orthophosphate to act is by decreasing the supersaturation of urine towards the calcium salts. Indeed ingestion of orthophosphate decreases the urinary excretion of calcium probably both by diminishing the intestinal absorption of calcium through the formation of insoluble calcium phosphate salts, and by increasing the renal tubular reabsorption of calcium (Bonjour, Hugi and Fleisch, unpublished observations). Such a decrease in supersaturation has been observed both for calcium oxalate and for calcium phosphate (9), the latter despite an increase in urinary orthophosphate.

Urinary Inhibitors

Another way of action by orthophosphate, which is perhaps the more important one is the increase of urinary excretion of inhibitors for crystallization and crystal aggregation. For a good understanding of such an effect a knowledge of these two processes is necessary. Thus this paper will sum up our present knowledge of urinary crystal inhibitors. For a more extensive review the reader is referrred to a recent publication (10).

A clear distinction must be made between the two processes, crystal formation and crystal aggregation. In the past attention was devoted merely to crystal formation. Only recently interest has shifted to aggregation, which is the process of crystals binding one to another leading to the formation of large clusters (11, 12,13,14,15). This process could possibly be the mechanism which distinguishes people excreting crystals in their urine (a normal phenomenon) to those forming stones. This hypothesis is strengthened by the fact that stone formers often excrete large aggregates of calcium oxalate in their urine while normal people excrete mostly only individual crystals (11).

Measurement of the Inhibitory Activity in Urine

Crystal formation. One of the first techniques used adapted the system described in the thirties to study calcification of cartilage (16). The effect of urine on the precipitation of calcium phosphate onto epiphyseal cartilage from rachitic rats is studied in vitro (17). However cartilage is enzymatically very active and is likely to destroy any inhibitors. Furthermore urine influences this enzymatic activity so that the results do not represent the amount of inhibitors present.

A better approach to this problem is the in vitro determination of the minimum ion concentration necessary for the formation of the solid phase (18,19,20,21). It is of great importance for the experimental conditions, especially the supersaturation to be well defined. This is difficult in full urine. One way, although tedious, is the chemical determination of all the ions and complexors involved and to calculate the relevant activities in the urine using the chemical stability constants described in the literature (6). This procedure is probably not without error since some of the stability constants are still doubtful. A simplified approach is to measure the relation of the measured concentration products to the solubility of the relevant salts in the individual urine (7). It seems that this ratio is equal to that obtained when using the true thermodynamic values (22). A non-negligeable weakness using this technique in full urine is that the effect of the inhibitors is often maximal, so that changes in their concentrations might not be measured.

To solve these various difficulties the same technique has been applied but using a standard solution with the addition of only a few per cent of urine. Unfortunately the results in diluted urine are not necessarily representative to whole urine. Indeed the inhibitory activity of a compound is often not related linearly with its concentration. Furthermore if the effects of each inhibitor should appear to be different, it can happen that certain inhibitors are relatively important in full urine but of minor importance or even not detected in diluted urine and vice versa. Thus there are doubts on the physiological relevance of the data obtained with diluted urine.

Another approach has been to analyze the kinetics of the precipitation of the mineral after addition of a seed. The latter can consist of crystals of the mineral which will precipitate or of crystals of another structurally related salt or even of an organic compound such as collagen. Again it is important that the saturation level is well defined, either by calculating the thermodynamic product or by using a constant ratio towards the solubility of the salt to be precipitated. For calcium oxalate the process is controlled by a biexponential reaction, so that the kinetic analysis is straight forward and the rate constants can be determined (23,24). Unfortunately the measurements have until now only been performed on diluted urines and it is not known whether extrapolation to full urine is possible. For calcium phosphate the precipitation curve is complex and cannot easily be analyzed quantitatively. Thus a simplified approach, also used for calcium oxalate (19,25), has to be employed which consists in determining the amount of calcium salts formed within one time period (25).

Recently we have developed a new method which allows to measure quantitatively the inhibitors in full urine (26). It is based on the determination of the amount of seed crystals needed to induce a certain amount of precipitation in the urine specimen. The Ca x P product of the urine is adjusted to the solubility of brushite in the respective urine specimen, bringing it therefore to a constant calcium phosphate activity product, a condition sine qua non for all inhibitory tests. Calcium phosphate precipitation is then initiated by adding calcium apatite which has a solubility below that of brushite. The amount of apatite needed to form a precipitation of 50 % of the calcium and phosphate present in the solution in a predetermined time is then measured. Since the inhibitors act through a binding on the surface of the growing crystals the technique is in a sense a titration: apatite crystals are added until their surface growth sites exceed the number of inhibitor molecules at which point precipitation occurs. The technique is reproducible and easy to perform. However, it has been until now developed only for calcium phosphate and not for calcium oxalate.

Crystal aggregation. All the known techniques (11, 12,13,14,15) make use of the ability of individual crystals to bind to larger clusters when incubated in metastable solutions. This process can be measured quantitatively by counting the number of larger particles formed at a predetermined time period using a Coulter counter. Urine slows down the aggregation of both calcium phosphate (13) and calcium oxalate (11,12,15). Unfortunately while this technique measures inhibitors very efficiently when urine is added to the solution at a few per cent, no technique exists yet for the measurement in whole urine. Indeed in whole urine precipitation of other salts occurs when the crystals of the phase the aggregation of which has to be measured are added, disturbing the measurements. Thus all the results obtained up to now are based on measurements in highly diluted urines and might quantitatively not be relevant to what occurs in full native urine.

Nature of the Various Inhibitors

Many studies have been devoted to the identification of the various inhibitors. This interest has evolved not only because of the possible relation to stone formation but also because of the inhibitors of calcium phosphate precipitation might be involved in normal and pathological calcification of other tissues. Again it is important to differentiate between the inhibitors of crystal formation and those of crystal aggregation and between the inhibitors affecting the various mineral phases.

Calcium phosphate formation. The first of these inhibitors to be isolated and identified from urine was inorganic pyrophosphate (21). This compound has proven to be very active in all of the systems tested. It increases the minimal Ca x P concentration necessary to form a precipitate (27), diminishes the rate of precipitation upon added seeds, such as brushite (28), octocalcium phosphate, apatite (26,29), and collagen (27), and inhibits the calcification of cartilage (30). The amount of pyrophosphate present in urine is in the range of 10^{-5} to 10^{-4} M (31,32), high enough to exert a strong, even maximal inhibition.

Other inhibitors are magnesium (33,34), zinc, stannous ions (35), citrate (26,33), and under certain conditions fluoride (35). In addition there are possibly other yet unidentified compounds (33,36). For a time they were thought to be peptides (33,36,37), a hypothesis which has recently been abandoned (33,38), the latest suggestion being phosphocitrate (38).

The relative quantitative role played by the various above mentioned compounds in the total inhibitory activity is not yet ascertained. Indeed results obtained in diluted urine cannot be extrapolated to full urine. Thus the fact that pyrophosphate is the main inhibitor when determined at 2 % urine (21) does not necessarily mean that this is also true in whole urine. We have recently found (26) that in whole urine 77 % of the inhibitory activity seems to be due to citrate, magnesium and pyrophosphate. From those, citrate is the most important one with 48 % followed by magnesium with 20 % and pyrophosphate with only 9 % of the total activity.

Calcium oxalate formation. The nature of the inhibitors is very similar to that of the compounds affecting calcium phosphate crystallization. Thus pyrophosphate (18,24), citrate (24) and magnesium (24) are efficient inhibitors. Furthermore many other substances, such as metals, dyes, polyelectrolytes (39) have been shown to be active. It is impossible to evaluate today the relative part played by the various compounds. This is especially so since it appears that the action of many of the inhibitors is diminished in the presence of urine itself (40). It would appear that the known inhibitors would represent only a small portion of the total inhibitory activity, the main part being exerted by macromolecules (19,24).

Calcium phosphate aggregation. We found various substances present in urine to inhibit efficiently the aggregation of calcium phosphate crystals. Thus citrate, pyrophosphate and interestingly various glycosaminoglycans, especially heparin, are active (13). In view of the fact that the inhibitory activity in urine is to a great extent not filtrable through a 50,000 MW filter, it is possible that the non-filtrable part is due to some type of glycosaminoglycans. Until now, since the test has been performed only in highly diluted urine, no conclusion can be drawn with respect to the relative quantitative role in full urine.

Calcium oxalate aggregation. It seems that the same compounds which inhibit the aggregation of calcium phosphate are also active on calcium oxalate. Thus pyrophosphate and glycosaminoglycans, especially heparin, were found to be extremely effective (12,14,15). As for calcium phosphate inhibitors it is difficult up to now to assess the part of the total inhibition played by the various parts. It appears, however, that pyrophosphate would account for only about 15 % of the total activity, the largest part being due again to macromolecules of large molecular weight (15,41). Since these are precipitated by cetyl pyridinium chloride they might well be glycosaminoglycans (41).

Mode of Action of the Inhibitors

Most of the studies done up to now have been performed with pyrophosphate and related compounds. These inhibitors are acting on the various processes of solid phase formation, such epitactic or heterogenous nucleation and crystal growth (18,24,26,27,28,29,33), crystal aggregation (12,13,14,15) and the further phase transformation (42,43). All these effects seem to be related to the strong binding of the inhibitors (44) on the surface of the crystals, a well known phenomenon in crystallization. It is not necessary for the whole surface to be covered, specific binding on certain sites of the crystals on less than 1 % of the surface being sufficient. The binding is not restricted to one type of binding sites, but the inhibitory activity seems to be related to one of them (44). For aggregation the change of the surface zeta potential which will alter attraction and repulsion between the crystals is probably the predominant mechanism.

Regulation of the Urinary Excretion of Inhibitors

Most of what is known on the regulation of urinary excretion of inhibitors is associated with pyrophosphate. The excretion of pyrophosphate is age and sex dependent (31,32). However, the most important parameter influencing its excretion is the intake of inorganic phosphate. An increase in the ingestion of orthophosphate enhances drastically the excretion of pyrophosphate (45,46). This parallism between the excretion of these two compounds appears to be due to a direct action on the kidney. Indeed administration of orthophosphate increases the renal clearance of pyrophosphate without changing the blood concentration (47). Furthermore, in dogs the unilateral infusion of orthophosphate in one kidney causes a greater and more rapid increase in the infused than in the contralateral organ (47). Finally, we have recently shown that during microperfusion of a proximal accessible rat tubule pyrophosphate is destroyed to about 70 % into orthophosphate. This hydrolysis is reduced by adding orthophosphate to the perfusing fluid (Boudry, Bonjour and Fleisch, unpublished results).

In view of the powerful effect of pyrophosphate on both crystal formation and aggregation of calcium phosphate and oxalate it is possible that the beneficial effects of orthophosphate (1,2,3,4) is due, at least partly, to the increase in pyrophosphate excretion.

Inhibitors in Stone Formers

Although the problem is not completely settled yet, it appears now that many patients with urinary stones do have some type of inhibitory deficiency. The uncertainty is explained by the multiplicity of the techniques used, many of them being probably not relevant, by the lack of differentiation between the inhibitors of crystal formation, aggregation and phase transformation, and by the lack of matched controls with respect to age, sex and especially diet.

A decrease in inhibitory activity has been described for calcium phosphate formation using the rat cartilage system (17,34) as well as the determination of the Ca x P formation product (25,48). For calcium oxalate a decrease was found using the formation product (25) as well as the rate of crystallization (25). Recently a decrease in the inhibition of calcium oxalate aggregation has also been described (11,49). This latter effect has been found especially in patients presenting a smaller calcium oxalate supersaturation so that when both parameters, supersaturation and inhibition of aggregation, are taken into account, stone formers and controls can be clearly separated (49).

Pyrophosphate appears to be frequently decreased in stone formers (48) especially in middle-aged men and in patients without hypocalciuria (32). The decrease in pyrophosphate becomes specially apparent when patients are matched with controls with respect to age, sex and diet (48), parameters which by themselves all influence pyrophosphate excretion. Increasing the phosphate intake can lead to a normalization of the urinary pyrophosphate.

Analogues of Physiological Inhibitors - the Diphosphonates

The therapeutical approach involving inhibitors has been centered along two lines: a) increasing the excretion of normally formed inhibitory compounds, such as pyrophosphate; b) synthesizing compounds related in structure to endogenous inhibitors, which after administration are excreted in the urine.

The most fruitful approach along the latter line has been the synthesis of diphosphonates, compounds related to pyrophosphate but characterized by a P-C-P bond. In contrary to pyrophosphate which is easily hydrolyzed enzymatically, the diphosphonates are resistant to both chemical and enzymatic destruction. They have furthermore the advantage of being excreted in urine when administered orally. The diphosphonates have been found to be powerful inhibitors of both calcium phosphate formation (43,50, 51) and aggregation (13), as well as calcium oxalate formation (20,52) and aggregation (14,15). In animal studies they were found, when given orally, to inhibit the experimental calcification of the kidneys and other tissues (51), and to decrease the formation of experimentally induced bladder stones (52). In man the oral administration of the diphosphonate disodium ethane-1-hydroxy-1,1-diphosphonate (EHDP) enhances the effect of urine to increase the minimum Ca x P concentration necessary to form crystals (53), decreases the growth of calcium phosphate in urine (54) and decreases the urinary excretion of calcium oxalate aggregates (55). Furthermore it induces an increase in urinary pyrophosphate which remains after discontinuation of the drug (53). In a pilot study we found that EHDP given four times a day at a total dose of 1100 mg/day, a mode of administration which ensures a steady urinary excretion over the day, appears to decrease the recurrence of the stones (53). However such a dose is likely to influence also bone turnover and mineralization, so that its administration does not seem to be warranted for general use. Nevertheless, the principle could be extended to the development of other diphosphonates or other compounds with the relevant physicochemical effects in urine but without effects on bone.

Conclusion

The clinical administration of orthophosphate has been described in the literature to prevent the formation of urinary calcium stones. This effect is likely to be due both to the decrease of urinary calcium as well as to the increase in the urinary excretion of inorganic pyrophosphate an inhibitor of crystal formation and crystal aggregation. The role of these latter two processes in relation to stone formation, and the relative importance of the various known physiological inhibitors as well as of the synthetic inhibitors have been reviewed.

Acknowledgments

This work has been supported by the Swiss National Science Foundation (3.725.76) and by the Procter and Gamble Company, USA.

References

1. Howard, J.E.: Urinary stone. Canad.Med.Ass.J. 86: 1001, 1962.
2. Thomas, W.C., and Miller, G.H.: Inorganic phosphates in the treatment of renal calculi. Modern Treatment 4: 494, 1967.
3. Smith, L.H., Thomas, W.C., and Arnaud, C.D.: Orthophosphate therapy in calcium renal lithiasis. In: Urinary Calculi. S. Karger, Basel, 188, 1973.
4. Bernstein, D.S., and Newton, R.: The effect of oral sodium phosphate on the formation of renal calculi and on idiopathic hypercalciuria. Lancet, 1105, 1966.
5. Ettinger, B.: Recurrent nephrolithiasis: Natural history and effect of phosphate therapy. Amer.J.Med. 61: 200, 1976.
6. Robertson, W.G., Peacock, M., and Nordin, B.E.C.: Activity products in stone-forming and non-stone forming urine. Clin.Sci. 34: 579, 1968.
7. Pak, C.Y.C., and Chu, S.: A simple technique for the determination of urinary state of saturation with

respect to brushite. Invest.Urol. 11: 211, 1973.

8. Pak, C.Y.C., Waters, O., Arnold, L.R., Holt, K., Cox, C., Barilla, D.: Mechanism for calcium urolithiasis among patients with hyperuricosuria: Supersaturation of urine with respect to monosodium urate. J.Clin. Invest., in press.
9. Robertson, W.G., Peacock, M., Marshall, R.W., Varnavides, C.K., Heyburn, P.J., and Nordin, B.E.C.: Effect of oral orthophosphate on calcium crystalluria in stone-formers. In: Urolithiasis Research. Plenum Press, New York, 339, 1976.
10. Fleisch, H.: Inhibitors and promotors of stone formation. Kidney Int., in press.
11. Robertson, W.G., and Peacock, M.: Calcium oxalate crystalluria and inhibitors of crystallization in recurrent renal stone-formers. Clin.Sci. 43: 499, 1972.
12. Fleisch, H., and Monod, A.: A new technique for measuring aggregation of calcium oxalate crystals in vitro: Effect of urine, magnesium, pyrophosphate and diphosphonates. In: Urinary Calculi. S. Karger, Basel, 53, 1973.
13. Hansen, N.M., Felix, R., Bisaz, S., and Fleisch, H.: Aggregation of hydroxyapatite crystals, Biochim. Biophys.Acta 451: 549, 1976.
14. Robertson, W.G., Peacock, M., and Nordin, B.E.C.: Inhibitors of the growth and aggregation of calcium oxalate crystals in vitro. Clin.Chim.Acta 43: 31, 1973.
15. Felix, R., Monod, A., Broge, L., Hansen, N.M., and Fleisch, H.: Aggregation of calcium oxalate crystals: effect of urine and various inhibitors. Urol.Res. 5: 21, 1977.
16. Gutman, A.B., and Yu, T.F.: Further studies of the relation between glycogenolysis and calcification in cartilage. In: Metabolic Interrelations. Josiah Macy Jr. Foundation, New York, 11, 1949.
17. Howard, J.E., and Thomas, W.C.: Some observations on rachitic rat cartilage of probably significance in the etiology of renal calculi. Trans.Amer.Clin.Chim. Ass. 70: 94, 1958.
18. Fleisch, H., and Bisaz, S.: The inhibitory effect of pyrophosphate on calcium oxalate precipitation and its relation to urolithiasis. Experientia 20: 276, 1964.
19. Gill, W.B., and Karesh, J.W.: Demonstration of protective (inhibitory) effects of urinary macromolecules on the crystallization of calcium oxalate. In:

Urolithiasis Research. Plenum Press, New York, 277, 1976.

20. Pak, C.Y.C., Ohata, M., and Holt, K.: Effect of diphosphonate on crystallization of calcium oxalate in vitro. Kidney Int. 7: 154, 1975.
21. Fleisch, H., and Bisaz, S.: Isolation from urine of pyrophosphate, a calcification inhibitor. Amer.J. Physiol. 203: 671, 1962.
22. Pak, C.Y.C., Hayashi, Y., Finlayson, B., and Chu, S.: Estimation of the state of saturation of brushite and calcium oxalate in urine: A comparison of three methods. J.Lab.Clin.Med. 89: 891, 1977.
23. Meyer, J.L., and Smith, L.H.: Growth of calcium oxalate crystals. I. A model for urinary stone growth. Invest.Urol. 13: 31, 1975.
24. Meyer, J.L., and Smith, L.H.: Growth of calcium oxalate crystals. II. Inhibition by natural urinary crystal growth inhibitors. Invest.Urol. 13: 36, 1975.
25. Pak, C.Y.C., and Holt, K.: Nucleation and growth of brushite and calcium oxalate in urine of stone-formers. Metabolism 25: 665, 1976.
26. Bisaz, S., Felix, R., Fleisch, H., and Neuman, W.F.: Quantitative determination of inhibitors of calcium phosphate precipitation in whole urine. Mineral & Electr.Metab., in press.
27. Fleisch, H., and Neuman, W.F.: Mechanisms of calcification: Role of collagen, polyphosphates, and phosphatase. Amer.J.Physiol. 200: 1296, 1961.
28. Marshall, R.W., and Nancollas, G.H.: The kinetics of crystal growth of dicalcium phosphate dihydrate. J.Phys.Chem. 73: 3838, 1969.
29. Fleisch, H., Russell, R.G.G., and Straumann, F.: Effect of pyrophosphate on hydroxyapatite and its implications in calcium homeostasis. Nature 212: 901, 1966.
30. Lewis, A.M., Thomas, W.C., and Tomita, A.: Pyrophosphate and the mineralizing potential of urine. Clin. Sci. 30: 389, 1966.
31. Fleisch, H., and Bisaz, S.: Die Pyrophosphatausscheidung im Harn beim gesunden Menschen. Helv.Physiol. Pharm.Acta 21: 88, 1963.
32. Russell, R.G.G., and Hodgkinson, H.: Urinary excretion of inorganic pyrophosphate by normal subjects and patients with renal calculus. Clin.Sci. 31: 51, 1966.
33. Smith, L.H., Meyer, J.L., and McCall, I.T.: Chemical nature of crystal inhibitors isolated from human

urine. In: Urinary Calculi. S. Karger, Basel, 318, 1973.

34. Mukai, T., and Howard, J.E.: Some observations on the calcification of rachitic cartilage by urine. Bull.Johns Hopkins Hospital 112: 279, 1963.
35. Meyer, J.L., and Nancollas, G.H.: Effect of stannous and fluoride ions on the rate of crystal growth of hydroxyapatite. J.Dent.Res. 51: 1443, 1972.
36. Howard, J.E., Thomas, W.C., Barker, L.M., Smith, L.H. and Wadkins, C.L.: The recognition and isolation from urine and serum of a peptide inhibitor to calcification. Johns Hopkins Med.J. 120: 119, 1967.
37. Smith, L.H., and McCall, J.T.: Chemical nature of peptide inhibitors isolated from urine. In: Renal Stone Res. Symp., Churchill, 153, 1969.
38. Howard, J.E.: Studies on urinary stone formation: A saga of clinical investigation. Johns Hopkins Med.J. 139: 239, 1976.
39. Sutor, D.J.: Growth studies of calcium oxalate in the presence of various ions and compounds. Brit.J. Urol. 41: 171, 1969.
40. Welshman, S.G., and McGeown, M.G.: A quantitative investigation of the effects on the growth of calcium oxalate crystals on potential inhibitors. Brit. J.Urol. 44: 677, 1972.
41. Robertson, W.G., Knowles, F., and Peacock, M.: Urinary acid mucopolysaccharide inhibitors of calcium oxalate crystallization. In: Urolithiasis Research. Plenum Press, New York, 331, 1976.
42. Fleisch, H., Russell, R.G.G., Bisaz, S., Termine, J.D., and Posner, A.S.: Influence of pyrophosphate on the transformation of amorphous to crystalline calcium phosphate. Calc.Tiss.Res. 2: 49, 1968.
43. Francis, M.D.: The inhibition of calcium hydroxyapatite crystal growth by polyphosphonates and polyphosphates. Calc.Tiss.Res. 3: 151, 1969.
44. Jung, A., Bisaz, S., and Fleisch, H.: The binding of pyrophosphate and two diphosphonates by hydroxyapatite crystals. Calc.Tiss.Res. 11: 269, 1973.
45. Fleisch, H., Bisaz, S., and Care, A.D.: Effect of orthophosphate on urinary pyrophosphate excretion and the prevention of urolithiasis. Lancet, 1065, 1964.
46. Russell, R.G.G., Edwards, N.A., and Hodgkinson, A.: Urinary pyrophosphate and urolithiasis. Lancet, 1446, 1964.
47. Russell, R.G.G., Bisaz, S., and Fleisch, H.: The in-

fluence of orthophosphate on the renal handling of inorganic pyrophosphate in man and dog. Clin.Sci. Mol.Med. 51: 435, 1976.
48. Baumann, J.M., Bisaz, S., Felix, R., Fleisch, H., Ganz, U., and Russell, R.G.G.: The role of inhibitors and other factors in the pathogenesis of recurrent calcium-containing renal stones. Clin.Sci.Mol.Med., in press.
49. Robertson, W.G., Peacock, M., Marshall, R.W., Marshall, D.H., and Nordin, B.E.C.: Saturation-inhibition index as a measure of the risk of calcium oxalate stone formation in the urinary tract. New Engl. J.Med. 294: 249, 1976.
50. Francis, M.D., Russell, R.G.G., and Fleisch, H.: Diphosphonates inhibit formation of calcium phosphate crystals in vitro and pathological calcification in vivo. Science 165: 1264, 1969.
51. Fleisch, H.A., Russell, R.G.G., Bisaz, S., Mühlbauer, R.C., and Williams, D.A.: The inhibitory effect of phosphonates on the formation of calcium phosphate crystals in vitro and on aortic and kidney calcification in vivo. Europ.J.Clin.Invest. 1: 12, 1970.
52. Fraser, D., Russell, R.G.G., Pohler, O., Robertson, W.G., and Fleisch, H.: The influence of disodium ethane-1-hydroxy-1,1-diphosphonate (EHDP) on the development of experimentally induced urinary stones in rats. Clin.Sci. 42: 197, 1972.
53. Baumann, J.M., Bisaz, S., Fleisch, H., and Wacker, M.: Biochemical and clinical effects of ethane-1-hydroxy-1,1-diphosphonate (EHDP) in calcium nephrolithiasis. Submitted.
54. Ohata, M., and Pak, C.Y.C.: Preliminary study of the treatment of nephrolithiasis (calcium stones) with diphosphonate. Metabolism 23: 1167, 1974.
55. Robertson, W.G., Peacock, M., Marshall, W.R., and Knowles, F.: The effect of ethane-1-hydroxy-1,1-diphosphonate (EHDP) on calcium oxalate crystalluria in recurrent renal stone-formers. Clin.Sci.Mol. Med. 47: 13, 1974.

FURTHER EVIDENCE SUPPORTING THE PHOSPHATE LEAK HYPOTHESIS OF IDIOPATHIC HYPERCALCIURIA

F.H. Shen, J.L. Ivey, D.J. Sherrard, R.L. Nielsen, M.R. Haussler, and D.J. Baylink
Seattle VA Hospital, Seattle, WA 98108; American Lake VA Hospital, Tacoma, WA 98493; Department of Medicine, University of Washington, Seattle, WA 98195; The Mason Clinic, Seattle, WA 98111; and Department of Biochemistry, College of Medicine, University of Arizona, Tucson, AZ 85724.

We have previously reported (1,2) that a group of patients with idiopathic hypercalciuria (IH) exhibited certain metabolic characteristics. Compared with age- and sex-matched control subjects, the IH patients were normocalcemic, but their serum phosphate and immunoreactive parathyroid hormone (PTH) concentrations were lower, serum 1,25-dihydroxyvitamin D (1,25-diOHD) concentration, urinary calcium excretion, and fractional enteral calcium absorption were higher. Even though their serum phosphate concentration was lower than that of the controls, urinary phosphate excretion was normal in the IH patients due to a lower TmP/GFR (2).

Many of the characteristics of these IH patients are also seen in the phosphate depletion syndrome (elevated 1,25-diOHD, increased fractional enteral calcium absorption, and urinary calcium excretion, and decreased PTH). The amount of phosphate excreted in the phosphate depletion syndrome decreases to almost nil (3), in contrast to the normal amount excreted by the IH patients (2).

Based on these observations we proposed (1,2) that the hypercalciuria in these patients was the result of an inappropriately low tubular reabsorption of phosphate, or renal leak of phosphate. The failure to reabsorb a normal amount of phosphate would produce a state of phosphate depletion which invokes several physiologic regulatory mechanisms to conserve phosphate (Fig. 1). One such physiologic response to phosphate depletion is an increase in 1,25-diOHD, which acts to increase the intestinal absorption of phosphate and to increase the tubular reabsorption of phosphate

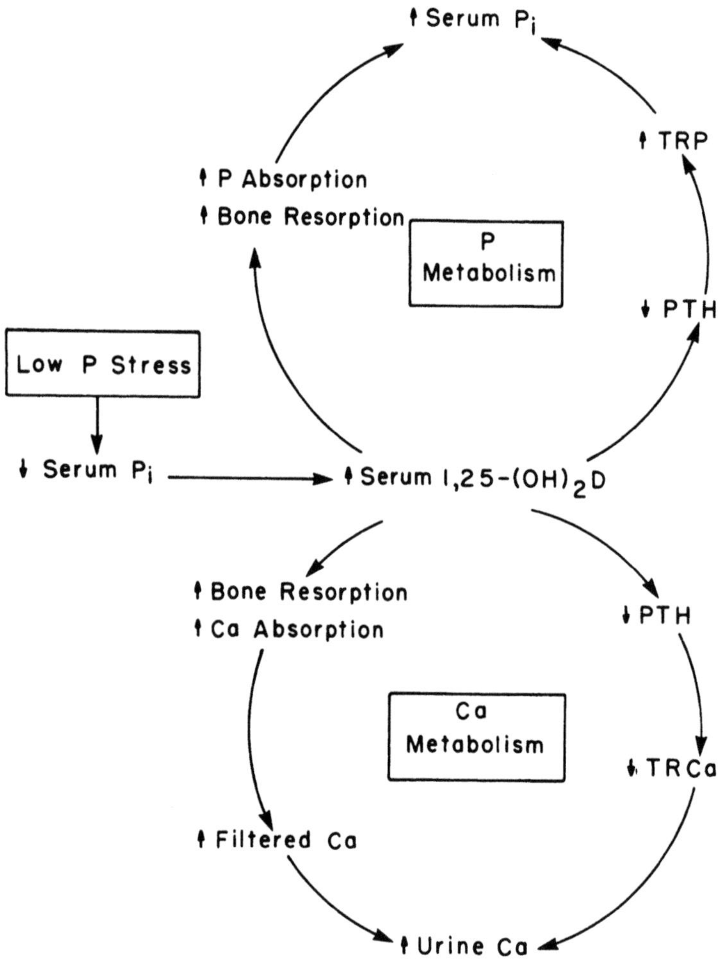

Figure 1. Changes in phosphate and calcium metabolism in response to a low phosphorus stress. The increase in serum 1,25-diOHD and the decrease in serum PTH act to conserve phosphate and dispose of the excess calcium by urine excretion (3,4,5,6). For simplicity, some responses have been omitted. For example, low serum phosphate and high serum 1,25-diOHD both probably inhibit bone calcium and phosphate deposition (7) and low serum phosphate alone probably inhibits PTH secretion (8) and PTH target organ response, viz., bone resorption (unpublished observation).

by decreasing PTH secretion (4). The postabsorptive increase in serum calcium (see below) may also directly promote renal tubular phosphate reabsorption (9), a possibility which is consistent with the previously demonstrated inverse relationship between serum phosphate and serum calcium (2). The increased serum 1,25-diOHD also acts to increase the intestinal absorption of calcium which increases postabsorptive renal filtered calcium load, while the decreased serum PTH reduces the tubular reabsorption of calcium. The increased filtered load of calcium combined with the decreased tubular reabsorption of calcium results in hypercalciuria (Fig. 1).

The latter occurs because of the nature of the serum calcium and phosphate regulatory mechanisms, i.e., both hormones simultaneously regulate both serum calcium and phosphate. Accordingly, in order to raise serum phosphate without raising serum calcium excessively, urine calcium must increase. If this hypothesis is correct, a therapeutic supplement of phosphate should compensate for the loss of phosphate due to the renal leak and thereby adjust the activities of the above regulatory mechanisms involved in phosphate conservation toward their normal basal levels. Thus, to further evaluate our hypothesis, patients with IH were treated with oral phosphate supplements, and their responses are described in this report.

METHODS

Ten, male patients with IH ranging from 26 to 59 years of age participated in this study, and nine completed the study with good compliance, as determined by a large increment in urine phosphate. The criteria for patient selection were: a history of renal stones, excretion of more than 300 mg of calcium in the urine per day on more than two occasions while on their regular diet, and no disease to which hypercalciuria is secondary. All available patients satisfying the above criteria and willing to participate were studied. Medication, such as hydrochlorothiazide, was discontinued at least two weeks prior to the study. Ten age-matched normal male employees of the Seattle V.A. Hospital served as controls.

On the first day of the study, morning fasting serum and 24 h urine samples were collected for chemical analysis and fractional enteral calcium absorption was determined. The IH patients were then treated with inorganic phosphate tablets p.o. for eight weeks (0.5 g of elemental phosphorus qid)* without changing their regular diets. Prior to discontinuation of therapy at eight weeks, serum and urine samples were collected for chemical analysis, and measurement of fractional enteral calcium absorption was repeated. Serum samples were collected at 10 a.m. 2 h after the first oral dose of phosphate.

*Phos-tabs tablets (Davies Rose Hoyt) kindly supplied by Mr. M. Grodberg.

Serum immunoreactive PTH was determined by a radioimmunoassay in which the specificity of the antibody is predominatly the N-terminal (1-34) sequence of native PTH (2). Serum 1,25-diOHD was determined by radioreceptor assay as previously described (5,10), and urine cyclic adenosine 3', 5'-monophosphate (cyclic AMP) was determined by the method of Gilman (11) and the cyclic AMP binding protein fraction from rabbit muscle. Fractional enteral calcium absorption was determined using the double-isotope method (2,12). Serum calcium was measured by atomic absorption spectrophotometry (4), and all other serum and urine chemistries were determined by conventional autoanalyzer techniques.

RESULTS AND DISCUSSION

Serum calcium in the IH group did not differ significantly from the control group throughout the study period (Table 1). Serum phosphate was significantly lower (decreased by 17%) in the IH group prior to phosphate supplementation, but did not differ significantly from the control group at eight weeks of phosphate supplementation.

In the IH group, urine calcium and fractional enteral calcium absorption were significantly elevated prior to phosphate supplementation, but did not differ significantly from the control group at the end of the eight week period.

In the IH group, phosphate treatment decreased serum 1,25-diOHD and increased serum immunoreactive PTH to levels which did not differ significantly from the control group (Table 1). To further document the PTH status of the IH patients during the study, urine cyclic AMP was measured. In the IH group prior to oral phosphate treatment, urine cyclic AMP, expressed per unit of urine creatinine, was significantly lower than that in the control group (Table 1). After eight weeks of oral phosphate treatment, however, urine cyclic AMP in the IH group was slightly, but not significantly, higher than that in the control group. Phosphate treatment produced an increase in urine cyclic AMP in each of the IH patients.

The effects of oral phosphate treatment are also evident when the data from the IH group at 0 and at 8 weeks are compared (Table 1). The latter comparison does not yield differences as great as the comparison of the control and the phosphate-treated IH group; however, all metabolic abnormalities were less at 8 than at 0 weeks, and several of these changes were statistically significant (Table 1).

The results of this study demonstrate that phosphate treatment either partially or completely corrects all of the metabolic abnormalities observed in this group of IH patients, and thus lend

Table 1. Serum, gut and urine parameters in IH patients prior to and at 8 weeks of oral phosphate treatment compared to control subjects.

	Control Group	IH Group Weeks of Oral Phosphate	
		0	8
Serum Ca, mg/dl	9.3±0.3*	9.6±0.4	9.3±0.4
Serum Pi, Mg/dl	3.5±0.4	3.0±0.6**	3.6±0.4¶
Serum 1,25-diOHD, ng/dl	3.4±1.0	4.9±1.6**	4.2±1.3
Serum iPTH, pg/ml	396±87	243±60**	353±96¶
Urine Ca, mg/24h	179±37	315±70**	210±58¶
Fractional Ca absorption, %	27±9	39±11**	34±11
Urine cyclic AMP, μmole/mg creatinine	3.3±0.6	2.5±0.6**	3.7±0.5¶

*Mean±SD
**Significantly different (P<0.05) from the control group.
¶Significantly different (P<0.05) from the IH group at 0 weeks.

further support for our hypothesis that IH is characterized by a state of mild phosphate depletion. We cannot definitely exclude the alternative possibility that phosphate treatment produces a nonspecific ameliorative effect in IH, analogus to the nonspecific therapeutic effect of digitalis in congestive heart failure. The improvement of all of the observed metabolic changes in the IH group by phosphate treatment, however, does not favor this possibility.

In addition, because the serum phosphate level in the IH group during phosphate treatment was obtained 2 h after an oral dose of phosphate, this value represents the maximum level obtained with oral phosphate treatment (unpublished). The integrated level over 24 h was probably lower than suggested by this value, yet the 24 h urine phosphate (2.0±0.5g/24h) was markedly increased on oral phosphate compared to the pretreatment level (1.1±0.2g/24h). The increased excretion of phosphate in the urine indicates that the state of phosphate depletion was not due to defective phosphate absorption from the gut, and is consistent with our concept that the primary defect (or at least the defect which cannot be explained by any of the other metabolic abnormalities) in IH is impaired renal tubular phosphate transport.

According to our hypothesis, the elevated urine calcium is an inherent consequence of the normal hormonal regulatory mechanisms (invoked by a low phosphate stress) which function not only to conserve phosphate but also to prevent excessive elevations of serum calcium (Fig. 1). This concept is supported by the marked increments in urine calcium that occur in normal subjects in response to low enteral phosphate absorption (3).

The above conclusions are based on the metabolic behavior of our IH patients when considered as a group. Based on the patient selection criteria employed, our patients are probably representative of IH patients in general. On the other hand, we cannot exclude the possibility that our group is pathogenically heterogeneous, and that the above conclusions do not hold for each IH patient. Although our study does not address this issue, such a possibility is favored by historical precedent, and has been suggested by otherworkers (13). Notwithstanding, there is *currently insufficient data to establish or refute such heterogeneity.*

ACKNOWLEDGMENTS

This work was supported in part by NIH Grants DE-02600 and HD-04872, and VA supported research, MRIS #0483.

REFERENCES

1. Shen, F., Baylink, D., Nielson, R., Hughes, M, and Haussler, M.: Increased serum 1,25-dihydroxycholecalciferol (1,25-diOHD$_3$) in patients with idiopathic hypercalciuria (IH). Clin. Res. 23:423A, 1975.

2. Shen, F., Baylink, D.J., Nielsen, R.L., Sherrard, D.J., Ivey, J.L., and Haussler, M.R.: Increased serum 1,25-dihydroxyvitamin D in idiopathic hypercalciuria. J Lab. Clin. Med., in press.

3. Dominguez, J.H., Gray, R.W., and Lemann, J., Jr: Dietary phosphate deprivation in women and men: Effects on mineral and acid balances, parathyroid hormone and the metabolism of 25-OH-vitamin D. J. Clin. Endocrinol. Metab. 43:1056, 1976.

4. Chertow, B.S., Baylink, D.J., Wergedal, J.E., Su, M.H.H., and Norman, A.W.: Decrease in serum iPTH in rats and in PTH secretion in vitro by 1,25-dihydroxycholecalciferol. J. Clin. Invest. 56:668, 1975

5. Haussler, M.R., Baylink, D.J., and Hughes, M.R.: The assay of 1α,25-dihydroxyvitamin D_3: Physiologic and pathologic modulation of circulating hormone levels. Clin. Endocrinol. 5:151s, 1976.

6. Baylink, D., Wergedal, J., and Stauffer, M.: Formation, mineralization, and resorption of bone in hypophosphatemic rats. J. Clin. Invest. 50:2519, 1971.

7. Ivey, J.L., Morey, E.R., Liu, C.-C., Rader, J.I. and Baylink, D.J.: Effects of vitamin D and its metabolites on bone. In Vitamin D: Biochemical, Chemical and Clinical Aspects Related to Calcium Metabolism. A.W. Norman, K. Schaefer, J.W. Coburn, H.F. DeLuca, D. Fraser, H.G. Grigoleit, and D.V. Merrath (Editors). de Gruyter. 349, 1977.

8. Ivey, J.L., Su,M., Feist, E., and Baylink, D.J.: Phosphate and vitamin D status on serum PTH in rats. Program and Abstracts of the 59th Annual Meeting of The Endocrine Society. 310, 1977.

9. Amiel, C., Kuntziger, H., Couette, S., Coureau, C., and Bergounioux, N.: Evidence for a parathyroid hormone-independent calcium modulation of phosphate transport along the nephron. J. Clin. Invest. 57:256, 1976.

10. Brumbaugh, P.F., Haussler, D.H., Bursac, K.M., and Haussler, M.R.: Filter assay for 1α,25-dihydroxyvitamin D_3. Utilization of the hormone's target tissue chromatin receptor. Biochemistry. 13:4091, 1974.

11. Gilman, A.G.: A protein binding assay for adenosine 3':5'-cyclic monophosphate. Proc. Natl. Acad. Sci. U.S.A. 67:305, 1970.

12. DeGrazia, J.A., Ivanovich, P., Fellows, H., and Rich, C.: A double isotope method for measurement of intestinal absorpion of calcium in man. J. Lab. Clin. Med. 66:822, 1965.

13. Pak, C.Y.C., Ohata, M., Lawrence, E.C., et al: The hypercalciurias. Causes, parathyroid functions, and diagnostic criteria. J. Clin. Invest. 54:387, 1974.

EVIDENCE FOR A RENAL PO_4 LEAK IN PATIENTS WITH CALCIUM NEPHROLITHIASIS

J. Lemann, Jr., R.W. Gray, and D.R. Wilz

Departments of Medicine and Biochemistry, Medical College of Wisconsin, Milwaukee, Wisconsin, U.S.A.

Patients having recurrent calcium oxalate and/or apatite nephrolithiasis demonstrate hypophosphatemia but normal rates of glomerular filtration and urinary phosphate excretion in comparison to healthy adults without a personal or family history of renal stones. These observations suggest that stone formers have a defect in net renal tubular reabsorption of filtered PO_4. We compared the responses of stone formers and of normal subjects to dietary PO_4 deprivation in order to assess whether the lower serum PO_4 levels in stone formers are the result of a renal PO_4 leak or a resetting of the level at which the kidneys regulate serum PO_4 levels. Nine male stone formers and 13 healthy male adults were studied while eating normal diets and then while eating a liquid diet providing only 2 mmol PO_4/day for 3 days. (Females were not studied because serum PO_4 falls in healthy women deprived of dietary PO_4.) During control, serum PO_4 averaged 1.30 ± 0.06 SE mmol/L in normals and 1.28 ± 0.06 mmol/L in stone formers, values that are not different for these small groups. Control $U_{PO_4}V$ averaged 32.4 ± 1.8 mmol/day in normals and 27.9 ± 2.3 mmol/day in the stone formers. These means are also not significantly different. However, after 3 days of dietary phosphate deprivation, mean serum PO_4 concentrations declined by -0.18 ± 0.04 mmol/L in stone formers ($p < 0.01$) but did not change from control in the normal men (+0.05 ± 0.05 mmol/L; NS). The mean change from control in serum PO_4 concentrations in stone formers was also significantly different from the change in normals ($p < 0.01$). In addition, $U_{PO_4}V$ on the 3rd day of dietary PO_4 deprivation fell to only

4.5 ± 1.0 mmol/day in stone formers, a value significantly higher than that observed in the normal men of 1.8 ± 0.5 mmol/day ($p < 0.02$). The observations that stone formers fail to achieve normal maximum renal PO_4 conservation and demonstrate a fall in serum PO_4 concentration in response to dietary PO_4 deprivation provides further support for the view that these patients have a renal PO_4 leak. The mechanism of such a leak remains to be determined. The suppression of PTH secretion that accompanies dietary PO_4 deprivation in normal subjects could be impaired or delayed among stone formers. Alternatively, stone formers may have a defect in a PTH-independent renal tubular PO_4 transport process.

INADEQUATE BONE RESPONSE TO PHOSPHATE AND VITAMIN D IN FAMILIAL HYPOPHOSPHATEMIC RICKETS (FHR)

F.H. Glorieux, P.J. Bordier, P. Marie, E.E. Delvin and R. Travers.
Genetics Unit, Shriners Hospital, McGill University, Montreal, Canada and Unité de Recherche André Lichtwitz INSERM, Hôpital Lariboisière, Paris, France.

With the almost complete disappearance of vitamin D deficiency in the North-American continent, most cases of rickets now encountered on the pediatric wards may be attributed to one of the several states of vitamin D resistance. The most common of them is familial hypophosphatemic rickets (FHR) a condition usually transmitted as a sex-linked dominant trait. It is characterized by a hypophosphatemia present at birth, bone changes resembling vitamin D deficiency rickets and growth retardation. Bony deformities of the lower limbs are frequent but myopathy is strikingly absent (1).

Recent theories to explain the basic defect in this condition have focused on a primary renal phosphate transport defect (2). The administration of phosphate salts in divided doses and large amounts of vitamin D have been shown to be efficient in correcting the hypophosphatemia during most of the nyctohemeral period and to promote catch-up growth (3). However, although improved, the radiological appearance of the bones is not completely normalized and coarsening of the trabeculation is a persistant finding. Several reports (4, 5, 6) have suggested that a metabolic defect in bone could contribute to the expression of this X-linked mutation. The present study was undertaken to evaluate the effect of current therapeutic approaches on bone in two female patients exibiting the typical features of FHR.

METHODS

The patients were studied on three consecutive occasions. First when untreated, then after a course of phosphate supplementation and finally after combined phosphate and vitamin D therapy.

In each occasion, biochemical parameters were measured from serum and early morning urine collections after an overnight fast. Standard methods were used for measuring calcium, phophorus, creatinine and alkaline phosphatases. 25-hydroxyvitamin D (25-OHD) was measured by radio-ligand assay and parathyroid hormone (PTH) by radioimmunoassay. Tubular reabsorption of phosphate (TmP/GFR) was calculated according to Bijvoet et al (7).

Bone was obtained by transilium trephine biopsy after oral administration of tetracycline 48 and 24 hours before the procedure (15 mg/kg/dose). Repeat biopsy was performed in a contralateral location. Quantitative histology was assessed on undecalcified sections. The parameters measured are listed on the adjacent tables.

RESULTS

All data are assembled in one table for each patient. The respective dosages of phosphate and vitamin D are indicated at the top, as well as the duration of each treatment period. Each vertical column corresponds to one study period.

-Biochemical

These appear in the upper parts of the tables. Normal serum calcium, low serum phosphorus, normal serum 25-OHD and PTH and low TmP/GFR characterize the untreated state (*). Rachitic changes on x-rays examination and growth retardation were also evident. After phosphate supplementation (**), correction of the hypophosphatemia was accompanied by decreased serum calcium and concomitant elevation of serum PTH. A positive effect on growth velocity was also recorded which was maintained during the combined phosphate and vitamin D therapy (***). The latter form of treatment appeared to restore normal serum calcium in both patients while serum PTH was normalized in CO but not in LM. During the two treatment periods the radiological appearance of the metaphyseal areas of the long bones was steadily improving.

-Histological

These are listed in the lower parts of the tables. Prior to any therapy, there was no osteopenia and osteomalacia was evident (osteoid tissue was increased in volume and surface, the extent of the calcification front was greatly reduced). The osteoblastic activity was also diminished. There was no sign of secondary hyperparathyroidsm. Phosphate administration has two striking effects. It stimulates osteoblastic activity: the proportion of osteoid tissue covered by osteoblasts is significantly increased. It also induces osteoclastic activity as a consequence of the secondary hyperparathyroidsm now present. Osteoid surface was decreased in LM but not in CO. In both cases, microradiography elicited mineral deposition distributed in a random fashion in the osteoid.

	Patient CO (Age:2,F)			Norm.
	<—125 days—>	<—171 days—>		
	*	**	***	
Phosphate salts	1.3 g/d —>			
Vit. D_2		25,000 I.U./d —>		
Serum: calcium (mg/dl)	9.6	8.8	9.5	>9.5
phophorus (")	2.5	4.1	2.35	>3.6
alkaline phosphatases (U/L)	875	550	380	<200
25-OHD (ng/ml)	31.6	25.2	70.3	20-30
PTH (μleq/ml)	45	165	50	25-100
TmP/GFR (mg/dl)	2.1	0.48	1.1	2.5-4.2
Height: (cm)	79	82	86	
Bone histomorphometry				
Amount of cancellous bone (% total bone vol.)	27	33.7	33.2	25-35
Amount of osteoid (% canc. bone)	26.8	26.2	20.3	5-8
Osteoid surface (2) (% total bone surf.)	72.4	72.6	60.5	<20
Calcification front (% osteoid surf.)	17.1	17.6	20	67-83
Osteoblastic surface (1) (% total bone surf.)	2.2	10.4	10.3	
Formation index (1)/(2) x 100	0.3	14.7	17	>10
Osteoclast count (no/mm^2)	0.12	0.33	0.23	
Resorption surface (% total bone surf.)	0.6	1.4	0.3	0.5-1.1

	Patient LM (Age:11,F)			
	<—166 days—>	<—165 days—>		Norm.
	*	**	***	
Phosphate salts		3.4 g/d ——————>		
Vit. D_2			50,000 I.U./d ——>	
Serum: calcium (mg/dl)	9.35	8.95	9.3	>9.5
phophorus (")	2.0	3.05	2.6	>3.6
alkaline phosphatases (U/L)	735	660	575	<200
25-OHD (ng/ml)	31.6	22.4	345	20-30
PTH (μleq/ml)	43	168	166	25-100
TmP/GFR (mg/dl)	1.52	0.6	0.9	2.5-4.2
Height: (cm)	121	124.5	129	
Bone histomorphometry				
Amount of cancellous bone (% total bone vol.)	29.6	25.8	32.8	25-35
Amount of osteoid (% canc. bone)	26.8	26.8	26.9	5-8
Osteoid surface (2) (% total bone surf.)	79	67.2	62.9	<20
Calcification front (% osteoid surf.)	12.3	17.3	17.9	67-83
Osteoblastic surface (1) (% total bone surf.)	6.7	9.2	9.5	
Formation index $^{(1)}/_{(2)}$ x 100	8	14	15	>10
Osteoclast count (no/mm^2)	0.1	0.76	1.6	
Resorption surface (% total bone surf.)	0.4	1.9	2.4	0.5-1.1

The calcification front is not significantly increased. Addition of vitamin D to the treatment resulted in a continuation of the osteoblastic hyperactivity, while osteoclastic activity was abated in CO but not in LM. The extent of the calcification front does not make any progress although osteoid surface and volume decrease slowly.

DISCUSSION

The effects of the two treatment schedules on serum biochemistry and growth rate are in line with those already reported (3). The histological findings, however show that bone from FHR patients does not react like bone of vit. D deficient patients similarly treated. In the latter case, it has been reported that the osteoid of patients treated with phosphate alone mineralized in a patchy manner with no formation of a calcification front, whereas vitamin D will rapidly induce the appearance of the normal mineralization process (8). The fact that formation of the calcification front was not promoted in our two FHR patients indicates that the cells responsible for this process may be resistant to the vitamin in the form it was administered. It is therefore conceivable that the transport defect evident in the renal tubular cell may also be present in bone. This would result, in FHR patients, in a genetically determined alteration of the ionic flux between the bone compartment and the extracellular fluid. Variable expressivity of this primary bone defect may explain that hypophosphatemia without bone disease (1) or with bone changes milder than rickets (9) may appear in discrete pedigrees.

REFERENCES

1. Winters, R.W., Graham, J.B., Williams, T.F., McFalls, V.W. and Burnett, C.M.: A genetic study of familial hypophosphatemia and vitamin D resistant rickets with a review of the literature. Medicine 37:97-142, 1958.

2. Glorieux, F.H. and Scriver, C.R.: Loss of a parathyroid hormone sensitive component of phosphate transport in X-linked hypophosphatemia. Science 175:997-1000, 1972.

3. Glorieux, F.H., Scriver, C.R., Reade, T.M., Goldman, H. and Roseborough, A.: Use of phosphate and vitamin D to prevent dwarfism and rickets in X-linked hypophosphatemia. New England J. of Med. 287:481-487, 1972.

4. Steendijk,R., van der Hooff, A., Niebsen, H.K.L. and Dowsey, J.: Lesion of the bone matrix in vitamin-D resistant rickets. Nature 207:426-427, 1965.

5. Steendijk,R. and Boyde, A.: Scanning electron microscopic observations on bone from patients with hypophosphatemic (vitamin D resistant) rickets. Calc. Tiss. Res. 11:242-250, 1973.

6. Frame, B., Arnstein, A.R., Frost, H.M. and Smith, R.W.: Resistant osteomalacia. Am. J. Med. 38:134-144, 1965.

7. Bijvoet, O.L.M., Morgan, D.B. and Fourman, P.: The assessment of phosphate reabsorption. Clin. Chim. Acta 26:15-24, 1969.

8. Bordier, P., Tun-Chot, S., Martin, J., Queillé, M.L. and Hioco, D.J: Mineralisation du tissu osteoide chez l'ostéomalacique induite par surcharge phosphorée ou par la vitamine D_3 In phosphate et métabolisme phosphocalcique. D. Hioco, Ed. Paris, Editions Sandoz 79-88, 1971.

9. Scriver, C.R., MacDonald, W., Reade, T.M., Glorieux, F.H. and Nogrady, B.: Hypophosphatemic non-rachitic bone disease; an entity distinct from X-linked hypophosphatemia in the renal defect bone involvement and inheritance. Amer. J. of Human Genetics. In press.

Supported by the Shriners of North America.

RENAL HANDLING OF PHOSPHATE IN VERY LOW BIRTHWEIGHT (VLBW) INFANTS (<1.3 kg): EFFECTS OF CALCIUM AND SODIUM INTAKE

I.C. Radde, R.F. Cifuentes, and G.W. Chance

Research Institute, Div. Perinatology & Endocrinology

The Hospital for Sick Children, Toronto, Canada

INTRODUCTION

In an extensive study of mineral requirements of very low birthweight (VLBW) infants we have examined in detail various aspects of phosphorus (P)-homeostasis, such as the effect of a higher (by 50%) P-intake on the renal clearance of phosphorus (C_P) and various indices of parathyroid function. This report deals with the effects of various intakes of calcium (ranging from 100 to 250 mg/kg/24 h) and of sodium (1.5 and 3.0 mEq/kg/24 h) on the C_P and urinary excretion of P (UP) in rapidly growing VLBW infants. The purpose of the study was to determine the C_P in infants (a) on a prolonged "low" Ca intake (100 mg/kg/24 h); (b) the effect of calcium supplementation to a total daily Ca-intake of 175, 210, or 250 mg/kg; and (c) the effect of Na-supplementation.

MATERIALS AND METHODS

The experimental protocol was as follows: birthweight of all infants was less than 1.3 kg and the infants were either pair- or group-matched according to birthweight and gestational age at birth into appropriate (AGA) or small for gestational age (SGA) infants. The infants entered the study at an age two to three weeks when they were able to tolerate at least 80% of the intended formula intake, which was either 200 ml/kg/24 h at 80 Kcal/dl (Groups 1-3, and 5 infants of Group 5) or 150 ml/kg/24 h at 100 Kcal/dl (Group 4 and 9 infants of Group 5). Infants were fed by gavage 2-hourly until they weighed approximately 1.5 kg and thereafter 3-hourly. They were nursed in incubators in an optimal thermal environment (1).

The daily intake per kg bodyweight from formula was: 100 mg Ca; 80 mg P, giving a Ca/P ratio of 1.25:1; 1.5 mEq Na and 2.5 μg vitamin D.

All infants, except those in Group 2 were supplemented with calcium lactate (100 mg/ml) in divided doses. Infants in Group 1 and 5 were also supplemented with Na to a total intake of 3 mEq/kg/24 h. This Na-supplement was in the form of $NaHCO_3$. All infants also received a vitamin supplement containing 12.5 μg of vitamin D in the daily dose.

Intake and output in urine and feces were measured weekly or every second week in all infants depending on the growth rate of the babies. Plasma samples were obtained at weekly intervals. Inorganic P concentrations were determined by an automated adaptation of the Gomori method (2) and Na concentrations by standard flame spectrophotometric techniques.

RESULTS

Patient Groups

Data on five groups of patients are included (Table I). Group 1 served as the control group with a Ca/P intake ratio of 2.6:1 (Ca 210 mg/200 ml, P 80 mg/200 ml). In this group the highest net retention rates of P were observed in the patients studied so far.

Table I

Group	n	Ca Intake mg/kg/24 h	P Intake mg/kg/24 h	Ca:P Intake	Na Intake mEq/kg/24 h
1	17	210	80	2.6:1	3
2	15	100	80	1.2:1	1.5
3	14	100→250	80	3.1:1	1.5
4	8	175	80	2.2:1	1.5
5	14	175	80	2.2:1	1.5→3

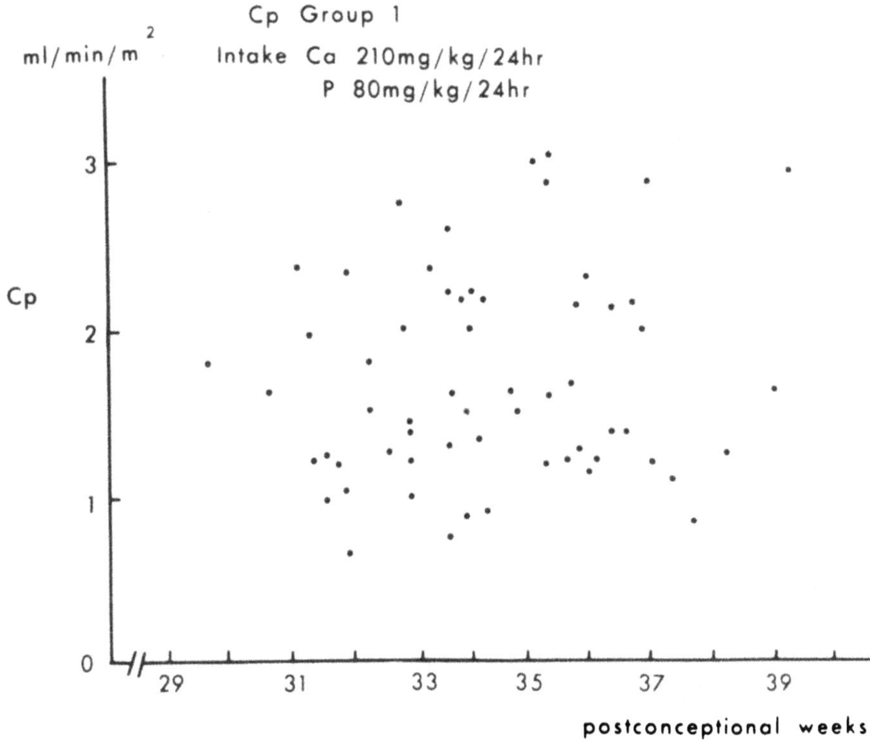

Fig. 1: Effect of postconceptional age (weeks) on C_P in Group 1

Age and C_P

On Figure 1, the C_P (ml/min/m^2) of infants in Group 1 has been plotted against the postconceptional age. No correlation was found between these two values. Figure 2 shows a plot of C_P against postnatal age in these same babies. There was a highly significant correlation between these two values and an increase in C_P with increasing postnatal age was noted until the infants were 42 days of age. Thereafter the C_P did not increase further. Plasma inorganic P decreased significantly with postnatal age in infants of Group 1.

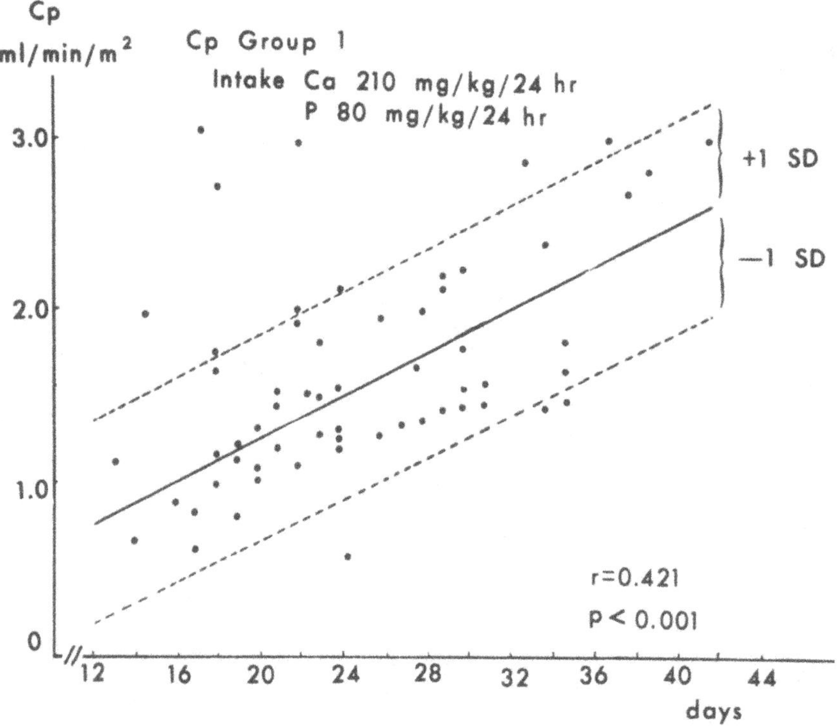

Fig. 2: Effect of postnatal age (days) on C_P in Group 1

Prolonged "Low" Ca Intake

The effect of prolonged (i.e. three to five weeks duration) relatively low calcium intake in infants of Group 2 on the Cp is depicted on Fig. 3. The Cp in these infants is two to four times as high as those of Group 1 at the same postnatal age and there is little age-related change until 42 days of age. Plasma inorganic P did not differ from values observed in Group 1. These infants developed skeletal demineralization on radiographs of long bones but no hypocalcemia. Their Ca accretion rate was considerably below that of the intrauterine accretion rate at the same post-conceptional age, i.e. 60 vs. 140 mg/kg/24 h. After 42 days of age, the Cp decreased significantly in Group 2 ($p<0.01$).

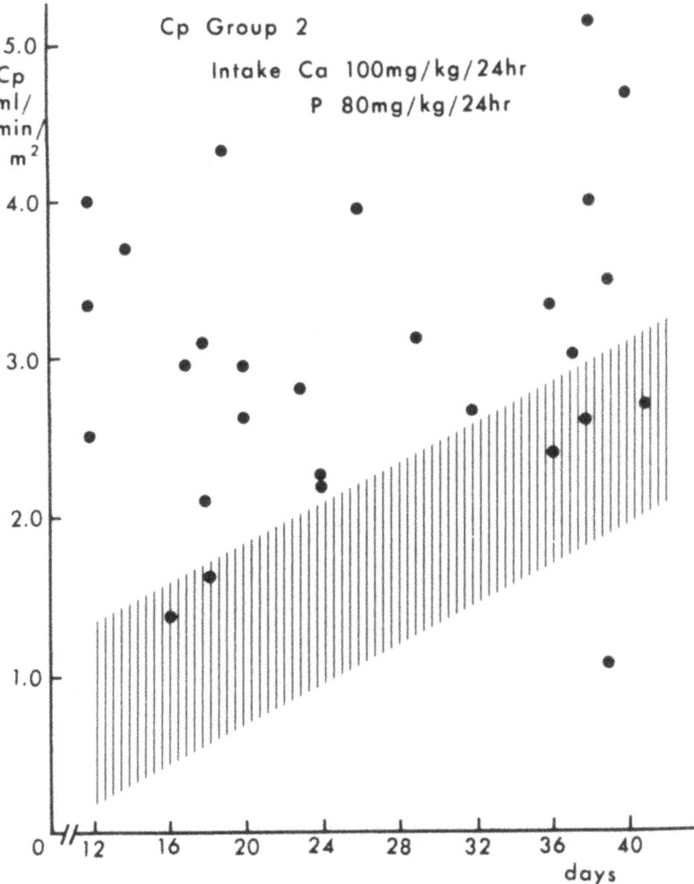

Fig. 3: C_P in Group 2 on "low" calcium intake. The shaded area indicates mean $\pm$ 1 SD of Group 1.

Effect of Ca Supplementation

Infants in Group 3 were supplemented with Ca to a total intake of 250 mg/kg/24 h after an initial urine and blood collection had been done while not supplemented with Ca. Figure 4 shows that the initial C_P was similar to that of Group 2, i.e. approximately twice as high as that of Group 1 at a similar postnatal age. With Ca

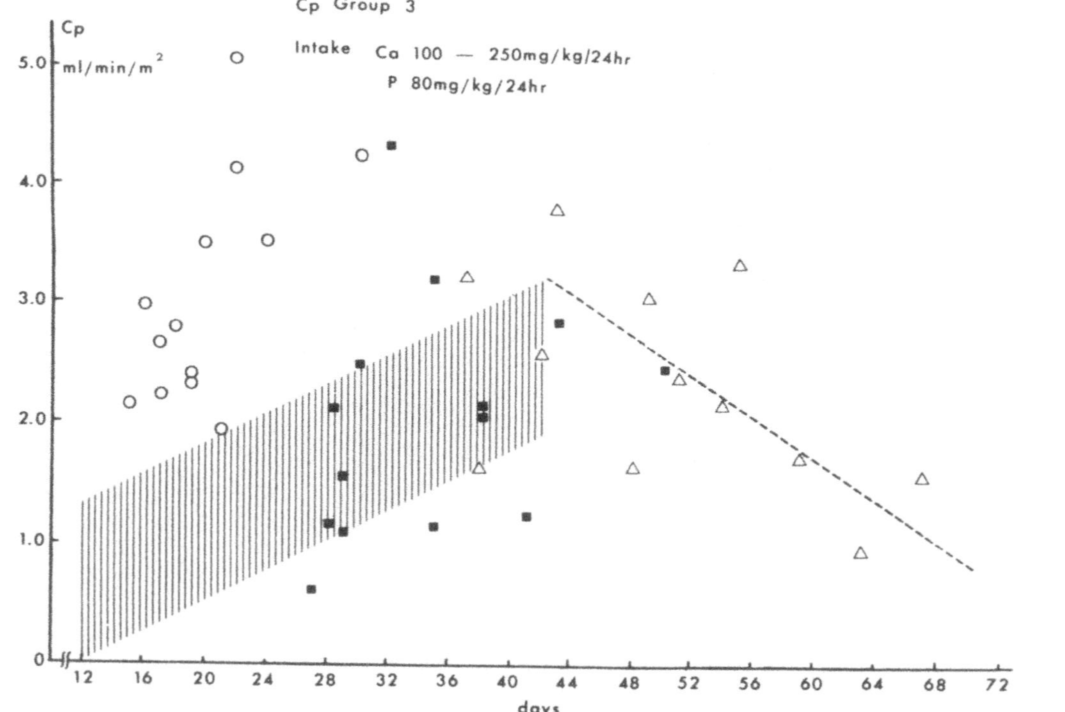

Fig. 4: Cp in Group 3. ○ = calcium intake of 100 mg/kg/24 h; ■ = calcium intake 250 mg/kg/24 h; for one to two weeks; Δ = calcium intake 250 mg/kg/24 h for three to four weeks. Regression line for collections after 42 days of age ($y = -0.073x + 6.223$, $r = 0.687$). The shaded area indicates mean $\pm$ 1 SD of Group 1 before 42 days of age.

supplementation the C_P decreased significantly ($p<0.02$). Most of the values were in the range observed in Group 1 at similar postnatal age although the Ca intake in Group 1 was somewhat lower (210 mg/kg/24 h). After the age of 42 days, there was a further progressive decline in the C_P in infants of Group 3, with a significant negative correlation between age and C_P ($p<0.01$). Thus, the C_P did not differ between infants fed 210 and those fed 250 mg/kg/24 h. Infants whose Ca intake was 175 mg/kg/24 h (Groups 4 and 5) showed C_P values similar to those of Group 2 at the same postnatal age (Table II).

Effect of Na-Supplementation

The C_P was compared between Groups 1+5 (supplemented with Na to a total intake of 3 mEq/kg/24 h) and Groups 3+4 (total Na-intake 1.5 mEq/kg/24 h). No significant differences in C_P were seen between the two groups when postnatal age was taken into consideration. When, however, the Ca intake was taken into consideration, Groups 3 and 4 (both not supplemented with Na, but with different Ca intakes) differed significantly.

Table II

Clearance of P: Effect of Ca, Na, and Age (m$\pm$SEm)

	Ca/Na	Age (days)	C_P
Group 3	250/1.5	42.4 $\pm$ 2.3	2.19 $\pm$ 0.18
Group 4	175/1.5	25.1 $\pm$ 2.8	2.93 $\pm$ 0.23
Group 5	175/3.0	37.1 $\pm$ 2.7	3.06 $\pm$ 0.36

There was no significant correlation between the urinary excretion of P and that of Na in either the non-supplemented or the Na-supplemented groups.

DISCUSSION

As McCrory (3) and Edelmann and his group (4,5) have pointed out it is postnatal age rather than postconceptional age which influences the degree of change in renal function of premature infants. Our results concerning the renal clearance of P are in agreement with this view. In Ca-supplemented infants with a daily total Ca intake of more than 200 mg/kg, we found an increase in the C_P with postnatal age until 6 weeks of age. This may be related to the increasing glomerular filtration rate and, therefore, to the increase in the filtered load of P. In a small series of ten VLBW infants reported elsewhere (6), we found a highly significant correlation between the glomerular filtration rate, as measured by the endogenous creatinine clearance, and the postnatal age. After the infants in the present series reached 6 weeks of age the C_P seemed to remain unchanged or even to decrease.

At approximately 36 weeks postconceptional age, new nephron formation ceases in the human fetus (7). In a previous study of the Na requirements of VLBW infants (8), we found improved Na-retention approximately at this age. Thus, we had expected a concomitant change in urinary excretion of P in the present study at this postconceptional age but failed to do so. Although the urinary excretion of P and Na are said to be closely related (9), we did not observe any increase in C_P with the change-over from a Na-intake of 1.5 to one of 3 mEq/kg/24 h.

Intestinal absorption, urinary excretion and net retention rates of Ca and P are said to be dependent on the intake ratio of these two elements (10,11). Other investigators (12) found no such relationship in humans unless the Ca or P intake was either very low or very high. In our present study the C_P seemed to be inversely correlated with the absolute amount of Ca ingested. Since the P-intake was constant in the five groups, the Ca:P changed directly with the calcium intake. Amiel *et al.* (13) observed effects of a calcium infusion on P excretion in thyroparathyroidectomized animals. They concluded that this action was a direct one and not necessarily mediated by cyclic AMP.

SUMMARY

Five patient groups of VLBW infants with the same P-intake but varying Ca and Na intake were examined as to their urinary excretion of P and Na and on their renal clearance of P. The effect of increasing the Na intake from 1.5 to 3 mEq/kg/24 h on C_P was also examined.

In the control group of infants with an intake of 210 mg Ca and 80 mg P/kg/24 h, the C_P was significantly correlated with postnatal, but not postconceptional age.

A relatively low Ca intake of 100 mg/kg/24 h led to age-related values two to three times as high, whereas Ca supplementation to a total intake of 250 mg/kg/24 h decreased the C_P significantly. A Ca intake of 175 mg/kg/24 h led to C_P similar to those seen with one of 100 mg/kg/24 h.

Changing the Na intake from 1.5 to 3 mEq/kg/24 h did not influence the C_P. There was no correlation between UP and UNa in any of the patient groups examined.

ACKNOWLEDGEMENTS

This work was supported in part by the Medical Research Council of Canada (Grant MA 4635).

REFERENCES

1. Hey,E.: Thermal neutrality. Br.Med.Bull. 31:69-74 (1975).

2. Gomori,G.: A modification of the colorimetric phosphorus determination for use with the photoelectric colorimeter. J. Lab. Clin. Med. 27: 955 (1942).

3. McCrory,W.W.: Developmental Nephrology. Harvard University Press, Cambridge, Mass. (1972).

4. Edelmann,C.M., Jr.,and Spitzer,A. J. Pediat. 75: 509-519 (1969). The maturing kidney. A modern view of well-balanced infants with imbalanced nephrons.

5. Nash,M.A. and Edelmann,C.M., Jr. Nephron 11: 71-90 (1973).The developing kidney. Immature function or inappropriate standard?

6. Cifuentes,R.F., Radde,I.C., Chance,G.W. Programme 6th Parathyroid Conference Vancouver, Canada, 1977,p.144.(Abstract). Phosphate handling in very low birthweight (VLBW) infants (<1.3 kg).

7. Potter,E.L. and Thierstein,S.T. J. Pediat. 22: 695 (1943). Glomerular development in the kidney as an index of fetal maturity.

8. Roy,R., Chance G.W.,Radde,I.C.,Hill,D.E.,Willis,D.M.,and Sheepers,J.: Pediat.Res. 10: 526-531 (1976). Late hyponatremia in very low birthweight (VLBW) infants (< 1.3 kg).

9. Schneider,E.G., Strandhoy,J.W., Willis,L.R. and Knox,F.G.: Kidney Int. 4: 369 (1973). Relationship between proximal sodium reabsorption and excretion of calcium,magnesium and phosphate.

10. Schryner,H.F., Hintz,H.F. and Craig,P.H.: J. Nutr. 101: 1257 (1971). Phosphorus metabolism in ponies fed varying levels of phosphorus.

11. Clark,I.: Am.J. Physiol. 217:871 (1969). Metabolic interrelations of calcium, magnesium and phosphate.

12. Hövels,O., Thilenius,O.G.,and Krafczyk,S.: Z. Kinderheilk. 83: 508 (1960). Untersuchungen Zum Calcium - und Phosphatstoffwechsel Frühgeborener .I. Der Einfluss des Angebotes, der Grundnahrung und des Calciumphosphorquotienten der Zufuhr auf die Calciumretention.

13. Amiel,C., Kuntziger,H., Couette,S., Coureau,C., and Bergounioux,N.:J. Clin. Invest. 57: 256-263 (1976). Evidence for a parathyroid hormone-independent calcium modulation of phosphate transport along the nephron.

ENDOCRINE REGULATION OF PLASMA PHOSPHATE IN SHEEP FETUSES WITH CATHETERS IMPLANTED IN UTERO

J.P. Barlet, Marie-Jeanne Davicco, J. Lefaivre and J.M. Garel*
I.N.R.A., Theix, F-63110 Beaumont
*Physiologie du Développement, Université P. et M. Curie, Paris.

Before term, in rodents (1, 2), ruminants (3, 4, 5, 6) and humans (7), phosphatemia is higher in the fetus than in the mother. This difference of concentration between both sides of the placenta is poorly understood. In rats, it has been demonstrated that the placental transfer of ^{32}P increased between the 19th day of gestation and term (1). In the same time fetal phosphatemia increased from 8.75 to 9.97 mg/dl (2). Calcitonin injection in fetal rats (8) and in fetal monkeys (9) induced a significant hypocalcemia and hypophosphatemia in the fetus. In rat fetuses treated with parathyroid extract intravenously or subcutaneously calcemia was increased while phosphatemia was lower than in fetuses injected with the vehicle alone (10). In acute preparations of sheep fetuses, the intravenous infusion of parathyroid extract (0.1 I.U./kg/mn during 1 hr) increased promptly and significantly the renal phosphate-glomerular filtration rate clearance ratio , while the glomerular filtration rate, serum calcium, serum phosphate and filtered load of phosphate did not change significantly (4). In fact the endocrine regulation of fetal phosphatemia remains obscure.The purpose of this investigation was to study the effects of calcitonin, parathyroid hormone, 1α-hydroxycholecalciferol and 5,6 trans-25 hydroxycholecalciferol, injected intravenously in unstressed fetal lambs, on fetal and maternal phosphatemia, calcemia and magnesemia.

MATERIALS AND METHODS

Animals. Limousine ewes, weighing 56 ± 3 kg, of known gestational age, mated with a Romanov ram, were used. In the

Limousine breed, the length of gestation is 155 days. Ewes bearing twin lambs were selected by radiography performed on the 80th day of gestation. During the experimental period each ewe was housed in an individual stall and fed daily 800 g luzerne hay and 200 g grain concentrate. They were starved for 16 hrs before surgery.

Surgery. Catheters were implanted in utero in sheep fetuses according to the method described by Mellor and Matheson (11). After laparotomy of the mother under halothane anesthesia at 90-110 days of gestation the pregnant uterine horn was exposed. A 2 cm incision was made in the uterus in the area of the neck of each fetus. The carotid artery and the jugular vein on one side were isolated and sterile polyvinyl catheters were fitted. Hormonal injections were done through the catheter implanted in the jugular vein and blood withdrawn through the catheter implanted in the carotid artery. Each catheter, in which the volume had been exactly measured, was filled with heparinized sterile 0.9 % NaCl. Then it was passed laterally under the skin and emerged about 30 cm from the incision which was closed with nylon suture. About 5 cm of each catheter was allowed to protrude from the skin and protected by a bandage passed around the abdomen of the ewe.

Blood samples were withdrawn under sterile conditions to minimize the risk of infection for the fetus. In this way 31 of the 34 chronically implanted catheters allowed to collect fetal blood from the 110th day of gestation until birth. The mean body weight at birth was similar in the 31 catheterized lambs (2.9 $\pm$ 0.3 kg) and in 30 unoperated controls (3.2 $\pm$ 0.1 kg).

Maternal blood samples were collected through a catheter implanted in the carotid artery of the ewe which had been anesthetized for fetal surgery.

Hormonal injections. Ewes bearing only twin lambs were selected for hormonal injections. One of the twin fetuses was injected between the 125th and the 135th day of gestation, the second was used as a control and injected simultaneously with the same volume of vehicle alone. In these experiments, it was shown that the fetal hematocrit did not change during the period of blood sampling.

1°) Three groups of 4 fetuses were injected either with purified porcine calcitonin (pCT ; Calcitar, Armour-Montagu ; 100 MRC mU/fetus) or with synthetic salmon calcitonin (sCT ; Armour-Montagu, lot K 600030 C-3 ; 100 MRC mU/fetus), or with synthetic 1-34 bovine parathyroid hormone (bPTH ; Beckman ; 200 IU/fetus). Each dose of pCT, sCT and bPTH was dissolved in 0.5 ml NaCl 0.9 % . To study the influence of synthetic analogs to 1,25 dihydroxycholecalciferol (1,25 diOHCC) on fetal calcemia and phosphatemia two groups of 4 fetuses were injected either with 5,6 trans-25-hydroxycholecalciferol (5,6 trans-25 OHCC ; RU 21016 : Roussel Laboratories ; 1 μg/fetus) or with 1α-hydroxycholecalciferol (1α-OHCC ; Leo Laboratories ; 0.1 μg/fetus). Each dose of 5,6 trans-25 OHCC and 1 α-OHCC was dissolved in 0.3 ml propylene glycol.

2°) To study the possible transplacental effects of active cholecalciferol metabolites four pregnant ewes with catheterized fetuses (3 bearing single lambs and 1 bearing triplets) were intravenously injected with 1α-OHCC (0.1 μg/kg body weight, dissolved in 0.2 ml propylene glycol). Three control ewes bearing single lambs were injected with the same volume of vehicle.

Blood analysis. After centrifugation, plasma phosphate level was measured by colorimetry (Technicon Autoanalyser) ; total plasma calcium and magnesium were measured by atomic absorption spectrophotometry (Perkin-Elmer 400). In some experiments fetal and maternal whole blood ionized calcium were measured using a calcium electrode (Orion SS-20).

RESULTS

During the 40 days before term, phosphatemia and calcemia in 30 sheep fetuses were always significantly higher than in the 19 mothers (11 bearing a single lamb, 5 with twin lambs and 3 with triplets). Similarly the whole blood ionized calcium level was higher in the fetuses than in the mother. Fetal plasma magnesium levels were also significantly higher than those found in the mother between 40 and 26 days before parturition, then this difference disappeared until birth. Any significant variation of these parameters occurred during the last 40 days of gestation neither in fetal nor in maternal arterial plasmas (fig. 1). Mean plasma phosphate and calcium levels tended to be lower in triplets (6.70 ± 0.28 mg/dl and 10.87 ± 0.13 mg/dl respectively) than in single lambs (7.11 ± 0.19 mg/dl and 11.09 ± 0.18 mg/dl respectively) but this difference was not statistically significant.

In the 4 fetuses injected with pCT a slight but significant hypophosphatemia and hypocalcemia occurred already after 30 mn and reached a nadir 60 mn after injection ($\Delta P = -0.64 \pm 0.11$ mg/dl , $P < 0.01$; $\Delta Ca = -0.42 \pm 0.07$ mg/dl , $P < 0.01$). No significant difference was observed between treated and control lambs at 180 mn (Fig. 2). sCT induced a more intense and more long lasting hypophosphatemia and hypocalcemia than pCT ($\Delta P = -0.92 \pm 0.14$ mg/dl, $P < 0.01$; $\Delta Ca = -1.09 \pm 0.26$ mg/dl, $P < 0.01$ 150 mn after injection) (Fig. 2). No significant effect was observed on maternal phosphatemia and calcemia in ewes when the fetuses were injected with pCT or sCT.

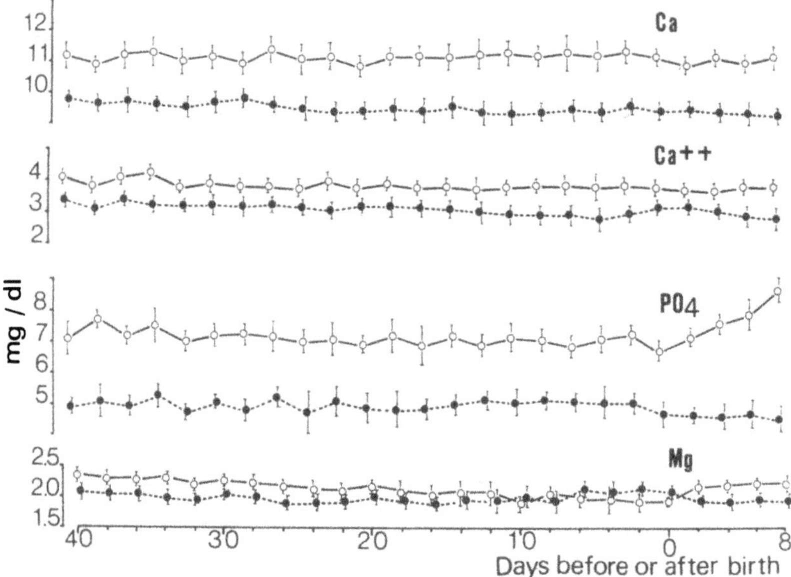

Fig. 1 : Plasma concentrations of calcium (Ca), phosphate (PO_4), magnesium (Mg) and whole blood ionized calcium (Ca^{++}) levels in 19 ewes (●------●) and their fetuses (○——○) during the last 40 days of gestation.

In 4 fetuses bPTH induced a significant hypophosphatemia ($\Delta P = -1.95 \pm 0.27$ mg/dl, $P < 0.01$ 180 mn after injection). The calcemia of these fetuses was slightly but significantly decreased 30 mn after injection (Fig. 3) and then rose up to 12.76 ± 0.36 mg/dl ($P < 0.01$) 150 mn later. No significant effect was observed on maternal calcemia or phosphatemia (Fig. 3).

At the doses used, bPTH, pCT and sCT had no significant effect either on fetal or maternal magnesemia.

In 4 fetuses 5,6 trans-25 OHCC had no significant effect on plasma phosphate, calcium, magnesium and whole blood ionized calcium levels during 72hrs after injection. Neither it has any effect on maternal plasma levels of these parameters.

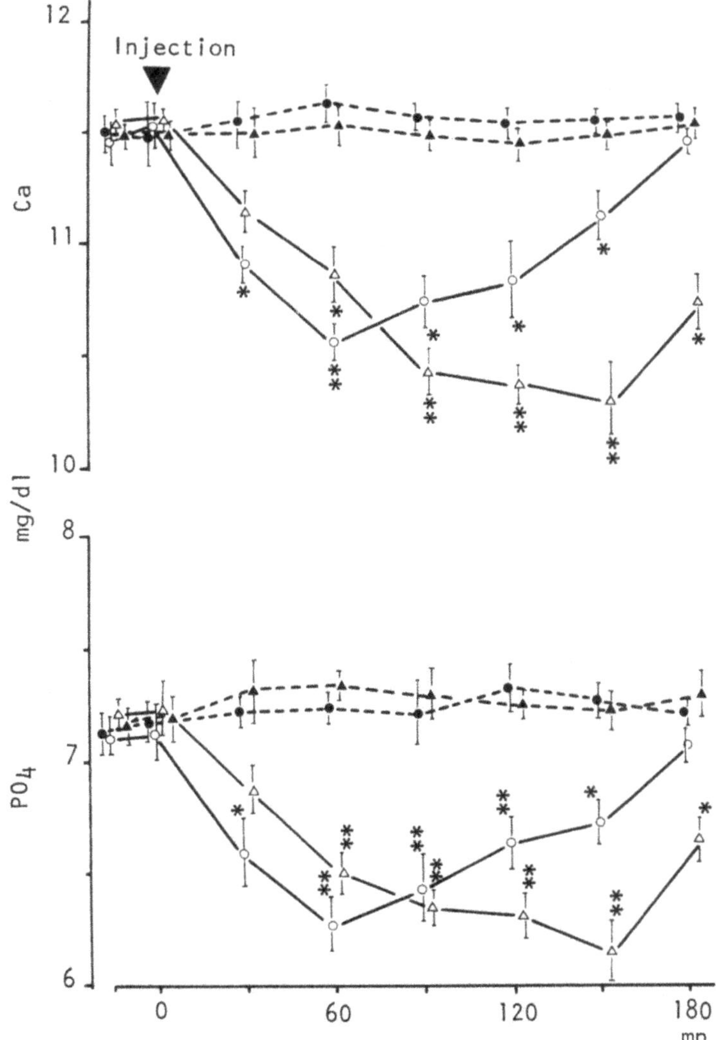

Fig. 2 : Plasma concentrations of calcium (Ca) and phosphate (PO_4) in fetuses injected with pCT (treated○——○; controls●– – – –●) or with sCT (treated△——△; controls▲– – –▲). Student's t test was used to compare treated and control animals (* $P < 0.05$; ** $P < 0.01$).

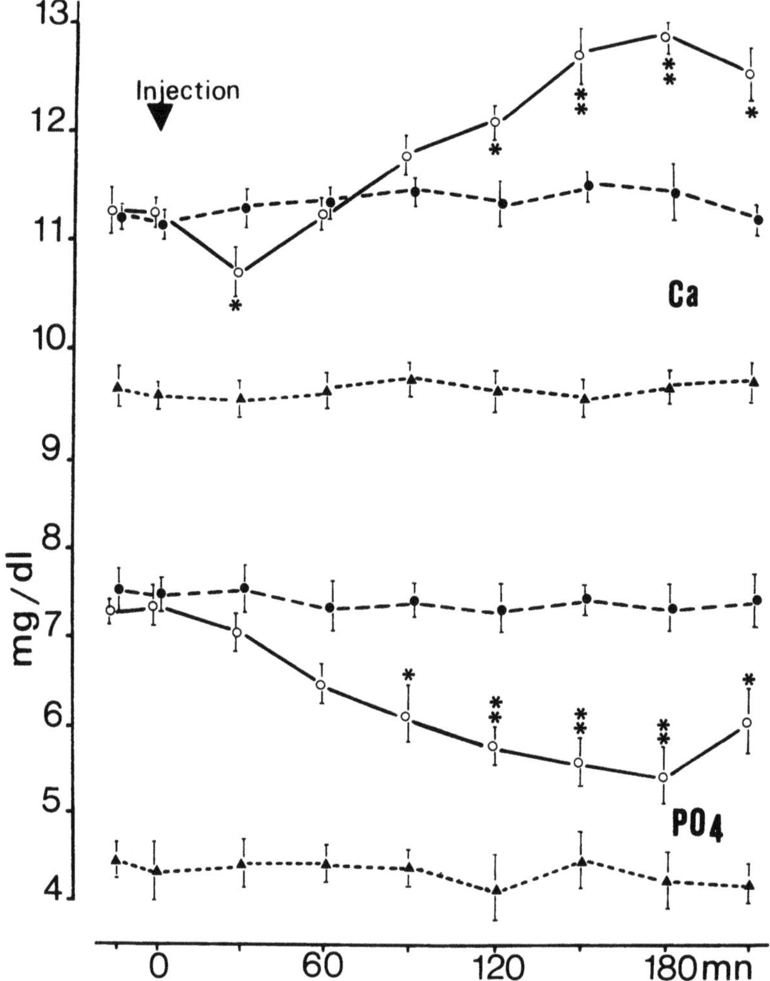

Fig. 3 : Plasma concentrations of calcium (Ca) and phosphate (PO_4) in fetuses injected with bPTH : treated :○——○; controls : ●— — —●; mothers :▲------▲. Student's t test was used to compare treated and control fetuses (* $P < 0.05$; ** $P < 0.01$).

In 4 fetuses 1α-OHCC increased significantly the fetal phosphatemia, calcemia and fetal whole blood ionized calcium level, the rise was maximum 48 hrs after injection. It has no significant effect on maternal plasma (Fig. 4). Fetal magnesemia was slightly but not significantly decreased during 72hrs after injection.

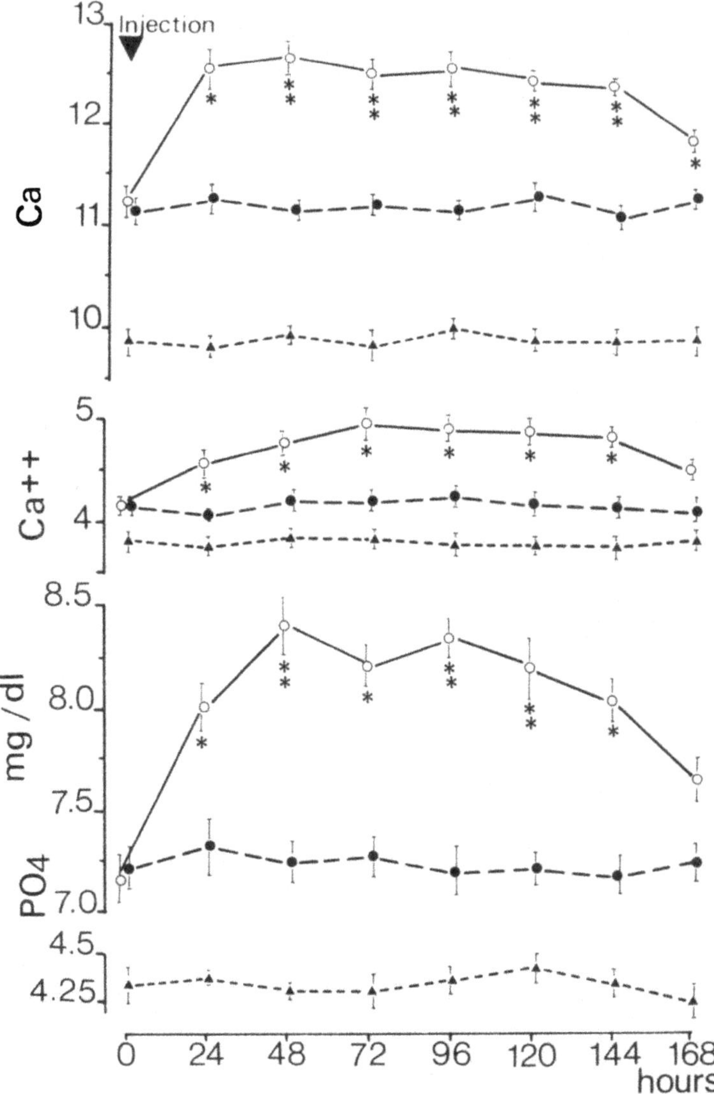

Fig. 4 : Plasma concentrations of calcium (Ca), phosphate (PO_4) in fetuses injected with 1α-OHCC:treated :○———○; controls :●— —●; mothers :▲- - - -▲. Student's t test was used to compare treated and control fetuses (* $P < 0.05$; ** $P < 0.01$).

In 4 ewes injected intravenously with 1α-OHCC a significant hyperphosphatemia and hypercalcemia occurred 12 hrs after injection and persisted during 120 hrs. In the 6 fetuses a significant hyperphosphatemia and hypercalcemia occurred from the 24th until the 96th hour following maternal injection (Fig. 5). Neither maternal nor fetal magnesemia was significantly changed.

DISCUSSION

It has been already reported in sheep fetuses that plasma concentrations of total and ultrafiltrable calcium were higher in the fetus than in the mother (12, 13). This was confirmed here using unstressed sheep fetuses since whole blood ionized calcium, plasma phosphate and magnesium levels were higher in the fetus than in the mother (Fig. 1). These differences between the fetus and dam were probably the result of active transports of ionized calcium, phosphate and magnesium across the placenta, according to a one-way process from the mother to the fetus (14, 15).

Subcutaneous injection of pCT (8 MRC mU/g body weight) decreased the plasma calcium concentration in rat fetuses older than 19.5 days (8) ; a larger dose (140 MRC mU/g body weight) of sCT must be given to decrease fetal plasma magnesium level (16). Preliminary experiments have shown in pig fetuses that pCT injected intravenously did not change plasma calcium (17). However, in Rhesus monkeys fetuses sCT produced a triphasic response in fetal plasma calcium concentration consisting of a prompt initial drop followed by a return to or above the baseline and then a more gradual decline (9). This effect on calcemia remains doubtful in the absence of control fetuses in this acute preparation. In growing mammals CT exerts its hypocalcemic and hypophosphatemic effects by inhibiting bone resorption and increasing urinary phosphate excretion (18). In sheep fetus the rate of calcium transfer from dam to fetus is equal to that of fetal bone accretion, indicating that bone resorption is low in sheep fetuses (15, 19). Since fetal hormones are probably not involved in the control of the placental transfer of calcium (20), the slight hypocalcemic effect of CT in fetal lambs might be due to a decrease in bone resorption or to an increase in bone accretion.

In our experimental conditions bPTH injected into sheep fetuses induced a biphasic response in fetal calcemia : a slight and transient hypocalcemia -probably the result of an increased bone accretion (21)- followed by hypercalcemia -probably the result of an increased bone resorption (18)-. Since we have not measured urinary phosphate excretion, definite conclusions concerning the renal effects of CT and PTH in sheep fetuses cannot be drawn. However, the hypophosphatemic effect of synthetic bPTH was

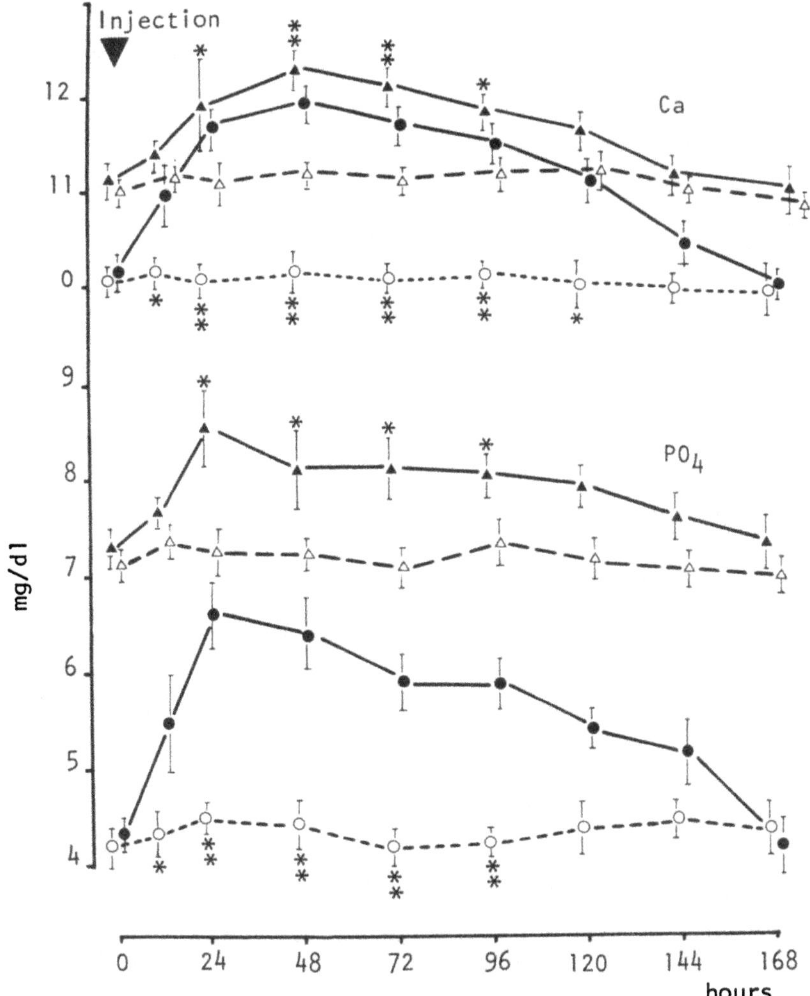

Fig. 5 : Plasma concentrations of calcium (Ca) and phosphate (PO_4) in four ewes injected with 1α-OHCC (●——●) and their six fetuses (▲——▲) and three control ewes (○- - -○) and their three fetuses (△— —△). Student's t test was used to compare treated and control ewes, and fetuses from treated and from control ewes. (* $P < 0.05$; ** $P < 0.01$).

in agreement with the increased renal phosphate excretion after parathyroid extract injection in sheep fetuses (4, 22).

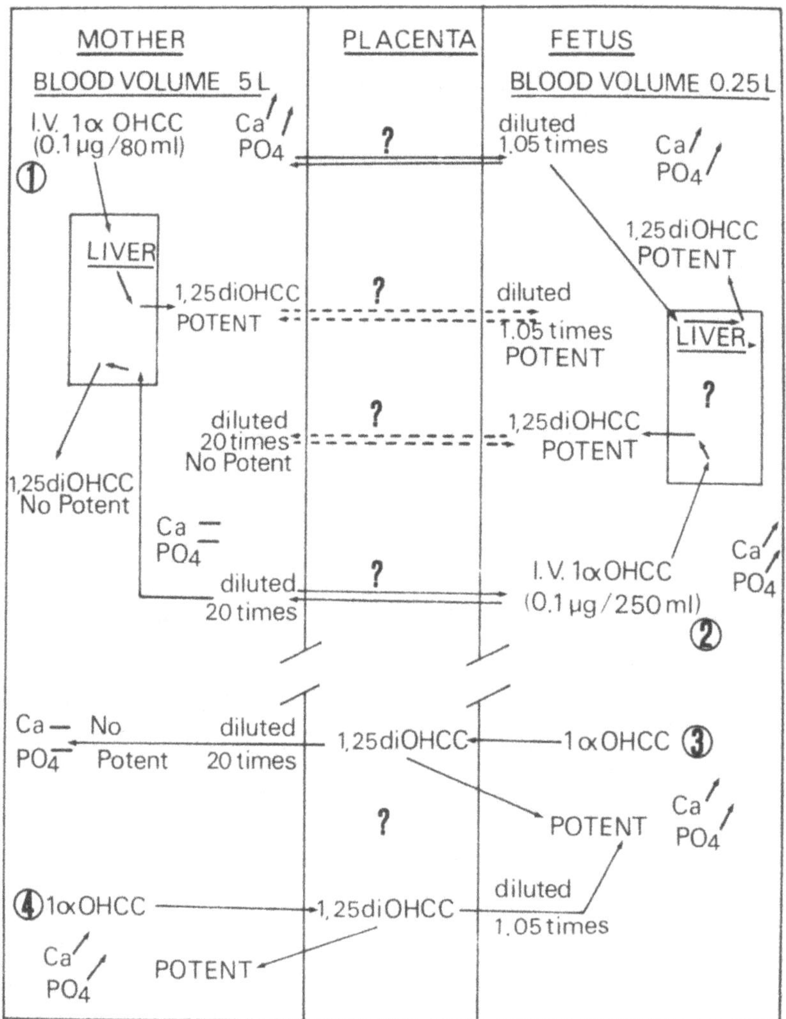

Fig. 6 : Tentative schedule to explain the mode of action of 1α-OHCC injected into the mother on fetal calcemia and phosphatemia and the lack of effect of 1α-OHCC on maternal calcemia and phosphatemia when this metabolite was injected to the fetus

- 1α-OHCC injected into the mother and hydroxylated into 1,25 di-OHCC in the maternal and (or) fetal liver ①
- 1α-OHCC injected into the fetus and hydroxylated into 1,25 di-OHCC in the fetal and (or) maternal liver ②
- 1α-OHCC injected into the fetus ③ or the mother ④ and hydroxylated into 1,25 di-OHCC in the placenta.

The lack of effect of 5,6 trans-25 OHCC on fetal calcemia and phosphatemia can be easily understood since it has been demonstrated that 5,6 trans-25 OHCC increased plasma calcium by stimulating calcium intestinal absorption (23).

When injected into ewes, 1α-OHCC induced hypercalcemia and hyperphosphatemia not only in the mother but also in the fetus (Fig. 5). It is well known that in rats, 1α-OHCC is rapidly metabolized into 1,25 diOHCC (24). Since maternal hypercalcemia in ewes does not affect fetal plasma calcium level (12, 25), our results suggest that 1α-OHCC injected into ewes could be metabolized into 1,25 diOHCC in the maternal liver. Subsquently 1,25 diOHCC might cross the placenta and act in the fetuses (Fig. 6); during the last month of gestation plasma 25-hydroxycholecalciferol levels in sheep fetuses seem relatively dependent upon maternal plasma 25-hydroxycholecalciferol levels (26). Another possibility would be that 1α-OHCC might cross the placenta and be metabolized into 1,25 diOHCC in the fetal liver. These two hypothesis would explain the fetal hypercalcemia and hyperphosphatemia when 1α-OHCC was injected into the mother (Fig. 6). They also may explain the absence of changes in maternal calcemia and phosphatemia when sheep fetuses were injected with 1α-OHCC, since this dose (0.1 μg) will be diluted 20 times in maternal blood after crossing the placenta (Fig. 6). If fetal liver converts 1α-OHCC into 1,25 diOHCC, this metabolite will be also diluted 20 times in maternal blood after crossing the placenta (Fig. 6). In these conditions it would be easy to understand that fetal injection of 1α-OHCC induced hypercalcemia and hyperphosphatemia in the fetus but no change in the mother (Fig. 6). However all our results obtained after injection of 1α-OHCC into the mother or into the fetus would be explained if the placenta is able to hydroxylate 1α-OHCC into 1,25 diOHCC (Fig. 6).

In conclusion, in the ovine species, during the last month of gestation, fetal blood phosphate, magnesium,total and ionized calcium levels were significantly higher than those found in the mother. Sheep fetuses responded to an intravenous injection of CT by a slight hypophosphatemia and hypocalcemia, while PTH injected into fetuses induced hypophosphatemia and hypercalcemia. Furthermore, since 1α-OHCC administration in sheep fetuses induced hyperphosphatemia and hypercalcemia without change in the mother, the ovine fetal liver is probably able to hydroxylate 1α-OHCC into 1,25 diOHCC except of the placenta can hydroxylate 1α-OHCC into 1,25 diOHCC. The rise in fetal plasma phosphate and calcium levels observed following injection of 1α-OHCC into the dam does not allow one to decide whether it is 1α-OHCC or 1,25 diOHCC which crosses the placenta. Nevertheless, the sheep fetus regulates its own phosphatemia and calcemia independently from maternal plasma phosphate and calcium concentrations.

Acknowledgements : The authors wish to thank Dr F. Caulin (Armour Montagu), Dr B. Mathieu de Fossey (Roussel Laboratories) and Dr J.L. Le Bossé (Leo Laboratories) for the generous gift of calcitonin, 5,6 trans-25 hydroxycholecalciferol and 1α-hydroxycholecalciferol. Pregnant ewes were supplied by M. Theriez and A. Brelurut (Station de l'Elevage).

REFERENCES

(1) Klem, K.K. :Placental transmission of ^{32}P in late pregnancy and in experimental prolongation of pregnancy in rats. Acta Obstet. Gynecol. Scand. 35 : 445, 1956.

(2) Garel, J.M.,and Pic, P. : Evolution of phosphatemia in the rat fetus during the late stages of gestation. Biol. Neonate 21 : 369, 1972.

(3) Malan, A.J. : Studies in mineral metabolism. VIII. Comparison of phosphorus partition in the blood of calf foetus, sheep foetus, and lambs, with corresponding maternal blood. J. Agric. Sci. 18 : 397, 1928.

(4) Smith, F.G., Tinglof, B.O., Meuli, J., and Borden, M. : Fetal response to parathyroid hormone in sheep. J. Applied Physiol. 27 : 276, 1969.

(5) Mellor, D.J.,and Matheson, I.C. : Variations in the distribution of calcium, magnesium and inorganic phosphorus within chronically sheep conceptuses during the last eight weeks of pregnancy. Quarterly J. Exper. Physiol. 62 : 55, 1977.

(6) Buckle, R.M., Smith, F.G.,and Alexander, D.P. : Assessment of parathyroid glandular activity in the foetus. In : Calcium, Parathyroid Hormone and the calcitonins, Talmage, R.V. and Munson, P.L. Eds., Excerpta Medica, Amsterdam, p. 197, 1972.

(7) Mull, J.W., and Bill, A.H. : Inorganic phosphorus content of prenatal and post-partum serum. Amer. J. Obstet. Gynecol. 23 : 807, 1932.

(8) Garel, J.M., Milhaud, G.,and Jost, A. : Action hypocalcémiante et hypophosphatémiante de la thyrocalcitonine chez le foetus de rat. C.R. Acad. Sci. Paris série D 267 : 344, 1968.

(9) Reynolds, W.A., Pitkin, R.M.,and Wezeman , F.H. : Calcitonin effects in primate pregnancy. Amer. J. Obstet. Gynecol. 122 : 212, 1975.

(10) Garel, J.M., Pic, P.,and Jost, A. : Action de la parathormone chez le foetus de Rat. Ann. Endocr. 32 : 253, 1971.

(11) Mellor, D.J., and Matheson, I.C. : Chronic catheterization of the aorta and umbilical vessels of foetal sheep. Res. Vet. Sci. 18 : 221, 1975.

(12) Bawden, J.W., Wolkoff, A.S., and Flowers, C.E. : Maternal-fetal blood calcium relationships in sheep. Obstet. Gynecol. 25 : 548, 1965.

(13) Delivoria-Papadopoulos, M., Battaglia, F.C., Bruns, P.D., and Meschia, G. : Total, protein-bound, and ultrafiltrable calcium in maternal and fetal plasma. Amer. J. Physiol. 213 : 263, 1967.

(14) Symonds, H.W., Sansom, B.F.,and Twardock, A.R. : The measurement of the transfer of calcium and phosphorus from foetus to dam in the sheep using a whole body counter. Res. Vet. Sci. 13 : 272, 1972.

(15) Braithwaite, G.D., Glascock, R.F.,and Riazuddin, Sh. : Studies on the transfer of calcium across the ovine placenta and incorporation into the foetal skeleton. Br. J. Nutr. 27 : 417, 1972.

(16) Garel, J.M.,and Barlet, J.P. : The effects of calcitonin and parathormone on plasma magnesium levels before and after birth in the rat. J. Endocr. 61 : 1, 1974.

(17) Littledike, E.T., Arnaud, C.D.,and Whipp, C.S. : Calcitonin secretion in the ovine, porcine and bovine fetuses. Proc. Soc. Exp. Biol. Med. 139 : 428, 1972.

(18) Milhaud, G.,and Moukhtar, M.S. : Antagonistic and synergistic actions of thyrocalcitonin and parathyroid hormone on the levels of calcium and phosphate in the rat. Nature (London) 211 : 1186, 1966.

(19) Ramberg, C.F., Delivoria-Papadopoulos, M., Crandall, E.D., and Kronfeld, D.S. : Kinetic analysis of calcium transport across the placenta. Amer. J. Physiol. 35 : 682, 1973.

(20) Twardock, A.R.,and Austin, M.K. : Calcium transfer in the perfused guinea-pig placenta. Amer. J. Physiol. 219 : 540, 1970.

(21) Parsons, J.A.,and Robinson, C.J. : Calcium shift into bone causing transient hypocalcemia after injection of parathyroid hormone. Nature (London) 230 : 581, 1971.

(22) Alexander, D.P., and Nixon, D.A. : Effect of parathyroid extract in foetal sheep. Biol. Neonate 14 : 117, 1969.

(23) Holick, M.F., Garabedian, M., and De Luca, H.F. : 5,6 trans-25 hydroxycholecalciferol : vitamin D analog active on intestine of anephric rats. Science 176 : 1247, 1972.

(24) Holick, M.F., Tavela, T.E., Holick, S.A., Schnoes, H.K., De Luca, H.F., and Gallagher, B.M. : Synthesis of 1α-hydroxy 6-^{3}H vitamin D_3 and its metabolism to 1α, 25-hydroxy 6-^{3}H vitamin D_3 in the Rat. J. Biol. Chem. 251 : 1020, 1976.

(25) Garel, J.M., Care, A.D., and Barlet, J.P. : A radioimmunoassay for ovine calcitonin : an evaluation of calcitonin secretion during gestation, lactation and foetal life. J. Endocr. 62 : 497, 1974.

(26) Ross, R., Care, A.D., Pickard, D.W., Peacock, M., and Robinson, J.S. : Plasma 25-hydroxy vitamin D levels in the sheep foetus and neonate. J. Endocr. 71 : 84P, 1976.

INTERRELATIONS BETWEEN PHOSPHORUS, CALCIUM, PARATHYROID HORMONE, AND PHOSPHATE EXCRETION IN THE NORMAL AND UREMIC DOG

Michael A. Kaplan, Janet M. Canterbury, George Gavellas, Eric Reiss, and Neal S. Bricker
University of Miami School of Medicine, Department of Medicine, Divisions of Nephrology and Endocrinology and Institute for Kidney Diseases
Miami, Florida, USA

INTRODUCTION

Phosphorus homeostasis is maintained in animals and man by excretion through the kidneys of the same amount of phosphorus absorbed from the intestines on an ongoing basis. There is apparently little impairment of gastrointestinal phosphorus absorption in uremia (1); yet phosphorus balance is well maintained in animals and man with advancing chronic renal disease. This balance is accomplished by progressive increases in fractional excretion of phosphate (FE_{PO_4}) by the kidneys and associated increases in parathyroid hormone (PTH) secretion (2-5).

Serum phosphorus concentration has no direct effect on PTH secretion; but it does modulate its rate of secretion via reciprocal changes in serum ionized calcium (6,7). Thus, as serum phosphorus concentration goes up, serum calcium concentration goes down. In uremic man and animals maintained on a constant high phosphorus intake, the continuing ability to maintain external phosphorus balance is associated with a progressive rise in PTH levels and fractional excretion of phosphate as glomerular filtration (GFR) falls. The hyperparathyroidism may function to dispose of ingested phosphorus despite diminished renal mass, but, recently, this role of hyperparathyroidism has been challenged (8).

In the present experiments, the interrelations between serum phosphorus, calcium, and PTH have been evaluated in the normal and uremic state, before and after challenging dogs with either 100 or 500 mg of oral phosphorus. In addition, the dynamic interrelationships between the phosphorus-calcium-PTH axis and regulation of renal phosphate excretion have been examined.

METHODS

Six normal and six uremic adult female mongrel dogs weighing 12-20 Kg and maintained on a diet containing 1500 mg of phosphorus daily were studied in the fasting unanesthetized state while standing quietly in slings. Experimental uremia was produced by ligation of most of the branches of the left renal artery coupled with contralateral nephrectomy. No studies were initiated for at least 3 weeks after the last surgical procedure.

A prime followed by a sustaining infusion of creatinine (blood levels 8-10 mg%) in 2.5% dextrose in water was administered through an indwelling venous catheter at the rate of 2 ml/min in the normal dogs and 0.3 ml/min in the uremic dogs. Urine was collected through a foley catheter and venous blood samples were obtained at the midpoint of the urine collection periods.

After starting the creatinine infusion, one hour was allowed for equilibration and three 20 min. control clearance periods were obtained. Thereafter either 100 or 500 mg of elemental phosphorus (as neutral sodium phosphate) were administered by oro-gastric tube and five consecutive 1-hr. clearance periods were obtained.

Urine and blood were analyzed for sodium and potassium by flame photometry (IL model 143) and phosphate and creatinine by modified autoanalyzer techniques (Technicon AutoAnalyzer II). Serum ionized calcium was determined with an orion flow through electrode system (Orion Biomedical model SS-20). Serum PTH was measured by radioimmunoassay (5,9).

RESULTS AND CONCLUSIONS

Control measurements for normal and uremic dogs respectively were as follows: GFR 68 vs 13 ml/min; PTH 68 vs 516 μl-eq/ml; and FE_{PO_4} 3 vs 46%. Values for serum phosphorus, ionized calcium, sodium and potassium were not significantly different in the two groups. Previous studies have shown that both intravenous and oral phosphorus will decrease serum calcium and thereby stimulate PTH secretion (6,7). However the quantitative interrelationships between phosphorus, calcium, and PTH in response to an oral phosphorus challenge have been only partially defined in normal animals and are essentially unexplored in the uremic state.

The present experiments demonstrate predictable and highly significant relationships between serum phosphorus, ionized calcium, and PTH. The linear correlation between the rise in serum phosphorus and the reciprocal depression of serum ionized calcium was identical in the normal and uremic dogs ($y=.001 + .10x$; $r=.9565$). Thus in both groups a 1 mg% rise in serum phosphorus produced a

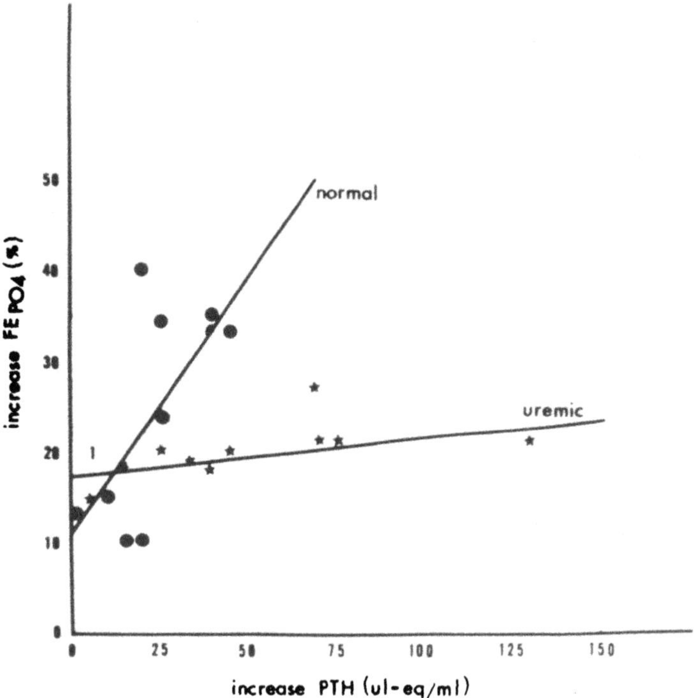

Fig. 1 Relationship between the increase in PTH and the associated rise in FE_{PO_4} produced by oral phosphorus in two normal (·) and two uremic (*) dogs.

0.1 mg% fall in serum ionized calcium over the range of serum phosphorus values extending from 4 to 10mg%.

The fall in ionized calcium, in turn, was associated with a rise in PTH levels, and for this function also, there was no significant difference between the response in the normal versus the uremic dogs. The linear regression equation relating the fall in ionized calcium (in mg%) to the rise in serum PTH (in ul-eq/ml) was $y=-6.4 + 269.8x$ ($r=.8079$).

Figure 1 shows the quantitative relationship between the rise in PTH produced by the oral phosphorus load and the change in FE_{PO_4} in two normal and two uremic dogs. This expresses the responsiveness of the nephrons to a rise in endogenous PTH. There was a

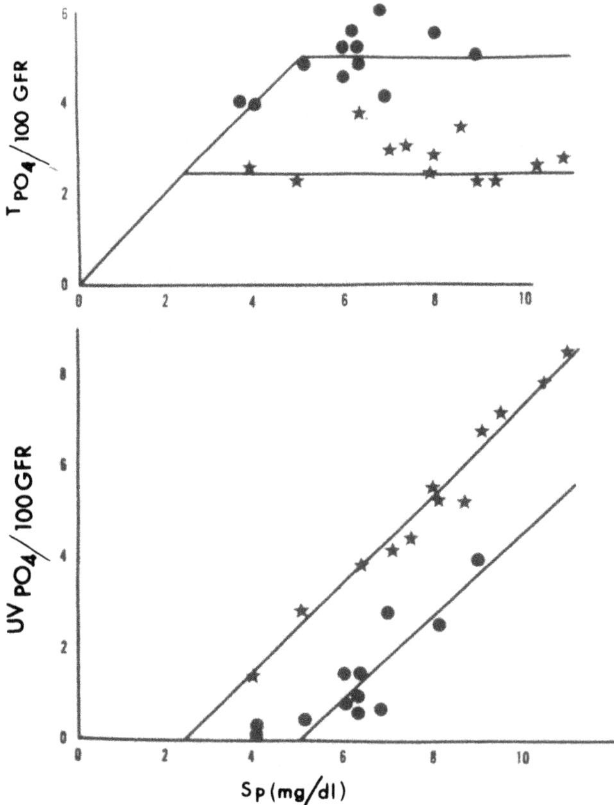

Fig. 2 Data for two normal (•) and two uremic (*) dogs relating increasing serum phosphorus and T_{PO_4}/GFR (upper panel) and UV_{PO_4}/GFR (lower panel).

significantly smaller increase in FE_{PO_4} for any given rise in PTH in the uremic as compared to the normal dogs ($p<.005$). This suggests a blunted renal tubular responsiveness.

Recently an increase in renal responsiveness to exogenous parathyroid hormone was reported in the uremic parathyroidectomized rat (10). In contrast, in the uremic dog with chronically high endogenous levels of PTH and high FE_{PO_4} values, there is no apparent enhanced end-organ sensitivity to exogenous hormone (11). These observations are not mutually exclusive since the parathyroid status of the animal is critical to the observed results (12). This is further suggested by plotting the present data in the form of a phosphate titration curve.

Figure 2 shows the effect of increasing serum phosphorus (equivalent to filtered load when factored by GFR) on tubular reabsorption of phosphate per GFR (T_{PO_4}/GFR: upper panel) and phosphate excretion per unit of GFR (UV_{PO_4}/GFR; lower panel) in two normal and two uremic dogs. At similar fasting control serum phosphorus concentrations the UV_{PO_4}/GFR is significantly higher in the uremic animals ($p<.001$). The uremic dogs are at Tm_{PO_4}/GFR at control fasting serum phosphorus while the normal dogs are in the splay area of the titration curve.

It has been reported that Tm_{PO_4}/GFR is lower in patients with hyperparathyroidism as compared to normal volunteers (13). This is attributed to the direct effect of parathyroid hormone on the renal tubular reabsorption of phosphate. A similar conclusion can be drawn from the present experiments where Tm_{PO_4}/GFR is significantly lower in uremic versus the normal dog. The blunted effect of endogenous PTH on FE_{PO_4} can be explained by the observation that the uremic dogs were already at Tm_{PO_4}/GFR in the control fasting state. The fact that the uremic dogs are at Tm_{PO_4}/GFR implies that as serum phosphorus concentration rises, the increment in filtered load of phosphorus will be excreted quantitatively and thus plays a major role in phosphorus homeostasis in these uremic hyperparathyroid animals.

In conclusion, the phosphorus, calcium, PTH axis functions in a sensitive, intact, and appropriate manner in the uremic dog. There is an apparently blunted end-organ response (as measured by FE_{PO_4}) to increases in endogenous PTH in the uremic dog which may be related to the observation that they are at Tm_{PO_4}/GFR in the control fasting state. The increment in serum phosphorus concentration and thus in the filtered load of phosphorus which follows addition of phosphorus to the ECF is the major variable in the excretion of an acute oral phosphorus load in the uremic hyperparathyroid dog.

ACKNOWLEDGMENTS

Supported by NIH grants 7 ROI AM 19822 and AM-16768.

REFERENCES

1. Coburn, J.W., Hartenbower, D.L., Brickman, A.S., Massry, S.G., and Kopple, J.D.: Intestinal absorption of calcium, magnesium, and phosphorus in chronic renal insufficiency. In Calcium Metabolism in Renal Failure and Nephrolithiasis. D. David (ed.), John Wiley and Sons, N.Y., 1977, p. 77.

2. Goldman, R. and Bassett, S.H.: Phosphorus excretion in renal failure. J. Clin. Invest. 33: 1623, 1954.

3. Slatopolsky, E., Gradowska, L., Kashemsant, C., Keltner, R., Manley, C., and Bricker, N.S.: The control of phosphate excretion in uremia. J. Clin. Invest. 45:672, 1966.

4. Slatopolsky, E., Robson, A.M., Elkan, I., and Bricker, N.S.: Control of phosphate excretion in uremic man. J. Clin. Invest. 47:1865, 1968.

5. Slatopolsky, E., Caglar, S., Pennell, J.P., Taggart, D.D., Canterbury, J.M., Reiss, E., and Bricker, N.S.: On the pathogenesis of hyperparathyroidism in chronic experimental renal insufficiency in the dog. J. Clin. Invest. 50:492, 1971.

6. Sherwood, L.M., Mayer, G.P., Romberg, C.F., Kronfeld, D.S., Aurbach, G.D., and Potts, J.T., Jr.: Regulation of parathyroid hormone secretion: proportional control by calcium, lack of effect of phosphate. Endocrinology 83:1043, 1968.

7. Reiss, E., Canterbury, J.M., Bercovitz, M.A., and Kaplan, E.L.: The role of phosphate in the secretion of parathyroid hormone in man. J. Clin. Invest. 49:2146, 1970.

8. Swenson, R.S., Weisinger, J.R., Ruggeri, J.L., and Reaven, G.M.: Evidence that parathyroid hormone is not required for phosphate homeostasis in renal failure. Metabolism 24:199, 1975.

9. Reiss, E. and Canterbury, J.M.: A radioimmunoassay for parathyroid hormone in man. Proc. Soc. Exp. Biol. Med. 128:501,1968.

10. Parkerson, M.L., Rolf, D., Miller, S., Slatopolsky, E., and Klahr, S.: Increased nephron sensitivity to parathyroid hormone as renal mass is decreased. Amer. Soc. Neph. Abst. 9:6A, 1976.

11. Kaplan, M.A., Canterbury, J.M., Gavellas, G., Bourgoignie, J.J., Reiss, E., and Bricker, N.S.: Resistance to calcemic with maintenance of phosphaturic effects of parathyroid hormone in the uremic dog. Clin. Res. 25:437A, 1977.

12. Kaplan, M.A., Canterbury, J.M., Gavellas, G., Reiss, E., and Bricker, N.S.: personal observation.

13. Bijvoet, O.L.M.: Relation of plasma phosphate concentration to renal tubular reabsorption of phosphate. Clin. Sci. 37:23, 1969.

THE HYPOCALCEMIA OF MAGNESIUM DEPLETION

E. Slatopolsky, R. Rosenbaum, P. Mennes and S. Klahr

Washington University School of Medicine, Department of Medicine, Renal Division, 4550 Scott Avenue, St. Louis, Missouri 63110 U.S.A.

Hypocalcemia has been observed in conjunction with severe magnesium depletion (1-8). This association is seen mainly in pathological conditions characterized by decreased absorption of magnesium from the gastrointestinal tract. The postulate that the hypocalcemia is the consequence of magnesium deficiency per se, and not calcium deficiency, is supported by studies showing that this syndrome can be reproduced by restricting magnesium in the diet or that hypocalcemia can be corrected by replacing magnesium alone without supplementation of calcium and/or vitamin D. The pathogenesis of hypocalcemia in magnesium depletion is multifactorial; however, recent studies have clarified previous controversial results regarding the role of PTH in this syndrome (2-5).

Individuals on a normal diet ingest approximately 300 mg of magnesium daily. Of this amount approximately 2/3 are excreted in the feces and 1/3 in the urine (Figure 1). If a human or an experimental animal is fed a low magnesium diet the kidney is capable of conserving magnesium maximally and negligible amounts of magnesium are excreted in the urine. Patients with profound magnesium depletion have been shown to excrete less than 1 mEq per 24 hours. However, the gastrointestinal tract does not adjust as well to a very low magnesium intake; magnesium secretion is likely to continue resulting in persistent magnesium losses in the stools and the development of magnesium depletion. Table I illustrates the most common causes responsible for the development of hypomagnesemia in clinical medicine. From a pathogenetic point of view the development of hypocalcemia in magnesium depletion may be due to 1) an increase in urinary calcium excretion, 2) a decrease in calcium absorption from the GI tract, and 3) a decrease in calcium mobilization from bone (Figure 2).

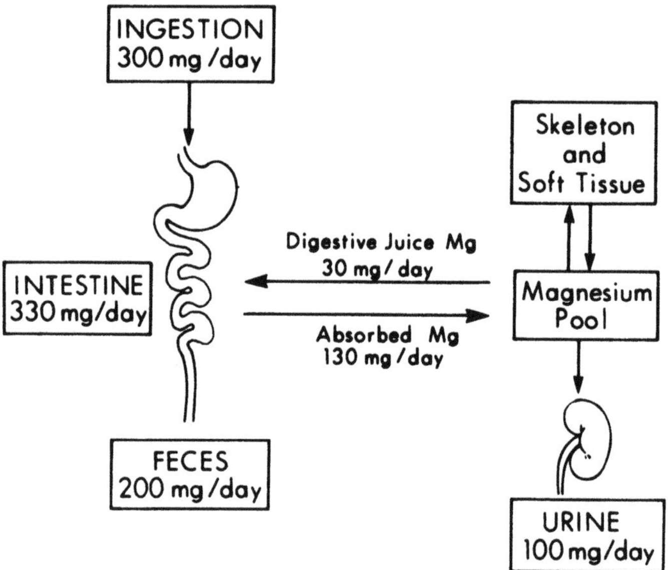

Figure 1. Schematic representation of magnesium metabolism in man

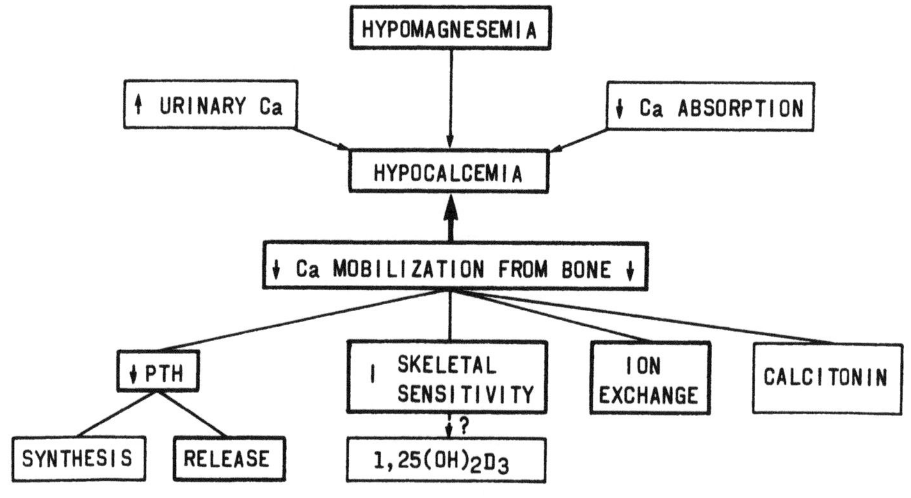

Figure 2. Pathogenetic mechanisms responsible for the development of hypocalcemia in magnesium depletion

TABLE I

CAUSES OF HYPOMAGNESEMIA

I. Decreased Intestinal Absorption

- Celiac Disease
- Tropical and Non-tropical Sprue
- Invasive and Infiltrative Process: Lymphomas
- Surgical Resection
- Intestinal Bypass
- Severe Diarrhea
- Prolonged Gastrointestinal Suction

II. Decreased Intake

- Protein-Caloric Malnutrition
- Starvation
- Prolonged Therapy with Intravenous Fluids Lacking Magnesium
- Chronic Alcoholism

III. Excessive Urinary Losses

- Diabetic Ketoacidosis
- Chronic Alcoholism
- Diuretic Therapy
- Diuretic Phase of ATN
- Post-Obstructive Diuresis
- Hypercalciuric States
- Primary or Secondary Hyperaldosteronism
- Inappropriate Antidiuretic Hormone Secretion
- Idiopathic Renal Magnesium Wasting
- Gentamicin Toxicity

The possibility that increased calcium excretion in the urine is responsible for the development of profound hypocalcemia in patients with hypomagnesemia is extremely remote. Patients with idiopathic hypercalciuria, in whom urinary calcium losses may be in the order of 300 to 500 mg daily, do not develop profound hypocalcemia. Moreover, there is evidence to indicate that the amount of calcium excreted in the urine is decreased in hypomagnesemia (4). The second possibility, that decreased calcium absorption from the GI tract is responsible for the hypocalcemia of magnesium depletion is also unlikely. Table II shows the results obtained in experimental animals fed a zero calcium diet. In

TABLE II

EFFECTS OF A ZERO CALCIUM DIET ON SERUM CALCIUM IN NORMAL CHICKENS, RATS, AND DOGS

	Chicken [1]	Rat	Dog
	serum calcium (mg/100 ml)		
Control Diet	n=10	n=16	n=15
	11.7	10.1	9.80
S.E.	±.21	±.07	±.21
Zero Calcium	n=10	n=15	n=6
Diet	11.3	9.94	9.50
S.E.	±.14	±.05	±.19

[1] From Reddy et al. (Reference 23)

chickens and rats fed a zero calcium diet for a period of a month and in dogs fed a calcium-free diet for 6 to 24 months, serum calcium did not decrease significantly as compared to controls. Of interest is the fact that some of the dogs were maintained on a zero calcium diet for a period of 2 years and serum calcium remained normal. It is known that when an animal is maintained on a low calcium diet, secondary hyperparathyroidism develops. In the presence of elevated concentrations of PTH in blood the rate of conversion of 25-hydroxycholecalciferol to 1,25-dihydroxycholecalciferol by the kidney increases. With an increase in the levels of $1,25(OH)_2D_3$ and parathyroid hormone, bone resorption increases and a greater amount of calcium is mobilized from bone. Thus, the experimental animal can maintain a fairly normal serum calcium despite a low calcium intake; however, the concentration of calcium in bone decreases substantially. It should be emphasized that although calcium malabsorption per se will be seldom responsible for the development of hypocalcemia for the reasons mentioned above, if calcium malabsorption is also accompanied by a decrease in the absorption of vitamin D or if the levels of 25-hydroxycholecalciferol in blood are low, it is then possible for calcium malabsorption to play a role in the development of hypocalcemia. The third and most likely explanation for the development of hypocalcemia in magnesium depletion in man is a decrease in calcium mobilization from bone as is depicted in Figure 2. Several factors may be responsible for decreased calcium mobilization from bone. The first one to be considered is the concentration of PTH in serum. Unfortunately, the literature is extremely controversial in this particular point, since high, normal, and low levels of PTH have been described in patients with profound hypomagnesemia. However, it seems that the degree of hypomagnesemia, and even more important magnesium depletion per se, may determine the level of PTH of blood. It is known that mild hypomagnesemia increases acutely the levels of PTH in vivo (9) or in vitro (10). On the other hand, profound hypomagnesemia decreases the levels of PTH in blood (2). It has been demonstrated that prior to the release of PTH from the parathyroid glands, a series of biochemical processes occur in which precursors of the native hormone (MW 9500) are cleaved inside the gland. A large peptide termed pre-pro-parathormone (pre-pro-PTH) is cleaved to pro-parathormone (pro-PTH), a peptide with six extra amino acids attached to the N-terminal region of the molecule. In the Golgi zone a proteolytic enzyme complex cleaves the amino terminal to yield native PTH (11). Several studies have shown that magnesium does not affect either the synthesis or the conversion of pro-parathyroid hormone to parathyroid hormone (12-13). On the other hand, studies in vivo indicated that the administration of magnesium intravenously to a hypomagnesemic patient increased the levels of circulating parathyroid hormone within two to five minutes (5). These studies suggest that the main defect in hypomagnesemia is due to a decrease in the release of PTH from the parathyroid gland. Studies performed in three hypomagnesemic uremic patients also indicated that the levels of circulating PTH are extremely low (14). After magnesium administration PTH levels rose rapidly in peripheral blood and serum calcium increased towards normal. A representative study is illustrated in Figure 3. Numerous studies, in humans and animals, have clearly indicated that in magnesium depletion in addition to altered release of PTH, the skeleton becomes resistant to the action of the hormone, thus aggravating the hypocalcemia (6-8, 15-17). On the other hand, other investigators have demonstrated that the response of the skeleton to the administration of PTH is normal (4,5,18,19). It is difficult to understand the conflicting results obtained by these two large groups of investigators. However, it seems that the conditions of the experiments, the age of the animal, the amount of PTH used in all of these experiments are quite different, which may in part explain the conflicting results. At this time, it would seem from the majority of the studies published in the literature that a form of skeletal resistance indeed is present in this syndrome. Moreover, there is evidence that the heteroionic exchange between the hydration shell of bone and the extracellular fluid is decreased in hypomagnesemia (20). Studies performed in vitro demonstrated that calcium exchange was less in bone from magnesium depleted rats than control animals (21). At the present time it is not known if alterations in the metabolites of vitamin D, such as decreased levels of $1,25(OH)_2D_3$ are responsible for the skeletal resistance observed in hypomagnesemia. Another possible explanation for the decreased mobilization of calcium from bone in hypomagnesemia is an increase in calcitonin. It is

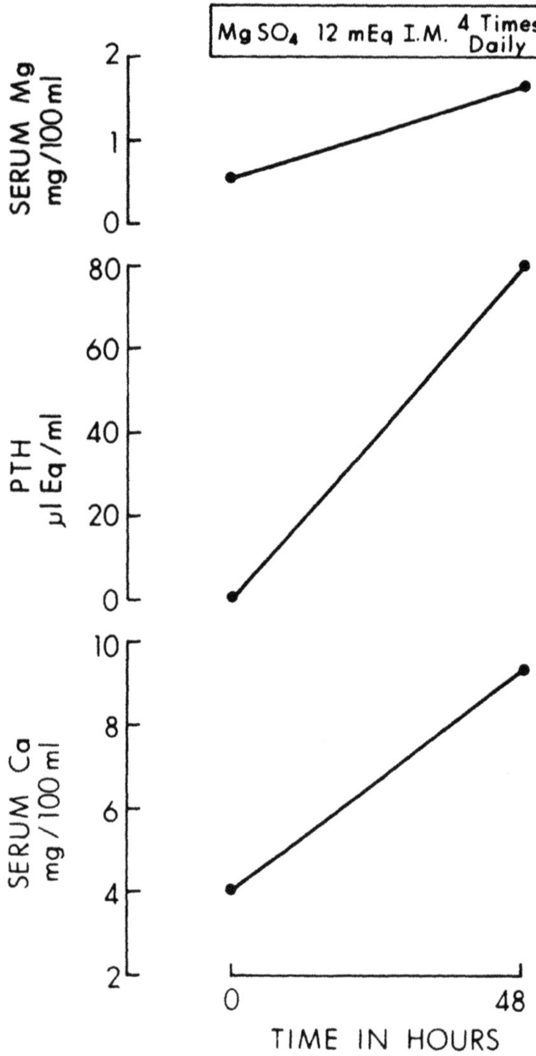

Figure 3. Serum magnesium, parathyroid hormone and calcium concentrations before and after the administration of magnesium to a uremic hypomagnesemic patient

known that calcitonin competes with PTH by blocking the activity of this hormone at the level of osteoclasts. However, it is known also that hypermagnesemia and not hypomagnesemia stimulates the release of calcitonin (22). Thus, the possibility that calcitonin plays a pathogenetic role in the hypocalcemia seen in the hypomagnesemic syndrome is unlikely.

In summary, the hypocalcemia observed in hypomagnesemia is the consequence of a decrease in calcium mobilization from bone, secondary to a defect in the release of PTH, a skeletal resistance to the action of PTH and a decrease in heteroionic exchange between the skeleton and the extracellular fluid.

ACKNOWLEDGMENTS

The original work reported in this manuscript was supported by U.S.P.H.S. NIAMDD grant AM-09976.

We would also like to thank Mrs. Patricia Verplancke for her assistance in the preparation of this manuscript.

REFERENCES

1. Shils, M.E.: Experimental human magnesium depletion. Medicine 48:61, 1969.

2. Anast, C.A., Mohs, J.M., Kaplan, S.L., et al: Evidence for parathyroid hormone failure in magnesium deficiency. Science 177:606, 1972.

3. Suh, S.M., Tashjian, A.H., Matsuo, N., et al: Pathogenesis of hypocalcemia in primary hypomagnesemia normal end organ responsiveness to parathyroid hormone, impaired parathyroid gland function. J. Clin. Invest. 52:153, 1973.

4. Chase, L.R., Slatopolsky, E.: Secretion and metabolic efficacy of parathyroid hormone in patients with severe hypomagnesemia. J. Clin. Endocrinol. Metab. 38:363, 1974.

5. Anast, C.A., Winnocker, J.L., Forte, L.R., et al: Impaired release of parathyroid hormone in magnesium deficiency. J. Clin. Endocrinol. Metab. 42:707, 1976.

6. Estep, H., Shaw, W.A., Waltington, C., et al: Hypocalcemia due to hypomagnesemia and reversible parathyroid hormone unresponsiveness. J. Clin. Endocrinol. Metab. 29:842, 1969.

7. Levi, J., Massry, S.G., Coburn, J.W., et al: Hypocalcemia in magnesium depleted dogs: Evidence for reduced responsiveness to parathyroid hormone and relative failure of parathyroid gland function. Metabolism 23:323, 1974.

8. Rude, R.K., Oldham, S.B., Singer, F.R.: Functional hypoparathyroidism and parathyroid hormone end-organ resistance in human magnesium deficiency. Clin. Endocrinol. 5:209, 1976.

9. Buckle, R.H., Care, A.D., Cooper, C.W. and Gitelman, H.J.: The influence of plasma magnesium concentration on parathyroid hormone secretion. J. Endocrinol. 42:529, 1968.

10. Targovnik, J.H., Rodman, J.S. and Sherwood, L.M.: Regulation of parathyroid hormone secretion in vitro: Quantitative aspects of calcium and magnesium ion control. Endocrinology 88:1477, 1971.

11. Cohn, D. and Hamilton, J.W.: Newer aspects of parathyroid chemistry and physiology. The Cornell Veterinarian 66:271, 1976.

12. Hamilton, J.W., Spierto, F.W., MacGregor, R.R. and Cohn, D.V.: Studies on the biosynthesis in vitro of parathyroid hormone. II. The effect of calcium and magnesium on synthesis of parathyroid hormone isolated from bovine parathyroid tissue and incubation medium. J. Biol. Chem. 246:3224, 1971.

13. Habener, J.F. and Potts, J.T., Jr.: Relative effectiveness of magnesium and calcium on the secretion and biosynthesis of parathyroid hormone in vitro. Endocrinology 98:197, 1976.

14. Mennes, P., Rosenbaum, R., Martin, K., and Slatopolsky, E: Impaired parathyroid hormone secretion in chronic renal disease secondary to hypomagnesemia. Ann. Intern. Med. (in press).

15. MacManus, J., Heaton, F.W., Lucas, P.W.: Decreased response to parathyroid hormone in magnesium deficiency. J. Endocrinol. 49:253, 1971.

16. Muldowney, F.P., McKenna, T.J., Kyle, L.H., Freaney, R., and Swan, M.: Parathormone-like effect of magnesium replenishment in steatorrhea. N. Engl. J. Med. 282:61, 1970.

17. Woodward, J.C., Webster, P.D., Carr, A.A.: Primary hypomagnesemia with secondary hypocalcemia, diarrhea and insensitivity to parathyroid hormone. Digestive Dis. 17:612, 1972.

18. Hahn, T.J., Chase, L.R., Avioli, L.V.: Effect of magnesium depletion on responsiveness to parathyroid hormone in parathyroidectomized rats. J. Clin. Invest. 51:886, 1972.

19. Suh, S.M., Csima, A., Fraser, D.: Pathogenesis of hypocalcemia in magnesium depletion. J. Clin. Invest. 50:2668, 1971.

20. Neuman, W.F., Neuman, M.W.: The Chemical Dynamics of Bone Mineral. Chicago, The University of Chicago Press, 1958, pp. 55-100.

21. MacManus, J., Heaton, F.W.: The influence of magnesium on calcium release from bone in vitro. Biochim. Biophys. Acta 215:360, 1970.

22. Littledike, E.T. and Arnaud, C.D.: The influence of plasma magnesium concentrations on calcitonin secretion in the pig. Proc. Soc. Exptl. Biol. Med. 136:1000, 1971.

23. Reddy, C.R., Coburn, J.W., Brickman, A.S., Hartenbower, D.L., Friedler, R.M., Massry, S.G., and Jowsey, J.: Studies on mechanism of hypocalemia of magnesium depletion. J. Clin. Invest. 52:3000, 1973.

THE EFFECT OF PTE INFUSION IN HYPOMAGNESEMIC STATES

M. Díaz Curiel, J.M. Castrillo, A. Rapado, P. Esbrit and M. Serrano
Unidad Metabólica, Fundación Jiménez Díaz, Universidad Autónoma de Madrid. Spain

The disorders of the parathyroid glands are probably the most frequent cause of hypocalcemia seen in hypomagnesemic states (1,2). The mechanisms reported in the literature are diverse: A) a defect in the secretion and/or formation of parathormone whose assessment by radioimmunoassay (iPTH) shows low serum levels, either absolute or relative to the degree of hypocalcemia (1, 3-5), and B) a failure in the peripheral action of the hormone (shown by the rise in iPTH) (6, 7) on the bone (8) and on the kidney, demonstrated by a deficient tubular response to the action of a parathyroid extract (PTE) (6, 9-11), measured by the tubular reabsorption of phosphate (TRP) and/or by the urinary excretion of cAMP.

Some other mechanisms have been suggested as responsible for the hypocalcemia of hypomagnesemia, such as a defect in the formation of vitamin D metabolites (6, 12, 13); an increase in the intestinal absorption of phosphate (14); abnormal distribution of calcium among diverse body compartments (15, 16) or an increase in serum calcitonin (3).

We were able to study the response of the renal tubule to the action of PTE as measured by the urinary phosphorus/creatinine (Up/Ucr) ratio and by cAMP in the urine in seven cases of hypomagnesemia. In a few cases serum levels of iPTH were also measured in an attempt to establish the relative significance of each of the mechanisms responsible for the PTH-dependent hypocalcemia observed in our patients.

MATERIAL AND METHODS

Seven patients in whom the basal values of serum magnesium ranged from 0.37 to 1.33 mg/dl were studied (Table I). The etiology of hypomagnesemia was renal in 4 cases (three of them with associated nephrocalcinosis), 2 had intestinal malabsorption (one lymphoma and one late-onset immunodeficiency) and 1 case chronic alcoholism. All the cases, but one, presented hypocalcemia (serum levels between 4.0 and 8.3 mg/dl) and 2 cases had radiological and pathological rickets.

The biochemical studies (Table II) revealed a functional hypoparathyroidism in 3 cases (TRP above 85%); in 2 of them iPTH was measured. The clinical data of some of these patients have been already published (13, 17, 18).

An infusion of 200 USP Lilly bovine parathyroid extract was administered by iv bolus injection and several urine samples were collected before and for the 120 following minutes. Blood samples were also taken before and after the test. In all the urine samples creatinine, phosphorus and cAMP were measured.

Creatinine was measured by Henry's method (19) and phosphorus by the method of Fiske and Subarow (20); a protein-binding method was employed for cAMP (21) and iPTH by a modification of Arnaud's method (22) with a C-terminal antibody. Calcium and magnesium were measured by atomic absorption spectrophotometry, and alkaline phosphatase by the method of Bessey and Lowry and it is expressed in King-Amstrong units.

TABLE I

CLINICAL DATA IN SEVEN CASES OF HYPOMAGNESEMIA

Case	Sex/Age	Tetany	Rickets/ Osteomal.	Nephro- calcinos.	Hypomagnes. pathogenesis
1	F/12	+	+	+	primary renal
2	M/26	+	+	+	primary renal
3	M/26	-	-	+	primary renal
4	M/31	+	-	-	intestinal malabsorption
5	F/31	+	-	-	intestinal malabsorption
6	M/50	-	-	-	chronic alcoholism
7	M/38	-	-	-	primary renal

TABLE II

BIOCHEMICAL DATA IN SEVEN CASES OF HYPOMAGNESEMIA

Case no.	Serum magnesium (mg/dl)	Serum calcium (mg/dl)	Serum phosphorus (mg/dl)	G.F.R. (ml/min)	T.R.P. %	Alkaline phosphatase (U.K.A.)	iPTH (pg/ml)
1	0.6	6.9	4.6	38	82	35.7	-
2	0.9	6.4	4.4	43	78	23.3	-
3	0.8	8.3	3.6	54	81	7.2	-
4	0.8	4.0	4.5	96	95	8.6	431
5	0.4	5.1	4.9	104	97	11.2	238
6	1.0	7.6	5.4	62	86	7.6	-
7	1.3	10.7	3.8	89	80	5.9	425
NORMAL VALUES	1.9	9.8	3.6	98	83	6.5	550
2 S.D.	0.2	0.8	0.7	20	8	2.5	

RESULTS

1. Hypomagnesemia associated with nephrocalcinosis (Table III):

The PTE infusion did not increase the Up/Ucr ratio in any of the cases. This response was also negative after intramuscular repletion of magnesium in 2 of the patients.

The urinary excretion of cAMP, measured in 2 of the patients, was normal after the PTE infusion, regardless of the magnesium serum values. All the 3 patients did not have clinical or biochemical signs of hypoparathyroidism.

2. Hypomagnesemia without nephrocalcinosis (Table IV):

In those cases with associated hypocalcemia and hypoparathyroidism biochemical pattern, the Up/Ucr ratio response to the PTE infusion was positive (increases ranging from 2.6 to 3.05 fold) (Normal: above 2.0 fold).

The same reponse was observed after magnesium repletion and correction of the hypocalcemia.

The urinary excretion of cAMP was normal before and after correction of the hypomagnesemia.

In 2 cases with hypocalcemia and hypomagnesemia the values of iPTH were within the low normal limits (Table II).

Case nunber 7 with hypomagnesemia and basal normocalcemia showed a normal response to the PTE infusion together with normal values of iPTH.

DISCUSSION

The low serum calcium values observed in most cases of hypomagnesemia have been ascribed to parathormone dysfunction (1, 2).

In subjects with hypomagnesemia the PTE infusion shows a normal response (3, 5, 7, 8, 17, 23). In other cases this response is low (6, 9, 10) which makes one assume certain absolute or relative insensitivity of the renal tubule to parathyroid hormone. Assessment of iPTH in these patients also show discordant values (3, 4, 5, 6, 16, 17, 24).

In our series when the hypomagnesemia was associated with nephrocalcinosis, the PTE infusion did not produce significant changes in the Up/Ucr ratio while the response could be considered normal in relation to the urinary excretion of cAMP, regardless of the serum magnesium levels. This behaviour is similar to what is

TABLE III

HYPOMAGNESEMIA WITH NEPHROCALCINOSIS

RESPONSE TO THE IV ADMINISTRATION OF PARATHYROID EXTRACT

CASE no.	SERUM MAGNESIUM (mg/dl)	Op/Ocr RATIO		cAMP (mmol/g Cr)	
		before PTE	after PTE	before PTE	after PTE
1	0.60	1.09	0.83	-	-
	1.75	1.13	1.11	-	-
2	0.90	0.60	0.59	3.28	416.4
	1.77	0.70	0.49	-	-
3	0.80	0.60	0.41	-	-
	1.33	0.60	0.40	1.65	95.7

TABLE IV

HYPOMAGNESEMIA WITHOUT NEPHROCALCINOSIS

RESPONSE TO THE IV ADMINISTRATION OF PARATHYROID EXTRACT

CASE no.	SERUM MAGNESIUM (mg/dl)	Op/Ocr RATIO		cAMP (mmol/g Cr)	
		before PTE	after PTE	before PTE	after PTE
4	0.84	0.21	0.56	-	-
5	0.37	0.18	0.52	8.2	649.6
	1.70	0.39	1.05	10.0	248.3
6	1.00	0.48	1.29	10.8	316.0
7	1.33	0.50	1.52	1.95	104.6

seen in pseudohypoparathyroidism type II (25).

This unresponsiveness to the phosphaturic action of the PTE when serum magnesium is corrected would favour the assumption that such a discordant effect may be related more to the nephrocalcinosis than to the existence of hypomagnesemia. In fact we have no evidence concerning the tubular response to PTE administration in other cases of nephrocalcinosis without hypomagnesemia.

Some other factors besides low serum magnesium values may be responsible for the hypocalcemia in the three cases of our series. All of them had chronic renal failure and 2 showed biochemical, radiological and pathological evidence of rickets (17), quite possible due to impaired vitamin D metabolism, mediated by the hypomagnesemia (26). In fact, the administration of magnesium alone to these patients, corrected the alkaline phosphatase levels and the radiological abnormalities without calcium or vitamin D supplementation (13).

In 3 other cases of our series we detected a pattern of hypoparathyroidism (low serum calcium levels with hyperphosphatemia and increased TRP). Those patients showed a positive phosphaturic response to the PTE infusion, which was not in accordance however with the serum calcium level and was below that observed in cases with postsurgical hypoparathyroidism (2)

That response might be caused by the hypomagnesemia, either by a resistance to the peripheral action of the PTE (8,9,10) or by partial blocking of the renal tubule PTH-receptors by the circulating hormone, a condition which will not be present in primary hypoparathyroidism. Accordingly, the assessment of iPTH in 2 of our cases showed values in the normal range but inappropiate to the level of serum calcium.

Thus these data support the assumption that in the hypomagnesemic states there might exist a resistence to the peripheral action of PTH (1, 6) together with an absence of its secretion and/or formation (5, 27) to explain the mechanism responsible for the hypocalcemia.

In case no. 5 the correction of the hypomagnesemia resulted in normalization of the serum calcium and phosphorus values while the renal tubule response to the PTE infusion became normal, thus confirming the etiologic role of serum magnesium levels in her previous hypoparathyroidism.

Case no. 7, a patient with hypomagnesemia due to renal hyperexcretion, who had normal calcium values (18), showed normal iPTH values and a normal response to PTE infusion, both in its phosphaturic action and in the urinary excretion of cAMP.

On the basis of all this evidence we believe that certain disorders in the production, secretion and peripheral action of the PTH play a significant but not the sole role in the production of hypocalcemia in hypomagnesemic states.

But there must be some other mechanisms, besides the low serum magnesium level, in the control of calcium metabolism which might prevent the development and presence of hypocalcemia in all the cases of hypomagnesemia (28).

REFERENCES

1. Rude, R.K., Oldham, S.B., and Singer, F.R.: Functional hypoparathyroidism and parathyroid hormone end-organ resistance in human magnesium deficiency. Clin.Endocrinol. 5:209, 1976

2. Schneider, A.B., and Sherwood, L.M.: Pathogenesis and management of hypoparathyroidism and other hypocalcemic disorders. Metabolism 24:871, 1975.

3. Suh, S.M., Tashjian, A.H., Matsuo, N., Parkin, D.K., and Fraser, D.: Pathogenesis of hypocalcemia in primary hypomagnesemia. Normal end-organ responsiveness to parathyroid hormone, impaired parathyroid gland function. J.Clin.Invest. 52:153, 1973.

4. Anast, C.S., Mohs, J.M., Kaplan, S.L., and Burns, T.W.: Evidence for parathyroid failure in magnesium deficiency. Science 177:606, 1972.

5. Anast, C.S., Winnacker, J.L., Forte, L.R. and Burns, T.W.: Impaired release of parathyroid hormone in magnesium deficiency. J.Clin.Endoc.Metab. 42:707, 1976.

6. Sherwood, L.M.: Magnesium ion and hypoparathyroid function. New Eng.J.Med. 282:752, 1970.

7. Medalle, R., Waterhouse, C., and Hahn, T.J.: Vitamin D resistance in magnesium deficiency. Am.J.Clin.Nutr. 29: 854, 1976.

8. Muldowney, F.P., McKenna, J.S., Kyle, L.H., Freaney, R., and Swan, M.: Parathormone-like effect of magnesium replenishment in steatorrhea. New Engl.J.Med. 282:61, 1970.

9. Estep, H.L., Martínez, G.R., and Jones, D.: Parathyroid hormone (PTH) unresponsiveness and 3',5'-cAMP secretion. Proc. 51st meet. of Endoc.Soc. New York, 1969.

10. Estep, H., Shaw, W.A., Watlington, C., Hobe, R., Holland, W., and Tucker, St G.: Hypocalcemia due to hypomagnesemia and reversible parathyroid hormone unresponsiveness. J. Clin.Endocrinol.Metab. 29:842, 1969.

11. Ashby, J.P., and Heaton, F.W.: Effect of magnesium deficiency and parathyroid hormone on cyclic AMP metabolism in rat renal cortex. J.Endocrinol. 67:105, 1975.

12. Harrison, H.E., and Harrison, H.C.: The interaction of vitamin D and parathyroid hormone on calcium, phosphorus and magnesium homeostasis in the rat. Metabolism 13:952, 1964.

13. Rapado, A., Castrillo, J.M., Arroyo, M., Traba, M.L., and Calle, H.: Magnesium-deficient rickets. A clinical study. In: Vitamin D and problems related to uremic bone disease. Ed. by Norman, A.W., Schaefer, K., Grigoleit, H.G., v. Herrath, D., and Ritz, E. W. de Gruyter. Berlin, 1975. p. 453.

14. Hahn, T.J., Chase, L.R., and Avioli, L.V.: Effect of magnesium depletion on responsiveness to parathyroid hormone in parathyroidectomized rats. J.Clin.Invest. 51:886, 1972.

15. Reddy, C.R., Coburn, J.W., Hartenbower, D.L., Friedler, R. M., Brickman, A.S., Massry, S.G., and Jowsey, J.: Studies on mechanism of hypocalcemia of magnesium depletion. J.Clin. Invest. 52:3000, 1973.

16. Chase, L.R., and Slatopolsky, E.: Secretion and metabolic efficacy of PTH in patients with severe hypomagnesemia. J. Clin.Endocrin.Met. 38:363, 1974.

17. Rapado, A., and Castrillo, J.M.: Hypomagnesemia associated with nephrocalcinosis. Abstract of 2nd International Symposium on Magnesium. Montreal, 1976. p. 70.

18. Rapado, A., and Castrillo, J.M.: Primary hypomagnesemia with hypokalemia and alkalosis associated with chondrocalcinosis. Abstract of 2nd International Symposium on magnesium. Montreal, 1976. p. 71.

19. Henry, R.J.: Clinical Chemistry. Harper & Row Pub. New York, 1964. p. 148.

20. Fiske, C.H., and Subarow, Y.: The colorimetric determination of phosphorus. J.Biol.Chem. 66:375, 1925.

21. Brown, B.L., Albano, J.D.M., Ekins, R.P., and Sgherzy, A.N.: A simple and sensitive saturation assay for measurement of adenosine 3',5'-cyclic monophosphate. Biochem. J. 121:561, 1971.

22. Arnaud, C.D., Tsao, H.S., and Littledike, T.: Radioimmunoassay of human parathyroid hormone in serum. J.Clin.Invest. 50:21, 1971.

23. Vainsel, M., Vandevelde, G., Smulders, J., Vosters, M., Hubain, P., and Loeb, H.: Tetany due to hypomagnesemia with secondary hypocalcemia. Arch.Dis.Child. 45:254, 1970.

24. Levi, J., Massry, S.G., Coburn, J.W., Llach, F., and Kleeman, C.R.: Hypocalcemia in magnesium-depleted dogs: evidence for reduced responsiveness to parathyroid hormone and relative failure of parathyroid gland function. Metabolism 23:323, 1974.

25. Drezner, M., Neelon, F.A., and Lebowitz, H.E.: Pseudohypoparathyroidism type II: A possible defect in the reception of the cyclic AMP signal. New Eng.J.Med. 289:900, 1973.

26. Norman, A.W., and Henry, H.: 1,25- dihydroxycholecalciferol. A hormonally active form of vitamin D. Rec.Prog.Horm.Res. 30:431, 1974.

27. Paunier, L., Radde, I.C., Kooh, S.W., Coven, P.E., and Fraser, D.: Primary hypomagnesemia with secondary hypocalcemia in an infant. Pediatrics 41:385, 1968.

28. Gitelman, H.J., Graham, J.B., and Welt, L.G.A.: Familial disorders characterized by hypokaliemia and hypomagnesemia. Ann.New York Acad.Sci. 162:856, 1969.

PROSTAGLANDINS AND DIVALENT CATION METABOLISM

Michael A. Kirschenbaum and Charles R. Kleeman
Department of Medicine
University of California, Los Angeles
Los Angeles, California 90024, U.S.A.

When von Euler (1) first described the prostaglandins thirty years ago, he could not have imagined that these lipids would be implicated in so many physiologic roles. With the rediscovery of these lipids and the elucidation of their chemical structure by Bergstrom and Samuelsson (2), a considerable volume of information has been generated. The prostaglandins are a group of 20-carbon acidic lipids generally resembling prostanoic acid. They are derived from the enzymatic conversion of either linolenic acid (the 1-series) or arachidonic acid (the 2-series) (3,4). During their synthesis, numerous short-lived cyclic endoperoxide intermediates are formed which by themselves are frequently more active than the prostaglandins (5). Almost every cell in the body has the capacity to synthesize prostaglandins although in the adult, the major organs of synthesis are the renal medulla, seminal vesicles, and uterus. The prostaglandins that are synthesized in the microsomes are probably not stored by the cell (6), but released into the cytoplasm and eventually into the extracellular fluid. The lung, liver, and renal cortex among other tissues, have the enzymatic ability to degrade prostaglandins (7). Although dozens of prostaglandins, intermediates, and metabolites have been identified, prostaglandin-E_2 (PGE_2) and prostaglandin-$F_{2\alpha}$ ($PGF_{2\alpha}$) appear to be implicated as the active naturally occurring agents. The prostaglandins can be identified and measured by various techniques with considerable variation in sensitivity and specificity (8). These methods include gas chromatography and mass spectrometry, thin layer chromatography, radioimmunoassay, membrane receptor assay, and bioassay.

There has been considerable speculation into the possible roles of these lipid compounds. It has been suggested that prostaglandins act as physiologic buffers preventing wide variations in body function. In this role, the prostaglandins have been postulated to act as hormones having their influence in three possible ways. Having access to the extracellular fluid, they could act as classic hormones affecting some distal target organ. Since almost all of the prostaglandins are degraded to inactive compounds through a single passage through the lungs and liver (7), the ability of prostaglandins to function as classic hormones would seem to be limited. However, under certain conditions, prostaglandins may be able to escape complete degradation (9) and circulate in concentrations capable of eliciting physiologic responses in distant target organs. Most available evidence suggests that prostaglandins function predominantly as local tissue hormones. Various stimuli are capable of inducing prostaglandin synthesis within cells. Once synthesized, prostaglandins are not stored but rather released into the pericellular area where they are able to accumulate in substantially higher concentrations than they could within the circulation. There are many examples of prostaglandins acting as local tissue hormones. The pregnant uterus releases prostaglandins which aid in the maintenance of normal uteroplacental blood flow (10). The renal medulla releases prostaglandins which may result in the antagonism of the hydro-osmotic effect of antidiuretic hormone (11). Prostaglandins released into inflammatory exudates increase vascular permeability (12). The final possible hormonal role of prostaglandins may be as an intracellular messenger capable of modifying either the formation or action of cyclic AMP by affecting adenyl cyclase, phosphodiesterase, protein kinases, the intracellular calcium pool, or other biologically active intracellular substances.

PROSTAGLANDINS AND SKELETAL CALCIUM FUNCTION

The relatively meager information available to us today suggests that prostaglandins play a role in the cellular processes which regulate the concentration of calcium or other divalent ions in body fluids. PGE was first shown to stimulate bone resorption *in vitro* by Klein and Raisz (13) in 1970 (Figure 1). These investigators administered ^{45}Ca to pregnant rats. The shafts of the radius or ulna of 19-day rat fetuses were removed and placed into culture medium. Then PGE, PTH, epinephrine or thyrocalcitonin was added to the culture medium and changes in ^{45}Ca in the medium were noted. PGE was able to stimulate bone resorption in a manner similar to PTH but was unable to increase serum calcium levels in intact rats when administered intravenously. At least in this study, PGE was more potent than PTH in equimolar concentrations, and the effect of both agents was greater than either agent administered by itself. Although not shown on this figure, thyrocalcitonin was able to blunt the bone resorbing effect of both PGE and PTH. Epi-

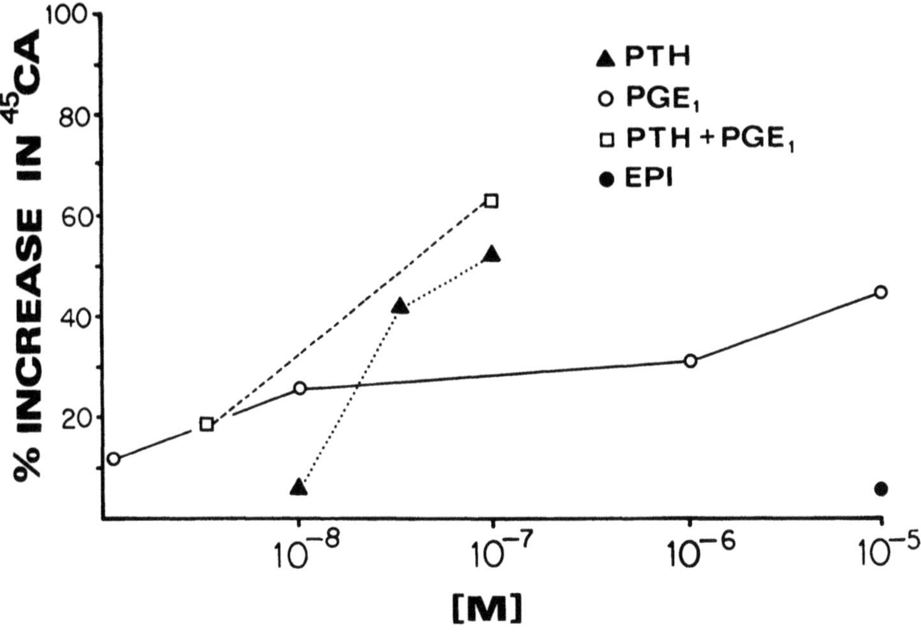

Figure 1 - Percent increase in ^{45}Ca release from fetal rat bones in culture induced by administration of PTH, PGE, and epinephrine as compared to administration of control culture medium. Adapted from Klein and Raisz (13).

nephrine, shown in the right-hand corner, was unable to stimulate bone resorption.

Subsequently, several other groups have administered prostaglandins to intact animals. In a study by Franklin and Tashjian (14) shown in Figure 2, a constant infusion of PGE_2 (65-260 ng/min) (probably a concentration approximating that seen at the tissue level) produced a significant elevation of plasma calcium and inorganic phosphorus levels in unanesthetized rats, suggesting that the effect of the prostaglandin was through enhanced bone resorption. The inability of PGE to consistently produce hypercalcemia in all strains of animals (13) is somewhat disturbing and may represent variations within individual groups of animals, an intrinsic lack of sensitivity of some species to the bone resorptive effects of prostaglandins, or the ability of prostaglandins to induce bone resorption only when in the physiologic setting of local

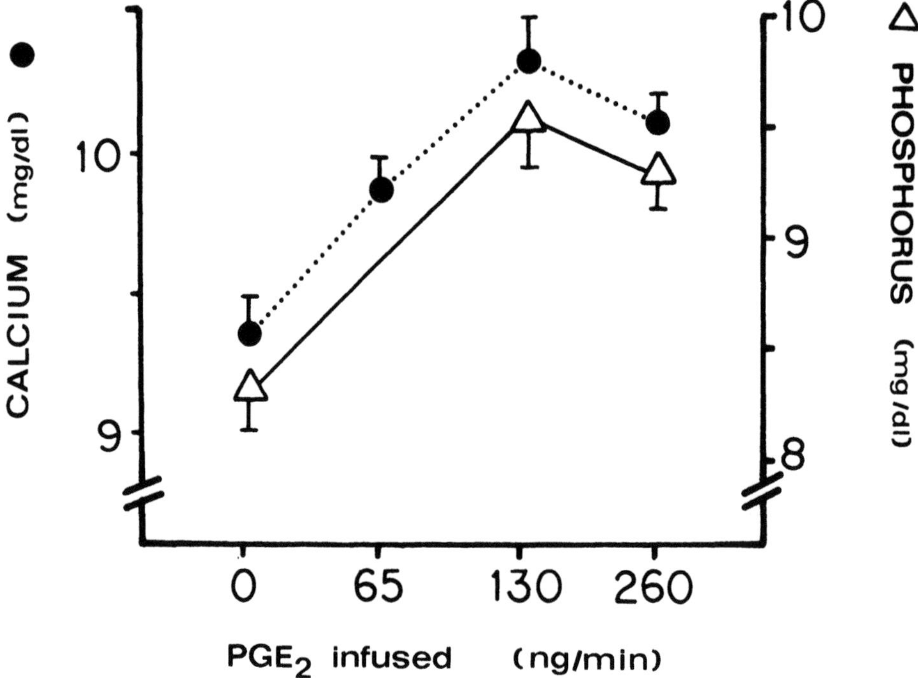

Figure 2 - Increase in plasma calcium and inorganic phosphorus after infusion of PGE_2 (65-260 ng/min) into normal rats. Adapted from Franklin and Tashjian (14).

endogenous release rather than with systemic infusion. Since the prostaglandin effect is inconsistent as compared to the effect of parathyroid hormone on bone, these studies suggest that these two agents may have their effect through different mechanisms.

Prostaglandins have also been postulated to participate in bone resorption under several other conditions. Goodson, Dewhirst, and Brunetti (15) have recently shown that PGE_2 levels as measured by radioimmunoassay are elevated in human gingiva and inflammatory exudates obtained from patients with necrotizing gingivitis when compared with gingiva from normal patients. They suggested that enhanced prostaglandin release resulted in the inflammatory changes and bone resorption related to the parodontal disease. These changes can be partially reversed by inhibiting prostaglandin synthesis with indomethacin. Benign dental cysts have also been associated with elevated prostaglandin levels and bone resorption. In a study by Harris and co-workers (16), homogenates of dental cysts were shown to synthesize a PGE_2-like material as measured by bioassay. Extracts of this material were able to induce bone resorption in a manner similar to PGE_2 itself. Indomethacin added to the dental cyst homogenates significantly reduced the capacity of the tissue to synthesize PGE and the ability to resorb bone. In 1971, Goldhaber (17) demonstrated that normal human gingival fragments were capable of stimulating bone resorption in organ culture. Gomes and his associates (18) have shown that these fragments, at least in the primate, were capable of releasing immunoreactive PGE. However the ability of these gingival fragments to release PGE and resorb bone does not imply a physiologic mechanism. In this regard, Feinblatt and his colleagues (19) have recently demonstrated that 20-day old chick embryos were capable of releasing a bone reabsorbing factor which was immunologically different than either PTH or thyroxine. This substance obtained from the thyroid was capable of resorbing bone and when added to a pharmacologic dose of PTH, increased the degree of bone resorption greater than the combined effect of either agent. Although not identified further, the effects of this agent were blunted by indomethacin, and thus it probably represents, in part, a prostaglandin. The effects of gingival fragments on bone resorption may not be unique and it is of interest to speculate that renal medulla, a tissue capable of active prostaglandin synthesis, when incubated with bone cells may also produce bone resorption.

The demonstration that PGE_2 can stimulate bone resorption has provoked considerable interest in the potential role of these lipids in the hypercalcemia associated with malignancy. The elevated serum calcium levels seen with malignancy have been thought to be related to local pressure or unknown metabolic effects of the skeletal metastases and to the secretion by the tumor of various humoral substances, including immunoreactive parathyroid hormone, vitamin D or its metabolites, a non-vitamin D steroid, and osteoclast activating factor capable of causing abnormal bone resorption by stimulating osteoclastic and osteocytic activity.

In 1972 Tashjian and co-workers (20) reported that a potent bone resorption-stimulating factor was produced by fibrosarcoma HSDM cells when grown in tissue culture. This factor was identified by radioimmunoassay to be PGE. The administration of these fibrosarcoma cells to mice resulted in a hypercalcemic syndrome which could be reversed by the administration of indomethacin, an inhibitor of prostaglandin synthesis. However, hypercalcemia in humans is more commonly associated with carcinoma and hematologic malignancies rather than sarcoma. Additional studies by Voelkel and his associates (21) in 1975 demonstrated that a strain of VX_2 carcinoma-bearing rabbits also developed profound hypercalcemia. Extracts of this VX_2 carcinoma obtained from normal animals had marked bone-resorbing activity which could be reversed by pretreating the animals with indomethacin. The ability of the tumor cells in culture to synthesize prostaglandins was also demonstrated.

Several groups of investigators have studied patients with various neoplasms to test the hypothesis that the hypercalcemia of malignancy is mediated by prostaglandins. Seyberth and his co-workers (22) studied 29 patients with solid tumors and compared them to 10 normocalcemic patients hospitalized for reasons other than malignancy, 6 patients with hyperparathyroidism, and 6 patients with hematologic malignancies and hypercalcemia. The urinary excretion levels of PGE-M, a stable metabolite of PGE_2 which does not designate the site of origin of the PGE_2 but rather the renal excretory rate of this metabolite, are shown in Figure 3 for all the patient groups. All of the normal patients fell within the two dashed lines. The patients with both hyperparathyroidism and hematologic malignancies had normal PGE-M excretion rates despite their elevated serum calcium levels. Of the 29 patients with cancer, 13 of 15 patients with hypercalcemia had increased PGE-M excretion rates whether or not they had evidence of bone involvement (as assessed by skeletal X-rays, bone scans, and autopsy) while the normocalcemic patients were all within the normal range (as compared with the control group of patients) or only slightly elevated above normal. Two patients had elevated PGE-M excretion rates although they were normocalcemic. Both of these two patients eventually became hypercalcemic. Immunoreactive parathyroid hormone levels were elevated only in the group of patients with primary hyperparathyroidism and were either undetectable or suppressed in all of the hypercalcemic patients with cancer. Treatment of these patients with indomethacin resulted in significant decreases in serum calcium and the urinary excretion of PGE-M (Figure 4). In another series of hypercalcemic patients with cancer, Robertson and associates (23) noted hyperprostaglandinemia as measured by radioimmunoassay in only 4 of 11 patients and noted that even though prostaglandin inhibitors could reduce prostaglandin synthesis, they reduced the serum calcium levels only in patients with hyperprostaglandinemia prior to treatment. Two other groups have studied the effect of inhibition of prostaglandin synthesis in patients with malignancy. Dindogru and associates (24) noted an inconsistent effect of indomethacin in 5 patients with hypercalcemia and Ito and co-workers (25) showed a decreased sensitivity of patients with hypercalcemia to indomethacin on repeated administration.

Two questions can be raised by these data: 1) where are these prostaglandins being synthesized? and 2) once synthesized, how do they cause clinical bone resorption and hypercalcemia? The site of the increased synthesis of prostaglandins in human hypercalcemic states is not known. The elevated serum levels might suggest that they may be synthesized at some distant tumor site or by

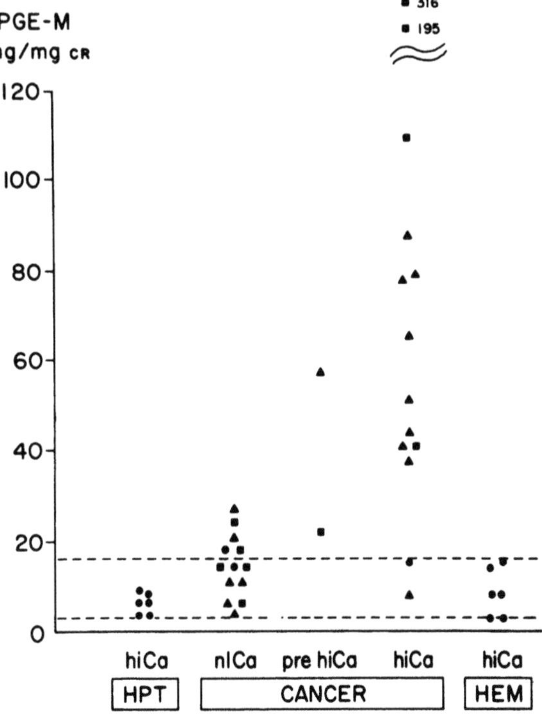

Figure 3 - PGE-M excretion rates in patients with hyperparathyroidism, cancer, and hematologic malignancies. Reproduced with permission from Seyberth et al. (22).

the tumor stimulating some other tissue to release prostaglandins by some yet undefined mechanism. Once synthesized, they could be carried to their target organ by the circulation. An alternate possibility might be a decrease in prostaglandin degradation associated with these malignancies allowing more of the lipids to circulate. A more reasonable explanation would be that the prostaglandins are synthesized locally in bone in response to some stimulus related to the tumor or by the tumor itself. The data obtained from the tumor cell cultures would suggest that the malignant cells themselves are capable of prostaglandin synthesis (20, 21).

Once the elevated serum or local tissue levels are produced, how do the prostaglandins cause bone resorption? It is unlikely that PGE, like pyrophosphate, acts directly on the solubility of calcium or other divalent ions in bone. Their action undoubtedly is in stimulating the activity of osteocytes and osteoclasts, with

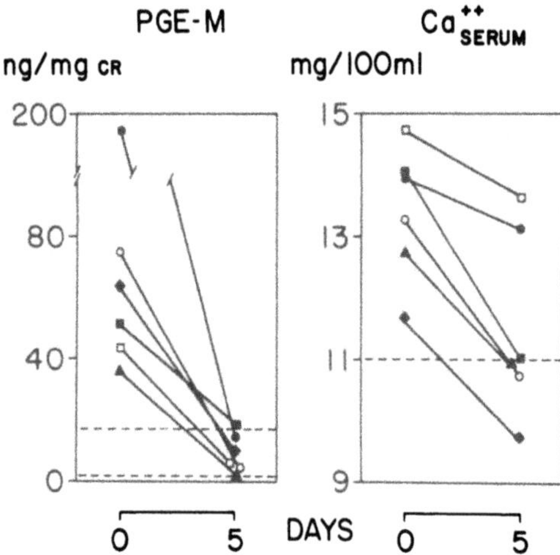

Figure 4 - Effect of indomethacin (75-150 mg/day) on PGE-M excretion rates and serum calcium levels in 6 patients with cancer. Reproduced with permission from Seyberth et al. (22).

possible inhibition of osteoblasts. Alternatively, prostaglandins might modulate the action of parathyroid hormone, vitamin D or thyrocalcitonin on bone. However, Vogel and co-workers (26) demonstrated that rabbits with VX_2 carcinoma can become hypercalcemic even after parathyroidectomy. Prostaglandins may have an action on bone similar to parathyroid hormone, stimulating cyclic AMP production and bone resorption. Interestingly, although hypercalcemia with malignancy can frequently be associated with hyperprostaglandinemia, conditions associated with elevated circulating prostaglandin levels, such as Bartter's Syndrome (27), are not usually associated with either alterations in bone metabolism or hypercalcemia.

A possible role of prostaglandins on the intracellular metabolism of bone cells in culture has been examined by Yu and co-workers (28). Both PGE_2 (10^{-6}M) and PTH (2 U/ml) increased cAMP levels within the cells and enhanced bone resorption. When administered together, the effect of PGE_2 and PTH on cAMP generation was greater than that produced by each agent alone. When PGE was administered concomitantly with theophylline (10^{-3}M) there was enhanced cAMP generation but bone resorption was comparable to PGE alone. Thyrocalcitonin (4.7 U/ml) resulted in enhanced cAMP generation but decreased bone resorption. When administered with PGE, thyrocalcitonin markedly enhanced cAMP generation but no effect on bone resorption was noted. A prostaglandin inhibitor, SC 19220, decreased both cAMP generation and bone resorption. Finally, a calcium antagonist, D_{600} (a methoxy-derivative of verapamil, a compound which interferes with transmembrane calcium movement) (29), was able to blunt the bone resorption induced by prostaglandin E_2 but did not alter the effect of the prostaglandin on cyclic AMP.

As has been observed in other tissues, it is attractive to suggest that prostaglandins affect bone cell function through the adenyl cyclase-cyclic AMP system. It is known that both parathyroid hormone and prostaglandin E_2 stimulate cyclic AMP content in fetal rat bones and that prostaglandin E_2 can stimulate cyclic AMP content in many other tissues including the renal tubular cell. However, epinephrine is capable of stimulating cyclic AMP release in bone cells but does not induce bone resorption (13,28). Also, at least in the studies by Yu and associates (28), thyrocalcitonin increased cyclic AMP levels but decreased bone resorption. It is clear from these and other data that there may be no direct association between prostaglandin E_2-related changes in cyclic AMP and bone resorption. Furthermore, it would appear that parathyroid hormone and prostaglandin E_2 bind to separate receptors since they produce a synergistic effect on cyclic AMP generation when used together (28).

Prostaglandins would appear to have two additional effects on bone. Raisz and Koolemans-Beynen (30) have shown that prostaglandin E_2 inhibited the incorporation of proline into bone collagen in organ cultures of fetal rat calveria suggesting that prostaglandins may block osteogenesis by inhibiting osteoblastic activity. Furthermore, Roos and his co-workers (31) have demonstrated that prostaglandins are capable of stimulating thyrocalcitonin release from cell cultures of C-cells derived from human medullary thyroid carcinoma.

Apart from its effect on skeletal calcium function, hyperprostaglandinemia in this setting may have broader physiologic effects. For example, in the kidney, the ADH-induced enhanced water permeability of the collecting duct appears to be antagonized by prostaglandin E_2 (11). It is possible that the polyuria and renal concentrating defect seen so commonly with hypercalcemia are due to enhanced prostaglandin synthesis in the renal medulla inhibiting ADH-induced water reabsorption and enhanced concentration or synthesis in the hypothalamus stimulating the thirst centers and water ingestion.

NON-SKELETAL CALCIUM FUNCTION

As previously mentioned, prostaglandins are synthesized by microsomes within cells. It has been suggested that prostaglandins act as intracellular messengers regulating some aspects of calcium function, either directly or indirectly through cyclic AMP. There is considerable evidence to suggest that prostaglandin E can alter the intracellular levels of cyclic AMP by affecting either adenyl cyclase of phosphodiesterase (32). The intracellular action of cyclic AMP may further be modified by an effect of prostaglandins on protein kinase and other enzyme systems (33). In many intracellular systems, calcium appears necessary for the biologic action of cyclic AMP and alterations in either cyclic AMP or intracellular calcium levels significantly affect cell action. Although there are data to suggest that prostaglandins both increase and decrease cyclic AMP generation within cells, the biological effects of prostaglandin E appear to be mediated by enhanced cyclic AMP production (34).

Because of the relationship between cyclic AMP and calcium, it is of interest that prostaglandins induce calcium release within cells probably through increasing cyclic AMP content. Moreover, cyclic AMP is also capable of increasing phospholipase A in brain, fat, and thyroid cells, thus increasing the concentration of prostaglandin substrate, arachidonic acid. Although highly speculative, prostaglandins may play a role in the dephosphorylation of ATP to form cyclic AMP.

Perhaps the most basic role of prostaglandins may be in facilitating the entry of calcium into cells. A calcium-ionophoretic action of prostaglandins has been demonstrated in mitochondrial and microsomal fractions (38) and prostaglandin-induced entry of calcium into muscle cells has been shown to stimulate excitation-contraction coupling in cardiac (39), uterine (38) and gastrointestinal muscle cells (40). Since the intracellular pool of free calcium ions appears to be critical in various essential intracellular biological reactions, prostaglandins may have a basic role affecting many metabolic cellular functions. These possible interrelationships are presented in Figure 5.

PROSTAGLANDINS AND PHOSPHORUS METABOLISM

Little is known of the relationship between prostaglandins and phosphorus metabolism although a recent study by Hilborn (41) suggests that phosphorus uptake, at least into 3T3 mouse fibroblast cells, is not dependent upon the presence of prostaglandin E_1. There are no data available to suggest that changes in serum phosphorus influence changes in prostaglandin metabolism. Similarly, there are no data to explain how changes in prostaglandin metabolism may influence the movement of inorganic phosphorus into cells or into subcellular structures to cause any specific physiologic effect. However, it is of interest to speculate that part of the hypophosphatemic syndrome may be dependent on altered prostaglandin metabolism. Hypercalciuria and, under some conditions hypercalcemia, may be seen in hypophosphatemia which may be dependent on elevated

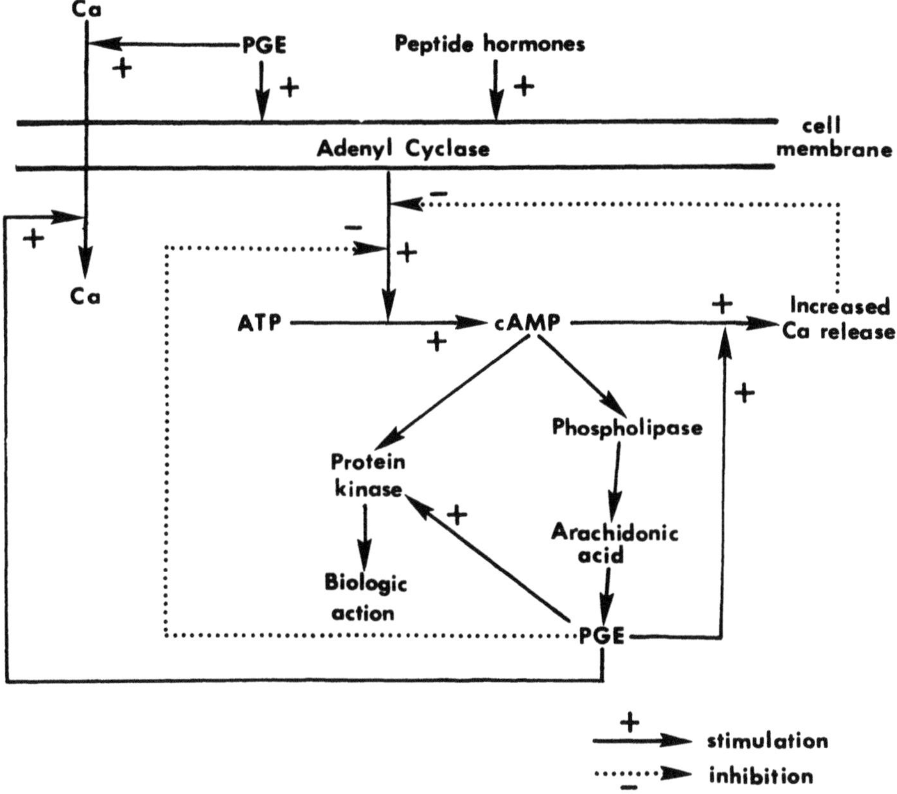

Figure 5 - Proposed interrelationships between PGE and calcium and other biologically active intracellular systems.

prostaglandin levels. Platelet dysfunction has been reported in hypophosphatemia as well as with a new prostaglandin, PGI_2 (42). Finally, the CNS, peripheral nerve, and muscle dysfunction observed in severe phosphate depletion (43) may involve a basic change in the prostaglandin availability to these tissues.

ACKNOWLEDGMENTS

This work was supported, in part, by National Institutes of Health Research Grant HL-21272-01 and a grant from the American Heart Association. Dr. Kirschenbaum is an Established Investigator of the American Heart Association.

REFERENCES

1. von Euler, U.S.: On the specific vasodilating and plain muscle stimulating substances from accessory genital glands in man and certain animals. J. Physiol. 88:213, 1937.

2. Bergstrom, S., Ryhage, R., Samuelsson, B., and Sjovall, J.: The structure of prostaglandin E, F, and F_2. Acta. Chem. Scand. 16:501, 1962.

3. Bergstrom, S., Danielsson, H., and Samuelsson, B.: The enzymatic formation of prostaglandin E_2 from arachidonic acid. Biochim. Biophys. Acta. 90:207, 1964.

4. Van Dorp, D.A., Beerthuis, R.K., Nugteren, D.H., and Vonkeman, H.: The biosynthesis of prostaglandins. Biochim. Biophys. Acta. 90:204, 1964.

5. Samuelsson, B. and Hamberg, M.: Role of endoperoxides in the biosynthesis and action of prostaglandins. In: Prostaglandin Synthetase Inhibitors, eds. H.J. Robinson and J.R. Vane, Raven Press, New York, 1974, p. 107-121.

6. Crowshaw, K.: The incorporation of $\{1-^{14}C\}$ arachidonic acid into the lipids of rabbit renal slices and conversion to prostaglandins E_2 and $F_{2\alpha}$. Prostaglandins. 3:607, 1973.

7. Ferreira, S.H. and Vane, J.R.: Prostaglandins: their disappearance from and release into the circulation. Nature (Lond.). 216:868, 1967.

8. Frolich, J.C., Williams, W.M., Sweetman, B.J., Smigel, M., Carr, K., Hollifield, J.W., Fleisher, S., Nies, A.S., Frisk-Holmberg, M., and Oates, J.A.: Analysis of renal prostaglandin synthesis by competitive protein binding assay and gas chromatography - mass spectrometry. In: Advances in Prostaglandin and Thromboxane Research, Vol. 1, eds. B. Samuelsson and R. Paoletti, Raven Press, New York, 1976.

9. Golub, M., Zia, P., Matsuno, M., and Horton, R.: Metabolism of prostaglandins A_1 and E_1 in man. J. Clin. Invest. 56:1404, 1975.

10. Venuto, R.C., O'Dorisio, T., Stein, J.H., and Ferris, T.F.: Uterine prostaglandin E secretion and uterine blood flow in the pregnant rabbit. J. Clin. Invest. 55:193, 1975.

11. Berl, T. and Schrier, R.W.: The mechanism of effect of prostaglandin E_1 on renal water excretion. J. Clin. Invest. 52:463, 1973.

12. Willis, A.L., Davison, P., Ramwell, P.W., Brocklehurst, W.E., and Smith, J.B.: Release and action of prostaglandins in inflammation and fever: Inhibition by anti-inflammatory and antipyretic drugs. In: Prostaglandins in Cellular Biology, eds. P.W. Ramwell and B.B. Pharriss, Plenum Press, New York, 1972, p. 227-259.

13. Klein, D.C. and Raisz, L.G.: Prostaglandins: Stimulation of bone resorption in tissue culture. Endocrinology. 86:1436, 1970.

14. Franklin, R.B. and Tashjian, A.H.: Intravenous infusion of prostaglandin E_2 raises plasma calcium concentration in the rat. Endocrinology. 97:240, 1975.

15. Goodson, J.M., Dewhirst, F.E., and Brunetti, A.: Prostaglandin E_2 levels and human periodontal disease. Prostaglandins. 6: 81, 1974.

16. Harris, M., Jenkins, M.U., Bennett, A., and Wills, M.R.: Prostaglandin production and bone resorption by dental cysts. Nature. 245:213, 1973.

17. Goldhaber, P., Rabadjija, L., Beyer, W.R., and Kornhauser, G.: Bone resorption in tissue culture and its relevance to periodontal disease. J. Amer. Dent. Assoc. (Special Issue). 87: 1027, 1973.

18. Gomes, B.C., Hausmann, E., Weinfeld, N., and De Luca, C.: Prostaglandins: bone resorption stimulating factors released from monkey gingiva. Calcif. Tiss. Res. 19:285, 1976.

19. Feinblatt, J.D., Tai, L.-R., and Leone, R.G.: Secretion of a bone resorbing factor by chick thyroid glands in organ culture. Endocrinology. 99:1363, 1976.

20. Tashjian, A.H., Voelkel, E.F., Levine, L., et al.: Evidence that the bone resorption-stimulating factor produced by mouse fibrosarcoma cells is prostaglandin E_2: a new model for the hypercalcemia of cancer. J. Exp. Med. 136:1329, 1972.

21. Voelkel, E.F., Tashjian, A.H., Franklin, R., Wasserman, E., and Levine, L.: Hypercalcemia and tumor-prostaglandins: the VX_2 carcinoma model in the rabbit. Metabolism. 24:973, 1975.

22. Seyberth, H.W., Segre, G.V., Morgan, J.L., Sweetman, B.J., Potts, J.T., and Oates, J.A.: Prostaglandins as mediators of hypercalcemia associated with certain types of cancer. N. Engl. J. Med. 293:1278, 1975.

23. Robertson, R.P., Baylink, D.J., Metz, S.A., and Cummings, K.B.: Plasma prostaglandin E in patients with cancer with and without hypercalcemia. J. Clin. Endocrinol. Metab. 43:1330, 1976.

24. Dindogru, A., Gailani, S., Henderson, F.S., Wallace, H.J., and Fitzpatrick, J.: Indomethacin in hypercalcemia. Lancet. 1: 1218, 1975.

25. Ito, H., Sanada, T., Katayama, T., and Shimazaki, J.: Indomethacin-responsive hypercalcemia. N. Engl. J. Med. 293:558, 1975.

26. Vogel, S.B., Enneking, W.F., and Thomas, W.C.: Effect of thyroparathyroidectomy in hypercalcemia associated with malignancy. Endocrinology. 80:404, 1967.

27. Gill, J.R., Frolich, J.C., Bowden, R.E., Taylor, A.A., Keiser, H.R., Seyberth, J., Hannsjorg, W., Oates, J.A., and Bartter, F.C.: Bartter's syndrome: a disorder characterized by high urinary prostaglandins and a dependence of hyperreninemia on prostaglandin synthesis. Am. J. Med. 61:43, 1976.

28. Yu, J.H., Wells, H., Ryan, W.J., and Lloyd, W.S.: Effects of prostaglandins and other drugs on the cyclic AMP content of cultured bone cells. Prostaglandins. 12:501, 1976.

29. Kohlhardt, M., Bauer, B., Krause, H., and Fleckenstein, A.: Differentiation of transmembrane Na and Ca channels in mammalian cardiac fibers by the use of specified inhibitors. Pflueger Arch. 335:309, 1972.

30. Raisz, L.G. and Koolemans-Beynen, A.R.: Inhibition of bone collagen synthesis by prostaglandin E_2 organ culture. Prostaglandins. 8:377, 1974.

31. Roos, B.A., Bundy, L.L., Miller, E.A., and Deftos, L.J.: Calcitonin secretion by monolayer cultures of human C-cells derived from medullary thyroid carcinoma. Endocrinology. 97:39, 1975.

32. Amer, M.A. and Marquis, N.R.: The effect of prostaglandins, epinephrine and aspirin on cyclic AMP phosphodiesterase activity of human blood platelets and their aggregation. In: _Prostaglandins in Cellular Biology_, eds. P.W. Ramwell and B.B. Pharris, Plenum Press, New York, 1972.

33. Johnson, M. and Ramwell, P.W.: Prostaglandin modification of membrane-bound enzyme activity: a possible mechanism of action. Prostaglandins. 3:703, 1973.

34. Hinman, J.W.: Prostaglandins. Ann. Rev. Biochem. 41:161, 1972.

35. Hamprecht, B., Jaffe, B.M., Philpott, A.W.: Prostaglandin production by neuroblastoma, glioma and fibroblast cell line. FEBS Lets. 36:193, 1973.

36. Dalton, C. and Hope, W.C.: Cyclic AMP regulation of PG biosynthesis in fat cells. Prostaglandins. 6:227, 1974.

37. Burke, G., Chang, L., and Szabo, M.: Thyrotropin and cyclic nucleotide effects on prostaglandin levels in isolated thyroid cells. Science. 180:872, 1973.

38. Carsten, M.E. and Miller, J.D.: Effect of prostaglandins and oxytocin on calcium release from a uterine microsomal fraction. J. Biol. Chem. 252:1576, 1977.

39. Moura, A.-M. and Simpkins, H.: The effects of hormones and prostaglandins on the calcium pools in cultured myocardial cells. Mol. Cell. Endocrinol. 5:349, 1976.

40. Ishizawa, M. and Miyazaki, E.: Calcium and the contractile response to prostaglandin in the smooth muscle of guinea-pig stomach. Experientia. 33:376, 1976.

41. Hilborn, D.A.: Serum stimulation of phosphate uptake into 3T3 cells. J. Cell. Physiol. 87:111, 1975.

42. Moncada, S., Higgs, E.A., and Vane, J.R.: Human arterial and venous tissues generate prostacyclin (prostaglandin X), a potent inhibitor of platelet aggregation. Lancet. 1:18, 1977.

43. Boelens, P.A., Norwood, W.K., and Kjellstrand, C.: Hypophosphatemia with muscle weakness due to antacids and hemodialysis. Am. J. Dis. Child. 120:350, 1970.

Metabolic Consequences of Phosphate Depletion

THE CLINICAL SYNDROME OF PHOSPHATE DEPLETION

Shaul G. Massry

Division of Nephrology and Department of Medicine,
The University of Southern California, Los Angeles,
California, USA

There are 600-700 grams of phosphorus in the human body, with 85% of it in the skeleton. Only 600-700 mg or 1/1000 of total body phosphorus is found in the extracellular fluid. About 15% of body phosphorus is located in soft tissues, mainly in the form of intermediary carbohydrate, lipid and protein compounds. The amount of inorganic phosphorus in the cell is very small, but it is very important since it is this fraction which provides the source of phosphorus for the resynthesis of adenosine triphosphate, ATP, (1).

Hypophosphatemia with and without phosphate depletion is encountered in a large number of clinical disorders. One study showed that 2% of hospital patients had levels of serum phosphorus below 2 mg/100 ml (2). Hypophosphatemia is noted more frequently among alcoholic patients, and it was reported that serum phosphorus levels of less than 2 mg/100 ml were observed in 10% of patients admitted to the hospital with alcoholism (3).

Three categories of disturbances may cause hypophosphatemia and/or phosphate depletion. These include decreased intestinal absorption of phosphorus, increased urinary losses of this ion, shift of phosphorus from extracellular to intracellular compartments, or a combination of these factors.

The clinical and metabolic consequences of hypophosphatemia and/or phosphate depletion are not well recognized. It must be emphasized, however, that phosphate depletion may result in disturbances of almost every organ system. This is not surprising, since inorganic phosphorus is essential for the resynthesis of ATP, which is an integral part of the energy-producing and energy-consuming systems of the living cell. The clinical signs and symptoms and the biochemical derangements that may accompany phosphate-depleted ion will depend on the rapidity with which the latter develops, as well as its severity or duration. The true incidence of phosphate depletion is not known.

Moderate hypophosphatemia may be defined as serum phosphorus between 2.5-1.0 mg/100 ml; it is not uncommon, and is usually not associated with signs and symptoms. Phosphate depletion may not be present in patients with moderate hypophosphatemia. Patients with blood phosphorus of less than 1.0 mg/100 ml are considered to have *severe hypophosphatemia*, and phosphate depletion may also be present. Such patients usually display the signs and symptoms of the syndrome of phosphate depletion. Table 1 presents the causes of moderate hypophosphatemia, while the clincal conditions which may be associated with severe hypophosphatemia are listed in Table 2.

Table 1: Causes and Mechanisms of Moderate Hypophosphatemia

CAUSE	MECHANISM
Hyperparathyroidism	↑ Urinary losses
Osteomalacia	↓ Intestinal absorption ↑ Urinary losses
Vitamin D deficiency	↓ Intestinal absorption ↑ Urinary losses
Malabsorption	↓ Intestinal absorption ↑ Urinary losses
Renal tubular defects	↑ Urinary losses
Extracellular volume expansion	↑ Urinary losses
Diuretic therapy	↑ Urinary losses
$NaHCO_3$	↑ Urinary losses
Chronic glucocorticoid effect	↑ Urinary losses
Recovery from hypothermia	↑ Urinary losses
Glucagon administration	↑ Urinary losses
Starvation	Lack of intake
Salicylate poisoning*	Shift of P into cells
Acute gout*	Shift of P into cells
Gram negative bacteremia*	Shift of P into cells
Insulin administration	Shift of P into cells
Glucose or fructose administration	Shift of P into cells
Androgen therapy	Incorption of P into cells

*These clinical conditions are associated with hyperventilation and respiratory alkalosis. The latter is associated with movement of phosphorus from extracellular fluid into cells.

Table 2: Causes of Severe Hypophosphatemia
Prolonged use of phosphate binding antacids
Hyperalimentation
Nutritional recovery syndrome
Recovery from severe burns
Severe respiratory alkalosis
Diabetes mellitus
Alcoholism

Various antacids, such as aluminum hydroxide or carbonate or magnesium hydroxide, bind phosphorus in the intestine and renders it unabsorbable. Therefore, severe hypophosphatemia and phosphate depletion may develop with the use of antacids. Indeed, severe hypophosphatemia has been noticed in patients with duodenal ulcer and in those with advanced renal failure who were treated with these compounds (4-6).

The hypophosphatemia in patients recovering from severe and extensive burns is probably related to two factors: 1) augmented urinary losses of phosphate during the diuresis period that follows the initial salt and water retention, and 2) phosphorus incorporation in newly formed tissue during the period of healing.

Marked hyperventilation causes respiratory alkalosis and profound hypophosphatemia (7-9). This is particularly important in conditions associated with prolonged and chronic alkalosis. Mollster and Tuttle (9) have shown that the fall in blood levels of inorganic phosphorus during respiratory alkalosis are not due to the rise in pH but due to the fall in pCO_2, since a similar increase in blood pH but without a change in pCO_2 produced by metabolic alkalosis, causes only a slight fall in blood phosphorus. In addition, phosphorus disappears from the urine during respiratory alkalosis indicating that the hypophosphatemia is due to a shift of phosphorus from extracellular sites into the cells. The sequence of events which lead to hypophosphatemia during respiratory alkalosis is depicted in Figure 1.

Several mechanisms may underlie the hypophosphatemia in patients with diabetes mellitus. It should be noted that serum phosphorus is usually normal when the disease is adequately controlled. However, hypophosphatemia of varying degree may develop in patients with untreated diabetes mellitus, and especially when the disease is complicated with ketoacidosis (10,11). Osmotic diuresis, metabolic acidosis, and insulin therapy may all be contributory in the genesis of the hypophosphatemia (Figure 2).

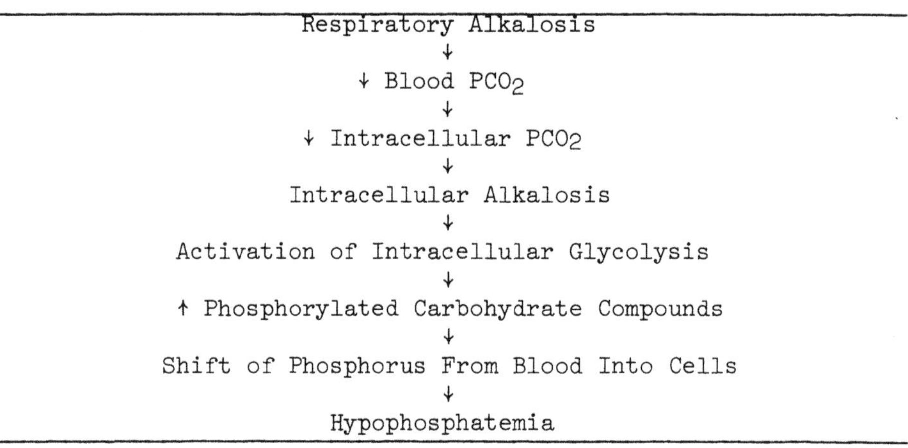

Figure 1: Mechanism of hypophosphatemia during respiratory alkalosis

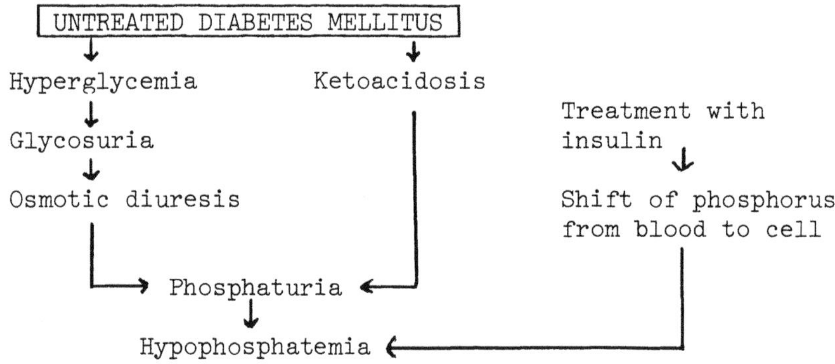

Figure 2: Mechanism of hypophosphatemia in patients with untreated diabetes mellitus

Hypophosphatemia is common in patients with chronic alcoholism. The factors responsible for the fall in serum phosphorus are multiple. They include poor dietary intake, use of antacids for the management of gastric disturbances, vomiting and diarrhea, alcohol ingestion, per se, metabolic acidosis (betahydroxybutyric and lactic acidosis) and hyperventilation associated with liver cirrhosis or acute withdrawal syndrome. The interaction between these factors and the pathways through which they may induce hypophosphatemia are depicted in Figure 3.

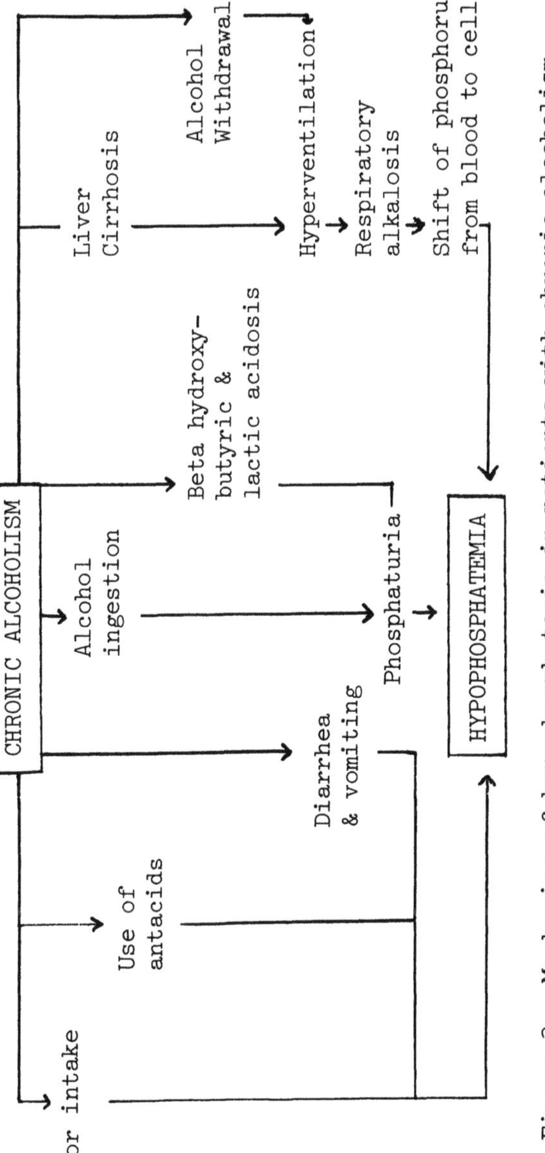

Figure 3: Mechanism of hypophosphatemia in patients with chronic alcoholism

Table 3: Effects of Severe Hypophosphatemia

1. Central Nervous System (12,13)
   Irritability, parasthesia, dysarthria, anisocoria, hyperreflexia, confusion, obtandation, convulsion, coma
2. Hematopoietic System
   Red blood cells (14-19): ↓ ATP content, ↓ hexokinase activity, ↑ fructokinase activity, ↓ 2,3 diphosphoglycerate, ↑ oxygen affinity, ↑ rigidity, ↓ life span, spherocytosis, hemolysis
   Leukocytes (20): ↓ chemotactic, phagocytic, and bacteriocidal activity
   Platelets (21): ↓ ATP content, thrombocytopenia, shortened platelets survival, impaired clot retraction, megakaryocytosis of the marrow
3. Hypofunction of the Parathyroid Glands (22-24)
4. Skeletal Abnormalities (5,6)
   Bone pain, pseudofractures, rickets or osteomalacia, bone resorption
5. Muscular Dysfunction (5, 25-27)
   Marked muscular weakness, rhabdomyolysis, ↑ blood creatine phosphokinase and aldolase, low transmembrane resting potential difference in muscle
6. Cardiac Function (28,29)
   ↓ myocardial stroke work, ↓ cardiac contractibility, ↑ left ventricular end diastolic pressure
7. Disturbances in Renal Function and Electrolyte Metabolism
   Elevation in serum calcium (5, 30-32)
   Hypomagnesemia (24,33,34)
   Metabolic acidosis (35-28)
   Fall in GFR (39)
   Hypercalciuria (5,32,33,38-41)
   Hypermagnesiuria (33,34)
   Hypophosphaturia (32,42-44)
   Blunted phosphaturic response to extracellular fluid volume expansion or PTH administration (43,45)
   Decreased proximal sodium reabsorption without natriuresis (46)
   Decreased Tm bicarbonate and bicarbonaturia (36,38)
   Decreased Tm glucose (47)
   Reduced titratable excretion
   Decreased renal content of inorganic phosphorus and ATP (32)
   Decreased intracellular hydrogen ion concentration (36)
   Decreased renal gluconeogenesis (48)
   Decreased urinary excretion of cyclic AMP (32)
   Stimulation of 25-hydroxycholecalciferol-1-α-hydroxylase and increased production of $1,25(OH)_2D_3$ (49,50)

The effects of severe hypophosphatemia on the functional integrity of various organs are listed in Table 3. It is evident that the consequences of profound hypophosphatemia and phosphate depletion are widespread. This is not surprising, since two critical disturbances occur during severe hypophosphatemia. First, a decrease in 2,3 diphosphoglycerate in the red blood cells, and this change is associated with increased affinity of hemoglobin to oxygen and, therefore, tissue hypoxia. Second, there is also a decrease in tissue content of ATP and, therefore, a decrease in the availability of energy rich phosphate compounds for cell function. Of course, other metabolic consequences may account for specific functional disturbances. For example, the hypercalciuria may be due to a humoral factor generated during phosphate depletion (51), and the decrease in Tm bicarbonate may be due to the rise in intracellular pH that may occur with phosphate depletion.

REFERENCES

1. Krebs, H.: Rate limiting factors in cell respiration. CIBA Foundation Symposium on Regulation of Cell Metabolism. Little, Brown Publishers, Boston, pp. 1-10, 1959.

2. Betro, M.G., and Pain, R.W.: Hypophosphatemia and hyperphosphatemia in a hospital population. Brit. Med. J. 1:273, 1972.

3. Stein, J.H., Smith, W.O., and Ginn, E.: Hypophosphatemia in acute alcoholism. Am. J. Med. Sci. 252:78, 1966.

4. Bloom, W.L., and Flinchum, D.: Osteomalacia with pseudofractures caused by the ingestion of aluminum hydroxide. JAMA 174:1327, 1960.

5. Lotz, M., Ney, R., and Bartter, F.C.: Osteomalacia and debility resulting from phosphorus depletion. Trans. Assoc. Amer. Physicians, 77:281, 1964.

6. Abrams, D.E., Silcott, R.B., Terry, R., Berne, T.V., and Barbour, B.H.: Antacid induction of phosphate depletion syndrome in renal failure. Western J. Med. 120:157, 1974.

7. Rapoport, S., Stevens, C.D., Engel, G.L., Ferris, E.P., and Logan, M.: The effect of voluntary overbreathing on the electrolyte equilibrium of arterial blood in man. J. Biol. Chem. 163:411, 1946.

8. Okel, B.B., and Hurst, J.W.: Prolonged hyperventilation in man. Associated electrolyte changes and subjective symptoms. Arch. Intern. Med. 108:757, 1961.

9. Mostellar, M.E., and Tuttle, E.P., Jr.: The effects of alkalosis on plasma concentration and urinary excretion of inorganic phosphate in man. J. Clin. Invest. 43:138, 1964.

10. Franks, M., Berris, R.F., Kaplan, N.O., and Myers, G.P.: Metabolic studies in diabetic acidosis. I. The effect of early administration of dextrose. Arch. Intern. Med. 80:739, 1947.

11. Franks, M., Berris, R.F., Kaplan, N.O., Myers, G.P.: Metabolic studies in diabetic acidosis. II. The effect of the administration of sodium phosphate. Arch. Intern. Med. 81:42, 1948.

12. Silvis, S.E., and Paragas, P.D., Jr.: Fatal hyperalimentation syndrome. Animal studies. J. Lab. Clin. Med. 78:918, 1971.

13. Silvis, S.E., and Paragas, P.D., Jr.: Parasthesias, weakness, seizures and hypophosphatemia in patients receiving hyperalimentation. Gastroenterol. 62:513, 1972.

14. Lichtman, M.A., Miller, D.R., and Freeman, R.B.: Erythrocyte adenosine triphosphate depletion during hypophosphatemia in a uremic subject. N. Engl. J. Med. 280:240, 1969.

15. Lichtman, M.A., Miller, D.R., Cohen, J., Waterhouse, C.: Reduced red cell glycolysis, 2,3-diphosphoglycerate and adenosine triphosphate concentration, and increased oxygen affinity caused by hypophosphatemia. Ann. Intern. Med. 74:562, 1971.

16. Travis, S.F., Sugarman, H.J., Rubergy, R.L., Dudrick, S.J., Delivoria-Papadopoulos, M., Miller, L.D., and Oski, F.A.: Alterations of red cell glycolytic intermediates and oxygen transport as a consequence of hypophosphatemia in patients receiving intravenous hyperalimentation. N. Engl. J. Med. 285:763, 1971.

17. Jacob, H.S., and Amsden, T.: Acute hemolytic anemia with rigid red cell hypophosphatemia. N. Engl. J. Med. 285:1446, 1971.

18. Klock, J.C., Williams, H.E., Mentzer, W.C.: Hemolytic anemia and somatic cell dysfunction in severe hypophosphatemia. Arch. Intern. Med. 134:360, 1974.

19. Territo, M.D., and Tanaka, K.R.: Hypophosphatemia in chronic alcoholism. Arch. Intern. Med. 134:445, 1974.

20. Craddock, P.R., Yawata, Y., Van Santen, L., Silverstadt, S., Silvis, S., and Jacob, H.S.: Acquired phagocyte dysfunction. A complication of the hypophosphatemia of parenteral hyperalimentation. N. Engl. J. Med. 290:1403, 1974.

21. Yawata, Y., Hebbel, R.P., Silvis, S., Howe, R., and Jacob, H.: Blood cell abnormalities complicating the hypophosphatemia of hyperalimentation: Erythrocytes and platelet ATP deficiency associated with hemolytic anemia and bleeding in hyperalimented dog. J. Lab. Clin. Med. 84:643, 1974.

22. Stoerk, H.C., and Carnes, W.H.: The relation of the dietary Ca: P ratio to serum Ca and to parathyroid volume. J. Nutr. 29:43, 1945.

23. Slatopolsky, E., Calger, S., Pennell, J.P., Taggart, D.D., Canterbury, J.M. Reiss, E., and Bricker, N.S.: On the pathogenesis of hyperparathyroidism in chronic experimental renal insufficiency in the dog. J. Clin. Invest. 50:492, 1971.

24. Dominguez, J.H., Fray, R.W., and Leman, J., Jr.: Dietary phosphate deprivation in women and men. Effects of mineral and acid balances, parathyroid hormone and the metabolism of 25-OH-vitamin D. J. Clin. Endocrinol. & Metab. 43:1056, 1976.

25. Tuller, M.A.: Myoglobinuria with or without drug usage. JAMA 217:1868, 1971.

26. Knochel, J.P., Bilbrey, G.L., Fuller, T.J., and Carter, N.W.: The muscle cell in chronic alcoholism. The possible role of phosphate depletion in alcoholic myopathy. Ann. N.Y. Acad. Sci. 252:274, 1975.

27. Fuller, T.J., Carter, N.W., Barcenas, C., and Knochel, J.P.: Reversible experimental myopathy associated with phosphorus depletion. J. Clin. Invest. 57:1019, 1976

28. O'Connor, L.R., Wheeler, W.S., and Bethune, J.E.: Effect of hypophosphatemia on myocardial performance in man. N. Engl. J. Med. 297:901, 1977.

29. Fuller, R.J., Nichols, W.W., Brenner, B.J., and Peterson, J.C.: Effects of phosphorus depletion on left ventricular energy generation. In Homeostasis of Phosphate and Other Minerals, eds. Massry, S.G., Ritz, E., and Rapado, A., Plenum Publishing Co., New York, In Press, 1978.

30. Freeman, S., and McLean, F.C.: Experimental rickets. Blood and tissue changes in puppies receiving a diet very low in phos-horus, with and without vitamin D. Arch. Pathol. 32:387, 1941.

31. Skikita, M., Tsurnfuji, S., and Ito, Y.: Adaptation in renal phosphorus excretion under the influence of parathyroids; a study of ureterally catheterized rats. Endocrinol. Jap. 9:171, 1962.

32. Kreusser, W.J., Kurokawa, K., Aznar, E., and Massry, S.G.: Phosphate depletion: Effect on renal inorganic phosphorus and adenine nucleotides, urinary phosphate and calcium, and calcium balance. Miner. Elect. Metab. 1:30, 1978.

33. Cuisinier-Gleizes, P., Thomasset, M., Sainteny-DeLove, I., and Mathieu, H.: Phosphorus deficiency, parathyroid hormone, and bone resorption in the growing rat. Calcif. Tiss. Res. 20:235, 1976.

34. Kreusser, W.J., Kurokawa, K., Aznar, E., Sachtjen, E., and Massry, S.G.: Effect of phosphate depletion on magnesium homeostasis. J. Clin. Invest. 61:In press, 1978.

35. Barzel, U.S.: Parathyroid hormone, blood phosphorus, and acid-base metabolism. Lancet, 1:1329, 1971.

36. Gold, L.W., Massry, S.G., Arieff, A.I., and Coburn, J.W.: Renal bicarbonate wasting during phosphate depletion: A possible cause of altered acid-base homeostasis in hyperparathyroidism. J. Clin. Invest. 52:2556, 1973.

37. Massry, S.G., Kurokawa, K., Arieff, A.I., and Ben-Isaac, C.: Metabolic acidosis of hyperparathyroidism. Arch. Intern. Med. 134:385, 1974.

38. Emmett, M., Goldfarb, S., Agus, Z.S., and Narins, R.C.: The pathophysiology of acid-base changes in chronically phosphate-depleted rats. Bone kidney interaction. J. Clin. Invest. 59:291, 1977.

39. Coburn, J.W., and Massry, S.G.: Changes in serum and urinary calcium during phosphate depletion: Studies on mechanisms. J. Clin. Invest. 49:1073, 1970.

40. Day, H.G., and McCollum, E.V.: Mineral metabolism, growth, and symptomatology of rats on a diet extremely deficient in phosphorus. J. Biol. Chem. 130:269, 1939.

41. Young, V.R., Lofgreen, G.P., and Luick, J.R.: The effects of phosphorus depletion and of calcium and phosphorus intake on the endogenous excretion of these elements by sheep. Brit. J. Nutr. 20:795, 1966.

42. Steele, T.H., Engle, J.E., Tanaka, Y., Lorenc, R.S., Dudgeson, K.L., and DeLuca, H.F.: On the phosphatemic action 1,25-dihydroxy vitamin D_3. Amer. J. Physiol. 229:489, 1975.

43. Steele, T.H., and DeLuca, H.F.: Influence of dietary phosphorus on renal phosphate reabsorption in the parathyroidectomized rats. J. Clin. Invest. 57:867, 1976.

44. Trohler, V., Bonjour, J.P., and Fleish, J.: Inorganic phosphate homeostasis: Renal adaptation to the dietary intake in intact and thyroparathyroidectomized rats. J. Clin. Invest. 57:264, 1976.

45. Beck, N.: Effect of dietary phosphorus (P) intake on renal actions of parathyroid hormone (PTH) and cyclic AMP (cAMP). Proc. Amer. Soc. Nephrol. 9:1, 1976.

46. Goldfarb, S., Westby, G.R., Goldberg, M., and Agus, Z.S.: Renal tubular effects of chronic phosphate depletion. J. Clin. Invest. 59:770, 1977.

47. Gold, L.W., Massry, S.G., and Friedler, R.M.: Effect of phosphate depletion on renal tubular reabsorption of glucose. J. Lab. Clin. Med. 89:554, 1977.

48. Kreusser, W.J., Descoeudres, C., Oda, Y., Aznar, E., and Massry, S.G.: Effects of phosphate depletion (PD) on renal gluconeogenesis (GNG). Proc. Amer. Soc. Nephrol. 10:90A, 1977.

49. Tanaka, Y., and DeLuca, H.F.: The control of 25-hydroxyvitamin D metabolism by inorganic phosphorus. Arch. Biochem. Biophys. 154:566, 1973.

50. Hughes, M.R., Haussler, M.R., Werdegal, J., and Baylink, D.J.: Regulation of serum 1α, dihydroxyvitamin D_3 by calcium and phosphate in the rat. Science, 190:578, 1975.

51. Ben-Isaac, C., Massry, S.G., Rosenfeld, S., Kleeman, C.R., and Bick, M.: Evidence for humoral factors responsible for the hypercalciuria of phosphate depletion. J. Clin. Invest. 53:5a, 1974.

DISTURBANCES IN ACID-BASE BALANCE DURING HYPOPHOSPHATEMIA AND PHOSPHATE DEPLETION

Michael Emmett and Donald W. Seldin

From the Department of Internal Medicine, The University of Texas Southwestern Medical School, Dallas, Texas

It is very difficult to produce appreciable phosphate depletion by simple dietary deprivation. During an 18-day study of normal men and women on a low phosphate diet (1), phosphate virtually disappeared from the urine by the twelfth day, but persistent stool losses resulted in a slight negative balance in both sexes. Nevertheless, serum phosphorus remained normal in men (perhaps because of greater soft tissue breakdown, as evidenced by more extensive potassium losses) but fell in women (where the large calcium losses suggest a skeletal origin). In both men and women, however, the loss of phosphate from the body was small. By contrast, severe hypophosphatemia may eventuate as a result of shifts of phosphate into cells without any appreciable loss from the body. To examine derangements in phosphate metabolism, therefore, a sharp distinction must be made between hypophosphatemia and disturbances in phosphate metabolism which may or may not be associated with it.

In Table I, hypophosphatemia is defined as a low concentration of serum phosphate with either normal or reduced cellular phosphate stores. Phosphate depletion means a reduction in the phosphate to nitrogen ratio (↓P/N) for the body as a whole. Redistribution refers to a transfer of phosphate from the extracellular space to certain tissues. Serum phosphorus may fall but the P/N ratio for the body as a whole remains unchanged. Finally, trapping refers to a block in the intracellular utilization of phosphate without any necessary change in the P/N ratio of the whole body or specific tissues.

The various disturbances leading to phosphate depletion, redistribution, and trapping are summarized in Table II, while Table III contrasts the possible intracellular phosphate

TABLE I

Deranged Phosphate Metabolism

Definitions	
Hypophosphatemia:	**Low concentration of serum phosphate; normal or low intracellular phosphate.**
Phosphate depletion:	**Loss of intracellular phosphate in excess of nitrogen (↓ P/N) for the body as a whole.**
Redistribution:	**Transfer of phosphate from certain tissues to sequestration sites (e.q., liver or muscle glycogen, growing bone, etc.). Total body phosphate is normal.**
Trapping:	**Intracellular block in utilization of phosphate. Total body and tissue phosphate normal.**

composition in uncomplicated malnutrition with that of the various derangements of phosphate metabolism. If pure starvation (malnutrition) is imposed without other associated stresses (Table III), the protein mass of the body shrinks, but cellular composition may remain relatively well preserved. It is, of course, recognized that the ketonemic acidosis of starvation, as well as other metabolic effects, may alter this picture, but it is important to emphasize the tendency of starvation to alter principally cellular mass, not cellular composition. Phosphate depletion always lowers the total body P/N ratio, although, as Table III indicates, total body phosphorus is depleted with urinary and stool losses but is actually increased if there is growth with relative phosphate deficiency. Redistribution (Table III) can cause profound hypophosphatemia and depletion of phosphorus in key organs, without necessarily altering total body phosphorus. Trapping (Table III) may cause serious lactic acidosis and rhabdomyolysis without altering in any way total body phosphorus. In evaluating clinical phosphorus homeostasis, therefore, the cellular phosphate stores of the total body as well as specific organs must be inferred or measured, if the significance of disturbed phosphate metabolism or hypophosphatemia or both is to be properly assessed.

TABLE II

Deranged Phosphate Metabolism

1. **Phosphate depletion (↓ total body P/N)**
   - a. **Urinary losses**
     - (1) **↑ parathyroid hormone**
     - (2) **↑ effective extracellular volume**
     - (3) **Fanconi lesions**
   - b. **Stool losses**
     - (1) **Malabsorption**
     - (2) **Amphojel during phosphate deprivation**
   - c. **Growth during phosphate deprivation**
2. **Redistribution (↓ P/N of only certain tissues)**
   - a. **Alkalosis**
   - b. **Liver glycogen deposition**
   - c. **Muscle glycogen deposition**
   - d. **Bone synthesis**
3. **Trapping (intracellular block in phosphate utilization)**
   - a. **Fructose loads**
   - b. **Hereditary fructose intolerance**

The most important causes of severe clinically significant hypophosphatemia have been examined in detail by Knochel (2) and are summarized in Table IV. Hypophosphatemia in alcoholics may result from phosphate depletion (perhaps resulting from starvation, magnesium depletion and ketonemic acidosis) on which is superimposed sudden redistribution of phosphate into tissues along with carbohydrate loads. Recovery from diabetic acidosis similarly appears to generate hypophosphatemia because rapid intracellular redistribution of phosphate under the impact of insulin is superimposed on a background of cellular deficit. By contrast, hyperalimentation with phosphate-free solutions and amphogel during phosphate deprivation represent forms of phosphate depletion owing to augmented stool losses.

The overall consequences of derangements in phosphate metabolism vary greatly, depending on the intensity and duration of the state, the specific tissue or tissues suffering the greatest assault, and concomitant stresses which tend to amplify the effects of phosphate disturbances. If, for example, severe exercise is superimposed on muscles depleted of phosphate, rhabdomyolysis may occur.

TABLE III

Derangements of Phosphate Metabolism

Body Composition	Total Body		Muscle & Kidney		Urine	Serum
	P	P/N	P	P/N	P	P
Malnutrition	↓	N	↓	N	N	N
Phosphate Depletion Urine (PTH, ↑ volume, Fanconi lesions) Stool (malabsorption, Amphojel)	↓	↓	↓	↓	N↑ 0	↓
Growth during Phosphate Deprivation	↑	↓	↑	↓	0	↓
Redistribution Alkalosis Liver glycogen Muscle glycogen Bone synthesis	N	N	↓	↓	0	↓
Trapping Fructose loads Hereditary fructose intolerance	N	N	N	N	N	N

TABLE IV

CLINICAL CAUSES OF SEVERE HYPOPHOSPHATEMIA

1. Alcoholics given carbohydrate loads
2. Hyperalimentation
3. Recovery from diabetic acidosis
4. Amphojel during phosphate deprivation

In the following discussion of acid-base disturbances druing derangements in phosphate metabolism, the effects of prolonged phosphate depletion on urine and plasma composition are examined, and cellular and renal contributions to the acid-base disturbances are first discussed. Second, acid-base disturbances in special forms of deranged phosphate metabolism are analyzed.

ACID-BASE BALANCE DURING PROLONGED PHOSPHATE DEPLETION

The studies of Emmett and his associates (3) provide long-term balance data on the effects of chronic phosphate deprivation in the rat. The results are summarized in Table V. During the first month, as phosphate disappeared from the urine, the excretion of bicarbonate and calcium increased greatly, but serum bicarbonate concentration remained unchanged, a finding suggesting extra-renal bicarbonate production. After one month, bicarbonate excretion had fallen sharply, but not to control levels; a mild metabolic acidosis supervened in plasma. The continued bicarbonate excretion in the presence of metabolic acidosis suggests both renal bicarbonate wasting, as well as lessened net extra-renal alkali production, as evidenced by falling calcium excretion (diminished bone breakdown) and rising serum and urine phosphorus (perhaps due to cell breakdown)

The sequence of events portrayed by these findings can be considered the consequence of cancelling and reinforcing tissue and renal responses to phosphate depletion, and is summarized in Table VI.

TABLE V

Acid-Base Pattern During Prolonged P Depletion

I. Early phase (constant low P diet) — < 1 month

- **A. Urine: ↑ HCO_3; ↑ Ca; ↓ P**
- **B. Plasma: stable HCO_3; ↑ Ca; ↓ P**
- **— .. alkali generation from bone breakdown**

II. Late phase (constant low P diet) — > 1 month

- **A. Urine: ↕ HCO_3 (less marked); ↑ Ca (less marked); ↑ P**
- **B. Plasma: mild acidosis; ↓ P (but rising)**
- **— .. continued, though lessening, alkali generation from bone breakdown; possible acid load from cell damage**

Bone Breakdown as a Source for Alkali Generation

Bone is a huge mineral reservoir containing 99% of the calcium, 80% of the phosphate, and 50% of the magnesium in the body. The major crystalline deposit is calcium-hydroxy apatite, $Ca_{10}(PO_4)_6CO_3$. When this salt dissolves at pH 7.4, the following results:

$$Ca_{10}(PO_4)_6CO_3 \xrightarrow{+8.2\ HOH} 10\ Ca^{++} + 4.8\ HPO_4^{=} + 1.2\ H_2PO_4^{-} + 9.2\ OH^{-} + CO_2$$

Thus, calcium-hydroxy apatite resorption adds calcium, phosphate and alkali to the extracellular fluids. In the intact animal, reduction of any one of these three components stimulates bone resorption, either by directly acting on the skeleton as in metabolic acidosis (4,5,6) and hypophosphatemia (7), by influencing hormone secretion (hypocalcemia stimulating parathyroid and inhibiting thyrocalcitonin release), or by activating vitamin D (phosphate depletion).

TABLE VI

Tissue and Renal Responses to P Depletion

- I. **Transcellular and cellular discharge of alkali and acid**
  - A. **Bone breakdown – alkali generation**
    - 1. **Ionization of apatite – alkali load**
    - 2. **↑ urinary Ca and HCO_3; constant plasma HCO_3**
  - B. **Cell breakdown – acid generation**
    - 1. **Lessening HCO_3 excretion with rising plasma P**
    - 2. **Potential sources of acid**
      - a. **↑ lactate production**
        - (1) **Hypoxia (↓ red cell 2-3DPG and ATP) → respiratory alkalosis → intracellular alkalosis**
        - (2) **↑ intracell. alkaline phosphate (stable pCO_2) → intracellular alkalosis**
      - b. **↓ Pi → ↓ ATP → rhabdomyolysis**
- II. **Renal responses**
  - A. **↓ bicarbonate reclamation – proximal tubule**
    - 1. **↓ HCO_3 Tm and threshold**
    - 2. **Fanconi disturbance**
    - – **? 2° to renal intracellular alkalosis or ATP depletion or both**
  - B. **↓ bicarbonate regeneration – distal nephron**
    - 1. **↑ HCO_3 delivery**
    - 2. **↓ urinary buffer (P)**
    - 3. **↓ NH_3 production**

The increased urinary calcium and bicarbonate excretion in the face of a normal serum bicarbonate is strong evidence for bone breakdown as the source of alkali. Despite this alkali load, metabolic alkalosis does not eventuate. However, when rats are nephrectomized during the first month of phosphate deprivation, distinct metabolic alkalosis develops (3), clearly indicating that the enhanced urinary bicarbonate excretion is the consequence, at least in part, of increased alkali generation. When colchicine was given to phosphate-depleted rats to inhibit bone resorption, a pronounced metabolic acidosis developed, yet urinary bicarbonate excretion still continued. This is clear evidence for impaired renal bicarbonate reabsorptive capacity, a defect that is masked by the alkali load derived from bone breakdown.

Cell Breakdown as a Possible Source for Acid Generation

After one month of phosphate depletion in the rat (3), bicarbonate excretion falls but not to normal, hypercalciuria lessens, and phosphate excretion increases. Metabolic acidosis develops and serum phosphorus rises (Table VI). Part of the fall in bicarbonate is clearly secondary to diminished renal reabsorptive capacity; part of the fall is also due to diminished bone breakdown caused by a shrinkage of bone mass, as evidenced by falling calcium excretion. But part of the fall in bicarbonate may be due to an acid load from soft tissues, as is suggested by the rising plasma phosphate. The acid load may originate from increased lactate production or mild rhabdomyolysis or both (Table VI).

Increased lactate produced may be the consequence of intracellular alkalosis. Phosphate deficiency, by diminishing red cell 2,3-DPG and ATP, impairs the release of oxygen, thereby tending to generate tissue hypoxia and respiratory alkalosis. In addition, intracellular alkalosis may result from increased intracellular alkaline phosphate salts, a conclusion suggested by the findings of Massry and his associates (8) that intracellular pH (as measured by DMO) is alkaline during phosphate depletion even when blood pCO_2 remains normal. The intracellular alkalosis resulting from these two mechanisms could activate the phosphofructokinase enzyme system, thereby accelerating glycolysis and enhancing lactate production. Furthermore, severe phosphate depletion may diminish hepatic cellular ATP, thereby stimulating glycolysis and lactate formation via a Pasteur effect.

In addition to lactate production, a profound reduction in intracellular phosphate may so reduce ATP as to lead to rhabdomyolysis, particularly if muscle phosphate depletion is associated with exercise (2,9).

Renal Responses to Phosphate Depletion

Impressive evidence exists that severe phosphate depletion causes diminished bicarbonate reabsorptive capacity and increased splay, suggesting impaired proximal tubular bicarbonate reabsorption (8). This could be the consequence of intracellular alkalosis. It is also possible that there is a diffuse disturbance in proximal tubular transport, as evidenced in clearance studies by a diminished Tm for glucose (10) and in micropuncture studies by a reduction in the reabsorption of sodium, calcium and water (11). This reduced proximal tubular reabsorptive capacity is not the consequence of increased parathyroid hormone, hyperkalemia, hypocapnea, or volume expansion (8,10,11,12). If renal ATP is reduced to the same extent that has been measured in other tissues, this may limit the net reabsorption in the proximal tubule of a wide variety of substances by impairing active transport.

Phosphate depletion results in the virtual elimination of phosphate from the final urine. The mechanism of this avid phosphate reabsorption is not understood. Phosphate reabsorption is not appreciably suppressed by parathyroid hormone, cyclic AMP, or an acute increase in the filtered load of phosphorus (13,14). The elimination of phosphate from the urine means that titratable acid excretion will be trivial. In consequence, urinary acid excretion is critically dependent on NH_3 excretion. However, the fact that ammonia excretion is low in phosphate-depleted animals cannot be construed as evidence that ammonia production is impaired, since the high urine pH resulting from diminished proximal bicarbonate reabsorption could sharply reduce ammonia trapping.

Two studies in human subjects suggest that ammonia production may be impaired. Infants recovering from protein-calorie malnutrition and phosphate depletion were found to have severe metabolic acidosis and a markedly reduced urinary excretion of phosphate and titratable acid; ammonia excretion was very low despite an acid urine pH. Phosphate repletion acutely increased the excretion of ammonia and titratable acid without altering urine pH (15). In malnourished adults (16) with very low rates of phosphate and titratable acid excretion, and an acid urine pH, ammonia excretion was nevertheless markedly reduced. Normalization of ammonia excretion was achieved with general recovery from malnutrition.

ACID-BASE DISTURBANCES RESULTING FROM PHOSPHATE TRAPPING

In special circumstances, deranged phosphate metabolism may be associated with lactic acidosis and rhabdomyolysis. It has already been pointed out that this may occur with phosphate depletion and exercise, where the low intracellular phosphate leads to ATP deficiency in liver and muscle. In the phosphate depletion associated with alcoholism, diabetic acidosis, or malnutrition, rapid utilization of carbohydrate resulting from glucose infusions or insulin administration may trap phosphate in the liver; rhabdomyolysis may result. These instances represent acute fulminant hypophosphatemia caused by the redistribution of phosphate during a chronic deficit. In such circumstances the clinical picture may be far more severe than in chronic phosphate depletion (2).

A very striking illustration of the effect of phosphate trapping occurs with fructose loads, even in normal subjects without any aldolase deficiency (17,18,19). Fructose metabolism in the liver is depicted in Figure 1, where fructose is seen to be metabolized via ketohexokinase to fructose-1-phosphate, a reaction that utilizes ATP and forms ADP. The rapid depletion of ATP and the fall in inorganic phosphate activates the enzyme adenylate deaminase, thereby catalyzing the conversion of adenosine monophosphate (AMP) to inosine monophosphate (IMP). The latter, in turn, inhibits the fructose-1-phosphate aldolase; fructose-1-phosphate therefore cannot be rapidly metabolized. In consequence, there is continued ATP and phosphate depletion with fructose-1-phosphate formation (17). In normal human subjects, large fructose infusions are associated with lactic acidosis (18,19). The lactic acidosis probably results from two effects of ATP depletion (Fig. 2). The phosphofructokinase enzyme system is activated by ATP depletion (Pasteur effect), causing increased hepatic lactate production. Second, it is likely that without adequate ATP, hepatic conversion of incoming lactate to glucose, a process requiring 6 ATPs, is impaired. The combination of increased production and diminished utilization of lactate by the liver generates lactic acidosis. In view of the evidence for concomitant rhabdomyolysis (2), it is possible that massive fructose loading can induce sufficient fructose to enter the muscle cell where its metabolism via hexokinase could result in ATP depletion.

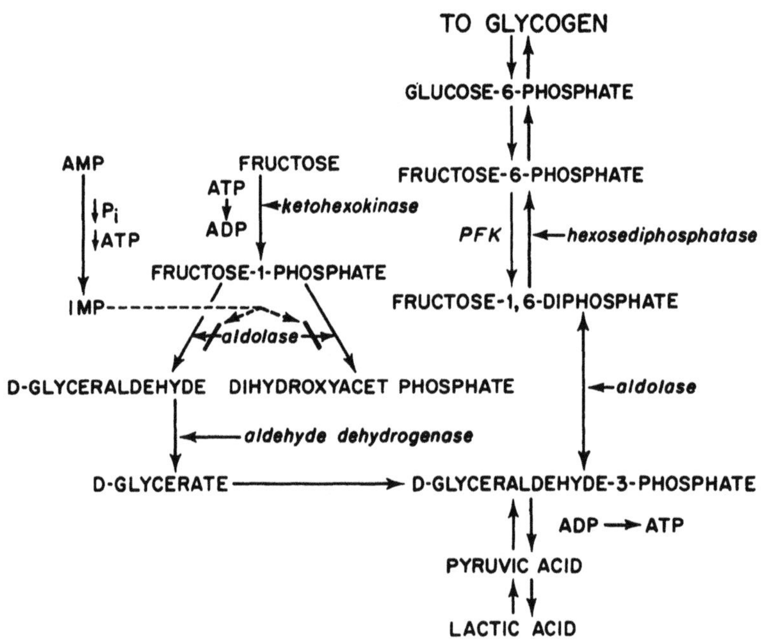

FIGURE 1

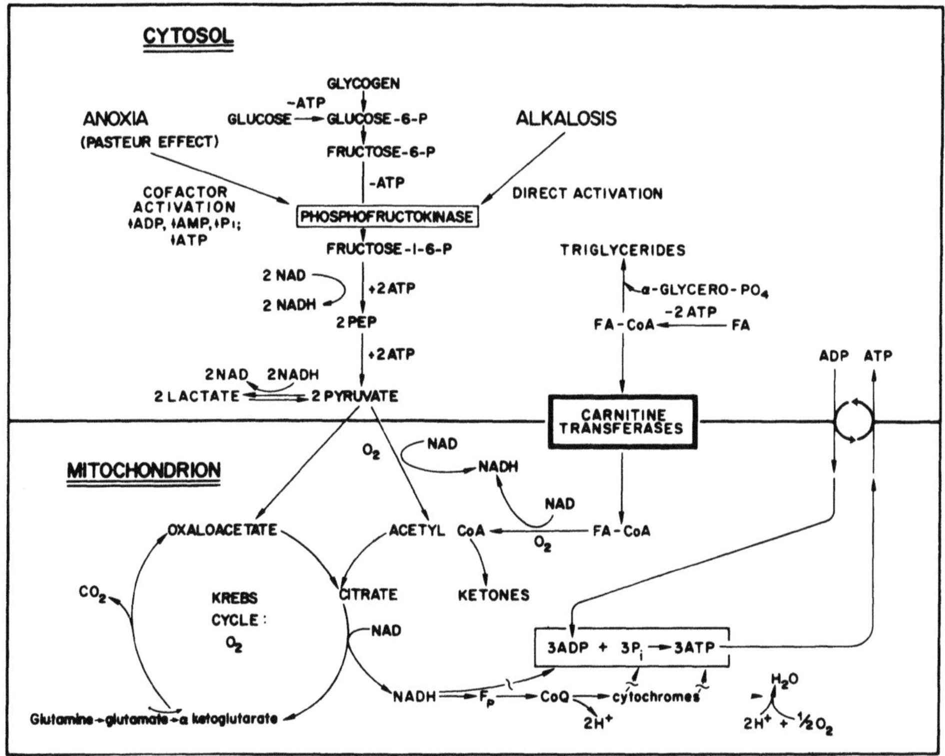

FIGURE 2

SUMMARY

Phosphate depletion leads to bone resorption, resulting in the accession of alkali to the blood and urine. There may also be a release of lactic acid from liver, resulting from ATP depletion and intracellular alkalosis. In general, the net result of these tissue effects is an alkali load discharged into the extracellular fluid.

In the kidneys, phosphate depletion causes impaired proximal tubular reabsorption of bicarbonate, and perhaps other substrates, owing in all likelihood to both intracellular alkalosis and depletion of ATP. This impaired proximal capacity to reclaim bicarbonate results in hyperchloremic acidosis. The distal nephron may contribute to acidosis by virtue of inability to produce titratable acid (phosphate-free urine) and perhaps impaired ammonia production.

Severe phosphate depletion, therefore, tends to produce hyperchloremic acidosis as a result of a diminished capacity for bicarbonate reclamation in the proximal tubule and probably some impairment of bicarbonate regeneration in the distal nephron. These effects, when marked, ultimately outweigh the contribution of alkali coming from bone breakdown.

In the liver, phosphate depletion may stimulate lactic acid production by reducing hepatic ATP stores (Pasteur effect) and producing intracellular alkalosis. ATP depletion may also limit hepatic uptake of lactate.

Finally, in muscle cells ATP depletion, resulting from either profound hypophosphatemia or the metabolism of massive fructose loads, may eventuate in frank rhabdomyolysis.

REFERENCES

1. Dominguez, J.H., Gray, R.W., and Lemann, J., Jr.: Dietary phosphate deprivation in women and men: effects on mineral and acid balances, parathyroid hormone and the metabolism of 25-OH-vitamin D. JCE & M 43:1056, 1976.
2. Knochel, J.P.: The pathophysiology and clinical characteristics of severe hypophosphatemia. Arch. Intern. Med. 137:203, 1977.
3. Emmett, M., Goldfarb, S., Agus, A., and Narins, R.G.: The pathophysiology of acid-base changes in chronically phosphate-depleted rats. J. Clin. Invest. 59:291, 1977.
4. Sherwood, L.M., Parris, E.E., and Raisz, L.G.: Physiologic and pharmacologic regulation of bone resorption. New Engl. J. Med. 282:909, 1970.
5. Goodman, A.D., Lemann, J., Jr., Lennon, E.J., and Relman, A.S.: Production, excretion, and net balance of fixed acid in patients with renal acidosis. J. Clin. Invest. 41:495, 1965.
6. Litzow, J.R., Lemann, Jr., Jr., and Lennon, E.J.: The effect of treatment of acidosis on calcium balance in patients with chronic azotemic renal disease. J. Clin. Invest. 46:280, 1967.
7. Raisz, L.G., and Niemann, I.: Effect of phosphate, calcium and magnesium on bone resorption and hormonal responses in tissue culture. Endocrinology 85:446, 1969.
8. Gold, L.W., Massry, S.G., Arieff, A.I., and Coburn, J.W.: Renal bicarbonate wasting during phosphate depletion. J. Clin. Invest. 52:2556, 1973.
9. Fuller, T.J., Carter, N.W., Barcenas, C., and Knochel, J.P.: Reversible changes of the muscle cell in experimental phosphorus deficiency. J. Clin. Invest. 57:1019, 1976.
10. Gold, L., Massry, S.G., and Friedler, R.M.: Effect of phosphate depletion on renal glucose reabsorption. Clin. Res. 24:400A, 1976.

11. Goldfarb, S., Westby, G.R., Goldberg, M., and Agus, Z.S.: Renal tubular effects of chronic phosphate depletion. J. Clin. Invest. 59:770, 1977.

12. Schmidt, R.W., and Fairfield, S.: On the pathogenesis of metabolic acidosis in phosphate depleted dogs. Clin. Res. 25: 449A, 1977.

13. Steele, T.H., Underwood, J.L., Stromberg, B.A., and Larmore, C.A.: Renal resistance to parathyroid hormone during phosphorus deprivation. J. Clin. Invest. 58:1461, 1976.

14. Steele, T.H., and Underwood, J.L.: Response to phosphorus depletion by the isolated rat kidney. J. Clin. Invest. 25:509A, 1977.

15. Kohaut, E.C., Klish, W.J., Beachler, C.W., and Hill, L.L.: Reduced renal acid excretion in malnutrition: a result of phosphate depletion. Am. J. Clin. Nutr. 30:861, 1977.

16. Klahr, S., Tripathy, K., and Lotero, H.: Renal regulation of A-B balance in malnourished man. Am. J. Med. 48:325, 1970.

17. Woods, H.F., Eggleston, L.V., and Krebs, H.A.: The cause of hepatic accumulation of fructose 1-phosphate on fructose loading. Biochem. J. 119:501, 1970.

18. Woods, H.F., and Alberti, K.G.M.M.: Dangers of intravenous fructose. Lancet 2:1354, 1972.

19. Sahebjami, H., and Scalettar, R.: Effects of fructose infusion on lactate and uric acid metabolism. Lancet 1:366, 1971.

PHOSPHATE DEPLETION AND ADENINE NUCLEOTIDE METABOLISM IN KIDNEY AND LIVER

K. Kurokawa, W.J. Kreusser, and S.G. Massry

University of Southern California School of Medicine,
Los Angeles, California U.S.A.

INTRODUCTION

Adenosine triphosphate (ATP) and other adenine nucleotides are the major energy coupling mechanism between the energy-producing and the energy-consuming systems in the cells. In a variety of diseased states, an altered metabolism of adenine nucleotides has been implicated in their pathogenesis. There are a few experimental model systems in which one can alter adenine nucleotide metabolism through a different mechanism and study the role of adenine nucleotides in cell functions as shown in Table 1 (1). Although studies using the first three models have been extensively performed, effects of phosphate depletion on the metabolism of adenosine triphosphate and other phosphate compounds in various organ systems have been studied rather to a lesser extent except in red cells, leukocytes, and platelets, where the relationship between a fall in plasma inorganic phosphate (Pi), a fall in tissue Pi, a decrease in tissue ATP, and some forms of cellular dysfunction have been demonstrated (2). Since a major portion of ATP is synthesized from ADP and Pi by oxidative phosphorylation in mitochondria, a deficiency of Pi will result in an impairment of ATP generation. Thus, various organ dysfunctions described in phosphate depletion have been attributed to a fall in the availability of energy-rich phosphate compounds such as ATP. Nevertheless, data on the changes in levels of adenine nucleotides and Pi in different organ systems are limited.

During phosphate depletion, there develops a variety of renal tubular dysfunctions, including altered tubular reabsorption of phosphate, calcium (Ca), sodium bicarbonate, and glucose (3-9). Some of these tubular dysfunctions may be due to a fall in ATP since transport mechanisms for these substances may partly depend on energy, the source of which could be ATP. Furthermore, renal conversion of 25-hydroxycholecalciferol (25-HCC) to 1,25-dihydroxycholecalciferol (1,25-DHCC) may be enhanced in phosphate depletion and this activation of 25-HCC-1-α-hydroxylase may be related to a fall in tissue Pi levels (10). Functional abnormality in liver cells during phosphate depletion has not been widely appreciated, but there have been a few reports implicating the presence of hepatic dysfunction in this diseased state (2).

In the present study, we evaluated the effects of phosphate depletion on adenine nucleotide metabolism and on changes in tissue Pi levels in kidney and liver to gain further insight into the mechanisms of some of the pathophysiology of phosphate depletion.

TABLE 1. Models to induce changes in adenine nucleotides in vivo

Mechanism	Procedure
1) Interference with oxidative generation of ATP	a) Temporary or permanent ligation of blood supply
	b) Injection of uncouplers of oxidative phosphorylation
2) Trapping of adenosine moiety as S-adenosyl derivative	a) Ethionine in rat, guinea pig, and so on--mainly liver
	b) Methionine in guinea pig--liver
3) Trapping of excess inorganic phosphate → deamination of AMP	a) Fructose or glycerol by injection--liver, kidney
	b) 2-Deoxyglucose
4) Deficiency of inorganic phosphate	a) Dietary phosphate restriction

METHODS

Male Sprague-Dawley rats, weighing 70-80 grams, were used. After several days of the equilibrium period when animals were fed a control diet containing 0.44% phosphate and 0.41% Ca, rats were divided into two groups. One group of rats was fed a diet containing low phosphorus (.03%-PD rats) ad libitum. They showed a retarded weight gain. The other group was fed control diet in an amount adequate to achieve a similar weight gain as PD rats (pair-weighed rats - PW rats). Both groups of rats had free access to de-ionized water throughout the study period. Rats were kept in metabolic cages on these dietary regimen for up to 8 weeks. After 8 weeks of phosphate depletion, some rats received the control diet ad libitum for 2 weeks (phosphate repletion). At various intervals of time during this experimental protocol, plasma and urine were collected for analyses of Pi, Ca, and Mg. At first, second, 4th, 6th and 8th weeks of phosphate depletion and at 10th week of study (8 weeks PD plus 2 weeks of phosphate repletion), kidney and liver were analyzed for Pi, Ca, Mg, and adenine nucleotides (ATP, ADP, and AMP), using the quick-freeze technique described below.

In separate experiments, besides PD and PW rats, another group of rats received 0.5% $MgCl_2.6H_2O$ as drinking water while they were fed low phosphorus diet. This procedure prevented a fall in plasma Mg. After 6 weeks they were sacrificed and kidney and liver were analyzed for Pi and adenine nucleotides.

Rats were lightly anesthetized with intraperitoneal injection of pentobarbital, 35 mg/kilogram body weight. The abdominal cavity was rapidly opened and the left kidney was avulsed and compressed between two plates of Dry Ice to a thin, frozen disc. Then, a piece of liver was frozen to a thin disc in the same manner. The time elapsing from opening the abdominal cavity until freezing the kidney was less than 7 seconds, and to freezing the liver less than 20 seconds. In preliminary studies, it was found that there was no difference in ATP levels between kidneys quick-frozen by the present method and those by compression with aluminum tongs pre-cooled in liquid nitrogen (11). Furthermore, when liver was frozen within 7 seconds after opening the abdomen and analyzed for ATP, the levels of hepatic ATP were not significantly different from those obtained by the present method. These data support the adequacy of the present procedure and are consistent with the relatively slow fall in hepatic ATP during acute ischemia induced during tissue sampling (12). Furthermore, the values obtained in the present study are comparable to those reported previously by several investigators (11-15). Frozen tissue, weighing 100-200 mg, was pulverized, weighed, and homogenized in 3.0 ml of 6% perchloric acid in 50% ethanol at $0^{o}C$. After removing the denatured protein, the supernatant was neutralized by careful dropwise addition of 3 M K_2CO_3 in 0.5 M triethanolamine as described by Nagata and Rasmussen (15). These neutralized perchloric acid extracts were analyzed for ATP, ADP, and AMP spectrophotometrically by the enzymatic method described by Williamson and Herczek (11). Tissue Pi was measured by the method described by Schulz _et al_ (16). Plasma Pi was measured by the method of Chen _et al_ (17), and Ca and Mg were measured by atomic absorption spectrometer.

RESULTS

Changes in Plasma and Urinary Phosphate, Calcium and Magnesium

As shown in Figure 1, there was a rapid fall in plasma Pi during the first few days of phosphate depletion, which was followed by more gradual decline throughout the study period. Plasma Ca rose from 10.2±0.11 to 12.4±0.20, 12.5±0.28, 12.0±0.36 mg/dl at 2nd, 3rd and 4th week of phosphate depletion, respectively, but returned to normal levels at 6th week of phosphate depletion. Plasma Mg level fell precipitously during the first day of phosphate depletion from 1.2±0.2 to 0.79±0.10 mEq/L, then maintained at low level. There was a marked fall in urinary phosphate excretion and marked rises in urinary excretion of Ca and Mg.

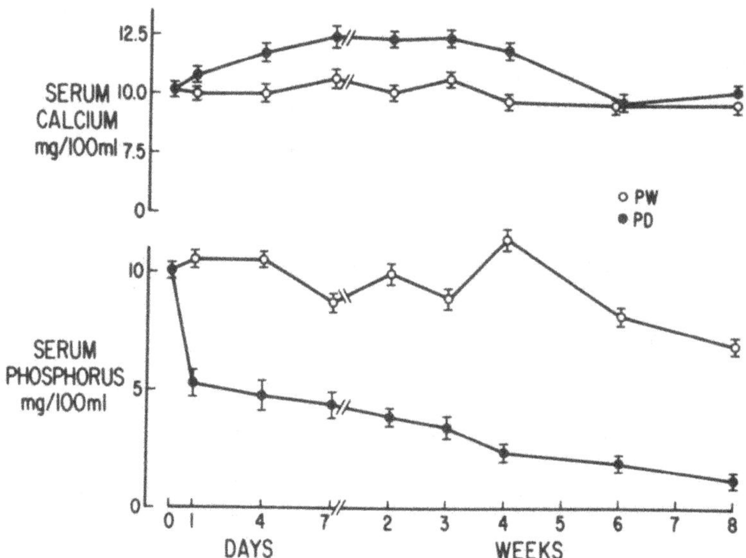

Figure 1: Changes in plasma calcium and inorganic phosphate during phosphate depletion for 8 weeks.

Changes in Tissue Inorganic Phosphate and Adenine Nucleotides in Kidney During Phosphate Depletion

Figures 2, 3, and 4 depict the changes in tissue Pi and adenine nucleotides in kidney during the course of phosphate depletion. Shaded areas represent 2-week course of phosphate repletion. Tissue Pi levels fell slightly during the first week of phosphate depletion, but became significantly lower ($p<0.05$) than control at second week of phosphate depletion. In both PD and PW rats, all adenine nucleotides were elevated during the first two weeks of phosphate depletion. A significant decrease in ATP in PD rats occurred at sixth week of phosphate depletion. After fourth week of study, renal ATP levels were higher in PW rats than those in PD rats. The ADP and AMP levels were essentially unchanged except for an increase in both nucleotides during the first two weeks in both PD and PW rats. The energy charge of adenylate, (ATP + ½ADP)/(ATP + ADP + AMP) (18), did not change significantly until 6th week of PD, but then fell significantly at 8th week of PD to 0.70±0.01 (control, 0.76±0.01). The equilibrium constant (Keq) for adenylate kinase, (ATP x AMP)/ADP^2, fell significantly from 1.67±0.10 to 1.40±0.08, 1.07±0.11, and 1.27±0.11, at 4th, 6th and 8th week of phosphate repletion, respectively (Fig 5). At 10th week of study after 2 weeks of phosphate repletion, renal Pi, ATP, ADP, AMP, and adenylate energy charge returned to normal, and Keq of adenylate kinase rose to a level higher than control both in PD and PW rats.

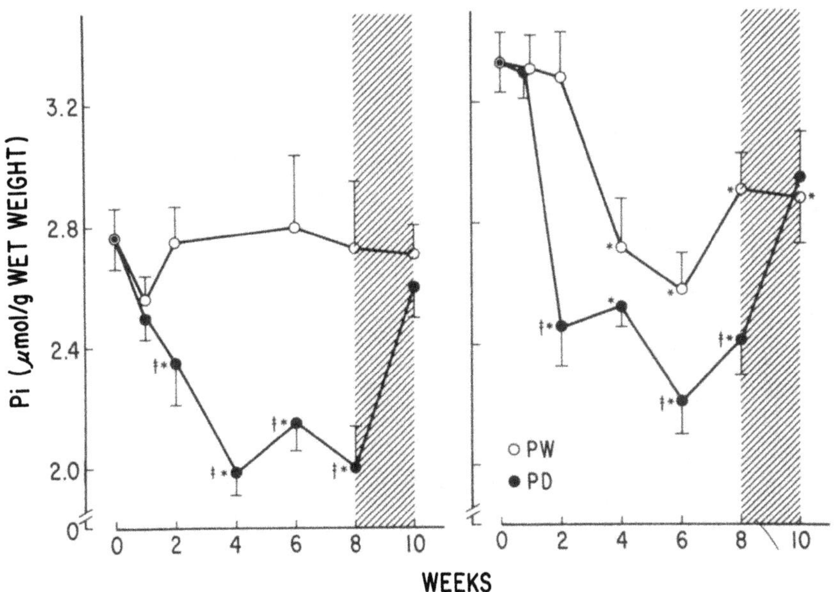

Figure 2: Effect of phosphate depletion and repletion on inorganic phosphorus of kidney (left panel) and liver (right panel). Data are the means ± SD for 6-13 rats at each point. Shaded area represents the phosphate repletion period. PW = pair-weighed rats; PD = phosphate-depleted rats.
* Significantly ($p<.05$) different from values at 0 time (normal).
‡ Significantly ($p<.05$) different from values of PW rats.

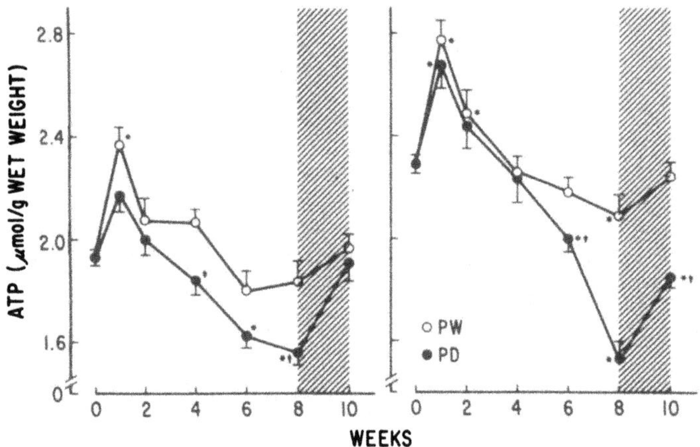

Figure 3: Effect of phosphate depletion and repletion on adenosine triphosphate (ATP) of kidney (left panel) and liver (right panel). Abbreviations as in Figure 2.

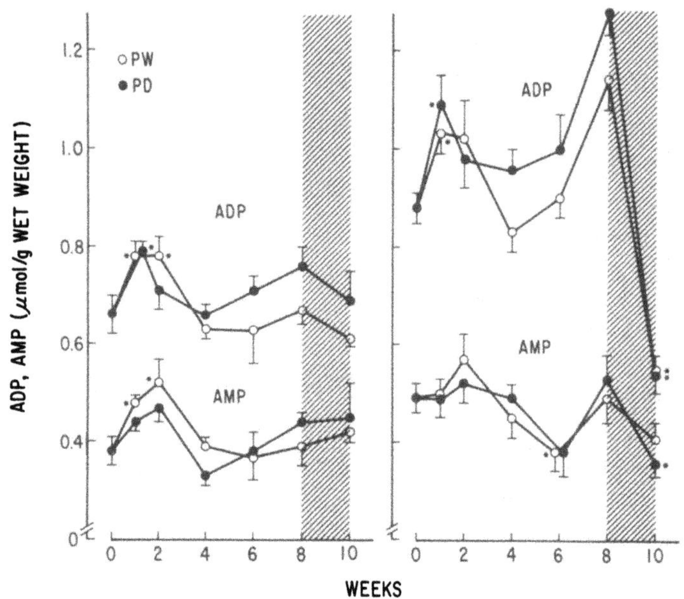

Figure 4: Effect of phosphate depletion and repletion on adenosine diphosphate (ADP) and adenosine monophosphate (AMP) of kidney (left panel) and liver (right panel). Abbreviations as in Figure 2.

Changes in Tissue Inorganic Phosphate and Adenine Nucleotides in Liver During Phosphate Depletion

As shown in Figures 2, 3, and 4 changes in the liver Pi and adenine nucleotides were similar to those in kidney except for the following few points. Liver Pi started to fall at second week of phosphate depletion, and it also started to fall in PW rats at 4th week of study. Nevertheless, liver Pi level remained higher in PW rats than in PD rats throughout the study. Liver ATP in PD rats fell at 6th week of PD, and it also fell slightly at 8th week in PW rats, though it remained higher than those in PD rats. The energy charge of adenylate did not fall until at 8th week in PD rats and it decreased to 0.50±0.01 (control, 0.74±0.01). Keq of adenylate kinase fell from 1.45±0.08 to 0.99±0.08, 0.78±0.12, and 0.51±0.06, at 4th, 6th and 8th week, respectively (Fig. 5). It also fell in PW rats in 6th and 8th week of study to 0.99±0.04 and 0.84±0.10, respectively. Upon the repletion of phosphate, liver ATP in PD rats returned halfway to normal, while there was a marked fall in ADP resulting in a rise in Keq. The energy charge also became slightly higher than control (0.74±0.01) in both PD (0.77±0.01) and PW (0.79±0.01) rats after repletion. These changes in the liver may suggest that liver is extremely "hungry" for Pi and rapidly synthesizing ATP upon phosphate repletion.

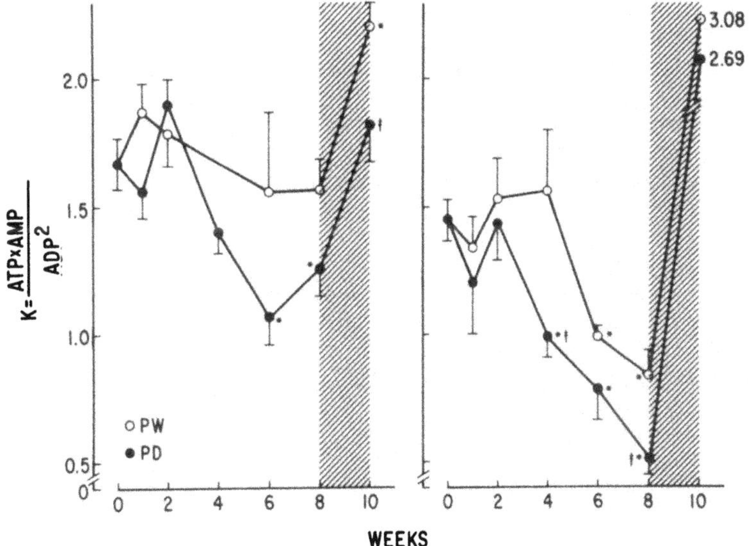

Figure 5: Changes in the equilibrium constant of adenylate kinase of kidney (left panel) and liver (right panel) during phosphate depletion. Abbreviations as in Figure 2.

There was no significant difference in water content of kidney and liver of PW, and PD rats at 0. 2, 4, 6 and 8 weeks of the study.

Effects of Magnesium Supplement on Equilibrium Constant of Adenylate Kinase

Changes in adenine nucleotides and Keq of adenylate kinase were compared at 6th week of study in PW, PD, and PD rats supplemented with Mg in drinking water throughout the course of the study. The supplement of Mg prevented a fall in plasma Mg occurring in phosphate depletion, but without effect on a fall in plasma Pi. As shown in Figure 6, Mg supplement did not prevent a fall in ATP but prevented a fall in Keq in the kidney. In the liver Mg supplement was, again, without effect on a fall in ATP, but Keq in this group (0.70±0.04) was between that in PW (0.89±0.07) and PD (0.54±0.06) rats.

DISCUSSION

The present results demonstrate that prolonged, severe phosphate depletion may cause a fall in ATP in kidney and liver, which may underlie some of the disturbances in functions of these organs. The time course study of phosphate depletion revealed that during the first week of phosphate depletion there was no significant fall in tissue Pi and ATP in liver and kidney while plasma Pi was falling rapidly (Figs. 1-4). At the second week of phosphate depletion, kidney and liver Pi decreased while renal and hepatic ATP started to fall after 6th week of phosphate depletion. Thus, there seems to be no direct correlation between plasma Pi, tissue Pi and ATP. By contrast, in erythrocytes for example, there is a good correlation between these parameters during PD (19,20). This is probably due to the lack of intracellular phosphate-storing organelles, mitochondria, in red blood cells and also due to the fact that Pi diffuses passively across the red cell membrane. In kidney and liver, however, a large portion of phosphate can be stored in mitochondria; thus, only prolonged phosphate depletion may result in significant depletion of the intracellular phosphate store. Furthermore, the transport of Pi across renal plasma membrane is, at least partly, an active process (21) which may help in preventing loss of Pi from cellular stores in the fact of low extracellular Pi. Because of its abundance within these cells, it may require a certain time for cell Pi to decrease to a rate-limiting level for ATP generation in mitochondria where the synthesis of ATP from ADP and Pi takes place. This may explain the time lag between a fall in tissue Pi at second week and a fall in ATP at sixth week, and may suggest that only after six weeks of phosphate depletion, intramitochondrial Pi might fall below the critical level for oxidative phosphorylation.

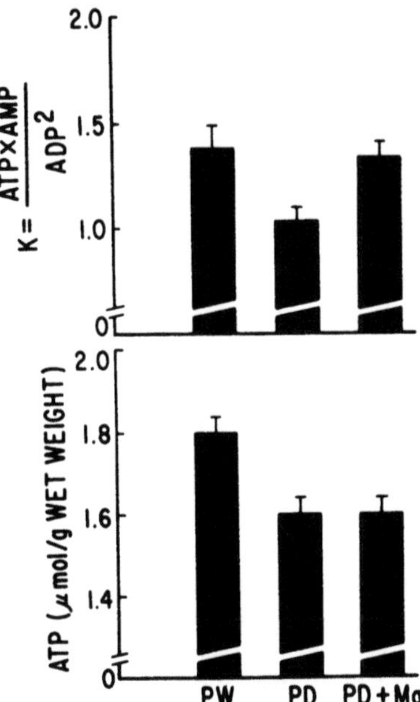

Figure 6: Effects of magnesium supplement on ATP levels and equilibrium constant of renal adenylate kinase. Values are means ± SD for 6 rats in each group. PD + Mg represents the group fed low phosphate diet with 0.5% $Mg_2Cl.6H_2O$ as drinking water. K value of PD rats and ATP levels of PD and PD + Mg groups were significantly ($p<.01$) different from those of PW rats.

Other factors may be operative to prevent a fall in renal and hepatic tissue Pi during phosphate depletion. One possible factor is an altered vitamin D metabolism or vitamin D metabolite. It has been shown that vitamin D may play an important role in extracellular and intracellular phosphate homeostasis through its action on intestine, bone, and perhaps kidney (22). The phosphate mobilizing action of vitamin D is primarily due to its active metabolite, 1,25-DHCC. A recent study by Birge and Haddad (23) indicates that vitamin D has a direct action on skeletal muscle phosphate uptake. They showed that vitamin D facilitates Pi entry into muscle cell of vitamin D-deficient rats, resulting in an increased ATP concentration and an accelerated incorporation of leucine into muscle protein. This action of vitamin D was shown to be due to 25-HCC, but not to 1,25-DHCC. The specific action of 25-HCC on muscle is further supported by the presence of the cytosol protein fraction in muscle which specifically bind to 25-HCC, with a lower affinity for 1,25-DHCC (23). It is possible that in kidney and liver the high plasma 1,25-DHCC levels seen in phosphate depletion (24) may enhance Pi uptake into cells, thus, helping to maintain cellular Pi and ATP against the low plasma Pi concentration as shown in **Figures 1 to 3.** Stated in another way, at any given extracellular Pi concentration, an elevated 1,25-DHCC may facilitate entry of Pi into cells and maintain ATP levels; thus, severe phosphate depletion is necessary to result in falls in cell Pi and ATP.

We did not measure specifically renal cortical Pi or adenine nucleotides. We assumed that changes observed in the whole kidney would reflect those in renal cortical tissue (12) since medullary tissue comprises only 10-15% of total renal tissue. One may argue that measurements of Pi and ATP in whole kidney may mask a fall in cortical Pi and ATP. However, if cortical Pi or ATP levels are to fall by 5%, medullary Pi or ATP has to rise approximately by 30% to make total renal Pi or ATP remain unchanged. This is an unlikely possibility. Tanaka and DeLuca have proposed that phosphate depletion stimulates renal 25-HCC-1-α-hydroxylase via a fall in renal cell Pi (10). We found a slight, but not significant, fall in renal tissue Pi during the first week of phosphate depletion. This does not exclude the possibility that the intracellular distribution and the intramitochondrial concentration of Pi may be altered despite no change in total Pi, and such changes might be of critical importance for the regulation of 1-α-hydroxylase activity.

The pattern of changes in adenine nucleotides during experimental phosphate depletion was different from that observed in other conditions shown in Table 1. In acute ischemia, there is a rapid fall in ATP with reciprocal rises in ADP and AMP, both in liver and kidney (12). A fall in ATP in kidney is very rapid, reaching 25% of normal at 30 seconds of ischemia (12). Trapping of excess inorganic phosphate by fructose injection causes an immediate fall in ATP with concomitant but transient rises in ADP and AMP, thus, a fall in the energy charge (25,26). Following this initial event, ADP and AMP fall and the energy charge returns toward normal despite a sustained low ATP level. This "adaptive" change in adenine nucleotide metabolism to restore the energy charge with further reduction of total adenylate pool may be of importance for the maintenance of cell integrity under such stressful conditions (27,28). This fall in AMP occurs due to stimulation of AMP deaminase and 5'-nucleotidase to cleave the accumulated AMP (28). It has been shown that AMP deaminase is inhibited by both ATP and Pi, and 5'-nucleotidase by ATP under normal conditions. A fall in ATP and/or Pi de-inhibits these enzyme activities, resulting in the degradation of AMP and the production of inosine monophosphate and adenosine. Inosine monophosphate is a potent inhibitor of fructose-1-phosphate aldolase, the enzyme which catalyzes the clearance of fructose-1-phosphate. The de-inhibition of 5'-nucleotidase may have a physiological significance in myocardium since adenosine may act as a potent coronary vasodilator. Thus, a rise in adenosine with a fall in ATP in myocardial ischemia may prevent further fall in ATP by increasing oxygen supply to the myocardium through vasodilatation. Inosine monophosphate and adenosine are further metabolized to inosine by 5'-nucleotidase and adenosine deaminase, respectively, and inosine will then be metabolized to uric acid, the level of which rises in plasma and in urine after fructose load (25). Thus, after fructose load, there is a net loss of adenine nucleotide, primarily in liver and kidney (25,26,28). It has been suggested that these biochemical findings in fructose loading in rats may resemble those seen in patients with hereditary fructose intolerance, a condition with defective fructose-1-phosphate aldolase in liver, kidney, and possibly gut, and part of the symptomatology of hereditary fructose intolerance may be due to ATP deficiency in these organs (29).

As shown in Figures 2 through 5, one of the major alterations in adenine nucleotide metabolism in the experimental phosphate depletion model was a fall in the equilibrium constant (Keq) of adenylate kinase which coincided with (in kidney) or preceded (in liver) a fall in ATP. Only at 8th week of phosphate depletion did the energy charge of adenylate fall significantly. The maintenance of the energy charge at 4th and 6th week of phosphate depletion with a fall in ATP and slight, but not significant, decrease in AMP may reflect the de-inhibition of AMP deaminase and 5'-nucleotidase by a fall in ATP and Pi. However, the striking change in Keq of adenylate kinase may be related to abnormal extracellular and intracellular distribution of Mg, a key ion for the regulation of this enzyme (30,31).

Hypomagnesemia with negative Mg balance due to excess urinary loss of this ion develops during PD in rats (32). Hypomagnesemia and hypermagnesuria was also noted during phosphate depletion in humans (33). In the present study, total Mg content in liver decreased at 6th and 8th week of phosphate depletion but did not change in kidney (34). However, this observation does not rule out a decrease in cytosolic Mg which comprises a portion of total cell Mg, a fraction of which is in ionized form (35). Since adenylate kinase is localized primarily in cytosol (36), a change in cytosolic Mg ion concentration will influence adenylate kinase significantly and may affedt the integrity of cell functions. It is of interest that the maintenance of serum Mg concentration during phosphate depletion by oral Mg supplementation prevented a fall in Keq of adenylate kinase though it was without effect on the fall in tissue Pi and ATP (Figure 6), supporting the role of Mg ion for an altered

Keq of the enzyme in phosphate depletion. The significance of this altered Keq of adenylate kinase on biochemical and physiological functions of these organs are to be evaluated.

Measurement of tissue levels of ATP at a steady state does not provide information on the turnover of this nucleotide. Considering the facts that Pi is necessary for the formation of ATP and that Mg is a co-factor for most of the ATP-catalyzing enzymes (such as kinases, ATP-ases), it is conceivable that in phosphate depletion both ATP synthesis and utilization are impaired due to a lack of Pi and due to a fall in Mg ion, respectively. Certainly, the evaluation of ATP turnover will provide further insight into the altered energy metabolism in phosphate depletion.

Rats do not ingest adequate amounts of food when they are fed low phosphorus diet, and their growth is impaired. Therefore, some of the abnormalities observed in the present study in phosphate depleted rats may be due to a prolonged low caloric intake, per se. Such effects may be seen in data obtained in pair-weighed rats which are not allowed to ingest adequate amounts of food. These include transient rises in ATP, ADP, and AMP at first week, a slight decrease in ATP at 8th week of study. Also, in liver Keq of adenylate kinase became lower in pair-weighed rats than in normal, but was still higher than in phosphate depleted rats at 6th and 8th week of the study.

Most of the biochemical changes seen in liver and kidney were reversible when rats were phosphate repleted for 2 weeks after 8 weeks of phosphate depletion. The blood chemistry was normalized. Kidney Pi and adenine nucleotide levels returned to normal except for slightly higher AMP, whereas, the abnormalities in liver were only partially restored after two weeks of phosphate repletion. The pattern of changes in adenine nucleotides, Keq of adenylate kinase higher than normal, and the energy charge, particularly in liver (Figure 2), may suggest the acceleration of oxidative phosphorylation with a rapid synthesis of ATP from ADP and Pi upon phosphate repletion.

REFERENCES

1. Farber, E.: ATP and cell integrity. Fed. Proc. 32:1534, 1973.

2. Knochel, J.P.: The pathophysiology and clinical characteristics of severe hypophosphatemia. Arch. Int. Med. 137:203, 1977.

3. Coburn, J.W., and Massry, S.G.: Changes in serum and urinary calcium during phosphate depletion: Studies on mechanisms. J. Clin. Invest. 49:1073, 1970.

4. Troehler, U., Bonjour, J.P., and Fleisch, H.: Inorganic phosphate homeostasis. Renal adaptation to the dietary intake in intact and thyroparathyroidectomized rats. J. Clin. Invest. 57:264, 1976.

5. Steele, T.H., and DeLuca, H.F.: Influence of dietary phosphate on renal phosphate reabsorption in the parathyroidectomized rat. J. Clin. Invest. 57:867, 1976.

6. Gold, L.M., Massry, S.G., Arieff, A.I., and Coburn, J.W.: Renal bicarbonate wasting during phosphate depldtion. A possible cause of altered acid-base homeostasis in hyperparathyroidism. J. Clin. Invest. 52:2556, 1973.

7. Harter, H.R., Mercado, A., Rutherford, W.E., Rodriguez, H., Slatopolsky, E., and Klahr, S.: Effects of phosphate depletion and parathyroid hormone on renal glucose reabsorption. Am. J. Physiol. 227:1422, 1974.

8. Goldfarb, S., Westby, G.R., Goldberg, M., and Agus, Z.S.: Renal tubular effects of chronic phosphate depletion. J. Clin. Invest. 59:770, 1977.

9. Gold, L.M., Massry, S.G., and Friedler, R.M.: Effect of phosphate depletion on renal tubular reabsorption of glucose. J. Lab. Clin. Med. 89:554, 1977.

10. Tanaka, Y., and DeLuca, H.F.: The control of 25-hydroxyvitamin D metabolism by inorganic phosphorus. Arch. Biochem. Biophys. 154:566, 1973.

11. Williamson, J.R., and Herczeg, B.E.: Assays of intermediates of the citric acid cycle and related compounds by fluorometric enzyme method; In, Lowenstein, J.M. 9ed.), Methods in Enzymology Vol 13, New York, Academic Press, p. 434, 1969.

12. Hems, D.A., and Brosnan, J.T.: Effects of ischaemia on content of metabolites in rat liver and kidney in vivo. Biochem. J. 120:105, 1970.

13. Hohorst, H.J., Kreutz, F.H., and Bücher, T.: Über Metabolitgehalte und Metabolit-Konzentrationen in der Leber der Ratte. Biochem. Z. 332:18, 1959.

14. Bucher, N.L.R., and Swaffield, M.M.: Nucleotide pools and $(6-^{14}C)$ orotic acid incorporation in early regenerating rat liver. Biochim. Biophys. Acta 129:445, 1966.

15. Nagata, N., and Rasmussen, H.: Parathyroid hormone and renal cell metabolism. Biochemistry 7:3728, 1968.

16. Schulz, D.W., Passonneau, J.V., and Lowry, O.H.: An enzymatic method for the measurement of inorganic phosphate. Anal. Biochem. 19:300, 1967.

17. Chen, P.S., Toribara, T.Y., and Warner, H.: Microdetermination of phosphorus. Anal. Chem. 28:1756, 1956.

18. Atkinson, D.E.: The energy charge of the adenylate pool as a regulatory parameter. Interaction with feedback modifiers. Biochemistry 7:4030, 1968.

19. Lichtman, M.A., Miller, D.R., and Freeman, R.B.: Erythrocyte adenosine triphosphate depletion during hypophosphatemia in a uremic subject. New Engl. J. Med. 280:240, 1969.

20. Lichtman, M.A., Miller, D.R., Cohen, J., and Waterhouse, C.: Reduced red cell glycolysis, 2,3-diphosphoglycerate and adenosine triphosphate concentration, and increased hemoglobin oxygen affinity caused by hypophosphatemia. Ann. Int. Med. 74: 562, 1971.

21. Wu, R.: Rate-limiting factors in glycolysis and inorganic orthophosphate transport in rat liver and kidney slices. J. Biol. Chem. 240:2373, 1965.

22. DeLuca, H.F.: Recent advances in our understanding of the vitamin D endocrine system. J. Lab. Clin. Med. 87:7, 1976.

23. Birge, S.J., and Haddad, J.G.: 25-hydroxycholecalciferol stimulation of muscle metabolism. J. Clin. Invest. 56:1100, 1975.

24. Hughes, M.R., Brumbaugh, P.F., Haussler, M.R., Wergedal, J.E., and Baylink, D.J.: Regulation of serum 1α,25-dihydroxyvitamin D_3 by calcium and phosphate in the rat. Science 190:578, 1975.

25. Maenpaa, P.H., Raivio, K.O., and Kekomaki, M.P.: Liver adenine nucleotides: Fructose-induced depletion and its effect on protein synthesis. Science 161:1253, 1968.

26. Burch, H.B., Lowry, O.H., Meinhardt, L., Max, P., and Chyu, K.: Effect of fructose, dihydroxyacetone, glycerol and glucose on metabolites and related compounds in liver and kidney. J. Biol. Chem. 245:5092, 1970.

27. Chapman, A.G., and Atkinson, D.E.: Stabilization of adenylate energy charge by the adenylate deaminase reaction. J. Biol. Chem. 248:8309, 1973.

28. Woods, H.F., Eggleston, L.V., and Krebs, H.A.: The cause of hepatic accumulation of fructose-1-phosphate on fructose loading. Biochem. J. 119:501, 1970.

29. Froesch, E.R.: Essential fructosuria and hereditary fructose intolerance. In, Stanbury, J.B., Syngaarden, J.B. and Fredrickson, D.S. (eds.), The Metabolic Basis of Inherited Disease, p. 131, McGraw-Hill, 1972.

30. Ross, I.A.: The state of magnesium in cells as estimated from the adenylate kinase equilibrium. Proc. Natl. Acad. Sci. U.S.A. 61:1079, 1968.

31. Blair, J.M.: Metal ions and enzyme equilibria. A mathematical treatment. FEBS Letters 1:100, 1968.

32. Kreusser, W.J., Kurokawa, K., Aznar, E., Sachtjen, E., and Massry, S.G.: Effect of phosphate depletion on magnesium homeostasis. J. Clin. Invest. 61:(in press), 1978.

33. Dominguez, J.H., Gray, R.W., and Lemann, J.J.: Dietary phosphate deprivation in women and men: Effects on mineral and acid balances, parathyroid hormone, and the metabolism of 25-OH-vitamin D. J. Clin. Endocrinol. Metab. 43:1056, 1976.

34. Kreusser, W.J., Kurokawa, K., and Massry, S.G.: Unpublished observation.

35. Thiers, R.E., and Vallee, B.L.: Distribution of metals in subcellular fractions of rat liver. J. Biol. Chem. 226:911, 1957.

36. Oscai, L.B., and Holloszy, J.O.: Biochemical adaption in muscle. II. Response of mitochondrial adenosine triphosphatase, creatine phosphokinase, and adenylate kinase activities in skeletal muscle to exercise. J. Biol. Chem. 246:6968, 1971.

EFFECT OF PHOSPHORUS DEPLETION ON THE RENAL TRANSPORT OF PHOSPHATE

Thomas H. Steele

Dept. of Medicine, University of Wisconsin

Madison, Wisconsin USA

Because phosphorus depletion is a condition with many adverse clinical consequences, it would seem desirable to have available a compensatory facility serving to promote inorganic phosphate (P_i) conservation and repletion. One very effective compensatory mechanism resides within the kidney.

It has long been known that phosphate-deprived persons or animals manifest profound hypophosphaturia, unless defective renal P_i reabsorption could be held responsible for phosphate depletion in the first place (1-4). Recent balance studies have confirmed this and indicated important sex differences in the response to phosphorus deprivation in humans (5). Also, phosphate loading studies in the rat have demonstrated an increased capacity for renal P_i reabsorption which is initiated during the very early stages of phosphate depletion (6,7). This "adaptive response" in renal P_i reabsorption to even modest phosphate deprivation is all the more remarkable, in that it occurs simultaneously with the defective or impaired reabsorption of certain other solutes filtered by the kidneys (8,9). The purpose of this article is to sketch briefly the development of our knowledge regarding the "adaptation" in P_i reabsorption to changes in the dietary phosphorus, and explore some recent developments in the field.

The response of the normal rat kidney to acute hyperphosphatemia was well characterized in the pioneering studies of Frick (10). In those experiments, the continued infusion of phosphate was accompanied by a subsequent decline in the maximum capacity for P_i reabsorption (Tm_{P_i}). Because phosphate loading may cause extracellular volume expansion and also can result in the increased secretion of parathyroid hormone (11), the so-called "self-depression" of Tm_{P_i} by phosphate infusion initially was ascribed, at least in part, to volume expansion and the stimulation by phosphate loading of parathyroid hormone (PTH) release and subsequent inhibition of renal P_i reabsorption.

Subsequently, in our laboratory, Engle (12) demonstrated that a similar phenomenon occurs in chronically parathyroidectomized (PTX) rats made acutely hyperphosphatemic by phosphate infusion (Figure 1). Engle's studies indicated that phosphate loading *per se* can inhibit Tm_{P_i}, independently of PTH, in rats stabilized on a normal dietary phosphorus intake. PTH and dibutyryl cyclic AMP infusion produced *further* decrements in Tm_{P_i} in the presence of phosphate loading, suggesting that

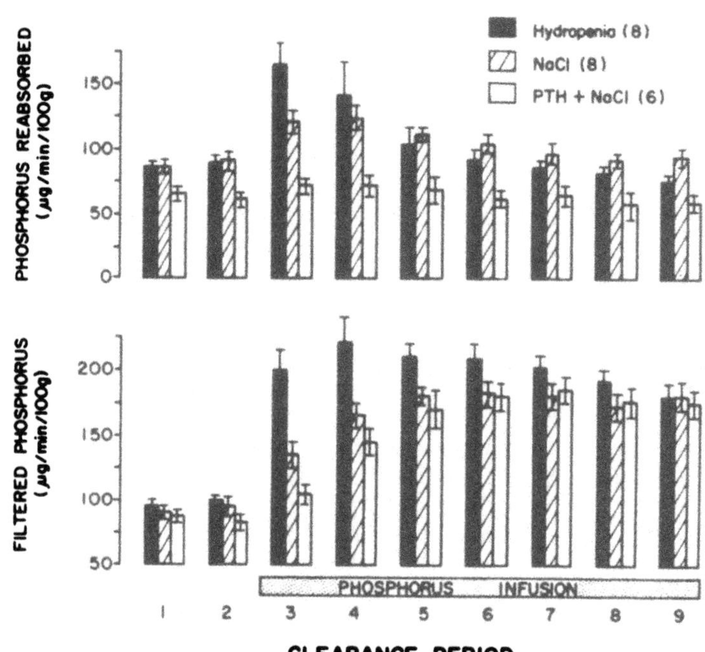

Figure 1: "Self-depression" of P_i reabsorption in parathyroidectomized rats during phosphate loading. From data of Engle (12).

the "self-depression" phenomenon occurred through an action on some component of P_i transport other than that affected by PTH or cyclic AMP (12). Acetazolamide, although phosphaturic at low plasma P_i levels, counteracted the depressive effect of phosphate infusion upon P_i transport during hyperphosphatemia. Thus, the response of the normal rat kidney to phosphate loading is to decrease P_i transport.

Almost simultaneously, studies by Tröhler et al (6) and work in our laboratory (7) indicated that the renal response to phosphate loading is very different in the phosphorus-depleted rat. Those studies demonstrated that renal P_i transport is accelerated in the rat following even very short-term dietary phosphorus deprivation (6). The adaptation in P_i reabsorption to a low phosphorus diet occurred in both intact and TPTX rats. In fact, in chronically thyroparathyroidectomized (TPTX) phosphate-depleted animals, when excessive extracellular volume expansion was avoided, fractional P_i excretion (FEp_i) remained less than 1% - even after the plasma P_i exceeded 20 mg/dl (7). A value of Tmp_i could not be attained in these animals. Thus, for practical purposes, P_i transport by the rat kidney is not saturable following phosphate depletion. A preliminary report of micropuncture studies has indicated that a portion of this adaptation may occur within the distal nephron (13), although other studies have demonstrated exceptionally avid P_i reabsorption by the proximal tubule of the phosphate-depleted dog (14).

Other investigations have revealed that vigorous volume expansion with sodium chloride could partially offset the accelerated P_i transport in phosphate-depleted animals, but P_i reabsorption in the depleted animals was always greater than values obtained in similarly treated rats which had not been deprived of phosphorus (15). In both normal and phosphorus-deprived TPTX rats, sodium bicarbonate loading had a greater inhibitory effect upon P_i reabsorption than did sodium chloride loading (15). Nevertheless, P_i reabsorption remained greater in phosphorus-deprived animals than in controls. Paradoxically, during combined bicarbonate and phosphate loading, intact phosphorus-deprived rats show a greater capacity for P_i reabsorption than did their TPTX counterparts (15). Although the biologic significance of this latter observation presently is not clear, it is consistent with other published data suggesting that PTH in small amounts may exert a permissive action serving to accelerate P_i transport under certain conditions (16). Finally experiments in vitamin D-deficient rats which had been maintained on a very low phosphorus intake also indicated that the adaptive P_i reabsorption response is not ameliorated or counteracted by vitamin D deficiency (17).

Because even small increases in the plasma P_i concentration can reciprocally decrease the plasma ionized calcium and result in stimulation of PTH secretion (11), the occurrence of the adaptive response in P_i transport in intact phosphate-depleted rats, suggested that resistance to at least the phosphaturic actions of PTH would likely be present following phosphorus deprivation (Figure 2). Indeed, the infusion of synthetic bovine PTH (1-34) tetratriacontapeptide in acutely TPTX short-term phosphorus-deprived rats failed to produce a phosphaturic response, but did so in animals which had been stabilized on a high dietary phosphorus intake (18). Yet, despite the absence of the phosphaturic response, the PTH-induced increase in urinary cyclic AMP excretion was as great in the phosphorus-deprived

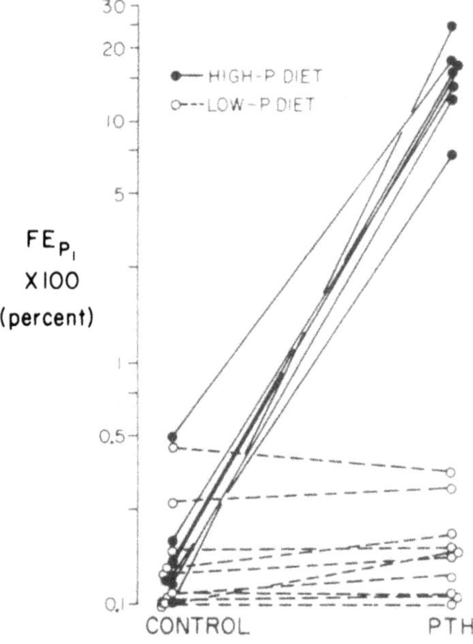

Figure 2. Refractoriness of phosphorus-deprived rats to the phosphaturic action of exogenous PTH. Data from (18).

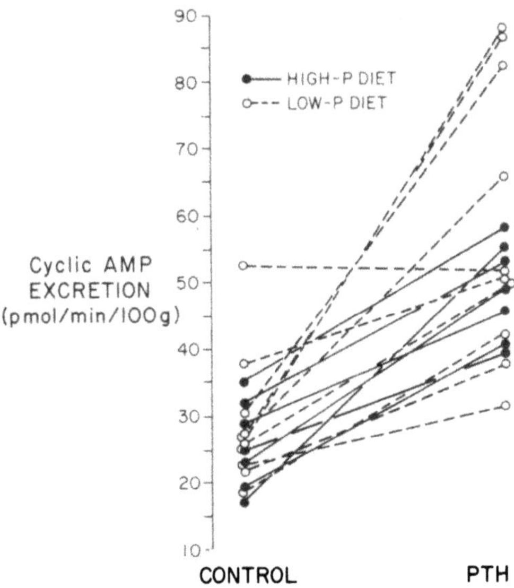

Figure 3. Normal urinary cyclic AMP response to exogenous PTH in phosphorus-deprived rats. Data from (18).

animals as in the controls (Figure 3). In addition, the phosphate-depleted rats manifested resistance to the phosphaturic action of dibutyryl cyclic AMP infusion (18). The resistance of P_i transport to PTH and dibutyryl cyclic AMP in phosphate depletion seems analogous to observations in patients with pseudohypoparathyroidism type II (19), and perhaps to other recent observations in the hamster (20). However, what, if any, common biologic thread may link the three conditions is not presently known.

In attempting to explain the mechanism underlying the diet-induced adaptive response in P_i transport, one obvious possibility is that diminished P_i within the renal cortex could allow the facilitation of P_i reabsorption. Although it has been demonstrated that extensive phosphate depletion can decrease tissue P_i and total phosphorus (21), the accelerated P_i reabsorption in the phosphorus-deprived rat occurs before measureable changes in tissue composition take place. In our hands, following short-term phosphorus deprivation in rats placed on a 0.07% phosphorus diet, renal cortical acid-extractable P_i and total phosphorus are not affected. Furthermore, tissue electrolyte composition was similar in these mildly phosphorus-deprived animals and controls. Thus, it seems unlikely that deficient tissue P_i *per se* is responsible for the increased P_i transport capacity in early dietary phosphorus deficiency. On the other hand, it remains conceivable that some subcellular component of tissue P_i could be depressed early in the course of phosphate depletion and could elicit the observed changes in P_i transport.

It has been suggested that a circulating humoral factor or factors may be responsible for some of the anomalies of renal transport occurring during phosphate depletion (22,23). Indeed, a recent preliminary observation has indicated that many of the abnormalities of renal function noted in phosphorus deprived rats, including hypophosphaturia, can be ameliorated or reversed by hypophysectomy (24). These data are suggestive of a humoral mechanism underlying some or all of the renal function changes in phosphate depletion. Thus, a humoral mechanism might be responsible for the augmented capacity for P_i reabsorption in phosphate depletion.

In order to examine the possibility that a circulating humoral substance mediates the accelerated P_i reabsorptive capacity of phosphate depletion, we have turned to the isolated perfused rat kidney. The preparation we utilize is similar to that developed and described by Bowman (25), whereas a recirculating albumin-containing cell-free perfusate is prepared by the method of Ross *et al* (26). Utilizing this "amalgamated" technique, glomerular filtration rate (GFR) values in the range of 0.5-0.8 ml/min can be attained, and fractional sodium reabsorption of 95-99% occurs consistently when the perfusate albumin concentration is 7.5 grams/dl. Yet, the function of the isolated kidney preparation admittedly is defective as compared to the organ functioning *in situ*. GFR and fractional sodium reabsorption both are less than in the intact rat. Furthermore, P_i reabsorption itself appears to be somewhat defective in the isolated perfused preparation. One would expect P_i reabsorption in this preparation to be similar to that observed in the acutely PTX or TPTX rat. Yet, FE_{P_i} at a perfusate P_i of 8 mg/dl averages 4-6% in the isolated rat kidney preparation, whereas FE_{P_i} averaged 1% in the acutely TPTX rat (7).

In order to determine if the presence (or absence) of a continuously circulating substance is necessary to effect the adaptive changes in P_i transport during phosphate depletion, we studied P_i transport in isolated

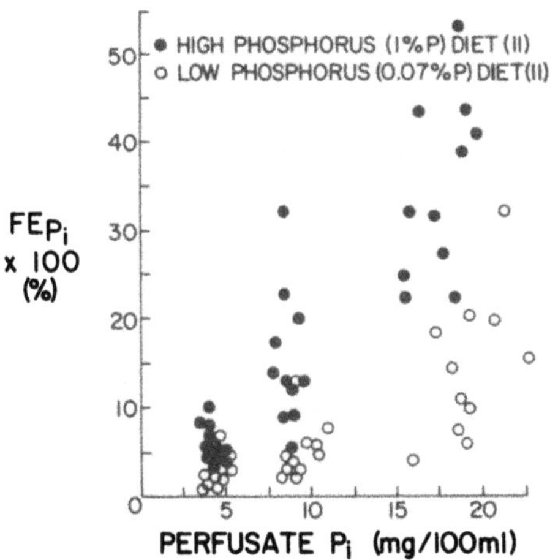

Figure 4. Diminished phosphaturia in isolated perfused rat kidneys harvested from phosphorus-deprived animals (27).

kidneys harvested from rats deprived of phosphorus for two weeks and compared the results with similar experiments on kidneys taken from normal controls (27). Each kidney was studied at three different perfusate P_i concentrations. As perfusate P_i was increased, FEP_i always was significantly less in the phosphorus-deprived kidneys (Figure 4), and absolute P_i reabsorption significantly greater (Figure 5) at any perfusate P_i concentration or filtered P_i load. Because the recirculating perfusate was identical for both types of preparations, the results indicate that it is unlikely that continuous circulation of any humoral substance is required to manifest the adaptive P_i transport phenomenon. Nevertheless, some as yet undefined circulating substance could be responsible for initiating intrarenal changes which then could cause and perpetuate the augmented P_i transport capacity during phosphate depletion.

In order to further examine the applicability of the isolated perfused rat kidney to the study of P_i reabsorption in phosphate depletion, we have examined the isolated preparation for PTH resistance. Prior PTX has little effect on P_i reabsorption in the preparation (Figure 6). In our hands, the isolated kidney requires large amounts of PTH in order to elicit a phosphaturic response. Nevertheless, in kidneys harvested from

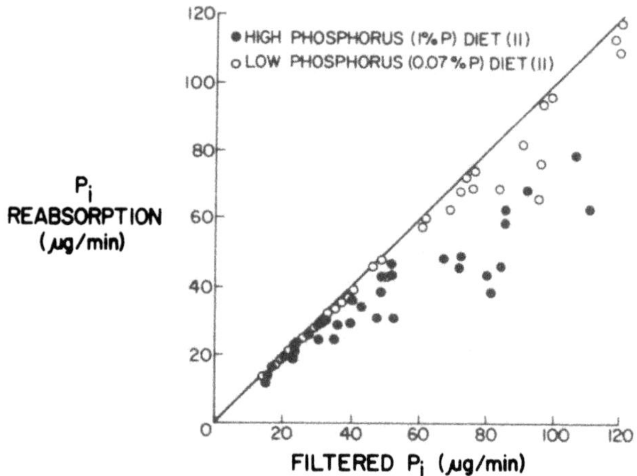

Figure 5. Accelerated P_i reabsorption in isolated perfused rat kidneys harvested from phosphorus-deprived animals (27).

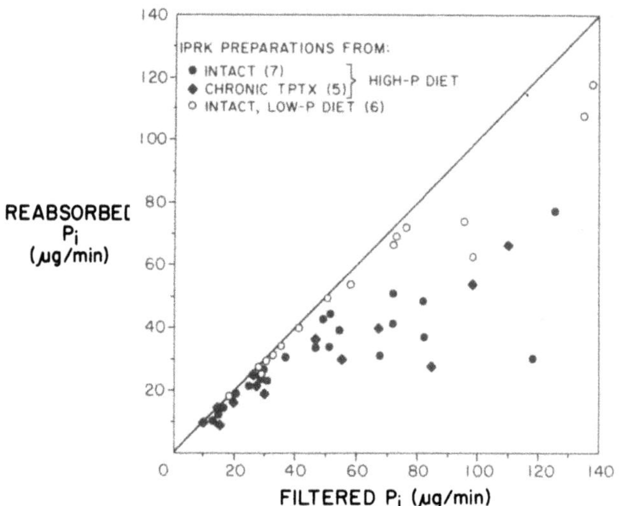

Figure 6. Lack of effect of prior parathyroidectomy on P_i reabsorption in isolated rat kidneys (27).

normal rats, FE_{P_i} at a perfusate P_i concentration of 8 mg/dl increased from a control value of 4%, to 10% after the addition of synthetic bovine PTH (1-34) tetratriacontapeptide to the perfusate at a concentration of 25 pg/ml. Yet, in kidneys harvested from phosphorus-deprived rats, the same amount of PTH increased FE_{P_i} from a control value of 2%, to only 3%, a significantly diminished increment (Figure 7).

Thus, although the isolated rat kidney preparation does exhibit defects both in solute transport and in hormonal responsiveness, it appears to be a useful preparation for studies on phosphate depletion. Perhaps this is underscored by the observation that diminished reabsorption of water, sodium, calcium, and magnesium occur in kidneys harvested from phosphorus-deprived rats, as compared to the values in organs harvested from normals (Figure 8). Yet, these defects in the reabsorption of filtered water and solute occur simultaneously with a capacity for enhanced P_i reabsorption. Such observations suggest that the isolated kidney is appropriate for studies of renal function in phosphate depletion, despite its functional limitations.

In summary, the mammalian kidney fortunately is able to respond to dietary phosphorus deprivation by rapidly increasing its capacity for P_i reabsorption. This serves a biologic function of allowing more rapid

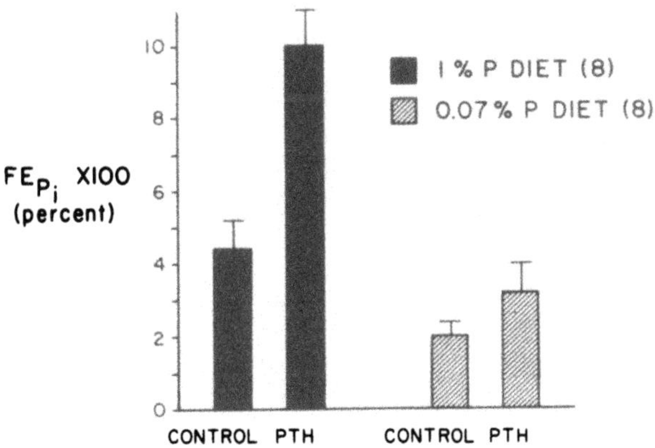

Figure 7. Resistance to synthetic PTH in isolated kidneys from phosphorus-deprived rats, as compared to responses in organs from animals stabilized on a high-phosphorus diet.

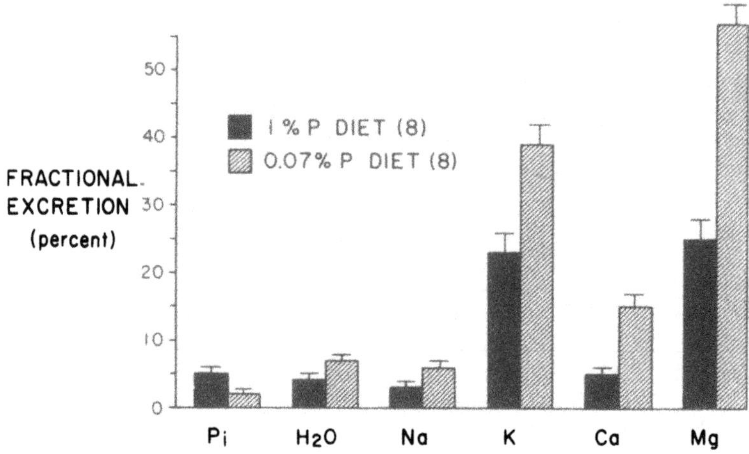

Figure 8. Defective net reabsorption of several solutes and water, in comparison to P_i, in isolated kidneys from phosphorus-deprived rats.

repletion of body phosphorus stores, once the opportunity for replenishment occurs. Crucial to this interpretation is the existence of renal resistance to the phosphaturic action of PTH during phosphate depletion. In the absence of this, any adaptive response in P_i transport soon would be aborted during the repletion process. At present, mechanisms underlying the augmented P_i reabsorption have yet to be established. Present evidence suggests that diminished acid-extractable P_i or renal cortical phosphorus is not required for the transport adaptation to occur, even though tissue compositional changes do occur following prolonged phosphorus deprivation. Although a circulating humoral factor, perhaps serving as the initiator of the adaptive response in P_i transport, seems a reasonable possibility, the existence of any such putative substance has yet to be demonstrated.

ACKNOWLEDGMENT

Some of the original investigations reported in this presentation were supported by grants from The Kroc Foundation.

REFERENCES

1. Shikita, M., Tsurufuji, S., and Ito, Y.: Adaptation in renal phosphorus excretion under the influence of parathyroids; a study of unilaterally catheterized rats. Endocrinol. Jpn. 9:171, 1962.

2. Thompson, D.D., and Hiatt, H.H.: Effects of phosphate loading and depletion on the renal excretion and reabsorption of inorganic phosphate. J. Clin. Invest. 36:566, 1957.

3. Lotz, M., Ney, R., and Bartter, F.C.: Osteomalacia and debility resulting from phosphorus depletion. Trans. Ass. Am. Physicians. 77:281, 1964.

4. Lotz, M., Zisman, E., and Bartter, F.C.: Evidence for a phosphorus-depletion syndrome in man. New Eng. J. Med. 278:409, 1968.

5. Dominguez, J.H., Gray, R.W., and Lemann, J., Jr.: Dietary phosphate deprivation in women and men: Effects on mineral and acid balance, parathyroid hormone and the metabolism of 25-OH-vitamin D. J. Clin. Endocrinol. Metab. 43:1056, 1976.

6. Tröhler, U., Bonjour, J.P., and Fleisch, H.: Inorganic phosphate homeostasis: Renal adaptation to the dietary intake in intact and thyroparathyroidectomized rats. J. Clin. Invest. 57:264, 1976.

7. Steele, T.H., and DeLuca, H.F.: Influence of the dietary phosphorus on renal phosphate reabsorption in the parathyroidectomized rat. J. Clin. Invest. 57:867, 1976.

8. Coburn, J.W., and Massry, S.G.: Changes in serum and urinary calcium during phosphate depletion: Studies on mechanisms. J. Clin. Invest. 49:1073, 1970.

9. Gold, L.W., Massry, S.G., Arieff, A.I., and Coburn, J.W.: Renal bicarbonate wasting during phosphate depletion: A possible cause of altered acid-base homeostasis in hyperparathyroidism. J. Clin. Invest. 52:2556, 1973.

10. Frick, A.: Reabsorption of inorganic phosphate in the rat kidney: I. Saturation of transport mechanism. II. Suppression of fractional phosphate reabsorption due to expansion of extracellular fluid volume. Pflügers Arch. Ges. Physiol. 34:351, 1968.

11. Reiss, E., Canterbury, J.M., Bercovitz, M.A., and Kaplan, E.L.: The role of phosphate in the secretion of parathyroid hormone in man. J. Clin. Invest. 49:2146, 1970.

12. Engle, J.E., and Steele, T.H.: Renal phosphate reabsorption in the rat: Effect of inhibitors. Kidney Int. 8:98-104, 1975.

13. Bonjour, J-P., Mühlbauer, R., Tröhler, U., and Fleisch, H.: Regulation and site of the tubular transport of inorganic phosphate in the rat kidney. In Urolithiasis Research. Fleisch, H., Robertson, G., Smith, L.H., and Vahlensieck, W., editors. Plenum, New York, 1976, p.377.

14. Wen, S-F., Boynar, J.W., Jr., and Stoll, R.W.: Renal phosphate transport in the phosphate-depleted dogs. In Phosphate Metabolism (Adv. Exper. Med. & Biology, vol. 81), Massry, S.G. and Ritz, E., editors. Plenum, New York, 1977, p. 101.

15. Steele, T.H.: Renal response to phosphorus deprivation: Effect of the parathyroids and bicarbonate. Kidney Int. 11:327, 1977.

16. Puschett, J.B., Beck, W.S., Jr., and Jelonek, A.: Parathyroid hormone and 25-hydroxy vitamin D_3: Synergistic and antagonistic effects on renal phosphate transport. Science. 190:473, 1975.

17. Steele, T.H., Engle, J.E., Tanaka, Y., Lorenc, R.S., Dudgeon, K.L., and DeLuca, H.F.: On the phosphatemic action of 1,25-dihydroxyvitamin D_3. Am. J. Physiol. 229:489, 1975.

18. Steele, T.H.: Renal resistance to parathyroid hormone during phosphorus deprivation. J. Clin. Invest. 58:1461, 1976.

19. Drezner, M., Neelon, F.A., and Lebovitz, H.E.: Pseudohypoparathyroidism type II: A possible defect in the reception of the cyclic AMP signal. New Eng. J. Med. 289:1056, 1973.

20. Knox, F.G., Preiss, J., Kim, J.K., and Dousa, T.P.: Mechanism of resistance to the phosphaturic effect of parathyroid hormone in the hamster. J. Clin. Invest. 59:675, 1977.

21. Kreusser, W.J., Kurokawa, K., and Massry, S.G.: Effects of phosphate depletion on levels of inorganic phosphorus and adenine nucleotides of renal cells. Clin. Res. 25:126A, 1977.

22. Ben-Isaac, C., Massry, S.G., Rosenfeld, S., Kleeman, C.R., and Bick, M.: Evidence for humoral factor responsible for the hypercalciuria of phosphate depletion. Clin. Res. 23:134A, (Abstract), 1975.

23. Massry, S.G.: Effect of phosphate depletion on renal tubular transport. In Phosphate Metabolism: Kidney and Bone. Avioli, L., Bordier, P., Fleisch, H., Massry, S., and Slatopolsky, E., editors. Nouvelle Imprimerie Fournié, Toulouse, 1976, p. 25.

24. Brautbar, N., Lee, D.B.N., Carlson, H.E., Coburn, J.W., and Kleeman, C.R.: Experimental phosphorus depletion: Attenuation of biochemical changes in hypophysectomized rats. Clin. Res. 25:165A, 1977.

25. Bowman, R.H.: The perfused rat kidney. In Methods in Enzymology. Hardmand, J.G., and O'Malley, B.W., editors, New York, Academic Press. 39:3, 1975.

26. Ross, B.D., Epstein, F.H., and Leaf, A.: Sodium reabsorption in the perfused rat kidney. Am. J. Physiol. 225:1165, 1973.

27. Steele, T.H., and Underwood, J.L.: Renal response to phosphorus deprivation in the isolated rat kidney. (submitted)

SKELETAL MUSCLE IN HYPOPHOSPHATEMIA AND PHOSPHORUS DEFICIENCY

James P. Knochel

Associate Chief of Staff for Research and Chief, Renal Section, VA Hospital, Dallas, Texas and Professor of Internal Medicine, University of Texas Medical School

The intentions of this presentation are to briefly review the clinical characteristics of acute rhabdomyolysis with hypophosphatemia; how this syndrome differs from the chronic hypophosphatemic myopathy and to provide a brief overview of our recent clinical and experimental work concerning cellular injury in phosphorus deficiency and hypophosphatemia.

At this workshop in 1975 we reported that there may be a relationship between rhabdomyolysis and acute hypophosphatemia (1). Rhabdomyolysis means lysis of skeletal muscle cells. In typical cases there will be acute pain, swelling and tenderness of skeletal muscle. Confirmatory chemical findings include abnormal elevations of serum creatine phosphokinase (CPK)or aldolase activity and identification of the muscle pigment myoglobin in the urine.

Hypophosphatemia occurs commonly in patients recovering from diabetic ketoacidosis, those treated with hyperalimentation and in severe, chronic alcoholics (2). The type of alcoholic patient most likely to become hypophosphatemic is one who drinks heavily and eats poorly. It is to be emphasized that such hypophosphatemia may not occur until the patient is admitted to the hospital for a variety of complications of his alcoholism. A normal serum phosphorus concentration at the time of admission may be rapidly supplanted by profound hypophosphatemia within one to four days in association with administration of nutrients without adequate phosphorus supplementation. To detect hypophosphatemia, it is often necessary to measure serum phosphorus concentration at the time of admission and at least daily for the first five days of hospitalization. In contrast, some patients demonstrate hypophosphatemia of modest degree at the time of admission to the hospital. Such patients are usually in active alcohol withdrawal and it is very likely that the hypophosphatemia is the result of respiratory alkalosis. In severe alcoholics and less commonly in other patients with hypophosphatemia, rhabdomyolysis may not appear until hypophosphatemia has existed for 24 or more hours. Those patients who demonstrate rhabdomyolysis at admission commonly give a history of convulsive seizures, total starvation for several days or severe intoxication.

It is to be emphasized that severe phosphorus deficiency, indicated by a marked depression of total muscle phosphorus content, may exist in the face of a normal serum phosphorus concentration. This could occur if active necrosis of tissue were underway. Presumably, necrotic tissue releases its content of phosphorus into the circulation (1). Alternatively, there could exist a biochemical defect in phosphorylation.

In contrast to rhabdomyolysis with acute hypophosphatemia, there appears to be a rather distinctive chronic myopathy associated with chronic hypophosphatemia (3). Certain differentiating characteristics of these disorders are illustrated in Table I. Patients with acute hypophosphatemia tend to develop rhabdomyolysis and often display myoglobinuria. They commonly have muscle

TABLE I

HYPOPHOSPHATEMIC MYOPATHY

ACUTE	CHRONIC
RHABDOMYOLYSIS	PROXIMAL WEAKNESS
MYOGLOBINURIA	WALKING DIFFICULTY
MUSCLE PAIN	OSTEOMALACIA USUAL
MUSCLE TENDERNESS	RHABDOMYOLYSIS ABSENT
GENERALIZED WEAKNESS	CPK, ALDOLASE NORMAL
ELEVATED CPK, ALDOLASE	ALKALINE PHOSPHATASE ELEVATED
HYPOPHOSPHATEMIA MARKED	HYPOPHOSPHATEMIA MODEST

pain and tenderness. Their weakness tends to be generalized. They show elevated CPK or aldolase activity and in most instances hypophosphatemia has been marked, implying a serum phosphorus concentration often less than 1.0 mg percent. In contrast to this disorder, muscular weakness in chronic hypophosphatemic myopathy is predominantly proximal. Distal muscular performance, such as grip strength may be normal. They experience great difficulty in walking and very often have osteomalacia. Acute rhabdomyolysis in these patients is not evident and accordingly, their CPK and aldolase activities are usually normal. Elevated alkaline phosphatase activity reflects osteomalacia. In these patients, hypophosphatemia is ordinarily not nearly so pronounced as it is in those with acute hypophosphatemic myopathy. The chronic myopathy related to a deficiency of Vitamin D appears to be clinically indistinguishable. However, that phosphate deficiency *per se* may cause such a myopathy is clearly evident from those instances in which phosphorus deficiency occurs after ingesting quantities of phosphate binding antacids. In such patients administration of elemental phosphorus by itself leads to complete recovery.

EVIDENCE FOR PHOSPHORUS DEFICIENCY IN THE CHRONIC ALCOHOLIC

Hypophosphatemia occurs in approximately one-half of patients hospitalized for treatment of severe alcoholism. Because of this finding, we measured phosphorus content, electrolyte content and in some patients, transmembrane electrical potential of muscle cells (1). The latter is a sensitive index of cellular permeability to monovalent ions and/or sodium transport. Altogether, studies have been conducted on 21 patients. Their serum CPK activity was elevated, ranging between 200 and 82,000 International units/ml. The normal value for total muscle phosphorus content in health is 29 mmoles/100 gm fat free dry solids (FFDS). The average value in the patients with chronic alcoholism we have studied to date is 17.7 mmoles/dg FFDS. The lowest was 12 mmoles/dg FFDS. Such values indicate severe phosphorus deficiency. In health, the mass of skeletal muscle in a 70 kg man averages 30 kg. The fat free dry solid fraction of skeletal muscle is about 25%. Thus, in health, muscle content of phosphorus is about 2,175 mmoles. If we allow for a shrinkage of muscle mass to 20 kg in a chronic alcoholic because of malnutrition, his total normal muscle phosphorus content should be 1,450 mmoles. In the chronic alcoholics with elevated CPK activity, the average total muscle phosphorus content was 17.7 mmoles/100 g FFDS. Thus, instead of 1,450 mmoles, their total muscle phosphorus content was about 885 mmoles. Therefore, their average phosphorus deficity was approximately 565 mmoles. Some individuals with the lowest values had deficits approaching 1000 mmoles. These do not include possible deficits in other tissues.

MECHANISMS OF PHOSPHORUS DEFICIENCY IN CHRONIC ALCOHOLISM

Factors that could cause phosphorus deficiency in alcoholism are shown in Table II. Many chronic alcoholics develop capricious appetites and therefore an inadequate dietary intake of phosphorus must play at least a partial role in some. In health, dietary phosphorus deficiency is exceptionally rare since all natural foods have a high phosphorus content. However, feeding

TABLE II

POSSIBLE FACTORS RESPONSIBLE FOR PHOSPHORUS DEFICIENCY IN THE ALCOHOLIC

1. INADEQUATE DIETARY INTAKE
2. VOMITING AND DIARRHEA
3. MAGNESIUM DEFICIENCY
4. DERANGED VITAMIN D METABOLISM
5. CALCITONIN
6. ACIDOSIS

a diet without phosphorus and especially if given in conjunction with phosphate binding antacids can in time lead to serious phosphorus deficiency.

Many chronic alcoholics have episodic vomiting and diarrhea. However, the phosphorus content of gastric contents is low and even voluminous diarrhea is not responsible for significant phosphorus losses in stools (4). Thus vomiting and diarrhea *per se* would probably not account for major losses of phosphorus.

Experimental magnesium deficiency in man induces a state of functional hypoparathyroidism (5). In association with this, serum phosphorus tends to become slightly elevated and phosphaturia occurs. Phosphaturia could well result from a slightly increased filtered load of phosphorus. Since alcoholics often become hypomagnesemic and magnesium deficient, such factors could well play a role in phosphorus deficiency.

In unreported studies by Matter and his co-workers (6) on human volunteers ingesting large amounts of bourbon whiskey each day for many weeks, phosphaturia appeared but not until serum magnesium concentration fell to abnormally low levels. In our most recent studies of skeletal muscle composition in patients with alcoholic myopathy, we have found that magnesium content, normally 8 mmoles/100 gm fat free dry solids, was significantly lower than normal ($p<0.01$), averaging 5.7 mmoles in the alcoholics (7). In the same muscle samples, muscle calcium content was elevated three times above the normal value. This finding has also been observed in experimental magnesium deficiency. Thus we do have evidence that in these patients, magnesium deficiency coexists with phosphate deficiency.

It was recently reported that plasma levels of 25-hydroxy vitamin D-3 are abnormally low in chronic alcoholics without liver disease (8). It seems possible that this could account for decreased formation of 1,25-hydroxy vitamin D-3 which could in turn decrease calcium absorption from the small intestine, cause hypocalcemia and lead to overproduction of parathormone. Such a mechanism could occur independently of magnesium deficiency. This then could account for phosphaturia. It is notable that when the severe alcoholics we studied were admitted to the hospital, before they developed severe hypophosphatemia, there was often abundant phosphorus in the urine. Some of these patients excreted up to 0.9 gm of phosphorus in their first 24 hour urine despite a poor preceding dietary intake and despite respiratory alkalosis. Both of the latter influences would ordinarily cause hypophosphaturia. However the phosphaturia disappeared rapidly with the appearance of hypophosphatemia. Whether the phosphaturia at the time of admission was related to overproduction of parathormone was not studied.

Recent studies have shown that ethanol is a potent factor stimulating release of calcitonin (9). In health, calcitonin induces a very slight decline of serum calcium concentration. It has been reported that it decreases intestinal absorption of phosphorus (10). It may also induce phosphaturia and magnesuria (11). Whether such effects play a role in phosphorus deficiency in the alcoholic have not been examined.

Acidosis leads to decomposition of intracellular organic phosphate compounds. The phosphorus so liberated readily diffuses into the serum and is excreted into the urine. Alcoholics often develop ketoacidosis while fasting during periods of hangover. They may also undergo transient CO_2 retention and respiratory acidosis as a result of acute severe alcoholic intoxication. It seems conceivably that either mechanism could cause intermittent phosphorus wasting.

The possible mechanism underlying phosphorus deficiency in remaining instances of hypophosphatemic rhabdomyolysis, such as diabetic ketoacidosis, are better understood than the cause of phosphorus deficiency in alcoholism. Besides the effects of acidosis *per se* on decreasing phosphorylation, recent evidence suggests that either acidosis (12) or insulin deficiency (13) independently interfere with synthesis of 1,25-dihydroxy vitamin D_3. The resulting malabsorption of calcium can lead to overproduction of parathormone with resulting phosphaturia and phosphorus depletion.

The mechanism of phosphorus deficiency in hyperalimentation is quite different. In this setting, the muscle cell has been starved but nevertheless is capable of responding to an anabolic stimulus. Its phosphorus content may be normal. Thus, with provision of nutrients a "hungry" cell could conceivably reconstruct protoplasm at least for a time and as a result of deficient supplies, phosphorus deficiency is inadvertently produced. It is also conceivable that the demand for phosphorus by other tissues, such as liver or bone, could be greater than that of skeletal muscle.

MECHANISMS OF ACUTE HYPOPHOSPHATEMIA

As pointed out earlier, some severe alcoholics have abundant inorganic phosphate in the urine at the time of admission to the hospital. Usually this disappears rapidly so that by the second or third hospital day, the urine has become virtually free of phosphorus as hypophosphatemia appears. Some of the possible mechanisms of acute hypophosphatemia are shown in Table III. It must be assumed that serum phosphorus is being incorporated

TABLE III

POSSIBLE MECHANISMS OF ACUTE HYPOPHOSPHATEMIA IN THE ALCOHOLIC

1. ADMINISTRATION OF NUTRIENTS
2. ACUTE RESPIRATORY ALKALOSIS
3. FRUCTOSE ADMINISTRATION
4. HYPERINSULINISM

into cells. This could occur by an anabolic stimulus provided by administration of nutrients. It could also occur as result of acute hyperventilation with respiratory alkalosis. Because of the rapid diffusibility of CO_2, acute hyperventilation is associated with a sharp rise in intracellular pH. This would activate phosphofructokinase thereby increasing phosphorylation. The source of phosphorus to form organic phosphates in the cells is cytoplasmic inorganic phosphate. Cytoplasmic inorganic phosphorus is in chemical equilibrium with inorganic serum phosphorus. Therefore, rapid phosphorylation during an anabolic state induced by administration of nutrients or that incident to respiratory alkalosis could well account for the severe hypophosphatemia seen in patients during treatment for chronic alcoholism.

Administration of fructose, still recommended by some physicians caring for patients with acute alcoholic withdrawal, may also lead to acute hypophosphatemia. Of importance, the hypophosphatemia associated with fructose can be more severe than that associated with administration of glucose. The mechanism of this response is related to the unregulated uptake of fructose by the cells of the liver (14). Specific kinases exist in the liver that catalyze phosphorylation of glucose (glucokinase) to glucose-6-phosphate and fructose (fructokinase) to fructose-1-phosphate. Increasing concentration of glucose-6-phosphate inhibits the activity of glucokinase, thereby regulating the uptake of both glucose and phosphorus. In contrast, increasing concentrations of fructose-1-phosphate do not inhibit fructokinase. Thus, fructose phosphorylation is unregulated and in consequence, hypophosphatemia is more pronounced after fructose than glucose. An additional problem related to intracellular phosphorus trapping mediated by fructose is the observation that it may be associated with acute hepatocellular damage (15). Thus when inorganic phosphorus or ATP concentrations inside the cytoplasm of liver cells fall sufficiently, AMP-deaminase and 5'-nucleotidase are activated. Adenylic compounds within the cell are irreversibly decomposed (14,16). The adenylic compounds are converted to inosine. Inosine impairs glycolysis by inhibiting aldolase (14). Inhibition of glycolysis commonly results in acute lactic acidosis. When the cellular content of ATP falls to a critical level, certain enzymes are released from the cell reflecting acute cellular injury (17). For such reasons, fructose should not be administered intravenously to any patient, especially one who is already apt to have liver damage because of alcoholism (15).

The final mechanism that could be implicated in the pathogenesis of acute hypophosphatemia in the withdrawing alcoholic is overproduction of insulin. It has been known for many years that patients with liver disease may develop a greater depression of serum phosphorus concentration after administration of glucose than a normal person (18). Recent studies (19) have shown that experimental phosphorus deficiency exaggerates insulin release in response to hyperglycemia. This has not been examined in the withdrawing alcoholic but certainly seems worthy of study.

EXPERIMENTAL HYPOPHOSPHATEMIC MYOPATHY

Acute rhabdomyolysis is common in patients with severe hypophosphatemia. In many instances this is not associated with overt clinical signs of rhabdomyolysis, such as muscle pain, swelling, tenderness or paralysis. However it may be severe and can be associated with myoglobinuria and acute renal failure. In such patients we have demonstrated not only acute severe hypophosphatemia but also, as discussed earlier, a marked deficiency of skeletal muscle phosphorus content. Experimental studies on dogs (20) have shown that feeding a phosphorus deficient diet in conjunction with phosphate-binding antacids for a period of 28 days leads to an electrochemical myopathy. This is characterized by a decline in resting membrane potential, a decline of muscle phosphorus content and increases in sodium and chloride contents. There also occurs a slight decline of magnesium and potassium content. In those studies malnutrition was prevented by gavage feeding the animals a complete diet except for its lack of phosphorus. Similar to some alcoholics who have not yet become acutely hypophosphatemic, there was no elevation of CPK activity and acute rhabdomyolysis did not occur.

In further attempts to establish a model more closely resembling that seen in the patient with chronic alcoholism, 17 additional dogs were fed a phosphorus deficient, calorie deficient but otherwise balanced diet so as to induce 30% weight loss. At this point the dogs were hyperalimented with a phosphorus deficient diet providing 140 calories per kg per day. These dogs developed rhabdomyolysis. This was characterized by sharp rises in CPK and in some, overt myoglobinuria. It was preceded by acute severe hypophosphatemia which correlated inversely with the peak CPK activity. Using additional dogs prepared in a similar manner, and then hyperalimented, provision of 4.6 grams of elemental phosphorus each day completely prevented acute rhabdomyolysis. We would tentatively conclude from these experimental studies that phosphorus deficiency per se produces an electrochemical myopathy which closely resembles the subclinical myopathy observed in many patients with chronic alcoholism before acute hypophosphatemia supervenes. Thus, without severe hypophosphatemia, CPK activity in both man and the dog with phosphorus deficiency was normal. However, with induction of acute severe hypophosphatemia in either man or the dog, with preceding phosphorus deficiency, led to acute necrosis of skeletal muscle. Finally, acute necrosis of skeletal muscle under these conditions apparently can be prevented by providing sufficient phosphorus in the diet to prevent hypophosphatemia.

REFERENCES

1. Knochel, J.P., Bilbrey, G.L., Fuller, T.J. and Carter, N.W.: The muscle cell in chronic alcoholism: The possible role of phosphate depletion in alcoholic myopathy. Annals NY Academy Sci 252:274-286, 1975.

2. Knochel, J.P.: The pathophysiology and clinical characteristics of severe hypophosphatemia. Arch Int Med 137:203-220, 1977.

3. Ravid, M. and Robson, M.: Proximal myopathy caused by iatrogenic phosphate depletion. JAMA 236:1380-1381, 1976.

4. Fordtran, J.: Personal communication, 1976.

5. Anast, C.S., Mohs, J.M., Kaplan, S.L., et al.: Evidence for parathyroid failure in magnesium deficiency. Science 177: 606-608, 1972.

6. Matter, B.J., Worona, M., Donat, P. et al: Effect of ethanol on phosphate excretion in man. Clin Res 12:255, 1964.

7. Knochel, J.P., Cohen, M., Anderson, R., Carter, N., Cotton, J. and Elms, J. Muscle composition in alcoholic myopathy. Clin Res 24:589A, 1976.

8. Velentizas, C., Oreopoulos, D.G., Brandes, L., Wilson, D.R., Marquez-Julio, A.: Abnormal vitamin-D levels in alcoholics. Annals Int Med 86:198, 1977.

9. Cohen, S.L., MacIntryre, I., Grahame-Smith, D. and Walker, J. S.: Alcohol-stimulated calcitonin release in medullary carcinoma of the thyroid. Lancet 1172-1174, 1973.

10. Tanzer, F.S. and Navia, J.M.: Calcitonin inhibition of intestinal phosphate absorption. Nature New Biology 242:221-222, 1973.

11. Ardaillou, R., Fallastre, J.P., Milhaud, G., Rosselet, F., Delaunay, F. and Richet, G. Renal excretion of phosphate, calcium and sodium during and after a prolonged thyrocalcitonin infusion in man.

12. Won Lee, S., Russell, J. and Avioli, LV: 25-Hydroxycholecalciferol to 1,25-Dihydroxycholecaciferol: conversion impaired by systemic metabolic acidosis. Science 195:994-995, 1977.

13. Schneider, L.E. and Schedl, H.P.: Experimental diabetes reduces circulating 1,25-dihydroxyvitamin D in the rat. Science 196:1452-1453, 1977.

14. Woods, H.F., Eggleston, L.V. and Krebs, H.A.: The cause of hepatic accumulation of fructose 1-phosphate on fructose loading. Biochem J 119:501-510, 1970.

15. Craig, W.M. and Crane, C.W.: Lactic acidosis complicating liver failure after intravenous fructose. Br Med J 4:211-212, 1971.

16. Farber, F: ATP and cell integrity. Fed Proc 32:1534-1539, 1973.

17. Sweetin, J.C. and Thomson, W.H.S.: Enzyme efflux and clearance. Clinica Chimica Acta 48:403-411, 1973.

18. Danowski, T.S., Gillespie, H.K,. Fergus, E.B. et al: Significance of blood sugar and serum electrolyte changes in cirrhosis following glucose, insulin, glucagon or epinephrine. Yale J Biol Med 29:361-375, 1957.

19. Harter, H.R., Santiago, J.V., Rutherford, W.E., Slatopolsky, E. and Klahr, S.: The relative roles of calcium, phosphorus and parathyroid hormone in glucose and tolbutamide-mediated insulin release. J Clin Invest 58:359-367, 1976.

20. Fuller, T.J., Carter, N.W., Barcenas, C. and Knochel, J.P.: Reversible changes of the muscle cell in experimental phosphorus deficiency. J Clin Invest 57:1019-1024, 1976.

PHOSPHOROUS DEPLETION AND VITAMIN D METABOLISM

Louis V. Avioli

Division of Bone and Mineral Metabolism, Washington University School of Medicine, The Jewish Hospital of St. Louis, 216 S. Kingshighway, St. Louis, Missouri

In man, phosphate deprivation (or depletion) is reportedly attended by decreased renal tubular reabsorption of sodium, magnesium, bicarbonate, uric acid and glucose, red cell dysfunction with decreased concentrations of 2,3-DPG and ATP, platelet abnormalities with thrombocytopenia, impairment of clot retraction, shortened survival time and decreased ATP levels, decreased leucocytic ATP concentrations with suppressed phagocytic, chemotactic and bacterocidal activities, central nervous system dysfunction characterized by varying degrees of numbness, dysarthria, paresthesiaes, convulsive diatheses, and coma, rhabdomyolysis and myalgia, abnormal hepatic cellular function, hypercalciuria, occasional hypercalcemia, augmentation of the intestinal absorption of calcium, hypophosphatemia and elevations in circulating $1{,}25(OH)_2D$ in women (1-5). These latter alterations in calcium metabolism when documented in phosphate deprived laboratory animals (predominantly rats), have been attended by increased bone resorption (6,7) and stimulated renal 1-hydroxylase activity with more rapid conversion of $25OHD_3$ to $1{,}25(OH)_2D_3$ (8-10). Stimulated 1-hydroxylase activity has also been documented <u>in vitro</u> using renal tubular mitochondrial preparations from hypophosphatemic chicks (11).

The relationship between dietary phosphate deprivation, calcium absorption, and bone metabolism had been under investigation for years prior to the discovery that calcium and phosphate conditioned the bioactivation of vitamin D, and increased calcium absorption during periods of phosphate deprivation documented in humans subjected to the rigors of calcium balance experimental procedures. Before it was recognized that vitamin D metabolism and bioactivation could be altered by chronic phosphate deprivation, the increased intestinal absorption of calcium and hypercalciuria were collectively ascribed primarily to decreased intestinal phosphate content, the latter resulting in a higher percentage of non-phosphate-bound dietary calcium available for transport (or absorption) by the intestine. Subsequent to the discovery of the renal 1-hydroxylating enzyme system which regulated the conversion of $25OHD_3$ to the most potent vitamin D_3 metabolite $1,25(OH)_2D_3$, studies were initially designed in animal models in order to evaluate the effect of pertubations in calcium and phosphate intake on the metabolism of vitamin D. In 1972, Haddad and Avioli first described the results of phosphate deprivation on vitamin D metabolism in the rat (12). Although phosphate deprivation resulted in increased intestinal calcium absorption, these investigators reported that they were unable to detect any changes in the hepatic uptake or release of an isotopic vitamin D_3 preparation, nor any "significant alteration" in the chromatographic profiles of an injected isotopically labeled form of $25OHD_3$ in plasma, kidney or intestinal mucosa (12). On repeat examination of these early studies which incorporated silicic acid chromatographic methodology (a separation procedure which has since been replaced by more definitive LH-20, celite and high pressure liquid chromatographic techniques), it now appears quite obvious that phosphorus deprivation did indeed result in an alteration in $25OHD_3$ metabolism in the phosphate deprived rat since phosphate-depleted animals demonstrated less $25OHD_3$ and increased amounts of at least one polar (unidentified) $25OHD_3$ metabolite in the intestinal mucosa. Subsequent to these preliminary observations, Tanaka and DeLuca concluded that phosphate deprivation stimulated the $25OHD_3$-1-hydroxylase in the rat since there was an increased accumulation of chromatographically-identified $1,25(OH)_2D_3$ in the blood and intestine under these conditions (8). These findings were later confirmed in the chick (11) and the rat (9-10,13) although the results in the chick were considered somewhat controversial (14).

After Bar and Wasserman reported that chicks fed low phosphorus diets responded like rats with stimulated intestinal calcium absorption (15), Ribovich and DeLuca reported that the administration of $1,25(OH)_2D_3$ did not eliminate the stimulation of intestinal calcium transport by low phosphate diets (9). The latter results were intriguing since, when 1-hydroxylase activity and calcium absorption was stimulated by calcium deprivation, exogenous $1,25(OH)_2D_3$ virtually eliminated the intestinal adaptation response (9). These results and those obtained in subsequent studies by Baxter and DeLuca (11), were consistent with the hypothesis that, whereas the stimulation of calcium absorption by calcium deprivation results primarily from increased $1,25(OH)_2D_3$ synthesis, the enhanced calcium absorption produced by low phosphate intake was only partly due to increased $1,25(OH)_2D_3$ synthesis.

In 1976, while studying the binding capacity of duodenal intestinal calcium binding proteins in the phosphate deprived rat, Thomasset _et al_ isolated a calcium binding protein which was independent of 1,25$(OH)_2D_3$ (16). In their studies, the appearance of this non-vitamin D dependent calcium binding protein correlated well with the associated increments in _in vivo_ calcium absorption and _in vitro_ calcium transport. In experiments designed to compare the effect of phosphate deprivation in vitamin D-deficient rats, Brautbar _et al_ concluded that the rise in serum calcium and hypercalciuria produced by phosphate deprivation did not require metabolic conversion of vitamin D_3 to 1,25$(OH)_2D_3$ (17), a conclusion consistent with an earlier report of Massry which ascribed the hypercalciuria of phosphate-deprived rabbits to a "humoral factor" (18).

Thus, the relationship between phosphate deprivation, calcium absorption and hypercalciuria in the mature animal appears to represent a combination of physiological events and cannot be ascribed solely to enhanced production of 1,25$(OH)_2D_3$. The results of experiments in younger weanling animals are even more convincing in this regard. Lee _et al_ have reported in this symposium, that phosphate deprivation leads to a decrease in _in vivo_ calcium absorption by the intestine and a correlated _decrease_ in the _in vitro_ duodenal uptake of calcium (19). Moreover, when male weanling rats were depleted of vitamin D and rendered hypophosphatemic by Edelstein _et al_., intestinal calcium binding protein(s) were also _decreased_, and 1,25$(OH)_2D_3$ virtually undetectable in the intestinal mucosa (20). In parallel studies of rats on low calcium diets, the young animals responded with an increase in intestinal calcium binding protein, and calcium absorption and a two-fold increment in the intestinal content of 1,25$(OH)_2D_3$ (20). These results are presently difficult to reconcile with those obtained in more mature animals although the relative sensitivity of the renal 1-hydroxylase in adult and immature animals to changes in circulating calcium (9,13,14), phosphate (8,10,11) pH, (10) and estrogens (4,5, 21) have yet to be completely elucidated.

The metabolic consequences of phosphate depletion in man is currently receiving increased attention (1,2). In 1960, Bloom and Finchum described a case of osteomalacia resulting from aluminum hydroxide ingestion (22). Later, Lotz and Bartter induced a variety of symptoms which were attended by hypercalciuria in normal volunteers by the administration of phosphate binding antacids (3). Two additional well documented cases of osteomalacia associated with chronic antacid ingestion have also appeared in the English literature (23,24). It has also recently been demonstrated that phosphate deprivation in humans accelerates the plasma turnover of $25OHD_3$ and is associated with a net increase in the intestinal absorption of calcium and phosphate, and a rise in circulating

$1,25(OH)_2D_3$ in women only (4,5). Phosphate deprived females develop progressive hypercalciuria and negative calcium balances in marked contrast to phosphate deprived males who remain in positive calcium balance despite the same degree of phosphate deprivation (4). This observation may represent the human correlate to avian studies wherein estrogens reportedly stimulate 1-hydroxylation of $25OHD_3$ (21). In this regard, it is noteworthy that the five patients who developed hypophosphatemia and calciuria during phosphate deprivation initially studied by Lotz and Bartter were females (3). In addition to these observations in phosphate-deprived normal individuals, Haussler _et al_ have reported elevations in circulating $1,25(OH)_2D_3$ in patients with "idiopathic hypercalciuria", a disorder characterized by hypophosphatemia, hypercalciuria, nephrolithiasis and increased intestinal calcium absorption (25).

It seems reasonable to conclude therefore that phosphate depletion in man and animals either directly or indirectly leads to a stimulated production (or decreased degradation) of $1,25(OH)_2D_3$ as well as a variety of cellular and functional disturbances attended by low tissue ATP concentrations (1,2). Although to date, the acquired alteration in vitamin D_3 metabolism appears limited to $1,25(OH)_2D_3$, more detailed analyses are essential in both man and experimental animals with specific emphasis on: (1) age-related changes in the intestinal and skeletal response to phosphate deprivation; (2) the relationship between maturity, serum calcium, estrogens, androgens and $1,25(OH)2D_3$ production in the phosphate-deprived state; and (3) the production and fate of heretofore unidentified circulating and tissue substance(s) which are increased by phosphate deprivation, and the effect of these agent(s) on calcium absorption, bone metabolism, calcium excretion, and the metabolism of biologically active vitamin D metabolites.

REFERENCES

1. Kreisberg, R.A.: Phosphate deficiency and hypophosphatemia. Hospital Practice 12:121, 1977.

2. Knochel, J.P.: The pathophysiology and clinical characteristics of severe hypophosphatemia. Arch. Int. Med. 137:203, 1977.

3. Lotz, M., Zisman, E. and Bartter, F.: Evidence for a phosphorus-depletion syndrome in man. N. Engl. J. Med. 278:409, 1968.

4. Dominguez, J.H., Gray, R.W. and Lemann, J., Jr.: Dietary phosphate deprivation in women and men: Effects on mineral and acid balances, parathyroid hormone and the metabolism of 25-OH vitamin D. J. Clin. Endo. Metab. 43:1056, 1976.

5. Gray, R.W., Wilz, D.R., Caldas, A.E. and Lemann, J., Jr.: Importance of phosphate in regulating plasma 1,25$(OH)_2$ vitamin D levels in humans: Studies in healthy subjects in calcium stone formers and in patients with primary hyperparathyroidism. J. Clin. Endocr. Metab. 45:299, 1977.

6. Baylink, D., Wergedal, J., Stauffer, M.: Formation, mineralization and resorption of bone in hypophosphatemic rats. J. Clin. Invest. 50:2519, 1971.

7. Bruin, W.J., Baylink, D.J. and Wergedal, J.E.: Acute inhibition of mineralization and stimulation of bone resorption mediated by hypophosphatemia. Endocrinology 96:394, 1975.

8. Tanaka, Y. and DeLuca, H.F.: The control of 25-hydroxyvitamin D metabolism by inorganic phosphorus. Arch. Biochem. Biophys. 154:566, 1973.

9. Ribovich, M.L. and DeLuca, H.F.: Influence of dietary calcium and phosphorus on intestinal calcium transport in rats given vitamin D metabolites. Arch. Biochem. Biophys. 170:529, 1975.

10. Lee, S.W., Russell, J. and Avioli, L.V.: 25-hydroxycholecalciferol to 1,25-dihydroxycholecalciferol: Conversion impaired by systemic metabolic acidosis. Science 195:994, 1977.

11. Baxter, L.A. and DeLuca, H.F.: Stimulation of 25-hydroxyvitamin D3-1α-hydroxylase by phosphate depletion. J. Biol. Chem. 251:3158, 1976.

12. Haddad, J.G., Jr. and Avioli, L.V.: Metabolism of vitamin D_3 during phosphate depletion. J. Nutr. 102:269, 1972.

13. Hughes, M.R., Brumbaugh, P.F., Haussler, M.R., Wergedal, J.E. and Baylink, D.J.: Regulation of serum 1α25-dihydroxyvitamin D_3 by calcium and phosphate in the rat. Science 190:578, 1975.

14. Henry, H.L., Midgett, R.J. and Norman, A.W.: Regulation of 25-hydroxyvitamin D_3-1-hydroxylase *in vivo*. J. Biol. Chem. 294:7584, 1974.

15. Bar, A. and Wasserman, R.H.: Control of calcium absorption and intestinal calcium-binding protein synthesis. Biochem. Biophys. Res. Comm. 54:191, 1973.

16. Thomasset, M., Cuisinier-Gleizes, P., Mathieu, H.: Duodenal calcium-binding protein (CaBP) and phosphorus deprivation in growing rats. Biomed. 25:345, 1976.

17. Brautbar, N., Walling, M.W. and Coburn, J.W.: Studies of experimental phosphate depletion: Effect of vitamin D deficiency and vitamin D sterols. In Program of the Endocrine Society (1977).

18. Massry, S.G.: Effect of phosphate depletion on renal tubular transport. In Phosphate Metabolism, Kidney and Bone. Ed. Avioli, L., Bordier, P., Fleisch, H., Massry, S. and Slatopolsky, E. Nouvelle, Imprieve Fournie, France, p. 25, 1976.

19. Lee, D.B.N., Brautbar, N., Walling, M.W., Carlson, H.E., Golvin, C., Coburn, J.W. and Kleeman, C.R.: Mineral balance and gut-sac transport studies in phosphorus depleted intact and hypophosphysectomized rats. Presented at 3rd Int. Workshop on phosphate and other minerals, Madrid, Spain, July 1977.

20. Edelstein, S., Noff, D., Puchett, J., Golub, E.E. and Bronner, F.: Low phosphorus intake and vitamin D metabolism and expression in rats. Presented at 3rd Int. Workshop on phosphate and other minerals, Madrid, Spain, July 1977.

21. Tanaka, Y., Castillo, L. and DeLuca, H.F.: Control of renal vitamin D hydroxylases in birds by sex hormones. Proc. Nat. Acad. Sci. 73:2701, 1976.

22. Bloom, W., Flinchum, D.: Osteomalacia with pseudofracture caused by the ingestion of aluminum hydroxide. JAMA 174: 1327, 1960.

23. Henneman, P.H., Benedict, P.H., Forbes, A.P. et al.: Idiopathic hypercalciuria. N. Engl. J. Med. 259:802, 1958.

24. Parfitt, A.M., Higgins, B.A., Nassim, J.R. et al.: Metabolic studies in patients with hypercalciuria. Clin. Sci. 27:463, 1964.

25. Haussler, M., Hughes, M., Baylink, D. et al.: Influence of phosphate depletion in the biosynthesis and circulating level of 1α,25-dihydroxyvitamin D. In Advances in Experimental Medicine and Biology 81:233, 1977.

THE EFFECTS OF PHOSPHATE DEPLETION ON BONE

Joel L. Ivey, Emily R. Morey, and David J. Baylink

American Lake Veterans Administration Hospital, Tacoma, WA 98493, and Department of Medicine, University of Washington, Seattle, WA 98195, and NASA-Ames Research Center, Moffett Field, CA 94035 USA

The importance of phosphate in the metabolism of an organism has been indicated by many of the other papers in this volume. Since phosphate is a major constituent of the mineralized phase of bone, this tissue can function as a reservoir for maintaining the extra-cellular fluid phosphate concentration during a period of phosphate depletion. In young, growing animals phosphate depletion results in decreased growth in general and decreased length of the long bones (1). Several workers have also shown that phosphate depletion results in an increased resorption of bone (1-3).

The effects of phosphate depletion on bone are discussed here with respect to the serum changes related to bone metabolism; the changes in bone formation and resorption produced by phosphate depletion; and the effects of phosphate depletion on bone in vitamin D deficiency. These effects are discussed in terms of what the changes are, the temporal relationships of the changes, and to the extent possible how they occur. All of the changes observed in bone during phosphate depletion are consistent with a response by bone to maintain serum and soft tissue phosphate concentrations, and thus constitute normal physiologic regulatory responses.

MATERIALS AND METHODS

The experiments described were performed on male weanling rats. The semi-synthetic diet used has been described previously (4). The diet used for intact control animals contained 0.6%

calcium and 0.6% phosphorus. For studying low concentrations of phosphorus in the diet, fibrin was used as the source of protein instead of casein, and with the phosphate salts omitted, the final concentration of phosphorus in this diet was 0.04%.

Blood was obtained by cardiac puncture at sacrifice, or from the tail vein when serial determinations were performed on the same animals, and total serum calcium and phosphorus determinations were made as previously described (5).

The histological methods used to quantitate the bone parameters have been described in detail elsewhere (5, 6, 7). Osteoclast numbers were determined from demineralized sections stained for acid phosphatase activity as described previously (8).

RESULTS AND DISCUSSION

Serum Parameters Related to Bone

In young, growing rats phosphate depletion results in decreases in serum phosphate and serum parathyroid hormone (PTH) and increases in total serum calcium and serum 1,25-diOH-D_3. Among the first changes in phosphate depletion are a marked reduction in serum phosphate and an increase in total serum calcium. A significant decrease in serum phosphate is observed within 6 h after the animals are placed on a low phosphorus (0.04% diet, and a nadir is observed by 12 h. The serum phosphate then rises slightly and remains relatively constant for an extended period (Figure 1). The rise in serum Ca, while smaller in magnitude, occurs over a similar time period and stabilizes at about 115% of the control value (10). The magnitudes of these changes, as well as the others that will be discussed, are dependent on the dietary phosphorus level. The changes in serum phosphate and calcium are observed in both intact and thyroparathyroidectomized (TPTX) animals, indicating that PTH is not required to produce the observed increase in total serum calcium (1). The increase in total serum calcium is due in part to an increase in ionized serum calcium (1).

An elevation in serum 1,25-diOH-D_3 is observed after 24 h of phosphate depletion (Figure 1), and increases by 4-fold after 14 d. Also shown in Figure 1 is the marked increase in endosteal osteoclast number observed in phosphate depletion. The increase in osteoclast number, however, occurs substantially later than the changes in serum phosphate or 1,25-diOH-D_3, with no detectable change until after 3 d of phosphate depletion (Figure 1).

To determine whether the initial rise in serum calcium

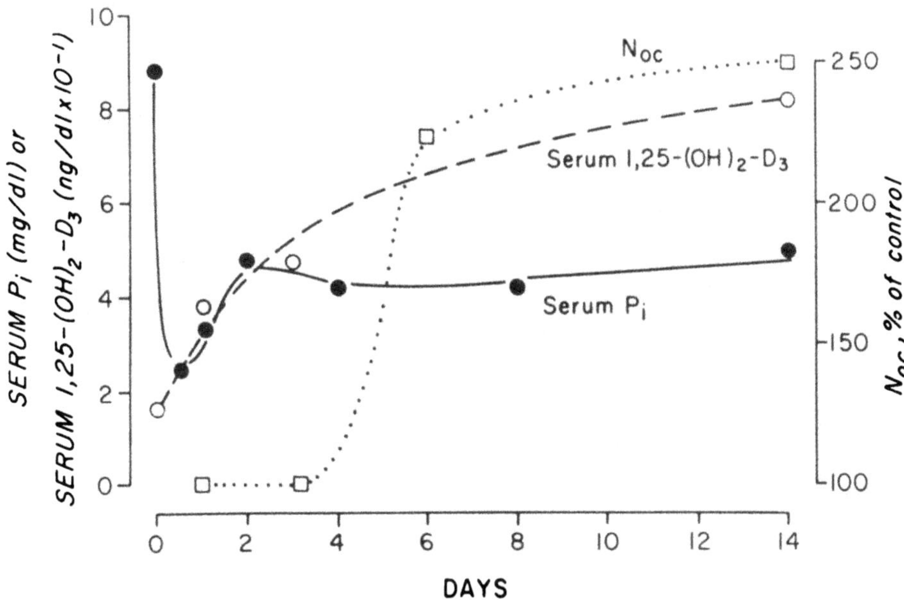

Figure 1. Effects of length of phosphate depletion on serum phosphate, serum 1,25-diOH-D_3, and endosteal osteoclast number (N_{OC}). These data were obtained from male weanling rats at the indicated times after they had been placed on a phosphate-deficient (0.04%P) diet. The values shown for serum 1,25-diOH-D_3 were obtained from a separate experiment published earlier (9).

observed in phosphate depletion was due to an early increase in the rate of bone resorption, Bruin et al. studied the ^{45}Ca kinetics of chronically and acutely ^{45}Ca-labeled bone. Their findings (10) suggest that there are several processes involved. When intact rats which had been previously labeled with ^{45}Ca were placed on a low phosphate (0.04%) diet, there was a rapid increase in total serum calcium, but an increase in the specific activity of serum ^{45}Ca observed after 48 h (10) indicated an increase in the rate of bone resorption, but since the number of endosteal osteoclasts is not increased by 72 h (Figure 1), this appears to represent an increase in the resorptive activity of the pre-existing osteoclast population. In contrast, in -P TPTX rats, serum ^{45}Ca specific activity is increased in 12 h, suggesting that in intact rats the effect of -P to increased A_{OC} is inhibited by calcitonin (10). Alternatively, there could have been an increase in N_{OC} by 48 h elsewhere in the skeleton, viz, the metaphysis, to account for the increase in serum ^{45}Ca specific activity after 48 h.

When intact rats were given ^{45}Ca at the time they were placed on the experimental diets and sacrificed 12 h later, the specific activity of bone ^{45}Ca was significantly lower and the specific activity of serum ^{45}Ca significantly higher in animals on a low (0.04%) phosphorus diet than in those on a normal (0.6%) phosphorus diet (10), indicating a decrease in calcium deposition in bone. Thus in phosphate depletion the rise in serum calcium appears to be initially due to a decrease in calcium deposition in bone, followed by an increase in the resorptive activity of pre-existing osteoclasts, and finally an increase in the number of osteoclasts.

Bone Formation

Phosphate depletion produces an inhibition of the processes involved in the formation of bone at both the periosteal and endosteal surfaces (Table 1) (1). The linear rate of matrix formation, which is the width of new matrix added per day and which reflects osteoblast activity, is decreased. The osteoid maturation rate, which is the rate at which the newly formed matrix is prepared for initiation of mineralization, is decreased. The initial mineralization rate, which is the rate at which initial mineralization proceeds, is decreased. Although the rate of matrix production is decreased, matrix production proceeds more rapidly than maturation of osteoid, resulting in a net increase in osteoid width during the period of phosphate depletion. At the endosteal surface much of the surface that would normally be involved in formation is converted to resorbing surface; as a consequence, the amount of endosteal bone formed is further reduced.

*Table 1. Periosteal bone matrix formation and mineralization**

	Dietary Phosphorus	
	0.6%	0.04%
Serum Ca, mg/dl	9.4±0.3**	11.2±0.5
Serum Pi, mg/dl	10.2±0.8	5.1±0.9
Linear rate of matrix formation, μ/d	7.7±1.4	3.2±0.4
Osteoid maturation rate, %/h	3.73±0.53	0.96±0.12
Initial mineralization rate, % of maximum/h	1.38±0.36	0.35±0.05
Osteoid width, μ	9.3±1.2	19.8±3.4

*Bone and serum parameters were determined after 14 d on diets containing the indicated amount of phosphorus (1).
**Mean SD, N=8 animal/group, all values for the 0.04% P(-P) group were significantly different (P<0.001) from the 0.6% P (control) group.

Table 2. Endosteal bone resorption parameters in phosphate depletion

	Dietary Phosphorus	
	0.6%	0.04%
Endosteal resorbing surface, mm^2	1.83±0.29*	4.55±0.22***
Linear bone resorption rate, μ/d	4.9±1.9	13.8±8.1**
Bone resorption rate, $(mm^3/d) \times 10^3$	11±4	50±29***
Medullary area, mm^2	0.93±0.10	1.54±0.11***
Cortical thickness, mm	0.34±0.02	0.14±0.01***

*Mean SD, N=8 animals/group
**P<0.05
***P<0.001
Bone resorption parameters were determined from the experiment shown in Table 1. (1).

Bone Resorption

As indicated above and shown in Table 2, chronic phosphate depletion produces an increase in the endosteal resorbing surface (which is the endosteal surface area involved in resorption and which reflects the number of osteoclasts on the endosteal surface), and the linear rate of bone resorption (which is the width of bone resorbed per day and which reflects the resorptive activities of the osteoclast population). The consequence of these effects is a marked increase in the bone resorption rate (the volume of bone resorbed per day, resulting in an increase in the size of the medullary cavity and a reduction in the cortical thickness. Because serum PTH is decreased in phosphate depletion (11), the observed increases in osteoclast activity and osteoclast number or resorbing surface might be due to either the depressed serum phosphate or the elevated serum 1,25-diOH-D_3. To evaluate the possible role of vitamin D in the bone changes associated with phosphate depletion, we have compared the effects of phosphate depletion on bone resorption in vitamin D-sufficient and -deficient rats.

Vitamin D Status and Bone Resorption in Phosphate Depletion

The results of an experiment in which young rats were fed a vitamin D-deficient (-D) or control (+D) diet for 4.5 weeks prior to placing one-half of each group on a low phosphorus diet are shown in Table 3. The bone resorption rate in each of the treatment groups (+D-P, -D+P, and -D-P) was significantly greater ($P<.025$) than in the control group (+D+P). Although significantly greater than in the control group, the bone resorption rate in the -D-P group was also significantly less than in either the +D-P or -D+P groups. The index of osteoclast activity, the linear bone resorption rate, was also significantly elevated ($P<0.05$) in each of the treatment groups compared to the +D+P control group. For this parameter, however, there were no significant differences between the treatment groups. The effect of the diet combinations on the endosteal resorbing surface showed a significant increase ($P<.001$) in only the +D-P group compared to the +D+P control group. These results indicate that some metabolite of vitamin D (possibly 1,25-diOH-D_3) is necessary to produce the marked increase in osteoclast number observed in phosphate depletion. The finding that the linear rate of bone resorption or osteoclast activity is significantly increased in the -D-P group could indicate a direct effect of low serum phosphate, or an effect of PTH which would be elevated in the -D-P group since serum calcium is also decreased in this group.

Table 3. Serum and bone parameters in vitamin D and phosphorus deficient rate.*

	Groups			
	+D+P	+D-P	-D+P	-D-P
Serum Ca, mg/dl	9.4±0.5**	11.6±0.6	5.8±0.6	8.4±0.7
Serum Pi, mg/dl	9.7±0.5	5.4±0.8	11.4±0.8	5.1±0.7
Endosteal Resorbing Surface, mm^2	1.2±0.9	3.6±1.3	1.7±0.6	1.2±0.7
Linear rate of bone resorption, μ/d	1.0±9.9	9.9±5.2	10.5±4.9	7.1±5.5
Bone resorption rate, $(mm^3/d) \times 10^3$	2.6±11.3	25.9±19.7	17.8±7.7	10.2±7.7

*Weanling rats were placed on diets which contained a 0.6% Ca and 0.6% P and normal D_3 (2IU/g) (+D) or no vitamin D_3 (-D) for a period of 4.5 weeks to ensure a vitamin D deficient state prior to initiating the phosphate depletion. One-half of the animals in each group were then placed on a diet containing 0.04% P (-P). The experiment was terminated after 14 d on the final diets.
**Mean±SD for 18-20 animals/group.

SUMMARY

Phosphate depletion causes significant changes in the composition of the cell population in bone and the metabolic activities of these cells. The data presented indicate that a vitamin D metabolite has a significant role in producing the increase in osteoclast number associated with phosphate depletion. The increased resorptive activity and number of osteoclasts leads to a marked increase in the rate of bone resorption resulting in the liberation of calcium phosphate, while the decrease in the rates of the processes involved in bone formation (matrix production, osteoid maturation, and mineralization) reduces the amount of phosphate which is removed from the circulation. Thus, all of the effects of phosphate depletion on bone are consistent with the interpretation that bone acts as a reservoir of phosphate and is used to maintain soft tissue and serum phosphate levels at the expense of bone.

ACKNOWLEDGMENTS

This work was supported in part by NIH Grants DE-02600 and HD-04872, and V.A. supported research, MRIS #0483.

REFERENCES

1. *Baylink, D., Wergedal, J., and Stauffer, M.: Formation, mineralization, and resorption of bone in hypophosphatemic rats. J. Clin. Invest. 50: 2519, 1971.*

2. *Day, H.G., and McCollum, E.V.: Mineral metabolism, growth, and symptomatology of rats on a diet extremely deficient in phosphorus. J. Biol. Chem. 130: 269, 1939.*

3. *Raisz, L.G., and Niemann, I.: Effect of phosphate, calcium, and magnesium on bone resorption and hormonal responses in tissue culture. Endocrinology. 85: 446, 1969.*

4. *Wergedal, J.: Enzymes of protein and phosphate catabolism in rat bone. I. Enyzme properties in normal rats. Calcified Tissue Res. 3: 55, 1969.*

5. *Baylink, D., Wergedal, J., Stauffer, M., and Rich, C.: Formation, mineralization, and resorption of bone in vitamin D-Deficient rats. J. Clin. Invest. 49: 1122, 1970.*

6. *Baylink, D., Wergedal, J., Stauffer, M., and Rich, C.: Effects of fluoride on bone formation, mineralization, and resorption in the rat. In Fluoride in Medicine. T. L. Vischer, editor. Hans Huber, Bern. 37, 1970.*

7. *Baylink, D., Morey, E., and Rich, C.: Effect of calcitonin on the rates of bone formation and resorption in the rat. Endocrinology. 84: 261, 1969.*

8. *Thompson, E., Baylink, D., and Wergedal, J.: Increases in number and size of osteoclasts in response to calcium or phosphorus deficiency in the rat. Endocrinology. 97: 283, 1975.*

9. *Haussler, M., Hughes, M., Baylink, D., Littledike, E.T., Cork, D., and Pitt, M.: Influence of phosphate depletion on the biosynthesis and circulating level of 1α,25-dihydroxyvitamin D. In Phosphate Metabolism. S. G. Massry and E. Ritz, editors. Plenum Press, New York. 233, 1977.*

10. *Bruin, W.J., Baylink, D.J., and Wergedal, J.E.: Acute inhibition of mineralization and stimulation of bone resorption mediated by hypophosphatemia. Endocrinology. 96: 394, 1975.*

11. *Ivey, J.L., Su, M., Feist, E., and Baylink, D.: Phosphate and vitamin D status on serum PTH in rats. Program and Abstracts of the 59th Annual Meeting of The Endocrine Society. 310, 1977.*

THE BIOCHEMICAL INDICES OF EXPERIMENTAL PHOSPHORUS DEPLETION (PD): A RE-EXAMINATION OF THEIR PHYSIOLOGICAL IMPLICATIONS

D. B. N. Lee, N. Brautbar, N. W. Walling,
H. E. Carlson, C. Golvin, J. W. Coburn, C. R. Kleeman

Departments of Medicine, UCLA Medical Center, and
Wadsworth V.A. Hospital Center, Los Angeles, California

The biochemical features observed in experimental phosphorus (P) depletion include hypercalcemia (↑P-Ca), hypophosphatemia (↓P-P), hypercalciuria (↑U-Ca), hypophosphaturia (↓U-P) and intestinal calcium (Ca) hyperabsorption (1-7). Exogenous P deprivation is the usual mode of inducing PD and has been considered fundamental in the generation of the various biochemical changes (Figure 1). However, it is entirely reasonable to postulate that these changes also may be induced or aborted by modifying the metabolic need for P. In the present study we observed that normal young rats maintained on normal P diets may develop biochemical features of PD if they undergo unusual and spontaneous acceleration in growth. On the other hand, in young rats with growth arrest induced by hypophysectomy, both the biochemical and clinical changes caused by low P diet may either be aborted or attenuated. These findings stress the importance of defining the prevailing anabolic need of experimental animals in interpreting both the adequacy of dietary P and the significance of the clinical and the biochemical changes of PD. Some relevant examples will be discussed. We also provide evidence demonstrating that in young rats PD results in a net reduction in intestinal Ca retention. Since both the synthesis of 1,25-dihydroxyvitamin D_3 ($1,25(OH)_2D_3$) and its accumulation in intestinal mucosa are increased in P deprived rats (8,9), this finding may represent an example in which the physiological interrelationship between the activity of $1,25(OH)_2D_3$ and net intestinal Ca retention is dissociated.

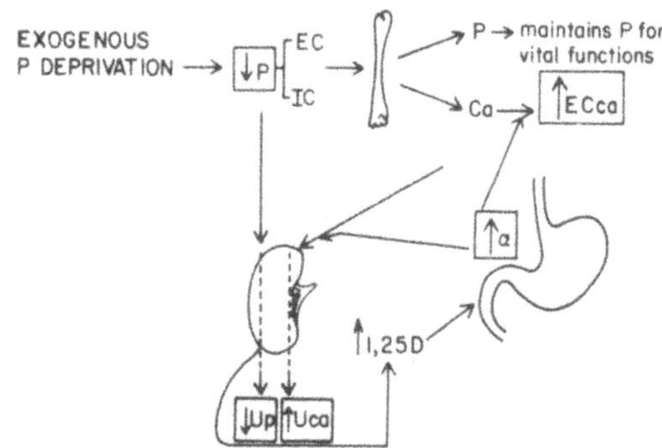

Figure 1. Biochemical indices of experimental phosphorus (P) depletion. P = phosphorus, Ca = calcium, EC = extracellular, IC = intracellular, α = intestinal Ca absorption, U = urinary, ↑ = increase, ↓ = decrease

MATERIALS AND METHODS

Sixty-70g intact (INT) and hypophysectomized* (HPX) male Sprague-Dawley rats were housed individually in metabolic cages. The effect of three different dietary groups was studied in both INT and HPX rats: normal phosphorus 0.3% *ad lib* (NP), low phosphorus 0.03% *ad lib* (LP), and normal phosphorus 0.3% pair-fed with LP mates (NP-PF). Each dietary group consisted of eight rats. Ca content was approximately 0.4%. The amino acid content of NP diet was made of casein whereas that for LP diet was made of a nutritionally equivalent amount of fibrin. Other constituents, including vitamin fortifications, were similar in both the NP and LP diets. The HPX rats received daily subcutaneous injections of L-Thyroxine, 800ng/100gm body weight (10), and Cortrosyn, 10μg/100gm body weight (11). INT rats received daily subcutaneous injections of euqal volumes of vehicle normal saline. Distilled water was given to all animals *ad lib*. All rats were weighted daily, as was the food consumed. Urines were collected daily and stools in 7-day pools. Blood was collected before and after the completion of the experiment by decapitation. The protocols of two studies were identical except that the dietary manipulation lasted two weeks in one and three weeks in the other.

Ca was analyzed by atomic absorption spectroscopy and P was measured by the Malachite Green micromethod of Hohenwallner and Wimmer (12). Intestinal mucosal ^{45}Ca uptake was measured by the method of everted gut sac (13).

*From Hormone Assay Laboratory, Inc., Chicago, Illinois, USA.

In two other experiments only INT rats were used. In one experiment three groups of rats on LP, NP, and high P 1.0% (HP) were studied. In this experiment the NP rats demonstrated spontaneous and unusual acceleration in growth. Weight gained per two weeks was 79.9± 16.0 (SD)gm vs our normal of 63.4± 9.9gm in several other similar studies ($p < 0.001$). In the remaining experiment only LP and NP-PF rats were studied. Two eight-rat groups were placed on LP diet and two additional groups on corresponding NP-PF diet. One LP group and its corresponding NP-PF group were sacrificed at the end of the first week and the remaining two groups were sacrificed at the end of the second week. In each instance *in vitro* duodenal and jejunal mucosal uptake of ^{45}Ca were measured. Two-3 cm of proximal duodenum and an approximately equal length of jejunum taken from around the midpoint of the small intestine were used in the construction of everted sacs.

RESULTS

The effect of PD on weight gain in INT and HPX young rats is illustrated with data obtained from one representative study (Figure 2). In INT rats weight gain is clearly retarded in the

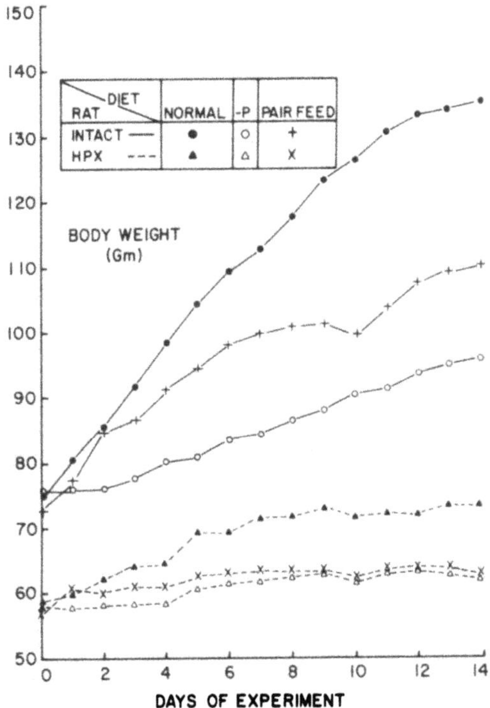

Figure 2

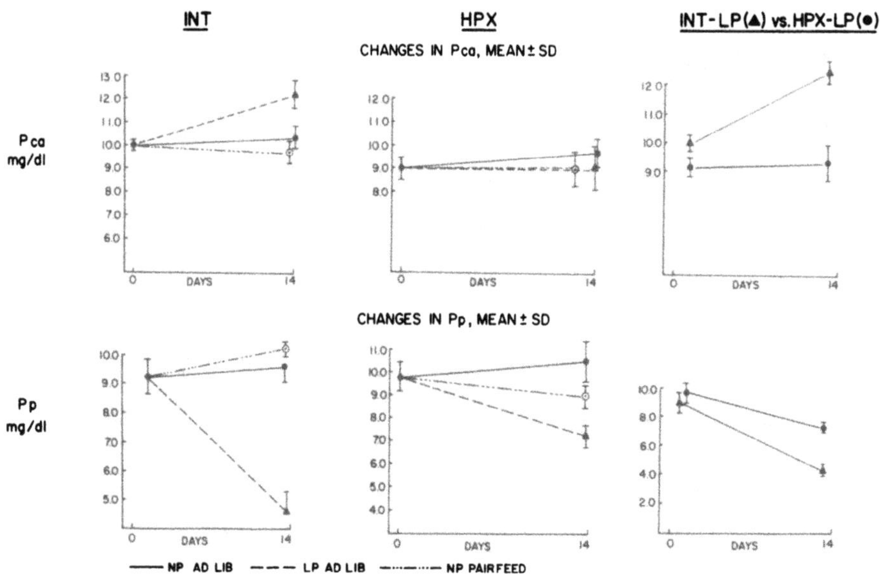

Figure 3. Changes in plasma calcium (Pca) and phosphorus (Pp) in intact (INT) and hypophysectomized (HPX) young rats maintained on normal 0.3% (NP) and low 0.03% (LP) phosphorus diet for 14 days. Each LP animal has a pair-fed mate eating NP diet.

LP group. The reduction in growth is attributable to both a reduction in food intake (as reflected by the difference between the growth curves of NP and NP-PF groups) and a specific effect of PD (as reflected by the difference between the growth curves of NP-PF and LP groups). Growth is clearly reduced in HPX rats. Weight gain in NP rats averaged under 1 gm per day and appeared to cease altogether when the mean weight reached 70 gm. Simple restriction of food intake (NP-PF) further stunted the growth and LP diet did not appear to cause any further discernible difference in weight gain.

LP diet resulted in the development of unequivocal $\uparrow$P-Ca in INT rats but was without effect on plasma Ca concentration in HPX rats (Figure 3). The initial plasma Ca concentration in HPX rats was lower than that found in INT rats ($p < 0.05$).

In INT rats plasma P concentration dropped precipitously in the LP group only. In HPX rats $\downarrow$P-P was seen in both the LP and the NP-PF groups, although the reduction was clearly more profound in the LP group. However, when compared with the INT rats, LP diet in HPX rats caused only a modest decrease in plasma P concentration. Figure 4 depicts the changes in urine Ca and P in both INT and HPX rats. $\uparrow$U-Ca was more marked in INT rats, both in absolute quantity and in relation to pre-depletion values. In both INT and HPX rats LP diet resulted in ↓U-P to negligible amounts.

In the study using INT rats maintained on LP, NP, and HP diets, the group consuming the NP diet demonstrated a spontaneous, but unusual, acceleration in weight gain (see Materials and Methods). Rats on HP diets demonstrated weight gain no different from INT rats on NP diets in other studies. Rats on LP diets gained little weight. The changes in plasma Ca and P concentrations and urinary Ca and P excretions are plotted in Figure 5. The limits of mean ± 2SD of each of these parameters obtained from two other studies using the same protocol and in rats demonstrating usual rates of growth are marked by shaded areas. Thus, in this study rats on both the NP and LP diets developed ↑P-Ca, ↑U-Ca and ↓U-P. The only difference is that rats on NP diets demonstrated all these features in the absence of ↓P-P.

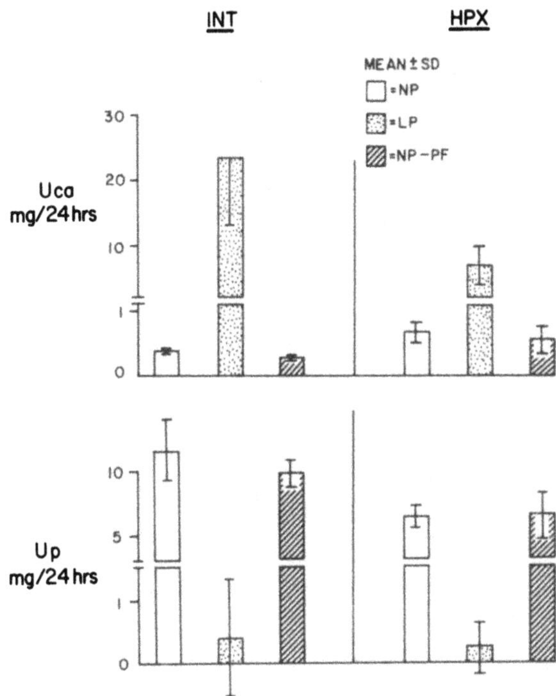

Figure 4. Urinary calcium (Uca), and phosphorus (Up) excretion in intact (INT) and hypophysectomized (HPX) young rats maintained for 14 days on normal 0.3% (NP) or low 0.03% (LP) phosphorus diet. Each LP rat has a pair-fed mate on NP diet (NP-PF)

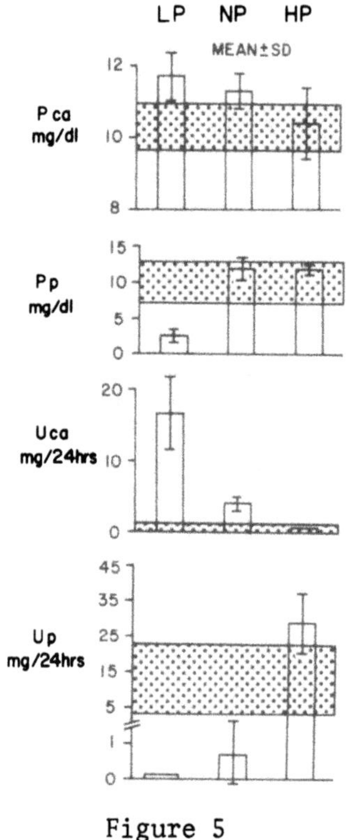

Figure 5

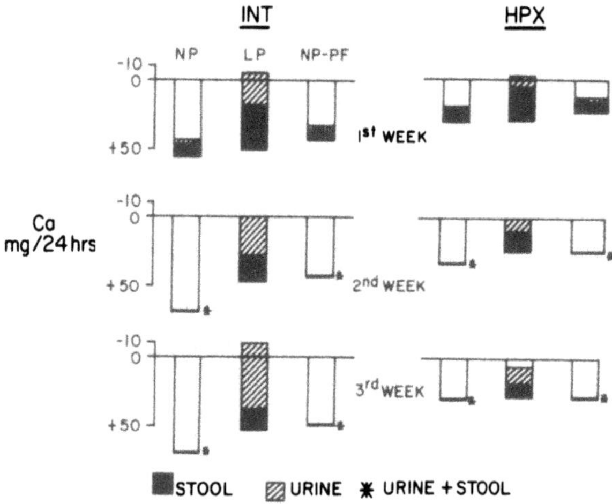

Figure 6. Calcium (Ca) balance studies in intact (INT) and hypophysectomized (HPX) young rats maintained on normal 0.03% (NP) or low 0.03% (LP) phosphorus diets. Each LP rat also has a pair-fed mate on NP diet (NP-PF).

Table 1

		$\frac{\text{Stool Ca}}{\text{Diet Ca}}$ X 100		
		NP	LP	NP-PF
Expt. 1-0676	1st week	14	38	21
	2nd week	13	30	14
Expt. 4-0377	1st week	--	64	58
	2nd week	--	60	56

The results of Ca balance studies are illustrated in Figure 6. LP diet in both INT and HPX rats led to a clear increase in fecal Ca, both in absolute quantities and in proportion to the dietary Ca intake. Decrease in net intestinal Ca retention following LP diet is also confirmed in two other studies. The ratio of stool Ca/diet Ca was either not decreased or clearly increased (Table 1).

The increased stool Ca coupled with ↑U-Ca resulted in a consistent zero or negative Ca balance in both INT and HPX rats on LP diets. This is in marked contrast to the distinct positive Ca balance seen in both NP and NP-PF rats, which, in this particular study, were able to reduce both stool and urinary Ca to negligible quantities. In vitro duodenal uptake of ^{45}Ca was measured towards the end of the third week and the results are illustrated in Figure 7. In INT rats ^{45}Ca uptake was not significantly different between animals on LP and NP-PF diets, although both groups demonstrated clear reduction in uptake when compared to rats on unrestrained NP diets. In HPX rats ^{45}Ca uptake was not different in

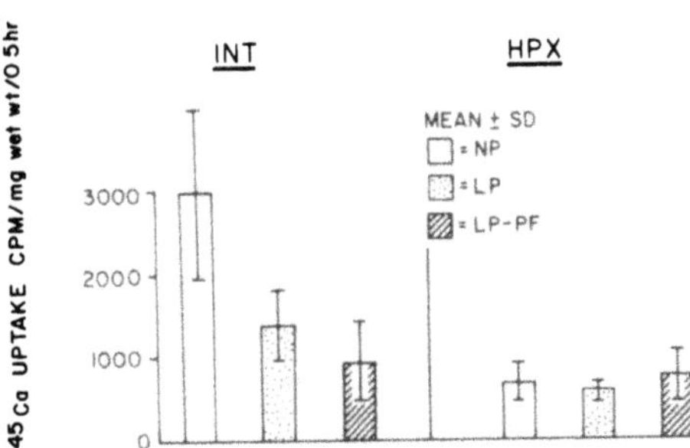

Figure 7. In vitro proximal duodenal uptake of ^{45}Ca in intact (INT) and hypophysectomized (HPX) young rats maintained for 18 days on normal 0.3% (NP) or low 0.03% (LP) phosphorus diet. Each LP rat has a pair-fed mate on NP diet (NP-PF).

all three dietary groups. With the exception of NP-PF group, HPX rats demonstrated significantly lower ^{45}Ca uptake when compared to the corresponding dietary groups in INT rats. In a separate study both duodenal and jejunal mucosal ^{45}Ca uptake were measured in similar INT young rats maintained either on LP or NP-PF diets. The measurements were made at the end of one and two weeks (Figure 8). Duodenal ^{45}Ca uptake between two groups was not different at the end of the first week but became clearly elevated in LP rats by the end of the second week. A reverse trend is seen in ^{45}Ca uptake by the jejunal mucosa. Increased uptake was seen in LP rats studied at the end of the first week, but by the end of the second week, the increment dissipated, and uptake between LP and NP-PF rats was no longer different.

DISCUSSION

The present study indicates that the response to an LP diet in young rats may be modified by hypophysectomy-induced growth retardation. Thus, ↑P-Ca was absent and the severity of ↑U-Ca, and ↓P-P was attenuated. The clinical effect of an LP diet in these animals was not dramatic, as was reflected by the similarity of weight curves between the LP and the NP-PF rats (Figure 2). The virtual arrest of growth would be expected to decrease the demand for P and therefore the amelioration of the deleterious effect of the LP diet. This may be the basis for the observation that PD develops readily and rapidly in young animals following simple dietary P deprivation, whereas the induction of a similar degree

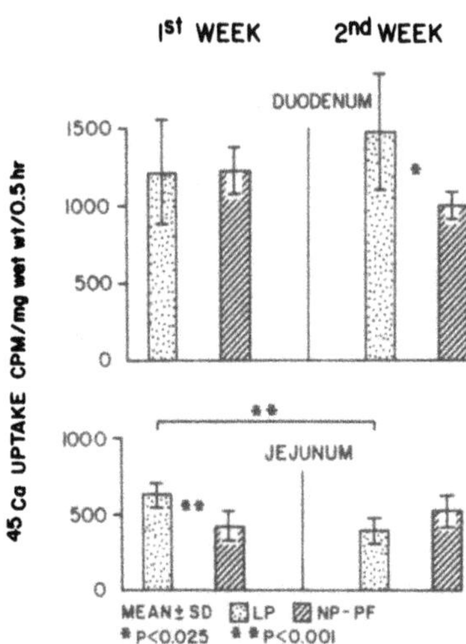

Figure 8. In vitro duodenal and jejunal uptake of ^{45}Ca in young rats maintained on low 0.03% phosphorus diet (LP) and pair-fed mates eating normal 0.3% phosphorus diet (NP-PF).

of P deficiency in grown animals requires longer duration of a low P diet and the additional use of phosphate-binding alkaline earth compounds such as Al(OH)3 (4). In one study PD developed within five weeks in young rats but took 26 weeks in adult rats (14). The observation that simple starvation (and therefore presumed cessation of growth) actually may lead to the healing of rickets in P-depleted rats also becomes more explicable (15). In clinical practice it has been noted that evidence of rickets is frequently absent in children who were expected to develop dietary rickets but in whom growth arrest was simultaneously present for various reasons (16). The absence of ↑P-Ca in non-growing HPX young rats fed with LP diets may account for the observation that ↑P-Ca was found in puppies (2) but not in adult dogs (4) in the state of PD.

While inhibition of growth, and therefore reduction in P demand, may ameliorate the adverse effect of P deprivation, the acceleration of growth may produce biochemical changes of PD in the absence of dietary P deprivation (Figure 5). In this study both the NP and LP rats developed ↑P-Ca, ↑U-Ca, and ↓U-P. The major difference however, was that the LP rats demonstrated poor growth and other clinical evidence of 'failure to thrive', whereas the NP rats demonstrated exceptional acceleration in growth and were clinically in perfect health. It therefore appears that under the conditions of this particular experiment, the body called forth similar responses in young rats fed with NP and LP diets. It is likely that the body 'sees' a similar state of relative excess of demand over supply. In the NP rats the normally ample P supply was exceeded only because of exceptional acceleration in growth, whereas in the LP rats the supply was exceeded simply to maintain life sustaining metabolic activities. In this connection it is particularly interesting to note that clinicians have previously observed radiological evidence of rickets in *normal* infants with rapid growth when no disturbance in mineral metabolism was detectable (16). In the unique syndrome of fatal hyperalimentation (17, 18) the constellation of features mimics PD with remarkable exactitude. The catastrophe is most likely the result of a sudden induction in anabolic activities creating a precipitous and often fatal imbalance between P demand and P supply.

It should be pointed out that the development of ↑P-Ca, ↑U-Ca, and ↓U-P in INT rats on NP diets (Figure 5) was not associated with perceptible changes in plasma P concentration. This suggests the existence of signal(s), other than ↓P-P, capable of eliciting adaptive changes to P deprivation. Figure 9 represents the more dramatic example of urinary P conservation induced by LP diet that we have encountered in our studies. Urinary P dropped precipitously on the very first day of the LP diet and virtually disappeared by the second day. This is true in both the normally growing rats and the growth retarded HPX rats indicating that ↓U-P is probably the earliest and the most sensitive reflection of threats to body P

URINARY P (INTACT RATS)
MEAN + SE
mg P/mg CR
24 hours
6.0
5.0
4.0
3.0
2.0
1.0
= NORMAL P
= LOW P
= NORMAL P PAIR FED.
1 2 3 4 5 6 7 8 9 10 11 12 13 14 15 16 17 18

URINARY P (HPX RATS)
MEAN + SE
mg P/mg CR
24 hours
6.0
5.0
4.0
3.0
2.0
1.0
= NORMAL P DIET
= LOW P DIET
= NORMAL P PAIR FED.
1 2 3 4 5 6 7 8 9 10 11 12 13 14 15 16 17 18

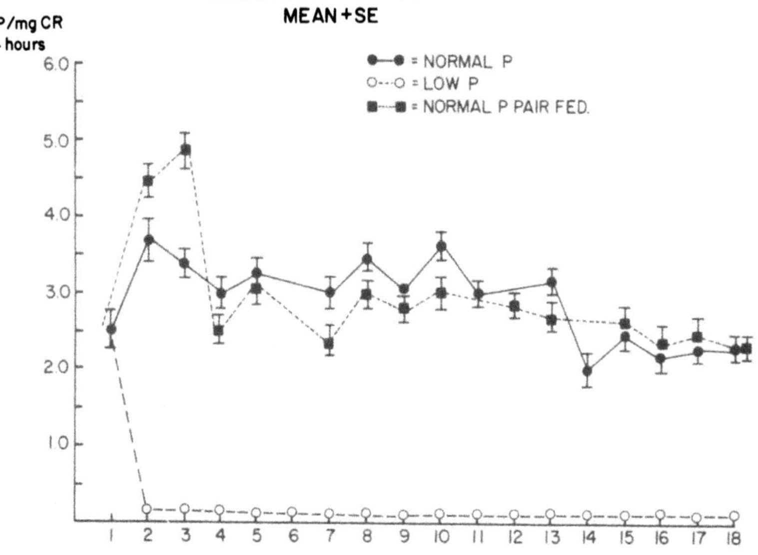

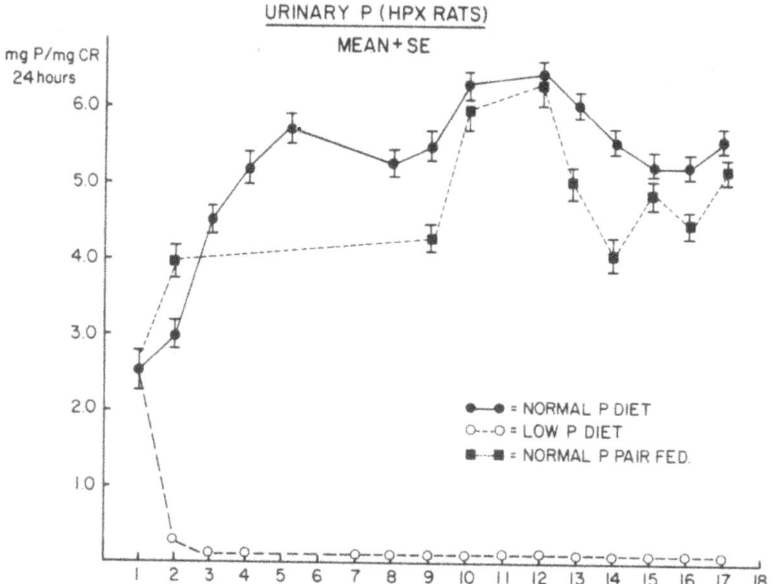

Figure 9

economy. This adaptive change in renal P conservation may occur before the development of discernible reduction in plasma P concentration. Beck (19) studied the effect of exogenous PTH on urine phosphate excretion in P-depleted TPTX rats. The rats were studied after being fed with either a normal or low-P diet for three days. Although the plasma P concentration was not different in the two groups after dietary manipulation, the phosphaturic effect of PTH administration was abolished in the low-P group. The data thus suggest that during PD the kidney becomes resistant to the acute effect of PTH on phosphate excretion, and that a change in this transport characteristic evolves before the development of a perceptible change in plasma P concentration. All these studies underscore the efficiency of the body P conserving mechanism(s) and suggest that the sensor which initiates these mechanisms is not necessarily hypophosphatemia but rather is more likely to be related to intracellular events and activities.

Increased intestinal Ca absorption is a recognized finding in animals fed with low P diet (5-7). The findings of elevated fecal Ca in both INT and HPX rats maintained on LP diet is therefore quite unexpected. However, further analysis of the published data indicates that most of the studies demonstrating an increase in intestinal Ca absorption under the condition of PD are based on data obtained from isotopic Ca uptake by isolated intestinal segments (5-7). In the few mineral balance studies reported, such as the classical study of Day and McCollum (1), the stool Ca was consistently higher in the P deficient rats when compared to the pair-fed mates on normal P diet. The 8-week balance data revealed a total stool Ca of 225 mg and a total dietary Ca intake of 850 mg (stool Ca/diet Ca = 26%) in PD rats, whereas the comparable figures for pair-fed mates were 125 mg, 822 mg and 14%, respectively. Of relevance may be the work of Henry and associates demonstating that in 1-month-old rats the retention of Ca from the diet is very much less in those fed with a low P diet than those fed with a diet adequate in P. The trend however is reversed in rats older than three months (20). The rats used by us, as well as those used by Day and McCollum, were all younger than three months.

Measurement of *in vitro* ^{45}Ca uptake by the proximal duodenal mucosa in INT rats was not different between rats on LP and NP-PF diets at the end of one week but became clearly elevated in LP rats at the end of the second week (Figure 8). In a separate study mucosal ^{45}Ca uptake was measured at the end of third week and again no clear difference was seen between the LP and NP-PF groups. These preliminary data suggest that in young rats an LP diet induces an increase in duodenal mucosal Ca uptake after a lag period. When an LP diet is administered over a more prolonged period and, therefore, presumably the degree of P depletion becomes more severe, the increase ability to accumulate Ca is lost. A similar sequence of events may occur in the jejunum following an LP diet, except the augmentation in uptake occurs and dissipates earlier (Figure 8). The decrease in ^{45}Ca accumulation by duodenal mucosa from HPX rats has been previously documented (21).

Thus, although it is quite clear that the net translocation of Ca from the intestinal lumen into the body is decreased in young rats (50-80 gm) maintained on LP diets, the transport characteristics of each segment of the intestine (duodenum, jejunum, ileum and colon) remain to be rigorously defined. Since both the synthesis of $1,25(OH)_2D_3$ and its intestinal mucosal accumulation are increased in P depleted rats (8,9), the potential exists for the development of a biological model in which the recognized interrelationship between the activity of $1,25(OH)_2D_3$ and net intestinal Ca absorption dissociates.

CONCLUSIONS

1. The biochemical changes of PD are reflections of a relative excess of demand over supply for P and are not invariably associated with overt clinical disruptions. They may develop in *normal* young rats maintained on NP diets, when growth is exceptionally accelerated; on the other hand, both the biochemical and clinical changes of PD may be attenuated in young rats maintained on LP diets if growth is arrested by hypophysectomy.

2. The evolution of the biochemical changes of PD does not always require the presence of hypophosphatemia.

3. In young rats LP diet leads to Ca 'wastage' in both the kidney and the intestine.

Acknowledgments: Vincent Silis, John O. Steppe, Maxine Domain, Wendy Adams, Sandy Brauner, Kitty Sullivan, Sandy Howard, Jr. This investigation was supported in part by UCLA Biomedical Research Support Grant RRO-5354 and a grant from the Kidney Foundation of Southern California (Dr. Brautbar). Dr. Lee is the recipient of a Veterans Administration Research Associateship. Dr. Walling is the recipient of a Veterans Administration Clinical Investigator Award.

References:

1. Day HG, McCollum EV: Mineral metabolism, growth, symptomatology of rats on diet extremely deficient in phosphorus. J. Biol. Chem. 130:269-283, 1939.

2. Freeman S, McLean FC: Experimental rickets. Blood and tissue changes in puppies receiving a diet very low in phosphorus with and without vitamin D. Arch. Path. 32:387-408, 1941.

3. Aubel CE: The effects of low phosphorus rations on growing pigs. J. Agricultural Res. 52:149-159, 1936.

4. Coburn JW, Massry SG: Changes in serum and urinary calcium during phosphate depletion: studies of mechanisms. J. Clin. Invest. 49:1073-1087, 1970.

5. Morrissey RL, Wasserman RH: Calcium absorption and calcium-binding protein in chicks on differing calcium and phosphorus intakes. Am. J. Physiol. 220(5):1509-1515, 1971.

6. Haddad JG, Jr., Boisseau V, Avioli LV: Phosphorus deprivation: the metabolism of vitamin D_3 and 25-hydroxycholecalciferol in rats. J. Nutr. 102:269-282, 1972.

7. Ribovich ML, DeLuca HF: The influence of dietary calcium and phosphorus on intestinal calcium transport in rats given vitamin D metabolites. Arch. Biochem. Biophys. 170:529-535, 1975.

8. Tanaka Y, Frank H, DeLuca HF: Intestinal calcium transport: stimulation by low phosphorus diets. Science 181:564-566, 1973.

9. Hughs MR, Brumbaugh PF, Haussler MR, Wergedal J, Baylink DJ: Regulation of serum 1 , 25-dihydroxyvitamin D_3 by calcium and phosphate in the rat. Science 190:578-579, 1973.

10. Frumess RD, Larsen PR: Correlation of serum triiodothyronine (T_3) and Thyroxine (T_4) with biologic effects of thyroid hormone replacement. Metabolism 24:547-554, 1975.

11. Colby HD, Malendowicz LK, Caffrey JL, Kitay JI: Effect of hypophysectomy and ACTH on adrenocortical function in the rat. Endocrinology 94:1346-1350, 1974.

12. Hohenwallner W, Wimmer E: The Malachite Green micromethod for the determination of inorganic phosphate. Clinica

Chimica Acta. 45:169-175, 1973.

13. Walling MW, Rothman SS: Adaptive uptake of calcium at the duodenal brush border. Am. J. Physiol. 225:618-623, 1973.

14. Copp DH, Snider AP: Study of calcium kinetics in calcium and phosphorus deficient rats with the aid of radiocalcium. In FC McLean, P Lacroix, AM Budy (Eds): Radioisotopes and Bone, Blackwell, Oxford, 1962.

15. McCollum EV, Simmonds N: Studies on experimental rickets. XV The effect of starvation on the healing of rickets. Johns Hopkins Hosp. Bull. 33:31-33, 1922.

16. Follis HR, Jr.: Diseases, particularly of bone, associated with derangements of calcium and phosphorus metabolism. In Reifenstein FC, Jr. (Ed): Metabolic Interrelations, Transactions of the Fifth Conference, The Josiah Macy, Jr. Foundation, January 5-6, 1953, pp 210-211.

17. Silvis SE, Paragas PV, Jr.: Fatal hyperalimentation syndrome. Animal studies. J. Lab. Clin. Med. 78:918-930, 1971.

18. Silvis SE, Paragas PV, Jr.: Paresthesias, weakness, seizures and hypophosphatemia in patients receiving hyperalimentation. Gastroenterology. 62:513-520, 1972.

19. Beck N: Effect of dietary phosphorus (P) intake on renal actions of parathyroid hormone (PTH) and cyclic AMP (cAMP). Am. Soc. of Nephrology, November 21-23, 1976, Washington, D.C. p1.

20. Henry KM, Kon SK, Todd PEE, Toothill J, Tomlin DH: Calcium and phosphorus metabolism in the rat: effect of age on rate of adaptation to a low calcium intake. Acta Biochimica Polonica 7:167-185, 1960.

21. Finkelstein JD, Schachter D: Active transport of calcium by intestine: effects of hypophysectomy and growth hormone. Am. J. Physiol. 203(5):873-880, 1962.

EFFECTS OF PHOSPHORUS DEPLETION ON LEFT VENTRICULAR ENERGY GENERATION

Thomas J. Fuller, Wilmer W. Nichols,
Bruce J. Brenner, and John C. Peterson
Department of Medicine, Veterans Administration Hospital, and the Department of Medicine,
University of Florida Medical School,
Gainesville, Florida 32610

Introduction

Recent studies have shown that phosphorus depletion has an adverse effect on skeletal muscle function and composition. Specifically, a symptom complex characterized by muscle stiffness, weakness and severe pain has been described in patients taking aluminum hydroxide containing antacids (1,2). These complaints were especially notable when serum phosphorus concentrations approached or fell below 1 mg/100 ml and improved rapidly with correction of the hypophosphotemia. In addition, phosphorus depletion in experimental animals is characterized by a low resting transmembrane electrical potential difference as well as changes in skeletal muscle composition consistent with a "sick" cell (3).

From the foregoing observations, it is clear that phosphorus depletion causes skeletal muscle dysfunction. Studies, however, designed to investigate the effects of phosphorus depletion on cardiac muscle have not been reported. The objectives, therefore, of the present study were to define the effects of chronic phosphorus deficiency on the energy generating ability of the left ventricle. Total external potential energy of the ventricle was obtained from serial measurements of left ventricular pressure and aortic root blood flow in awake dogs during phosphorus depletion and repletion accomplished by changes in dietary phosphorus intake.

Methods

Five healthy adult male dogs, weighing 16 to 23 Kg were used for the study. Under aseptic conditions and general anesthesia (halothane), a left thoracotomy was performed. The ascending aorta was isolated and an appropriate size electromagnetic flow probe installed (Biotronex Laboratory, Inc., Kensington, Maryland) by the technique outlined by Khouri (4). A solid state high fidelity pressure transducer (Konigsberg Instrument, Inc., Pasadena, California) was inserted into the left ventricle at the apex using the procedure described by Stone (5). The leads of the two transducers were exteriorized at the back of the neck between the scapulae; the chest was closed and the animal allowed to recover.

Ascending aortic blood flow and left ventricular pressure were recorded on magnetic tape (Hewlett-Packard, Model 3960) beginning after a post-surgical recovery period of 12 to 15 days and continued on a weekly basis for the period of the study. Total external potential energy or power of the left ventricle was obtained by continuous multiplication of the ventricular pressure and aortic blood flow signals (6) using a mini computer (Hewlett-Packard, Model 9820). Integration of the pulsatile power curve gives mean or average energy and division by the heart rate gives stroke work.

Phosphorus depletion was produced following surgical recovery over a 35 day period by feeding the animals 20 g/Kg of a synthetic phosphorus-deficient but otherwise nutritionally adequate diet. Each 450 g contains 90 g of protein, 270 g of carbohydrate and 45 g of fat (ICN Nutritional Biochemicals Div., International Chemical and Nuclear Corp., Cleveland, Ohio). They were also given aluminum carbonate gel (Basaljel extra strength (R), Wyeth Laboratories, Philadelphia), 60 cm^3/day. Upon chemical analysis each 450 g of this diet contained 117 mg of elemental phosphorus and 160 mEq of potassium. During the period of post surgical recovery and during the 3 week period of repletion, the same synthetic diet was used except that phosphorus was added as Na_2HPO_4 to provide a total elemental phosphorus intake of 1.87 g.

In each dog, in addition to the cardiac studies, sequential measurements of skeletal muscle content of phosphorus and serum inorganic phosphorus concentration were obtained by methods previously published (3). This was done in order to ascertain the level of phosphorus depletion. These studies were performed initially at the end of the post surgical recovery period before phosphorus depletion was induced. Repeat studies were then performed after 5 weeks of phosphorus restriction and again after 3 weeks of phosphorus repletion. Throughout the study plasma samples were collected for measurement of electrolytes and blood gases. No histologic studies were obtained.

Results

Serum electrolytes and blood gases

After five weeks of phosphorus depletion, there were no significant differences in serum Na^+, K^+, Cl^-, Mg^{++}, and Ca^{++} concentrations. Serum phosphorus fell significantly from an average control value of 5.2 ± 0.3 to 0.9 ± 0.2 mg/dl ($p < .001$) after 5 weeks of phosphorus depletion.

Skeletal muscle composition

After 5 weeks of phosphorus depletion, muscle phosphorus content had dropped approximately 22% from 28.1 ± 0.4 to 22.2 ± 0.8 mmPi/100 g fat-free dry weight (FFDW) ($p < .001$). With repletion muscle phosphorus content increased to 26.3 mmPi/100 g FFDW.

Cardiac muscle studies

The effects of phosphorus depletion and repletion on the external energy generated by the left ventricle are shown in Table I. Although measurements were made weekly after surgical recovery, only those during control (day 0), and late (35 days) phosphorus depletion and late (56 days) phosphorus repletion periods are given. During the period of the study, heart rate and peak systolic and diastolic aortic pressures did not change significantly. During phosphorus depletion left ventricular end diastolic pressure increased from a resting control value of 4.2 ± 0.9 mmHg to 7.2 ± 1.0 mmHg ($p < .001$) while stroke work decreased an average of 34% ($p < .01$). Also, both average and peak external left ventricular potential energy decreased 28% ($p < .005$) and 24% ($p < .01$) respectively. During phosphorus repletion all four variables returned toward their control values.

Discussion

It is evident from these studies that chronic phosphorus deficiency reduces the energy generating ability of the left ventricle. Measurements after 5 weeks of phosphorus depletion showed no significant change in heart rate, peak systolic and diastolic aortic pressure but did show a rise in left ventricular end diastolic pressure and a fall in average and peak external potential energy and stroke work. This was at a time when peripheral stores of phosphate as measured by skeletal muscle content were decreased by 22%. Phosphorus depletion, therefore, causes a reduction in myocardial stroke work independent of the Frank-Starling effect. Upon restoring phosphorus to the diet, all abnormalities cleared rapidly.

TABLE I

EFFECTS OF PHOSPHORUS DEPLETION ON LEFT VENTRICULAR ENERGY GENERATION

	Day		HR b/Min	Systolic mmHg	Diastolic mmHg	LVEDP mmHg	Average Energy mwatts	Peak Energy mwatts	Stroke Work mjoules
Control	0	Mean	100	126	87	4.2	612	3867	376
N = 5		SEM	9	3	4	0.9	62	148	36
Late PO_4 Deficiency	35	Mean	109	115	81	7.2	443	2934	249
		SEM	9	6	6	1.0	48	217	35
N = 5		P	NS	NS	NS	< .001	< .005	< .01	< .01
Late PO_4 Repletion	56	Mean	114	116	81	5.0	607	3710	324
		SEM	6	5	4	0.8	68	138	39
N = 5		P	NS	NS	NS	NS	NS	NS	NS

Definition of Terms:
HR - Heart rate; LVEDP - left ventricular end diastolic pressure

There are at least 2 hypothetical explanations for these changes in resting cardiac function. The first could be a defect in the production or utilization of the key energy sources for myocardial contractile force - the high energy phosphates, adenosine triphosphate (ATP) and creatine phosphate. It is well known that an inadequate supply of inorganic phosphorus may impair the resynthesis of ATP (7). Phosphorus depletion might also affect the level of myofibrillar ATP-ase activity thereby decreasing available energy. Such a defect, although not evaluated in this study, has been noted in a human study characterized by a decrease in muscle work (8).

The second possibility is that phosphorus depletion impairs Ca^{++} metabolism. In contrast to skeletal muscle which will contract in the absence of calcium in the external medium, cardiac muscle contraction ceases almost immediately when extracellular calcium is withdrawn (9). There is no significant difference in serum Ca^{++} concentration throughout this study. However, a decrease in inorganic phosphate effects both the uptake of Ca^{++} by the cell as well as it effects the intracellular distribution (10). In addition, in certain animal models, a decrease in cardiac function has been associated with an abnormality of calcium pumping by the sarcoplasmic reticulum (11). This pump is dependent upon ATP which requires the availability of adequate stores of inorganic phosphate for resynthesis.

References

1. Mordehai, R., and Robson, M.: Proximal myopathy caused by iatrogenic phosphate depletion. J.A.M.A. 236:1380, 1976.
2. Lotz, M., Zisman, E., and Bartter, F.C.: Evidence for a phosphorus depletion syndrome in man. N. Engl. J. Med. 278:409, 1968.
3. Fuller, T.J., Carter, N.W., Barcenas, C., and Knochel, J.P.: Reversible changes of the muscle cell in experimental phosphorus deficiency. J. Clin. Invest. 57:1019, 1976.
4. Khouri, E.M.: Implantation of flow transducers on the left coronary artery and central aorta. In Chronically Implanted Cardiovascular Instrumentation. McCutcheon, E.P., editor. Academic Press, New York 1st edition 257, 1973.
5. Stone, H.L.: Implantation of solid state pressure transducers. In Chronically Implanted Cardiovascular Instrumentation. McCutcheon, E.P., editor. Academic Press, New York 1st edition 229, 1973.
6. McDonald, D.A.: Blood Flow In Arteries. Williams and Wilkins, Baltimore 2nd edition, 1974.

7. Krebs, H.: Rate limiting factors in cell respiration. In Ciba Foundation Symposium on the Regulation of Cell Metabolism. Little, Brown & Co., Inc., Boston, 1-10, 1959.
8. Alpert, N.R., and Gordon, M.G.: Myofibrillar adenosine triphosphatase activity in congestive heart failure. Am. J. Physiol. 202:940, 1962.
9. Chidsey, C.A.: Calcium metabolism in the normal and failing heart. In the Myocardium Failure and Infarction. Braunwald, E., editor, H.P. Publishing Co., Inc., New York, 37, 1974.
10. Rasmussen, H.: Ionic and hormonal control of calcium homeostasis. Am. J. Med. 50:567, 1971.
11. Suko, J., Vogel, J.H.K., and Chidsey, C.A.: Intracellular calcium and myocardial contractility. Circ. Res. 27, 235, 1970.

EFFECT OF DIETARY PHOSPHORUS DEPRIVATION ON RENAL HANDLING OF CALCIUM AND PHOSPHORUS

Nama Beck

The University of Texas Health Science Center

San Antonio, Texas, U.S.A.

It has been shown (1-6) that chronic Pi deprivation decreases urinary Pi excretion, but increases Ca excretion, suggesting a close relationship between Ca and Pi in renal adaptation to a variation in dietary Pi intake. However, in chronic Pi deprivation, plasma concentrations of Pi and Ca, and filtered loads of these ions are altered. It is therefore difficult to differentiate whether changes in urinary excretion of these ions were due to changes in filtered loads, or due to changes in tubular reabsorption of these ions independent of filtered loads.

In the present experiments dietary Pi intake was restricted for a short duration, 3 days, and therefore, neither plasma concentrations, nor filtered loads of Ca and Pi were altered, making it possible to evaluate the effect of a variation in dietary Pi intake per se on renal tubular handling of Ca as well as Pi, and on PTH actions in the kidney.

Sprague-Dawley rats were fed low Pi diet containing 0.02% Pi or the matching control diet which had been supplemented with 0.22% Pi for 3 days ad libitum. The rats of both groups were thyro-parathyroidectomized 14 to 16 hours before the studies. All experiments were initiated at 8 a.m. to minimize diurnal variation in renal handling of Ca or Pi. After anesthesia with Nembutal, catheters were placed into the trachea, the jugular vein for iv infusion, and the urinary bladder for collection of urine samples. Then saline was infused at a rate of 0.25 ml/min throughout the experiments. Three hours after the initiation of iv infusion, urinary flow rate and urinary excretion rates of Ca and Pi became stable. Then, after obtaining the first blood sample, three 10 min urine samples were collected for basal values.

Plasma Pi and Ca concentrations, and glomerular filtration rate measured by inulin clearance were not measurably different between the control diet and the low Pi diet groups, $p > 0.05$ each. As a result, the filtered load of Pi was also not measurably different between the two groups, $p > 0.05$. However, urinary Pi excretion was markedly less in the low Pi diet group. In contrast, urinary Ca excretion was significantly greater in the low Pi diet group, $p < 0.01$ each.

Table I. Effect of low Pi diet on renal functions in TPTXed rats.

	Control Diet	Low Pi Diet
Number of rats studied	9	9
Plasma Pi (mM)	1.82±0.18	1.91±0.13
Plasma Ca (mM)	0.90±0.05	0.91±0.05
GFR (ml/min-100 g b.w.)	1.09±0.14	0.94±0.13
FL-Pi (μmol/min-100 g b.w.)	1.98±0.18	1.80±0.20
FL-Ca (μmol/min-100 g b.w.)	0.98±0.05	0.86±0.05
Pi excretion (nmol/min-100 g b.w.)	95±31	0.9±0.1
Ca excretion (nmol/min-100 g b.w.)	31.6±4.2	148.8±14.2

Values are means±SE.

In contrast to the findings in chronic Pi deprivation, the changes in urinary excretion of Pi and Ca in the present experiments were due mainly to changes in tubular reabsorption independent of changes in filtered loads of these ions: the fractional tubular Pi reabsorption rate, 95.23 ± 2.46% vs 99.95 ± 0.02%; and the fractional tubular Ca reabsorption rate, 95.81 ± 0.45% vs 82.59 ± 0.39%.

The results in the present experiments also suggest that the observed changes in tubular reabsorption of Ca as well as Pi are probably independent of PTH or calcitonin, because the rats were TPTXed; blood pH was not measurably different, pH 7.39 ± 0.01 vs 7.36 ± 0.01, which does not support the possibility that change in renal handling of Ca and Pi is due to acidosis (7,8); or to changes in plasma concentration of Pi or Ca, since they were not different between the two groups of rats.

It is possible that although plasma Pi concentration was not measurably decreased, intracellular Pi might have been depleted by dietary Pi deprivation, which in turn may lead to an alteration in renal handling of Pi and Ca. However, inorganic Pi concentration in renal cortical homogenates was not measurably different between the two groups: 14.0 ± 0.9 vs 13.5 ± 0.7 μmol/g of wet tissue, $p > 0.05$.

A further interesting observation is that urinary excretion of Ca as well as Pi alters in response to a variation in dietary Pi intake within 24 hours. In the low Pi diet group, urinary Pi excretion decreased 91 ± 2% in the 1st day, and 98 ± 1% in the 2nd day; and urinary Ca excretion increased 226 ± 95% in the 1st day, and 249 ± 88% in the 2nd day. This prompt change in renal response suggests that the alteration in renal handling of Ca and Pi is an adaptation to a variation in dietary Pi intake, independent of chronic Pi depletion. The primary signal to the kidney for this adaptation remains unknown.

After these basal observations, 10 U of PTH were injected as a single venous injection, and four 10 min urine samples were collected. In the control diet group, PTH promptly increased urinary Pi excretion, but in the low Pi diet group, PTH failed to increase Pi excretion. These findings are consistent with those of other investigators (9).

Table II Renal response to PTH 10 U.

		Control Diet	Low Pi Diet
Number of rats studied		9	9
Pi excretion:	basal	95±31	0.9±0.1
	PTH 10 U	274±42	1.1±0.1
Ca excretion:	basal	31.6±4.2	148.8±14.2
	PTH 10 U	3.7±0.8	68.5±10.1

Values are means±SE, nmol/min-100 g b.w.

In contrast, urinary Ca excretion was promptly decreased in response to PTH in both groups. Since the basal values of urinary Ca excretion were markedly different between the two groups, the response to PTH cannot be compared quantitatively. However, these findings show that renal response to PTH for Ca and for Pi are different, suggesting the possibility that the mechanisms involved in renal adaptation to a variation in dietary Pi intake for Ca and Pi may also be different.

In conclusion, restriction of dietary Pi intake for only 3 days decreases urinary Pi excretion, and increases Ca excretion, which are independent of PTH or calcitonin secretion, plasma concentration of Pi or Ca, or filtered load of these ions, suggesting that Pi deprivation alters tubular reabsorption of these ions through as yet unrecognized mechanisms. In the Pi deprived rats, the phosphaturic response to PTH is abolished, but not the Ca-reabsorptive response to the hormone, suggesting that the mechanisms involved in renal adaptation for Ca and for Pi may be different.

Acknowledgments

The work is supported by the grants from National Institute of Heart, Lung and Blood (NHL 19057) and Veterans Administration Research Fund.

References

1. Crawford, J.D., Osborne, M.M., Jr., Talbot, N.B., Terry, M.L., and Morrill, M.F.: The parathyroid glands and phosphorus homeostasis. J. Clin. Invest. 29: 1448, 1950.

2. Steele, T.H., and DeLuca, H.F.: Influence of dietary phosphorus on renal phosphate reabsorption in the parathyroidectomized rats. J. Clin. Invest. 57: 867, 1976.

3. Trohler, U., Bonjour, J-P, and Fleisch, H.: Inorganic phosphate homeostasis: renal adaptation to the dietary intake in intact and thyroparathyroidectomized rats. J. Clin. Invest. 57: 264, 1976.

4. Coburn, J.W., and Massry, S.G.: Changes in sodium and urinary calcium during phosphate depletion: studies on mechanisms. J. Clin. Invest. 49: 1073, 1970.

5. Dominguez, J.H., Gray, R.W., and Lemann, J., Jr.: Dietary phosphate deprivation in women and men: Effects on mineral and acid balances, parathyroid hormone and the metabolism of 25 (OH)-vitamin D. J. Clin. Endocrin. Metab. 43: 1056, 1976.

6. Goldfarb, S., Westby, G.R., Goldberg, M., and Agus, Z.S.: Renal tubular effects of chronic phosphate depletion. J. Clin. Invest. 59: 770, 1977.

7. Beck, N., Kim, H.P., and Kim, K.S.: Effect of metabolic acidosis on renal action of parathyroid hormone. Amer. J. Physiol. 228: 1483, 1975.

8. Beck, N., and Webster, S.K.: Effects of acute metabolic acidosis on parathyroid hormone action and calcium mobilization. Amer. J. Physiol. 230: 127, 1976.

9. Steele, T.H.: Renal resistance to parathyroid hormone during phosphorus deprivation. J. Clin. Invest. 58: 1461, 1976.

RENAL TUBULAR PHOSPHATE REABSORPTION IN THE PHOSPHATE DEPLETED DOG

R.A.L. SUTTON, G.A. QUAMME, T. O'CALLAGHAN,
N.L.M. WONG, J.H. DIRKS
University of British Columbia, Vancouver and
McGill University, Montreal, Canada

Phosphate depletion has been shown to produce a variety of alterations in renal tubular function. Filtered phosphate is avidly reabsorbed, and the phosphaturic responses to volume expansion, parathyroid hormone and bicarbonate infusion are diminished or abolished (1,2). Renal tubular reabsorption of calcium (3) is impaired, leading to impressive hypercalciuria, and evidence has been presented which suggests that phosphate depletion is associated with impairment of tubular glucose (4) and bicarbonate (5) reabsorption, and alteration of proximal fluid reabsorption (6).

In the present micropuncture studies, we have examined the renal tubular handling of inorganic phosphate (Pi) in chronically Pi depleted dogs, and its response to parathyroid hormone (PTH) and to Pi infusion. Data obtained from Pi infused, phosphate replete thyroparathyroidectomised (TPTX) dogs are also presented, for comparison with the data from Pi depleted dogs.

METHODS

A. 14 dogs were chronically Pi depleted by means of a low Pi diet and oral aluminium hydroxide (amphogel) for periods of 6-8 weeks. These dogs were subjected to standard 3 phase re-collection micropuncture experiments consisting of

1. Control Phase - Late proximal and distal tubule and clearance collections obtained.
2. PTH Phase. Purified bovine PTH, 60U/hour infused. After 1 hour for equilibration, recollections obtained.
3. PTH and Pi Phase. PTH infusion continued, and neutral sodium phosphate infused 100 μmol prime and then 40 μmol/min. After 1 hour for equilibration, further

recollections obtained.

B. 10 normal, phosphate replete dogs were TPTX 1-3 days prior to experiments and then maintained on Lilly parathormone 50U I.M. twice daily until 24 hours before experiment. 3-phase recollection micropuncture experiments were performed, consisting of

1. Control Phase. Tubule and clearance collections.
2. Low Pi Infusion. Neutral phosphate 40 μmol/min was infused, and after 1 hour for equilibration, recollections obtained.
3. High Pi Infusion. The infusion rate was increased to 80 μmol/min., and after a further hour for equilibration, recollections were again obtained.

The micropuncture and analytical methods were as previously described from this laboratory (7); tubule fluid samples were analysed for phosphorus as well as other elements (Na, Ca, Mg, K, and Cl) using the Camebax electron microprobe.

RESULTS

A. Phosphate Depleted Dogs.

The plasma and clearance data (from the left, micropunctured kidney) are shown in Table 1, and the micropuncture data in Table 2.

TABLE 1

PHOSPHATE DEPLETION
CLEARANCE DATA (LEFT KIDNEY)

	Control	PTH	PTH + Pi
P_{Pi} mg/100 ml.	1.29 ±0.23	1.78 ±0.29**	5.71 ±0.68**
V ml/min.	0.32 ±0.05	0.38 ±0.10	0.37 ±0.05
C_{In} ml/min.	22.9 ±2.0	20.7 ±2.0	21.3 ±2.3
P_{Na} mEq/L	147 ±1.3	148 ±1.0	150 ±0.7
UF_{Ca} mEq/L	2.87 ±0.10	2.96 ±0.07	2.74 ±0.11
FE_{Na} %	1.0 ±0.2	1.1 ±0.3	1.5 ±0.3
FE_{Ca} %	4.0 ±0.8	2.2 ±0.7**	1.6 ±0.5*
FE_{Pi} %	1.4 ±0.3	1.2 ±0.3	17.7 ±5.6*

*p <0.05 **p <0.001 compared with preceding phase

TABLE 2

PHOSPHATE DEPLETION

MICROPUNCTURE DATA: PROXIMAL TUBULE

	Control	PTH	PTH + Pi
TF/P_{In}	1.52 ±0.02	1.43 ±0.04	1.50 ±0.07
TF_{Pi} (mg/100 ml)	0.37 ±0.02	0.77 ±0.09*	5.05 ±0.42*
TF/UF_{Pi}	0.28 ±0.04	0.35 ±0.03	0.88 ±0.05*
$TF/UF_{Pi/In}$x100%	19 ±3	26 ±3	59 ±4*

*p <0.01 compared with preceding phase

MICROPUNCTURE DATA: DISTAL TUBULE

	Control	PTH	PTH + Pi
TF/P_{In}	5.6 ±0.3	4.7 ±0.3	4.6 ±0.3
TF_{Pi} (mg/100 ml)	0.31 ±0.02	0.46 ±0.05	6.43 ±1.07*
TF/UF_{Pi}	0.50 ±0.08	0.42 ±0.07	0.90 ±0.09*
$TF/UF_{Pi/In}$x100%	8.8 ±1.4	8.8 ±2.2	19.2 ±2.3*

*p <0.01 compared with preceding phase

Following PTH infusion in these Pi-depleted dogs, plasma Pi increased significantly (1.29 to 1.78). There was no change in inulin clearance, UF_{Ca}, FE_{Na} or FE_{Pi}, but FE_{Ca} fell significantly (4.0 to 2.2%). At the late proximal tubule, although mean tubule fluid Pi concentration increased significantly (0.37 to 0.77 mg/100 ml) fractional Pi rejection was unchanged (19 to 26%). At the distal tubule, TF_{Pi}, TF/UF_{Pi} and fractional rejection of Pi were all unchanged.

Figure 1 shows that the mean tubule fluid Pi concentration at both proximal and distal tubules was in the range of 0.2 - 0.5 ml/100 ml in each animal and was unrelated to the plasma Pi concentration, which varied from 0.3 to 3 mg/100 ml.

Table 3 shows the calculated segmental Pi reabsorption in the 3 phases. Filtered load was calculated from P_{Pi} and whole kidney GFR (C_{In}) and proximal reabsorption from the mean $TF/UF_{Pi/In}$ data (fractional rejection). 'Loop' reabsorption was calculated from the mean proximal and distal rejected fractions, and represents reabsorption between late proximal and distal puncture sites, including the later part of the proximal tubule with the pars

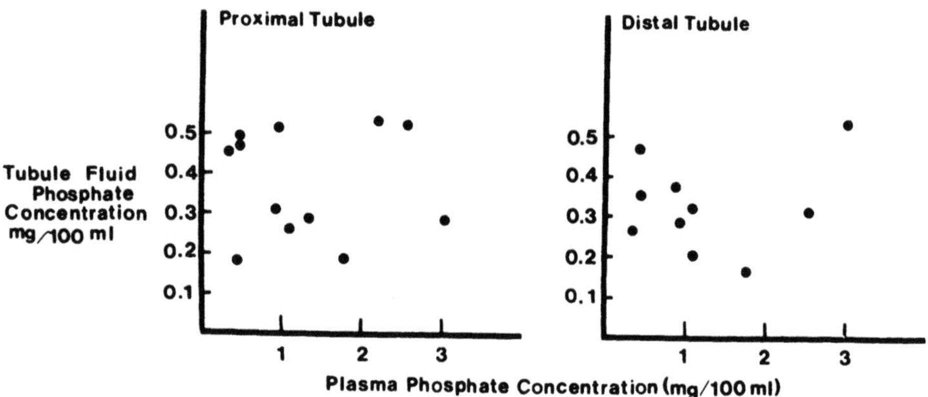

Figure 1. Relationship between tubule fluid and plasma phosphate concentrations in phosphate-depleted dogs.

recta together with the loop of Henle and part of the distal tubule. Terminal reabsorption is the difference between distal delivery and urinary excretion, and ignores the possibility of important heterogeneity between the punctured superficial and other nephrons. Fractional reabsorption of the load delivered to each segment is also shown in Table 3 (figures in parenthesis).

B. Phosphate Infusion Data (TPTX Dogs).

Table 4 shows the plasma and clearance data, and Table 5 the micropuncture data from these experiments.

Table 6 shows the calculated absolute segmental Pi reabsorption in each phase, as well as the fractional reabsorption of the load delivered to each segment in each phase. Fractional Pi excretion in the urine increased from 2.8 to 23.7 to 62.1% as P_{Pi} increased from 4.15 to 4.86 to 6.62 mg/100 ml. Proximal TF/UF_{Pi} increased from 0.63 to 0.98 to 1.29 and distal TF/UF_{Pi} increased from 0.27 to 1.09 to 2.40. Calculated absolute proximal Pi reabsorption decreased from 491 to 317 to 173 μg/min., representing 56, 34 and 15% of filtered load respectively. Absolute 'loop' reabsorption changed little, but the proportion of the delivered load absorbed by the loop decreased from 86 to 62 to 36%. Calculated terminal absorption decreased from 25 to 8 μg/min with the low Pi load, and in the third phase urinary Pi exceeded distal delivery by 92 μg/min., suggesting phosphate secretion in this segment.

TABLE 3
PHOSPHATE DEPLETION

CALCULATED ABSOLUTE SEGMENTAL Pi REABSORPTION (μg/min) AND FRACTIONAL REABSORPTION OF SEGMENTAL LOAD (% in parentheses)

	Control	PTH	PTH + Pi
Filtered load	295	368	1216
'Proximal' absorption	238 (81)	272 (74)	498 (41)
'Loop' absorption	30 (52	63 (66)	486 (68)
'Terminal absorption'	22 (81)	28 (84)	18 (8)
Excreted	3.8	4.4	215

TABLE 4
PHOSPHATE LOADING
CLEARANCE DATA (LEFT KIDNEY)

	Control	Low Pi	High Pi
P_{Pi} mg/100 ml	4.15 ±0.4	4.86 ±0.5**	6.62 ±0.5**
UF_{Ca} mEq/L	2.07 ±0.2	2.01 ±0.2*	1.96 ±0.2
FE_{Na} %	1.50 ±0.4	2.04 ±0.8	2.84 ±0.8
FE_{Ca} %	2.3 ±0.6	2.4 ±0.9	2.6 ±0.8
FE_{Pi} %	2.8 ±1.1	23.7 ±5.9**	62.1 ±6.6**

* p <0.05 ** p <0.01
compared with preceding phase.

TABLE 5

PHOSPHATE LOADING
MICROPUNCTURE DATA

Proximal			
TF/P_{In}	1.45 ±0.04	1.32 ±0.04	1.33 ±0.05
TF/UF_{Pi}	0.63 ±0.05	0.98 ±0.09**	1.29 ±0.11**
$TF/UF_{Pi/In} x100\%$	44.3 ±3.5	65.6 ±6.4**	85.3 ±8.2**
Distal			
TF/P_{In}	4.97 ±0.33	5.06 ±0.52	4.51 ±0.26
TF/UF_{Pi}	0.27 ±0.04	1.09 ±0.20	2.40 ±0.21**
$TF/UF_{Pi/In} x100\%$	5.8 ±1.1	24.6 ±5.4	54.2 ±4.7**

**p <0.01 compared with previous phase

TABLE 6

TPTX DOGS - PHOSPHATE LOADING

CALCULATED ABSOLUTE SEGMENTAL Pi REABSORPTION (μg/min) AND FRACTIONAL REABSORPTION OF SEGMENTAL LOAD (% in parentheses)

	Control	Low Pi	High Pi
Filtered load	876	933	1152
'Proximal' absorption	491 (56)	317 (34)	173 (15)
'Loop absorption	333 (86)	383 (62)	357 (36)
'Terminal' absorption	25 (48)	8 (3.5)	-92 (secreted)
Excreted	27	225	714

DISCUSSION

Proximal fluid reabsorption in Pi depletion, as reflected by the mean TF/P inulin ratio for selected 'late' superficial proximal tubule samples (1.52 ±0.02) was not different from that which we have observed under other circumstances. We are not able therefore, to confirm the recent report (6) that proximal fluid reabsorption is decreased in the phosphate depleted dog. In control Pi depletion, Pi concentration was extremely low both at the proximal and distal tubule in all dogs, and was not apparently related to plasma Pi concentration. Mean proximal Pi reabsorption was 81% of filtered load. Only 9% of filtered load reached the distal puncture site, and only 1.3% was excreted in the urine. Although these data suggest the presence of Pi absorption in post-proximal segments, the reabsorption between proximal and distal puncture sites may have been in the pars recta and the differences between distal delivery and urinary excretion may in part reflect heterogeneity of nephrons with more avid reabsorption in the deeper nephrons. PTH infusion did not significantly increase fractional Pi delivery to the proximal or distal tubule or fractional urinary excretion, despite a significant rise in mean P_{Pi}, indicating an almost total refractoriness to the phosphaturic effect of PTH. Calcium excretion did however, decrease significantly, as previously reported by some authors (3), but not by others (6). Infusion of phosphate, together with PTH, resulted in a significant rise in proximal, distal and urinary fractional phosphate delivery. Proximal fractional Pi reabsorption decreased to 41%, though calculated absolute reabsorption increased from 238 and 272 μg/min. in the first and second phases to 498 μg/min.. Calculated loop reabsorption was proportionately similar to the previous phases but absolute reabsorption increased very markedly. In the terminal segment, although delivery increased about 10-fold, Pi reabsorption decreased slightly, suggesting a marked inhibition of reabsorption in this segment following Pi infusion.

In the Pi infused TPTX dogs, Table 5 shows that the calculated absolute and fractional proximal reabsorption were sharply decreased in response to Pi loading. It is of interest that the 'loop' segment, which may mainly reflect the later proximal tubule including pars recta, also showed a decrease in fractional reabsorption of filtered load, but calculated absolute reabsorption remained virtually unchanged. In the terminal segment the calculated modest absorption of Pi prior to Pi loading changed to substantial apparent secretion of Pi after the higher Pi load. These data confirm the existence of 'self-suppression' of proximal Pi reabsorption, independent of PTH, with Pi loading in the dog and suggest that the phenomenon may occur primarily in the earlier part of the proximal tubule, prior to the puncture site. The loop segment does not increase its reabsorption in response to increased load but an absolute decrease in absorption was not observed in this segment. It is of interest to compare the high Pi load (third phase) in these experiments with the Pi loading and PTH phase in the experiments in the Pi depleted dogs. Calculated filtered Pi loads were similar (1152 and 1216 μg/min.). Despite PTH infusion calculated absolute proximal reabsorption was much greater in the Pi depleted than in the Pi replete TPTX dogs, fractional reabsorption of delivered load to the loop was also higner in the Pi depleted dogs, and apparent Pi secretion in the terminal segment was seen only in the Pi replete dogs.

These data confirm previous observations that antecedent diet markedly influences overall renal phosphate reabsorption (8, 9) and indicates that in the depleted dog, even in the presence of PTH all segments of the nephron absorb Pi very much more avidly than those of the TPTX Pi replete dog.

REFERENCES

1. Wen, S.F. Phosphate transport in the phosphate-depleted dog. Abstracts 8th Annual Meeting of American Society of Nephrology, p. 9, 1975.

2. Steele, T.H. Renal response to phosphorus deprivation: Effect of the parathyroid and bicarbonate. Kidney International 11: 327, 1977.

3. Coburn, J.W. and Massry, S.G. Changes in serum and urinary calcium during phosphate depletion, studies on mechanisms. J. Clin. Invest. 49: 1073, 1970.

4. Gold, L.W., Massry, S.G. and Friedler, R.M. Effect of phosphate depletion on renal tubular reabsorption of glucose. J. Lab. Med. 89: 554, 1977.

5. Gold, L.W., Massry, S.G., Arieff, A.I. and Coburn, J.W. Renal bicarbonate wasting during phosphate depletion: a possible cause of altered acid-base homeostatis in hyperparathyroidism. J. Clin. Invest. 52: 2556, 1973.

6. Goldfarb, S., Westby, G.R., Goldberg, M., and Agus, Z.S. Renal tubular effects of chronic phosphate depletion. J. Clin. Invest. 59: 770, 1977.

7. Edwards, B.R., Baer, P.G., Sutton, R.A.L. and Dirks, J.H. Micropuncture study of diuretic effects on sodium and calcium reabsorption in the dog nephron. J. Clin. Invest. 52: 2418, 1973.

8. Steele, T.H. and DeLuca, H.F. Influence of dietary phosphorus on renal phosphate reabsorption in the parathyroidectomized rat. J. Clin. Invest. 57: 867, 1976.

9. Trohler, U., Bonjour, J.P. and Fleisch, H.F. Inorganic phosphate homeostasis, renal adaption to the dietary intake in intact and thyroparathyroidectomized rats. J. Clin. Invest. 57: 264, 1976.

LOW PHOSPHORUS INTAKE AND VITAMIN D METABOLISM AND EXPRESSION IN RATS

S. Edelstein[1] and D. Noff
Municipal Government Medical Center
Ichilov Hospital
Tel Aviv - Jaffo (Israel)
J. Puschett
Allegheny General Hospital
Pittsburgh, Pennsylvania 15212 (U.S.A.) and
E. E. Golub[2] and F. Bronner
The University of Connecticut Health Center
Farmington, Connecticut 06032 (U.S.A.)

Male weanling rats, depleted of vitamin D for 4 wks., were repleted for 4 wks. with 1,2 - [^{3}H]-4-[^{14}C]-vitamin D_3 and then placed on three regimens: normal mineral intake (0.4% Ca, 0.3% P); low-Ca (0.004% Ca, 0.3% P) and low-P (0.4% Ca, 0.13% P). Three weeks later 1,25-dihydroxyvitamin D_3 (1,25-$(OH)_2$-D_3) levels were determined in plasma and intestine on the basis of the $^{3}H/^{14}C$ radioactivity ratios. Calcium-binding protein (CaBP) was estimated in parallel experiments with 4 groups of rats that had been on semi-synthetic regimens containing 1.5% Ca, 1.5% P; 1.5% Ca, 0.2% P; 0.06% Ca, 0.2% P; and 1.5% Ca, 0.03% P for 7 - 10 days. In comparison with the controls, the low Ca diets led to a doubling in 1,25-$(OH)_2$-D_3 levels in intestinal mucosa, and to detectable levels of 1,25-$(OH)_2$-D_3 in plasma. CaBP was markedly elevated. On the other hand, in the low P groups, in spite of hypophosphatemia, 1,25-$(OH)_2$-D_3 was undetectable in plasma and virtually undetectable in intestine. Moreover, CaBP levels were unchanged on 0.2% P intakes and markedly depressed on 0.03% P. Hypophosphatemia became more pronounced as P intake decreased, while plasma Ca increased. It therefore appears that in rats, as contrasted with chickens, hypophosphatemis is not a major factor regulating metabolism and expression of 1,25-$(OH)_2$-D_3.

[1] Present address: Biochemistry Department, The Weizmann Institute of Science, Rehovot (Israel).
[2] Present address: Department of Biochemistry, The University of Pennsylvania School of Dental Medicine, Philadelphia, Pennsylvania 19174 (U.S.A.).

INTRODUCTION

The active vitamin D metabolite, 1,25-dihydroxyvitamin D_3 (1,25-$(OH)_2$-D_3), is produced in kidney mitochondria from the circulating form of vitamin D, 25-hydroxyvitamin D_3 (1, 2). C-1 hydroxylation is thought to be rate-limiting and subject to biological regulation (1, 2). In states of low-calcium intake, there occurs an increase in the amount of 1,25-$(OH)_2$-D_3 formed and a corresponding decrease in the amount of 24,25-dihydroxyvitamin D_3 (3). This increase in circulating 1,25-$(OH)_2$-D_3 is thought to be responsible for the increase in duodenal calcium-binding protein (CaBP), the best known molecular expression of vitamin D action (4-8). In the chick low phosphate intake has also been found associated with increased 1,25-$(OH)_2$-D_3 levels in the blood and target tissues and with increased production of CaBP (9). In the rat, however, the effects of low phosphate intake and hypophosphatemia on vitamin metabolism are less clearcut. Thus while DeLuca and collaborators (10,11) have reported that hypophosphatemia in rats is associated with increased calcium absorption and Haussler and colleagues (12) have reported increased plasma levels of 1,25-$(OH)_2$-D_3 in rats on low-phosphate diets, Hurwitz _et al_. (13) found that their hypophosphatemic, vitamin D-replete rats absorbed less calcium than normophosphatemic controls. Moreover, Freund and Bronner (5) found no increase in CaBP in hypophosphatemic, vitamin D-replete rats, as compared to normophosphatemic controls, whereas Thomasset _et al_. (14) reported an increase in duodenal CaBP in phosphate deficiency.

Accordingly, the effect of hypophosphatemia on the concentration of 1,25-$(OH)_2$-D_3 in plasma and in target tissues was studied and CaBP was measured in the duodenum under these conditions. As will be shown, hypophosphatemia in rats, resulting from low phosphate intake, was not associated with an increase in 1,25-$(OH)_2$-D_3 in intestine or plasma, nor with increased CaBP. On the other hand, low calcium intake led to the expected increase in target tissue concentration of 1,25-$(OH)_2$-D_3 and in its expression in intestinal mucosa.

EXPERIMENTAL

Male Wistars rats that had been maintained on a vitamin D-deficient diet (0.4% Ca, 0.3% P, Teklad Mills, Madison, WI., TD No. 72081) for 4 weeks from weaning were repleted with radiolabeled vitamin D_3 (0.75 μg 1,2-^{3}H, 4-^{14}C-vitamin D_3 administered by subcutaneous injection every 5-7 days) for 4 weeks and then divided into three diet groups: (a) 0.4% Ca, 0.3% P; (b) low-Ca diet 0.004% Ca, 0.3% P (Teklad Mills, TD No. 96292 with added P); (c) low-P 0.4% Ca, 0.13% P (Teklad Mills, TD No. 96292 with added Ca). The animals continued to receive radioactive vitamin D by injection for 20 days when they were killed. Intestinal mucosa and plasma were analyzed for vitamin D_3 metabolites.

CaBP measurements were carried out on mucosal scrapings obtained from 120 g Sprague-Dawley rats that had been placed on four regimens for 7-14 days: High Ca, high P (1.5% Ca, 1.5% P, Teklad Mills, TD No. 67207); high-Ca, low-P (1.5% Ca, 0.2% P, Teklad Mills, TD No. 70389); high-Ca, very low P (1.5% Ca, 0.03% P, Teklad Mills, TD No. 75087) and low-Ca, low-P (0.06% Ca, 0.2% P, Teklad Mills, TD No. 67205A).

Vitamin D_3 metabolite analysis was on chloroform-methanol (15) extracts which, in the case of the mucosa, were analyzed by thin-layer chromatography (16) and, in the case of plasma, by column chromatography (Sephadex LH-20, equilibrated and developed in chloroform/petroleum ether, 17). The latter procedure permits separation of the dihydroxylated metabolites of vitamin D_3. The amount of 1,25-$(OH)_2$-D_3 was calculated from the $^3H/^{14}C$ specific radioactivity ratios (18), with care taken to differentiate between 1,25-$(OH)_2$-D_3 and other polar derivatives that cochromatograph with 1,25-$(OH)_2$-D_3.

Mucosal tissue for CaBP analysis was processed and the supernate chromatographed as previously described (5, 7), except that the Sephadex G-50 columns had been equilibrated with ^{45}Ca and ^{40}Ca (0.03 μCi/ml, 0.005 mM). The area of the second elution peak ($v_e/v_o \simeq 1.5$) corresponds to the amount of calcium bound by the vitamin D-dependent CaBP (5).

Plasma Ca was analyzed by atomic absorptiometry (13) and plasma P by the method of Ames (19).

RESULTS

Table 1 shows that low-calcium or low-phosphorus intakes led to a decrease in circulating 24,25-dihydroxyvitamin D_3 (24,25-$(OH)_2$-D_3) and an increase in a more polar peak which co-elutes with 1,25-$(OH)_2$-D_3. Tritium loss, indicating the presence of 1,25-$(OH)_2$-D_3, was observed only in the plasma of rats fed the low-calcium diet.

As shown in Fig. 1, lipid extracts prepared from the intestinal mucosa of animals fed the low-calcium diet showed increased content of 1,25-$(OH)_2$-D_3, whereas similar extracts from the intestinal mucosa of animals fed the low-phosphorus diet contained virtually no 1,25-$(OH)_2$-D_3. Thus a low-phosphorus regimen led to a virtual suppression of the intestinal accumulation of 1,25-$(OH)_2$-D_3.

Table I

Plasma levels of dihydroxylated metabolites of vitamin

Diet Group % Ca	% P	Plasma Ca mg/dl (SE)	Plasma P mg/dl (SE)	24,25-$(OH)_2$-D_3 pmol/ml	polar peak pmol/ml	1,25-$(OH)_2$-D_3 pmol/ml
0.4 (Normal Mineral)	0.3	10.0 (0.2)	6.8 (0.1)	15.3	0.4	undetectable
0.004 (Low-Ca)	0.3	8.1 (0.3)	5.5 (0.3)	5.9	0.8	0.2
0.4 (Low-P)	0.13	9.1 (0.4)	4.5 (0.3)	7.7	0.6	undetectable

The polar peak is eluted at v_e of 1,25-$(OH)_2$-D_3. 1,25-$(OH)_2$-D_3 content was calculated from tritium loss.

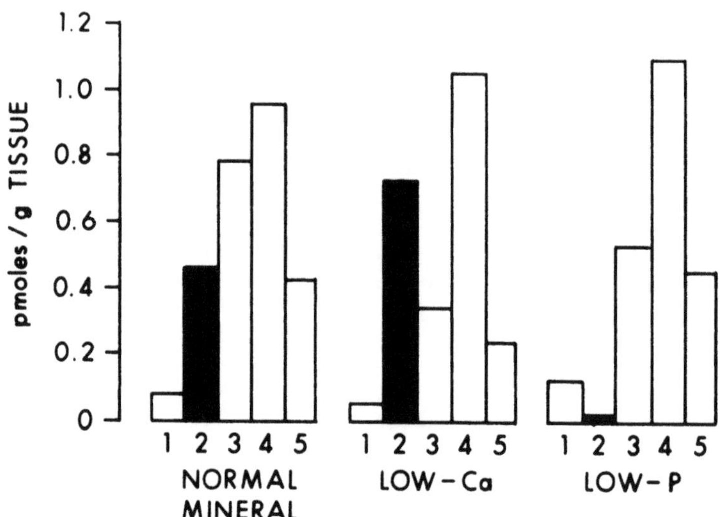

Figure 1 - The distribution of vitamin D_3 metabolites in the intestinal mucosa of rats fed normal-mineral, low-calcium and low-phosphorous diets. 1. Polar metabolites; 2. 1,25-$(OH_2D_3$; 3. 24,25-$(OH)_2D_3$; 4. 25-OH-D_3; 5. vitamin D_3.

Table 2 indicates that progressive lowering of the dietary phosphate was associated with a progressive drop in plasma P levels, and a smaller, but significant and progressive rise in plasma Ca. The CaBP content of the mucosa was unaffected when plasma P dropped to 6.4 mg/dl, but was reduced to 40% of the control value in animals on the very low P intake. On the other hand, when comparable animals were fed 0.2% P with only 0.06% Ca in the diet, the intestinal CaBP level was much higher than when their Ca intake was 1.5%. Indeed, the duodenal CaBP content of these animals was, as previously reported (5), the highest of the four groups studied. Thus, lowering of dietary P to 0.2% had no effect on CaBP, whereas lowering the Ca intake to 0.06% more than doubled the mucosal CaBP content.

Table II

Mucosal CaBP content

Diet Group % Ca	% P	Plasma Ca (SE) (mg/dl)	Plasma P (SE) (mg/dl)	Intestinal Calcium-binding protein (natoms Ca bound/g mucosa) (SE)
1.5 (High-Ca, High-P)	1.5	10.55 (0.17)	9.60 (0.27)	24.2 (3.2)
1.5 (High-Ca, Low-P)	0.2	11.71 (0.01)	6.37 (0.04)	24.9 (1.1)
0.06 (Low-Ca, Low-P)	0.2	10.02 (0.38)	not done	53.3
1.5 (High-Ca, Very Low-P)	0.03	12.69 (0.38)	4.59 (0.06)	10.1 (2.5)

DISCUSSION

Our experimental protocol enabled us to replace body stores of vitamin D with doubly-labeled vitamin D_3 and to measure the steady-state effects of dietary maneuvers on vitamin D metabolism and action. Restriction of calcium intake led, as in the chick (9), to increased accumulation of 1,25-$(OH)_2$-D_3 in intestinal tissue and to the expected increase in intestinal CaBP (5, 9, 20). But, unlike the chick, and contrary to the report of increased plasma levels of 1,25-$(OH)_2$-D_3 in the rat (12), our animals on low-P intakes exhibited no increase in 1,25-$(OH)_2$-D_3 in plasma and intestine. They also did not exhibit increased levels of CaBP, in contrast with the report of Thomasset et al. (14). Rather, low-P intakes were associated with decreased or undetectable levels of 1,25-$(OH)_2$-D_3 in plasma and intestine and with a depression of CaBP.

It is well-known that the phosphorus-deficient rat is hypercalcemic and hypercalciuric (13, 21). This situation has been interpreted as having resulted from the body's great need for phosphate and its willingness to compromise calcium homeostasis in order to obtain scarce phosphorus from the only source, the skeleton (22). Whatever the cause of the hypercalcemia and hypercalciuria, an increase in calcium absorption would seem antihomeostatic, i.e. it would compromise calcium homeostasis even further. Apparently this situation occurs in the chick, but does not occur commonly in the rat, since in our hands phosphate deficiency has not been associated with increased calcium absorption (13) nor with increased CaBP levels (Table 2).

The data reported by us indicate a correlation between intestinal 1,25-$(OH)_2$-D_3 levels and CaBP. However, Bar et al (20) have shown that in the chick the intestinal response to low-phosphorus treatment in terms of CaBP and calcium transport is only partially correlated with 1,25-$(OH)_2$-D_3 metabolism. Moreover, Freund and Bronner (6) have suggested that cellular calcium levels regulate the expression of 1,25-$(OH)_2$-D_3 in the enterocyte, a suggestion confirmed in vitro (23).

What then emerges is that low calcium intakes are associated in both chicks and rats with an apparent increase in the production of 1,25-$(OH)_2$-D_3 and increased levels of this metabolite in the enterocyte. In turn this is associated with a marked increase in CaBP.

Hypophosphatemia, on the other hand, does not seem to lead to an increased production of 1,25-$(OH)_2$-D_3 in the rat nor to its augmented expression in the form of intestinal CaBP. On the contrary, very low-P intake and pronounced hypophosphatemia were associated with depressed 1,25-$(OH)_2$-D_3 levels and lowered CaBP in the intestine. Thus low plasma phosphate does not appear to play a direct role in the rat in the regulation of 25-hydroxyvitamin D-1-hydroxylase activity, nor in the expression of its product in the intestine.

ACKNOWLEDGMENTS

Supported in part by USPHS grant AM 14251 (F.B.), AM 17575 (J. P.) and RR05709 (J.P.) and The University of Connecticut Research Foundation (F.B.).

REFERENCES

1. DeLuca, H.F. and Schnoes, H.K. Metabolism and mechanism of action of vitamin D. Ann. Rev. Biochem. 45:631, 1976.

2. Norman, A.W. and Henry, H. 1,25-dihydroxycholecalciferol-a hormonally active form of vitamin D_3. Rec. Progr. Horm. Res. 30:431, 1974.

3. Boyle, I.T., Gray, R.W. and DeLuca, H.F. Regulation by calcium of in vivo synthesis of 1,25-dihydroxycholecalciferol and 21,25-dihydroxycholecalciferol. Proc. Natl. Acad. Sci., U.S.A. 68:2131, 1971.

4. Wasserman, R.H., Corradino, R.A., Fullmer, C.S. and Taylor, A. N. Some aspects of vitamin D action; calcium absorption and the vitamin D-dependent calcium binding protein. Vit. Horm. 32:299, 1974.

5. Freund, T. and Bronner, F. Regulation of intestinal calcium-binding protein by calcium intake in the rat. Am. J. Physiol. 228:861, 1975.

6. Freund, T. and Bronner, F. Stimulation in vitro by 1,25-dihydroxyvitamin D_3 of intestinal cell calcium uptake and calcium-binding protein. Science 190:1300, 1975.

7. Bronner, F. and Freund, T.S. Intestinal CaBP: a new quantitative index of vitamin D deficiency in the rat. Am. J. Physiol. 228:689, 1975.

8. Bar, A. and Wasserman, R.H. Duodenal calcium-binding protein in the chick: A new bioassay for vitamin D. J. Nutr. 104:1202, 1974.

9. Edelstein, S., Harell, A., Bar, A. and Hurwitz, S. The functional metabolism of vitamin D in chicks fed low-calcium and low-phosphorus diets. Biochim. Biophys. Acta 385:438, 1975.

10. Tanaka, Y., Frank, H. and DeLuca, H.F. Intestinal calcium transport: Stimulation by low phosphorus diets. Science 181: 564, 1973.

11. Ribovich, M.L. and DeLuca, H.F. The influence of dietary calcium and phosphorus on intestinal calcium transport of rats given vitamin D metabolites. Arch. Biochem. Biophys. 170: 529, 1975.

12. Hughes, M.R., Haussler, M.R., Wergedal, J. and Baylink, D. Regulation of serum 1α,25-dihydroxyvitamin D_3 by calcium and phosphate in the rat. Science 190:578, 1975.

13. Hurwitz, S., Stacey, R.E. and Bronner, F. Role of vitamin D in plasma calcium regulation. Am. J. Physiol. 216:254, 1969.

14. Thomasset, M., Cuisinier-Gleizes, P. and Mathieu, H. Duodenal calcium-binding protein (CaBP) and phosphorus deprivation in growing rats. Biomedicine 25:345, 1976.

15. Bligh, E.G. and Dyer, W.J. A rapid method of total lipid extraction and purification. Can. J. Biochem. Physiol. 37:911, 1959.

16. Lawson, D.E.M., Bell, P.A., Pelc, B., Wilson, P.W. and Kodicek, E. Synthesis of [1,2-$^3H_2$]cholecalciferol and metabolism of [4-^{14}C, 1,2-$^3H_2$]-and [4-^{14}C, 1-^3H]-cholecalciferol in rachitic rats and chicks. Biochem. J. 121:673, 1971.

17. Weisman, Y., Sapir, R., Harell, A. and Edelstein, S. Maternal-perinatal interrelationships of vitamin D metabolism in rats. Biochim. Biophys. Acta 428:388, 1976.

18. Weber, J.C., Pons, V. and Kodicek, E. The localization of 1,25-dihydroxycholecalciferol in bone cell nuclei of rachitic chicks. Biochem. J. 125:147, 1971.

19. Ames, B.N. Assay of inorganic phosphate, total phosphate and phosphatases. Adv. Enzymol. 8:114, 1966.

20. Bar, A., Hurwitz, S. and Edelstein, S. Response of renal calcium-binding protein. Independence of kidney vitamin D hydroxylation. Biochim. Biophys. Acta 411:106, 1975.

21. Cuisinier-Gleizes, P., Thomasset, M., Sainteny-Debove, F. and Mathieu, H. Phosphorus deficiency. Parathyroid hormone and bone resorption in the growing rat. Calcif. Tiss. Res. 20: 235, 1976.

22. Bronner, F. Vitamin D deficiency and rickets. Am. J. Clin. Nutr. 29:1307, 1976.

23. Golub, E.E., Reid, M., Bossak, C., Wolpert, L. and Bronner, F. The effect of calcium on calcium binding protein induction _in vitro_. Fed. Proc. 36:456, 1977 (abstract).

Topics on Bone

PATHOGENESIS OF RENAL OSTEODYSTROPHY: ROLES OF PHOSPHATE AND SKELETAL RESISTANCE TO PTH

E. Ritz, H.H. Malluche,* B. Krempien, W. Tschope and S.G. Massry*
Dept. Int. Med. and Pathology, Univ. of Heidelberg, Heidelberg/Germany and LAC/USC Medical Center, Div. Nephrology, Los Angeles/Calif.*

The different pathogenetic mechanisms responsible for uremic bone disease are still not fully understood. However, as some of the factors involved in the development of renal osteodystrophy have been clarified, it became apparent that abnormalities in phosphate homeostasis play an important role in the control of PTH secretion and in modifying the skeletal response to PTH.

Phosphate retention which may occur with loss of renal function has been implicated in the genesis of secondary hyperparathyroidism of incipient renal failure. It is accepted that this effect is mediated by lowering the concentration of ionized serum Ca in blood. However, there is no consensus as to the mechanism through which P retention induces hypocalcemia.

Interesting observations on the role of P in provoking secondary hyperparathyroidism have accrued from veterinarian pathology. In the 19th century, a German veterinarian (1) described a peculiar disease in piglets, ingesting high P-low Ca diets. The disease was called "sneezing disease". It is characterized by laboured respiration and sneezing resulting from deformities in the turbinate nasal bones. These deformities are caused by generalized osteitis fibrosa, which leads to the collapse of the snout skeleton. Similar observations have also been made in other species (e.g. horse, cat, monkey), when high P diets were given in the presence of low Ca intake. However, analgous findings have not been reported in human beings.

The seminal paper in the study of the role of P in the genesis of renal secondary hyperparathyroidism has been the communication of Slatopolsky et al (2). These authors showed that development of secondary hyperparathyroidism in renal failure was dependent upon the magnitude of dietary P intake. As functional renal mass was reduced, PTH levels in the blood rose when the dietary intake of P was maintained constant, but blood PTH did not increase when dietary intake of P was reduced.

In patients with terminal renal failure, it has been demonstrated that hyperphosphatemia is an important stimulus for PTH secretion. As a case in point, Fournier et al (3), found a positive correlation between the levels of PTH and serum P in hemodialyzed patients.

Thus, the available data would indicate that hyperphosphatemia can cause secondary hyperparathyroidism in the absence or presence of impaired renal function. However, convincing evidence is lacking that such hyperphosphatemia does occur in incipient renal failure.

In order to describe the changes in incipient renal failure, Bricker and Slatopolsky advanced the hypothesis which implies that a transient and possibly undetectable increase in serum P occurs early in renal failure with each decrement in renal function. Such transient hyperphosphatemia would directly decrease the blood level of ionized Ca in the extracellular fluid which then stimulates the parathyroid glands to release more hormone. PTH would decrease tubular reabsorption of P and would return both serum P and ionized serum Ca into the normal range, but at the expense of elevated serum PTH levels. Such a sequence would provide a mechanism to maintain the constancy of P levels in the extracellular fluid.

There is some controversy to what extent changes in tubular reabsorption of P are necessary to maintain the constancy of serum P in renal failure. Bijvoet (4) recommended the use of TmP/GFR for the evaluation of renal handling of P. Since TmP/GFR is invariant to changes in GFR and changes of load, it is a more useful mathematical expression of tubular handling of P than is TRP which varies in response to changes of both GFR and load.

If we assume for the moment that the rate of tubular reabsorption be at its maximum, then the filtered load of phosphate (L) is the sum of the rate of tubular reabsorption (TP) and the rate of urinary excretion (UV_P). Serum P (P) can, therefore, be given as the sum of two terms, a threshold term ($\frac{TmP}{GFR}$) and a load term ($\frac{UV_P}{GFR}$).

$$L = P \times GFR - TP + UV_P$$

$$P = \frac{TmP}{GFR} + \frac{UV_P}{GFR}$$

Based on data of Morgan (5), Figure 1 describes the changes of serum P when GFR decreases but when the tubular threshold (TmP/GFR) remains

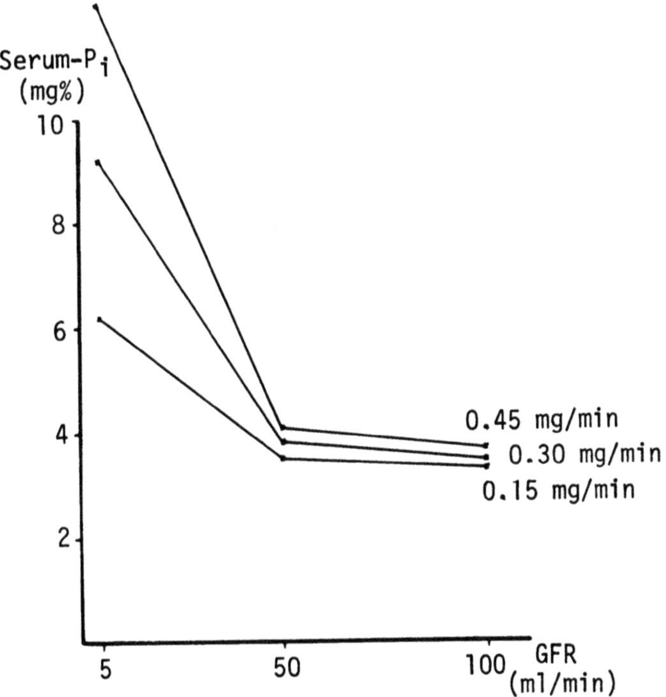

Figure 1. Relation between P_i load and serum $[P_i]$ at constant tubular threshold (T_{M_P}/GFR 3,2 mg/100 ml).

unchanged, e.g. in the absence of a secretory PTH response. A decrease in GFR initially causes little change in serum P (or in TRP for that matter) but a further decrease in GFR causes a large increase in serum P and a decrease in TRP.

In early renal failure, serum P is relatively insensitive to the P load, whereas in advanced renal failure it is exquisitely sensitive to changes in phosphate load. For arithmetical reasons, changes of serum P in incipient renal failure must, therefore, be minute even in the absence of changes of the renal threshold.

On the other hand, as shown in Figure 2, at a constant rate of urinary P excretion, variations in the threshold (TmP/GFR) have a large effect on serum P when GFR is high but a small effect when GFR is low. These mathematical relationships have the following implications for serum P homeostasis: in incipient renal failure, serum P increases only marginally and only minute adjustments of the threshold, if any, are necessary while in advanced renal failure an increase in serum P is due to the further decrease in GFR and cannot be prevented by a decrease in the threshold, even to zero.

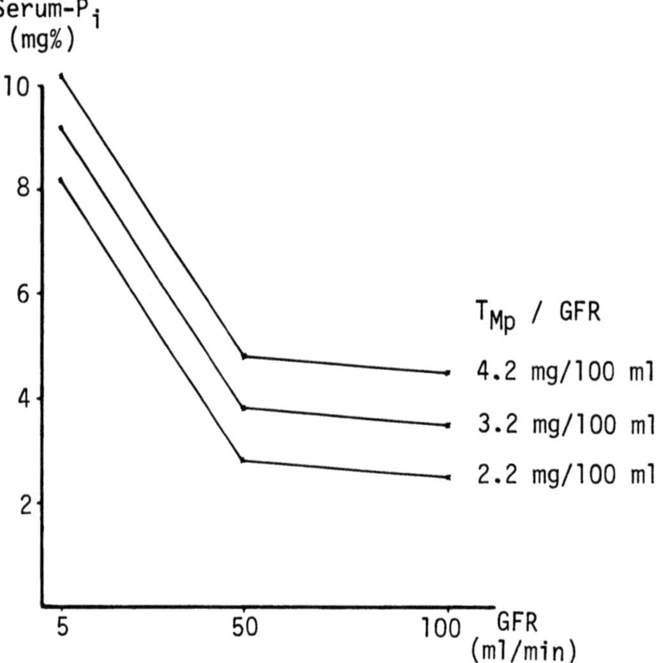

Figure 2. Relation between tubular threshold and serum [P_i] at constant P_i load (0,3 mg/min).

In view of the above arithmetical relationship, it is not surprising that Swenson et al (6), found the fraction of filtered phosphate excreted increased and the concentration of P in blood remained virtually normal, despite progressive renal failure in TXPTX dogs in whom blood levels of serum Ca were maintained normal with vitamin D supplementation. Phosphate homeostasis in the absence of PTH effects in the kidney was also shown by Loreau et al (7), who immunized rats against tubular basement membranes thus, abolishing the stimulatory effect of PTH on renal adenylate cyclase. The animals developed interstitial nephritis and renal failure as well, but fractional excretion of P still increased markedly.

An important mechanism of renal adaptation to dietary intake of P was demonstrated by Trohler et al (8), who showed that at any given level of serum P, P depleted rats reabsorb more P than P loaded rats. The diet induced modulation of the renal tubular capacity to transport P was independent of PTH, calcitonin, serum calcium (at least at the time of the clearance measurement), of the state of extracellular fluid expansion, of urinary pH and occurred even in vitamin D depleted animals.

If the sequence of events described by the phosphate retention theory does occur, the following constellations of serum chemistry would be predicted:

a) elevated serum P and diminished serum Ca (absence of full compensation)
b) normal serum P and normal Ca (full compensation)
c) diminished serum P and elevated serum Ca (exaggeration of the adaptive response of the parathyroids)

Friis, Hahnemann and Week (9), found low serum P levels in the presence of low serum Ca levels in patients with incipient renal failure. Such a combination cannot be explained by the above theory.

Hypophosphatemia in these patients results from a fall in TmP/GFR, as reported by Morgan (5) and, as confirmed by our own calculations. It might well be argued, that fasting serum P is lower in these patients as a result of parathyroid oversecretion, outlasting the postprandial hyperphosphatemic stimulus. However, we were unable to demonstrate more pronounced circadian swings of serum P in patients with incipient renal failure; circadian variations of serum P, if anything, were even diminished. The coefficient of variation of 6 sequential measurements throughout the day was 12.4±4.37% in 18 normal controls and 9.5±4.66% in 7 patients with incipient renal failure (p 0.10, 0.05). In addition, Massry, Ritz and Verberckmoes (10) and our group (Figure 3), failed to find an exaggerated rise in serum P after an oral P load.

Secondary hyperparathyroidism occurs early in renal failure, as indicated by serum PTH measurements of Reiss (11) and by histological studies of Malluche et al (12) (Figure 4). Such hyperparathyroidism is due to hypocalcemia. Other mechanisms, in addition to phosphate retention, have been advanced to explain the hypocalcemia.

A state of PTH resistance in patients with renal failure is suggested by the simple clinical observation that decreased ionized serum Ca concentrations occur in the presence of elevated PTH concentrations. This points to an error in the blood bone equilibrium which is not corrected by PTH. The magnitude of this error is unrelated to the level of bone turnover, as documented by the radiokinetic studies of Letteri (13), in which no correlation was found between serum Ca levels and bone accretion rate. Skeletal resistance to the acute Ca mobilizing action of parathyroid hormone has been demonstrated by Massry in a series of clinical and experimental studies (14-16). The factors that have been implicated in the genesis of PTH resistance are summarized in Table 1. Skeletal resistance to PTH also exists in pseudohypoparathyroidism. The analogy is of more than passing interest and may point to some underlying common pathogenetic mechanism. Pseudohypoparathyroidism patients, as well as those with renal failure, exhibit hypocalcemia, hyperphosphatemia, elevation of serum PTH, decreased urinary excretion of calcium, reduced intestinal absorption of Ca and osteitis fibrosa (Table 2).

PTH acts in the skeleton on two different systems: 1) the osteocytic Ca transfer system, which is presumably involved in the homeostasis of serum Ca and, more specifically, in the correction of an acute hypocalcemic stimulus, and 2) osteoclastic resorption which is primarily involved in skeletal remodeling. It is of note that the calcemic effect of PTH, which presumably involves osteocytic Ca transfer from a hypothetical bone fluid compartment to the extracellular fluid space, is defective in both states. In pseudohypoparathyroidism, the resistance to the calcemic effect of PTH can be abolished by the administration of vitamin D or 1,25-

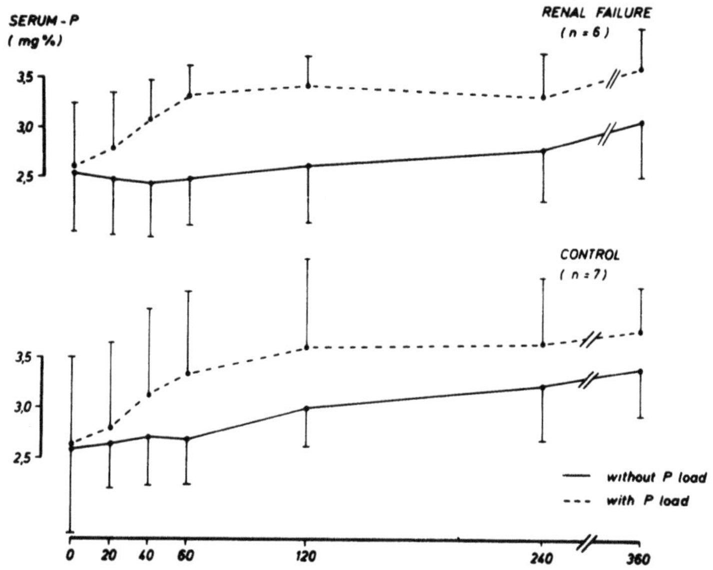

Figure 3
6 patients with incipient renal failure (C_{Cr} 65±1.25 ml/min) and 6 healthy controls (C_{Cr} 148±12.8) were studied between 9 a.m. and 3 p.m., on the first day without, and on the second day with an oral P load administered at 9 a.m. (1 g P/70 kg given as Na-K-phosphate buffered at pH 7.4 and dissolved in 100 ml water). Serum PTH was elevated in the patients with renal failure. At the time of the investigation the rate of urinary P excretion was not different in the two groups (controls without P load 232±37.8 mg/6h; with P load 340±120; renal failure - without P load 210±28.3; with P load 337±71.3). The rise in serum P was no more pronounced in the patients with incipient renal failure.

Table 1
Possible mechanisms of PTH resistance

- $1,25\ (OH)_2$VITAMIN D DEFICIENCY
- DEFECT OF PERIPHERAL PTH RECEPTORS
- SATURATION OF RECEPTORS BY INERT PTH FRAGMENTS
- DEFECT IN ADENYLATE-CYCLASE OR POST ADENYLATE-CYCLASE STEPS
- RETENTION OF TOXIN
- CALCITONIN EXCESS
- SURFEIT OF OSTEOID
- HYPOMAGNESEMIA

Table 2
As pointed out by Frame and Parfitt (17) there exists an interesting analogy with respect to Ca Metabolism between renal failure on the one hand, and the variety of pseudohypoparathyroidism with osteitis fibrosa (PHPOF) on the other hand.

PSEUDOHYPOPARATHYROIDISM WITH OSTEITIS FIBROSA		RENAL OSTEODYSTROPHY
+	HYPOCALCEMIA	+
+	HYPERPHOSPHATEMIA	+
+	SERUM PTH ELEVATED	+
+	UV_{Ca} DECREASED	+
+	A_{Ca} DECREASED	+
+	OSTEITIS FIBROSA	
	PTH RESISTANCE	
+	-OSTEOCYTIC Ca TRANSFER	+
-	-OSTEOCLASTIC RESORPTION	?
+	-RENAL P EXCRETION	-

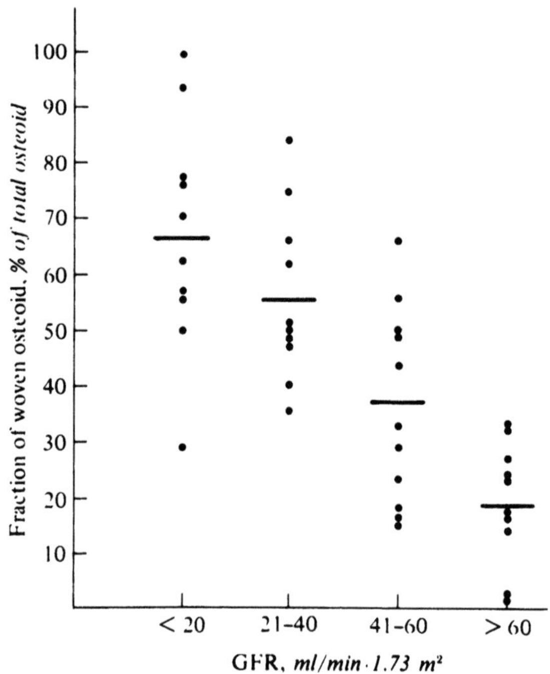

Figure 4
Prevalence of woven osteoid at various levels of GFR (Ref. 12; with the permission of Springer-Verlag). Woven osteoid (characterized by disordered collagen texture and warp-and-woof pattern under polarized light) is evidence of hyperparathyroidism and was seen even at a GFR 60 ml/min x 1.73 m^2.

dihydroxy-vitamin D (18). In pseudohypoparathyroidism the stimulatory effect of PTH on osteoclasts and on the remodeling system is not impaired as documented by the common presence of osteitis fibrosa. As one point of distinction, in pseudohypoparathyroidism the phosphaturic effect of PTH is blunted (at least in the absence of 1,25-dihydroxycholecalciferol) whereas, the effect of PTH in increasing fractional urinary phosphate and cAMP excretion is still present in uremia.

Resistance to the action of PTH in activating osteoprogenitor cells and in inducing the appearance of osteoclasts is suggested by the studies of Bordier (19) who found less osteoclasts at any given level of serum PTH in bone of patients with secondary renal hyperparathyroidism as opposed to patients with primary hyperparathyroidism. The interpretation of these findings hinge critically on the

PTH radioimmunoassay which is notoriously prone to interference from inactive PTH fragments in patients with renal failure. Within the error of the method, no such defect of PTH in inducing the appearance of osteoclasts was noted in out preliminary experimental studies in the proximal tibial metaphysis of uremic rats (unpublished studies). As pointed out by Baylink (20) this may indicate that the presumed absence of 1,25-dihydroxycholecalciferol does not impair the osteoclastic response to PTH in the presence of circulating 25-OH-vitamin D_3.

Since a diminished calcemic response implies malfunction of the osteocytic Ca transfer system, it is of interest that histologically osteocytes in Haversian bone of uremic individuals show evidence of activation, as reported by Krempien, Geiger and Ritz (21). The response of osteocytes of PTX uremic dogs to the infusion of PTH was studied directly by electron microscopy. In agreement with previous experiments (15), serum calcium rose conspicuously in sham operated dogs, but only slightly in bilaterally nephrectomized dogs.

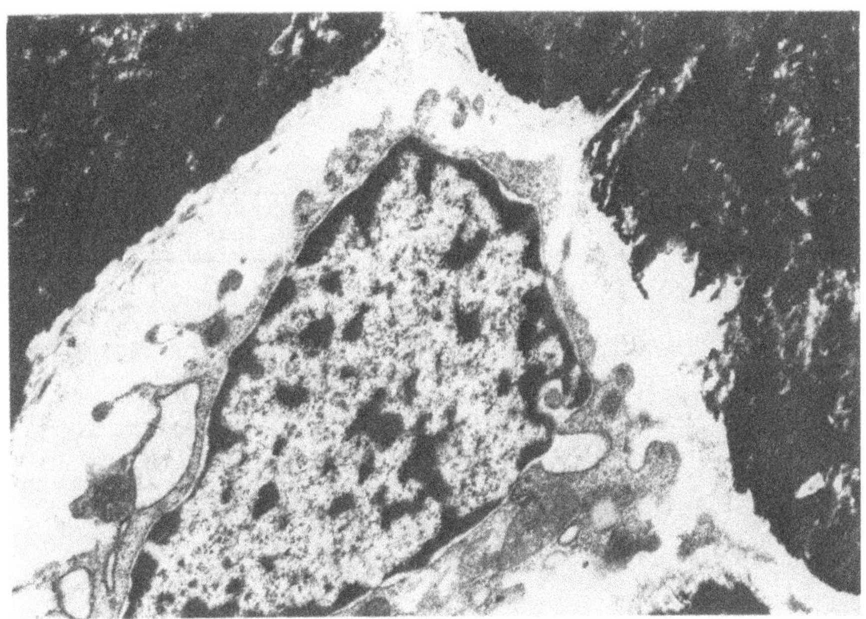

Figure 5
Osteocyte of PTX control dog infused with PTH. Enlargement x 18600. PTX beagle puppies were bilaterally nephrectomized (or sham operated). 20 h after nephrectomy, 200 IU PTE (Parathormone Lilly) were infused for 20 h. Note extensive ruffling of the cellular membrane with vesicle formation.

As shown in Figures 5-7, activation of osteocytes, assessed by the criteria described elsewhere in this book (Krempien, B., Friedrich, G., Ritz, E.: Effect of PTH on Osteocyte Ultrastructure) was seen both in PTX-control dogs and in PTX-uremic dogs. The changes may be somewhat less pronounced in uremic dogs, but this certainly cannot account for the profound impairment of the calcemic response to PTH.

Massry et al (15), have shown that the acute calcemic response to PTH in uremic dogs is partially restored by the administration of 1,25-dihydroxycholecalciferol. In analogy to pseudohypoparathyroidism, PTH resistance in renal failure seems to be due, at least partially, to low circulating levels of 1,25-dihydroxycholecalciferol.

In an unpublished study, Massry evaluated the effect of restriction of dietary phosphate in proportion to the reduction of the glomerular filtration rate in patients with incipient renal failure (10). He found that this procedure resulted in enhanced intestinal absorption of Ca, improvement in the calcemic response to PTH and a fall in the blood levels of parathyroid hormone. These findings

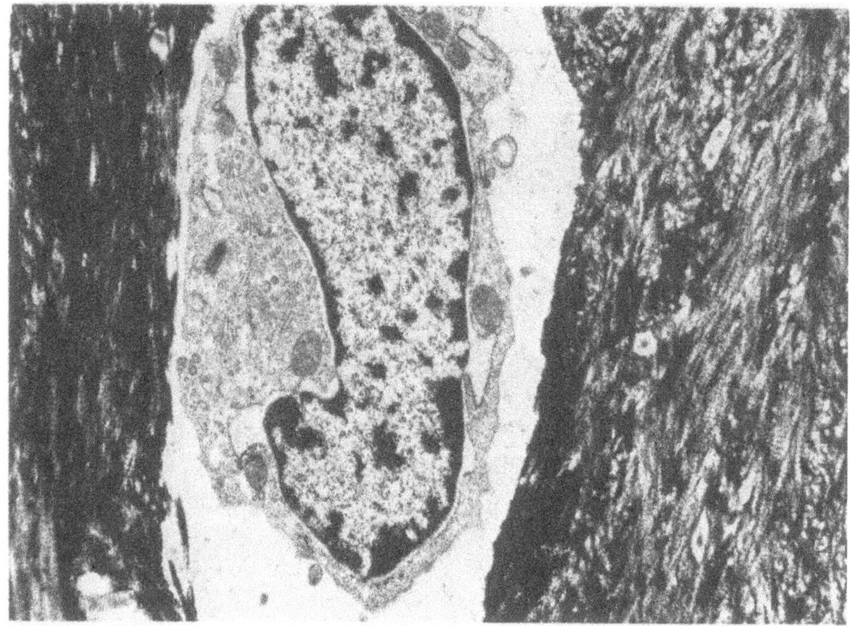

Figure 6
Osteocyte of PTX nephrectomized dog infused with PTH. Enlargement x 12400. Note wide cytoplasm, large Golgi apparatus and vesicles close to the plasma membrane.

would imply a role of P in the development of PTH resistance in early renal failure, but the observations are consistent with the notion that phosphate restriction was associated with enhanced production of $1,25(OH)_2D_3$.

Information on circulating 1,25-dihydroxycholecalciferol levels in early renal failure is currently of preliminary nature. Normal serum levels, as reported by some investigators, may still be inappropriate for the prevailing level of PTH. Perhaps intestinal absorption of Ca can be used as an in vivo bioassay for circulating 1,25-dihydroxycholecalciferol activity. In a previous study (22), fractional absorption for Ca was found to be dminished in some patients with incipient renal failure even at a GFR of 60-80 ml/min x 1.73 m^2, i.e. much earlier than reported before. Such a finding would be consistent with a reduction of circulating 1,25-dihydroxycholecalciferol.

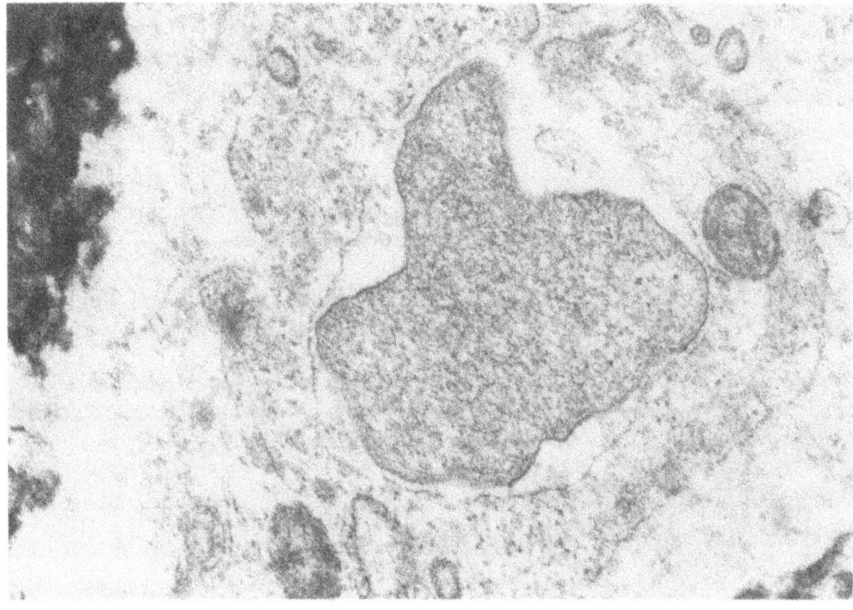

Figure 7

Same as Figure 6. Detail of osteocyte with formation of vesicles which fuse with the plasma membrane.

It appears that the factors underlying the hypocalcemia, secondary hyperparathyroidism and PTH resistance in incipient renal failure are multiple. Phosphate retention apparently plays an important role in this process, although its action is probably not that of a direct effect on the ionic concentrations in the extracellular fluid, but an indirect one. We would like to advance the working hypothesis, that this indirect effect is mediated through derangements in the production of 1,25-dihydroxycholecalciferol. The hypothesis would be in agreement with available data but direct confirmatory evidence is needed.

LITERATURE

1. Rehn, E.: Die schnuffelkrankheit des schweines und ihre Beziehung zue Osteitis fibrosa infantilis des Menschen. Beitr. Path. Anat. Allg. Path. 44:274, 1908.

2. Slatopolsky, E.; Cagler, S.; Pennel, J.P.; Tagart, D.B.; Canterbury, J.M.; Reiss, E., and Bricker, N.S.: On the pathogenesis of hyperparathyroidism in chronic experimental renal insufficiency in the dog. J. Clin. Invest. 50:492, 1971.

3. Fournier, A.E.; Arnaud, C.D.; Johnson, W.J.; Taylor, W.F., and Goldsmith, R.S.: Etiology of hyperparathyroidism and bone disease during chronic hemodialysis. II. Factors affecting serum immunoreactive parathyroid hormone. J. Clin. Invest. 50:599, 1971.

4. Bijvoet, O.L.M.: Relation of plasma phosphate concentration to renal tubular reabsorption of phosphate. Clin. Sci. 37:23, 1969.

5. Morgan, B.: Osteomalacia, Renal Osteodystrophy and Osteoporosis. Charles C. Thomas, Springfield, Illinois. 1973.

6. Swenson, R.S.; Weishinger, J.R.; Ruggi, J.L., and Reaven, G.M.: Evidence that parathyroid hormone is not required for phosphate homeostasis in renal failure. Metabolism 24:199, 1975.

7. Loreau, N.; Cosyns, J.P.; Lepreux, C., and Ardaillou, R.: Renal adenylate cyclase, calcitonin receptors and phosphate excretion in rats immunized against tubular basement membranes. In Phosphate Metabolism Proc. 2nd Int. Workshop on Phosphate (Plenum, New York), p. 71, 1977.

8. Trohler, U.; Bonjour, J.P.; Fleisch, H.: Inorganic phosphate homeostasis. Renal adaptation to the dietary intake in intact and thyroideoparathyroidectomized rats. J. Clin. Invest. 57:264, 1976.

9. Friis, Th.; Hahnemann, S.; Weeke, E.: Serum Ca and serum phosphorus in uremia during administration of sodium phytate and aluminum hydroxide. Acta Med. Scand. 183:497, 1968.

10. Massry, S.G.; Ritz, E.; Verberckmoes, R.: Role of phosphate in the genesis of secondary hyperparathyroidism of renal failure. Nephron 18:77, 1977.

11. Reiss, E.; Canterbury, J.M.; Kanter, A.: Circulating parathyroid hormone concentration in chronic renal insufficiency. Arch. Int. Med. 124:417, 1969.

12. Malluche, H.H.; Ritz, E.; Lange, H.P.; Kutschera, J.; Hodgson, M.; Seiffert, U., and Schoeppe, W.: Bone histology in incipient and advanced renal failure. Kidney Int. 9:355, 1975.

13. Letteri, J.M.; Cohn, S.H.: Total body neutron activation analysis in the study of mineral homeostasis in chronic renal disease. In Calcium Metabolism in Renal Failure and Nephrolithiasis, John Wiley, New York, 1977.

14. Massry, S.G.; Coburn, J.W.; Lee, D.B.N.; Jowsey, J., and Kleeman, C.R.: Skeletal resistance to parathyroid hormone in renal failure. Study in 105 human subjects. Ann. Intern. Med. 78:357, 1973.

15. Massry, S.G.; Stein, R.; Garty, J.; Arieff, A.I.; Norman, A.W.; Coburn, J.W., and Friedler, R.M.: Skeletal resistance to the calcemic action of PTH in uremia. Role of 1,25$(OH)_2D_3$. Kidney Int. 9:467, 1976.

16. Llach, F.; Massry, S.G.; Singer, F.R.; Kurokawa, J.; Kaye, J.H., and Coburn, J.W.: Skeletal resistance to endogenous parathyroid hormone in patients with early renal failure. A possible cause for secondary hyperparathyroidism. J. Clin. Endocrin. Metab. 41:339, 1975.

17. Frame, B.; Parfitt, A.M.: The syndrome of parathyroid hormone resistance. In Clinical Aspects of Metabolic Bone Disease, Frame, B., et al., eds., Excerpta Medica, Amsterdam, 1973, p. 454.

18. Drezner, M.K.; Neelon, F.A.; Haussler, M.; McPherson, H.T., and Lebovitz, H.E.: 1,25 Dihydroxycholecalciferol deficiency: The probable cause of hypocalcemia and metabolic bone disease in pseudohypoparathyroidism. J. Clin. Endocrin. Metab. 42:621, 1976.

19. Bordier, P.J.; Marie, P.J.; Arnaud, C.D.: Evolution of renal osteodystrophy. Kidney Int. Suppl. 2:102, 1975.

20. Ivey, J.L.; Morey, E.R.; Liu, C.C.; Rader, J.I.; Baylink, D.J.: Effects of vitamin D and its metabolites on bone. In Vitamin D, Biochemical, Chemical and Clinical Aspects Related to Vitamin D Metabolism, Norman, A.W., et al., eds., de Gruyter, p. 349, 1977.

21. Krempien, B.; Ritz, E., and Geiger, G.: Behavior of osteocytes in various ages and uremia morphological studies in human cortical bone. In. Proc. First Workshop on Bone Morphometry, Jaworsky, Z.E.G., and Klosevych, S., eds. Univ. of Ottawa Press, p. 288, 1976.

22. Werner, E.; Malluche, H.H., and Ritz, E.: Intestinale Ca-Absorption im Fruhstadium der Niereninsuffizienz und ihre Beeinflussung durch 5,6-trans-25-OH-CC Verh. Dtsch. Ges. Inn. Med. Vol 83 1977 (in press).

EFFECT OF PTH ON OSTEOCYTE ULTRASTRUCTURE

B. Krempien, E. Friedrich, and E. Ritz

Depts. of Pathol. and Int. Med.,
University of Heidelberg,
69 Heidelberg, Germany (FRG)

Parathyroid hormone (PTH) has been shown to cause an increase in the fraction of activated osteocytes, to induce periosteocytic osteolysis, to produce histochemical changes in osteocytes and to affect osteocyte ultrastructure (1,2,3). Analogous findings have been observed in osteocytes of patients suffering from primary or secondary hyperparathyroidism (4,5,6,7).

However, certain aspects of the action of PTH on osteocytes remain poorly defined. In the present investigation, the effects of PTH on osteocytes in cortical bone of rats (acute and chronic administration of supraphysiological doses of PTH) were studied. It was the purpose of the investigation to define the mechanisms underlying the conformational changes of the plasma membrane, to characterize the topography of periosteocytic osteolysis and to study the changes leading to cell death.

MATERIALS AND METHODS

Male 150g Wistar rats (Fa. Ivanovas, Kisslegg/Allgäu) were kept in single cages on Altromin C 1000 (0,95% Ca, 0,8% P, 500 IU vitamin D3/1000g) ad lib. Demineralized water was given as drinking fluid.

In the acute experiment, the animals were given synthetic 1,34-tetratriacontapeptide of bovine parathyroid hormone (Beckman Co.) intraperitoneally in a dose of 30 IU 24h and 8h prior to being sacrificed.Controls were given solvent injection.

In the chronic experiment, animals received 2x200 IU Parathormone Lilly/day for a total period of 21 days. Control animals received solvent injection.

Cortical bone of the proximal metaphysis of the tibia was removed immediately after death, fixed with glutaraldehyde-cacodylate buffer and fixed subsequently in osmium tetraoxyde. The specimens were then washed in cacodylate buffer and embedded. Undecalcified sections were stained with uranylactate and lead citrate and examined by transmission electron microscopy.

RESULTS AND DISCUSSION

In contrast to osteocytes of solvent injected control animals (fig. 1), osteocytes of PTH injected animals (fig. 2) were characterized by a broad cytoplasm and by the appearance of numerous thin cytoplasmic processes.

There was a striking increase in the rough endoplasmic reticulum (fig. 6) and in the Golgi apparatus (fig. 2) pointing to enhanced synthesis of protein. Within the cytoplasm, numerous lysosomal vesicles were visible, which fused with the plasma membrane and emptied their contents into the lacunar space (fig. 3). The finding underlines the importance of lysosomal enzymes in the digestion of perilacunar bone matrix.

Numerous microtubuli were seen close to the plasma membrane and in close contact with lysosomal vesicles, documenting the role of this cellular structure in the movement and the exocytosis of lysosomes. In addition to microtubuli, densely packed microfilaments were seen. These structures were often virtually "filling up" the cytoplasmic processes. In the cytoplasm, the microfilaments were frequently running parallel to the plasma membrane. The appearance of microfilaments, not reported heretofore, points to the role of the cytoskeleton in changing the conformation of the membrane and in forming cytoplasmic processes. Such an ultrastructural appearance would be compatible with undulating movements of the plasma membrane or with amoeboid motility of the osteocyte within the lacuna.

Within the enlarged lacunar space (fig. 4, fig. 7), numerous cellular processes, debris of collagen fibers and floccular material were clearly visible. Osteolysis

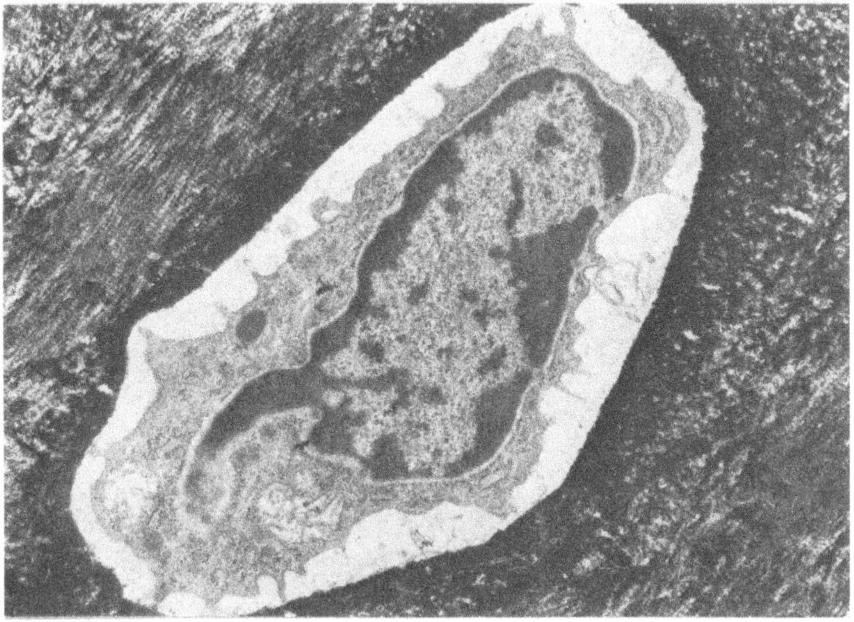

Figure 1
Osteocyte of control animal. Metaphyseal cortex of proximal tibia of solvent injected control rat. Transmission electron micrograph. Enlargement.

Note narrow cytoplasmic rim; no cytoplasmic processes; scanty ergastoplasmic reticulum and Golgi apparatus; narrow lacunar space; smooth lacunar border without signs of peristeocytic osteolysis.

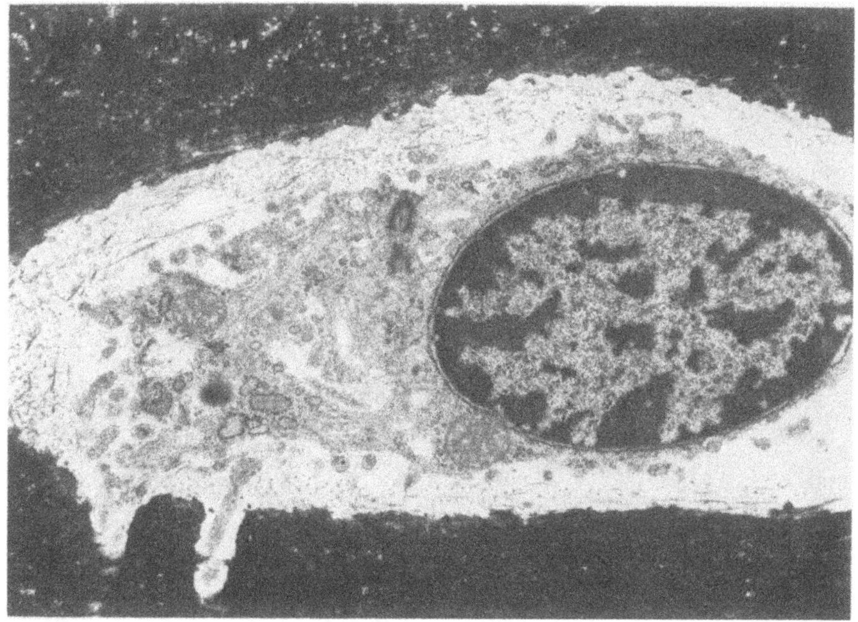

Figure 2
Osteocyte of PTH injected animal. (in this and all subsequent figures 2x200 IU PTE/day for 21 days). Transmission electron micrograph. Enlargement x 18600.

Note broad cytoplasma with numerous thin cytoplasmic processes which are concentrated at the cell pole opposite to the nucleus; cell nucleus in excentric position; prominent and enlarged Golgi apparatus; big mitochondria; large lacunar space containing flocculous and fibrous material.

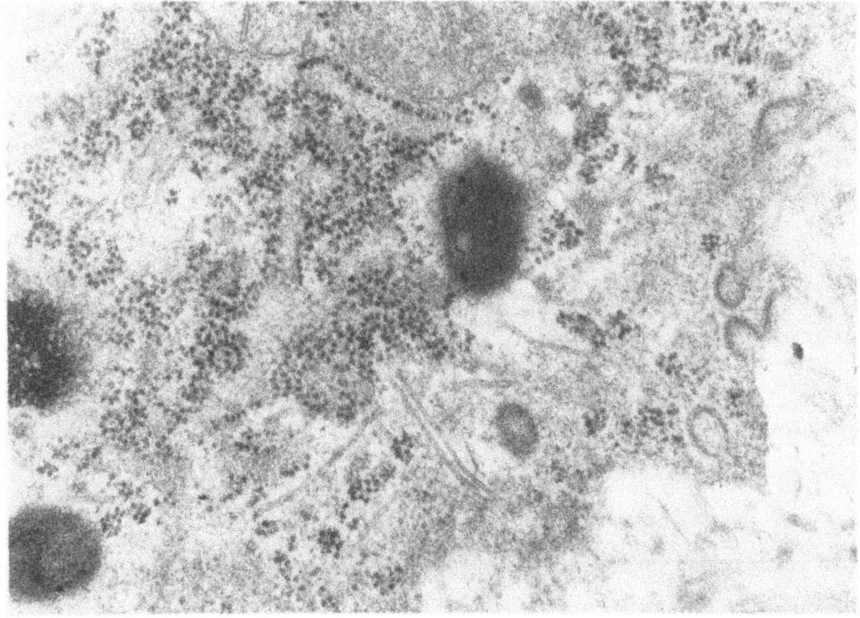

Figure 3
Osteocyte of PTH treated animal exhibiting exocytosis of lysomes. Enlargement x 54000.

Note plasma membrane fusing with lysosoma vesicles which empty their contents into the lacunar space; numerous microtubuli close to plasma membrane and to lysosomal vesicles.

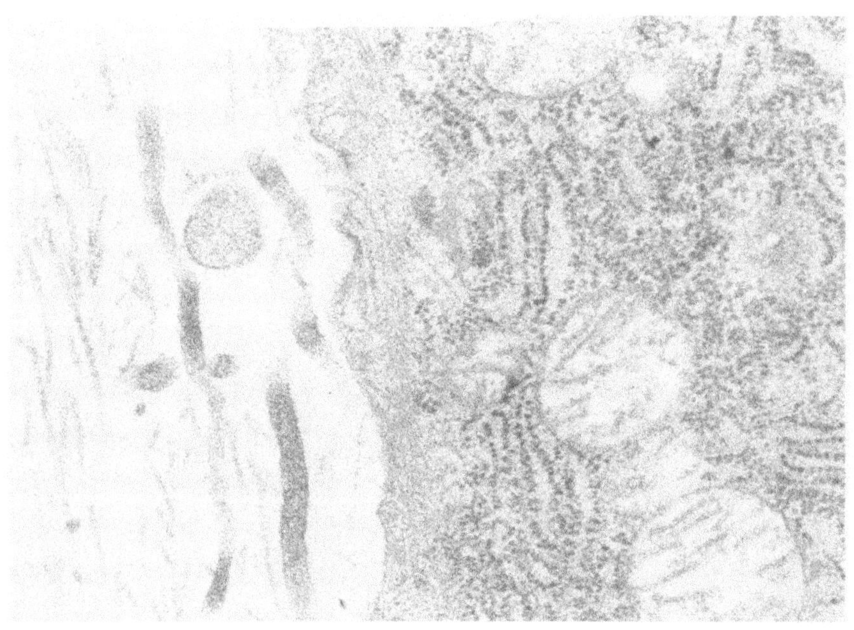

Figure 4
Osteocyte of PTH treated animal exhibiting microfilaments parallel to plasma membrane. Enlargement x 54000.

Note densely packed microfilaments located underneath of and running parallel to the plasma membrane; lacunar space filled with cellular processes and collagen fibers; within the cytoplasm abundant ergastoplasmic reticulum and two mitochondria.

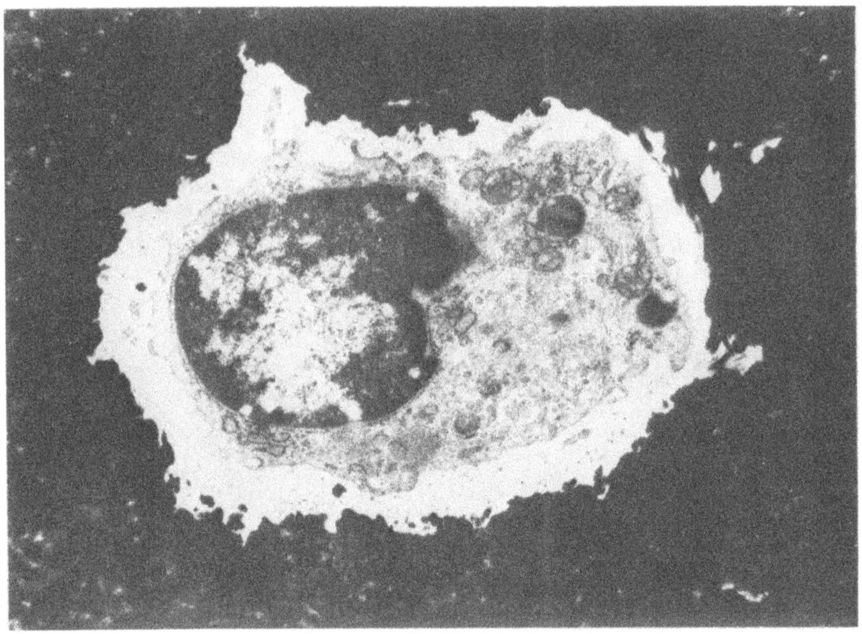

Figure 5
Osteocyte of PTH treated animal exhibiting lysosomes. Enlargement x 18600.

Note numerous lysosomes (so called "dense bodies") within the cytoplasm in proximity to the Golgi apparatus; nucleus located in excentric position; numerous cytoplasmic processes; osteolysis of the lacunar wall ("brush border" after Bonucci).

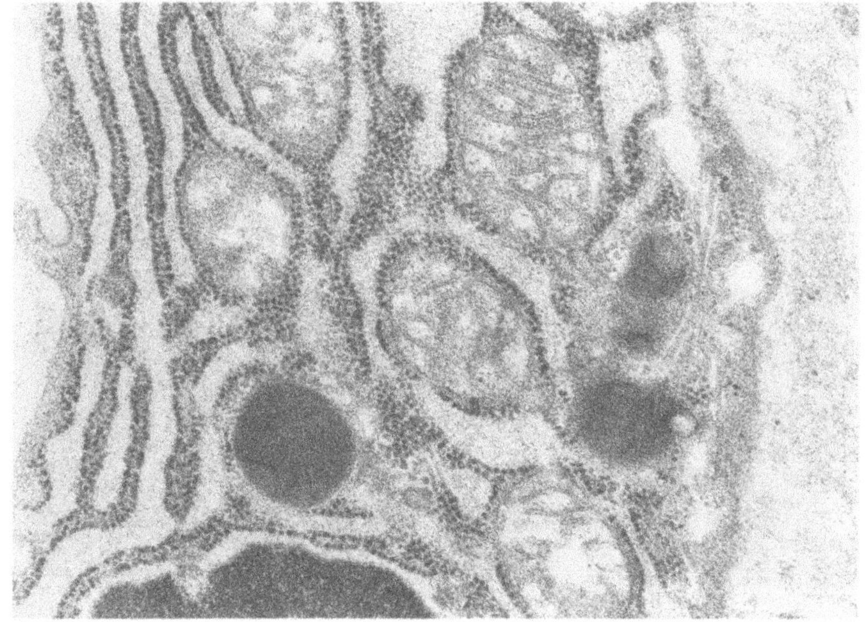

Figure 6
Osteocyte of PTH treated animal exhibiting ergastoplasmic reticulum. Enlargement x 54000.

Note rough endoplasmic reticulum (to the left) and large mitochondria. To the lower right several lysosomes (so called "dense bodies") in close contact with microtubuli.

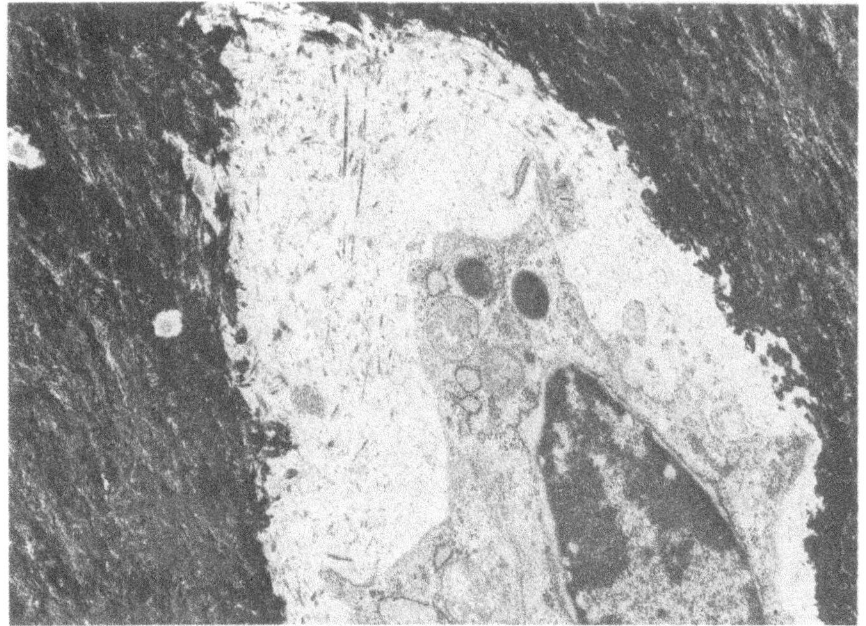

Figure 7
Osteocyte of PTH treated animal exhibiting osteolysis.
Enlargement x 18600.

Note numerous cytoplasmic processes with active exocytosis of lyosomes; enlargement of lacunar space with formation of a cisterna; cisterna filled with floccular material and debris of collagen fibers; lacunar wall irregularly eroded by osteolysis with needle shaped crystal material jutting into the lacunar space; on top denuded collagen fibers.

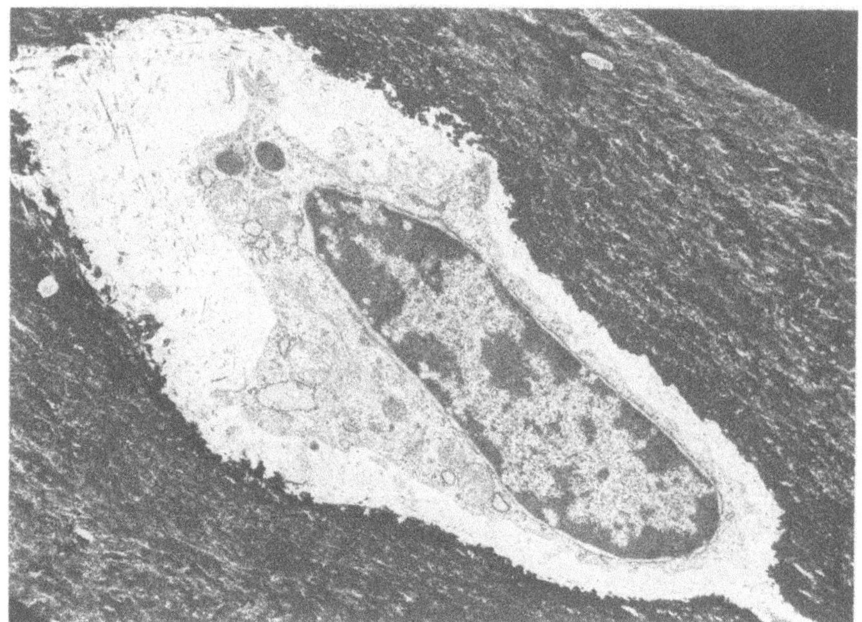

Figure 8
Osteocyte of PTH treated animal exhibiting asymmetry of osteocytic osteolysis. Enlargement x 10200.

Note relatively quiescent lacunar wall to the lower right and intense osteolysis to the upper left. For detail see Figure 7.

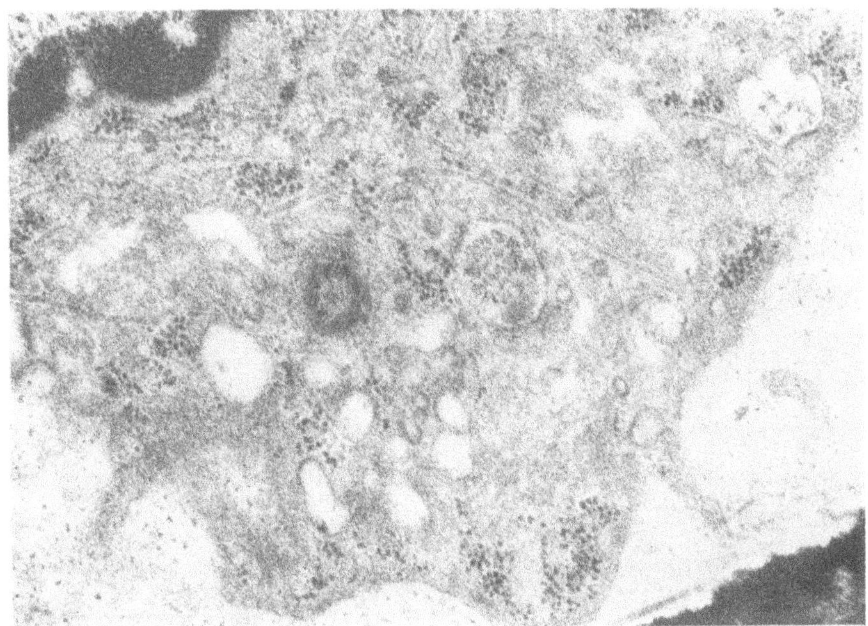

Figure 9
Osteocyte of PTH treated animal exhibiting microtubuli within the Golgi apparatus. Enlargement x 54000.

Note cisternae of the Golgi apparatus, interspersed between rough endoplasmic reticulum; numerous microtubuli (particularly on top).

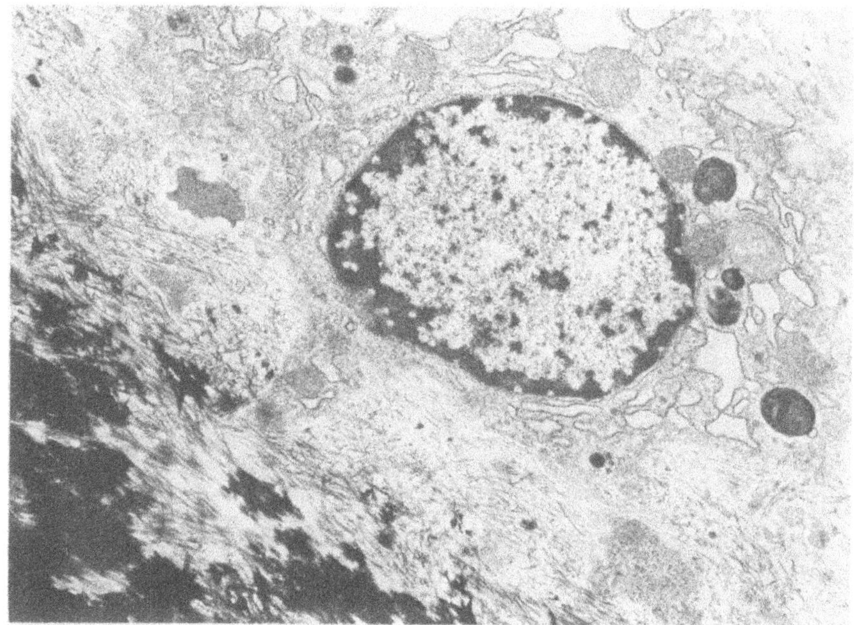

Figure 10
Osteocyte of PTH treated animal exhibiting autolysis. Enlargement x 18600.

Note extreme lysis of lacunar wall with mineral fragments and loose collagen fibers; lacunar space filled with debris; complete dissolution of plasma membrane; extremely wide cisternae in the cytoplasm which presumably represent remnants of the ergastoplasmic reticulum and Golgi apparatus; several lysosomes, occasionally in the form of autophagosomes (to the right).

of the lacunar wall with the formation of a "brush border" (after Bonucci;7) was noticeable. The lacunar wall was irregularly eroded, with needle shaped crystal material jutting into the lacunar space. Numereous denuded collagen fibers and debris of collagen fibers appeared in these sites (fig. 7). A striking finding, which has not been reported before, was the marked asymmetry of osteolysis around the lacunar perimeter (fig. 8). Somewhat analogous to osteoclasts, osteocytes appeared polarized with respect to lytic activity, which apparently was restricted to one cell pole. At the "lytic cell pole", cytoplasmic processes formed a huge cisterna, into which active exocytosis of lysosomes took place. This situation is reminiscent of osteoclasts, where a microenvironment is also formed underneath the ruffled border.

In some osteocytes, extreme lysis of the lacunar wall was accompanied by signs of osteocyte autolysis (fig. 10), as documented by the complete dissolution of the plasma membrane, the extreme widening of ergastoplasmic reticulum or Golgi apparatus and the appearance of autophagosomes. This finding is compatible with exhaustion of cells subsequent to excessive stimulation of cellular metabolism by PTH. An increase in the fraction of dead osteocytes has also been noted in patients with hyperparathyroidism (5) and may represent a dead end of the osteocyte life cycle (8).

SUMMARY

Osteocyte ultrastructure was studied in the cortical bone of the tibia of rats after acute or chronic administration of supraphysiological doses of PTH. Confirming previous reports, an increase in the width of the cytoplasm with the appearance of numerous thin cytoplasmic processes, an increase in rough ergastoplasmic reticulum and Golgi apparatus, an increase in lacunar width and lysis of the lacunar wall ("brush border" after Bonucci) were observed. Particularly striking was the appearance of numerous microfilaments and microtubules in the cytoplasm of activated osteocytes. The appearance of microfilaments, often densely packed in cytoplasmic processes or running parallel to the plasma membrane, points to a role of the cytoskeleton in mediating the effects of PTH on conformational changes of the plasma membrane (and possible on cell motility); microtubules were particularly prominent in the Golgi field and are presumably involved in the exocytosis of lysosomes. Another striking feature was the non-random distribution of periosteocytic osteolysis along the lacunar perimeter. Osteolysis was particularly pronounced at the cell pole opposite to the cell nucleus. After chronic administration of PTH, autolysis of osteocytes,associated with signs of excessive periosteocytic osteolysis,was frequently encountered.

REFERENCES

1. Porte, J., Meunier, P., Bernard, J., Roche, M.: L'ostéolyse periostéocytaire dans l'hyperparathyréo-idisme experimental induit par l'EDTA. Influence de la calcitonine Path.Biol. 20, 775-779, 1972
2. Jande, S.S.: Effects of Parathormone on Osteocytes and their Surrounding Matrix. Z. Zellforsch. 130, 463, 1972
3. Bélanger, L.F.: Osteolysis: an Outlook on its Mechanism and Causation. In: Gaillard, P.J., Talmage R.V., Budy, A.M., eds.: The Parathyroid Glands: Ultrastructure, Secretion and Function, p. 137, Chicago Univ. Press, 1965
4. Recklinghausen, F.: Untersuchungen über Rachitis und Osteomalacie, Jena: G. Fischer 1910
5. Krempien, B., E. Ritz, G. Geiger: Behaviour of Osteo-cytes in Various Ages in Chronic Uremia. Morpholo-gical Studies in Human Cortical Bone, in: Proc. Ist Workshop on Bone Morphometry, Z.F.G. Jaworsky, S. Klosevyck eds., Univ. of Ottawa Press, 1976
6. Bonucci, E.: Ultrastructural Aspects of Bone Mineralisation in Renal Osteodystrophy, in: Phospha-te Metabolism eds.: Shaul Massry, E. Ritz, Advances in Experimental Medicine and Biology, vol. 81, 477, Plenum Press, New York-London, 1977
7. Bonucci, E., G. Gherardi: Osteocyte Ultrastructure in Renal Osteodystrophy, Virchows Arch. A 373, 213-231, 1977
8. Rasmussen, H., P. Bordier: The Physiological and Cellular Basis of Metabolic Bone Disease, Williams and Wilkins Co., Baltimore, 1974

BONE LINING CELLS AND THE BONE FLUID COMPARTMENT, AN ULTRA-STRUCTURAL STUDY

J.L. Matthews, C. Vander Wiel, R.V. Talmage

Department of Pathology, Department of Orthopedic Surgery, Baylor University Medical Center, Dallas, TX
University of North Carolina, Chapel Hill, NC

Critical data has been developed in recent years that supports the hypothesis that ion concentrations in bone fluid and general extracellular fluid are modulated by a functional membrane that separates the fluid of bone from the general ECF. The evidence for the postulated functional membrane in bone is based on the experiments of Geisler and Neuman[1], and Ramp and Neuman[2], Scarpace and Neuman[3,4]. The prime points of the data are that potassium is concentrated in the bone fluid and that mineralization of the matrix is increased when bone cells are disrupted or poisoned inferring that the cells serve to partition these fluids, excluding excess calcium from the matrix surfaces. The actual "membrane" and mechanisms of its action are not clearly established. Talmage has suggested that the cells lining the bone surface (osteoblasts) serve this partitioning function[5]. The Talmage model proposes that calcium enters the bone fluid compartment by passive diffusion from the general ECF to the bone fluid compartment by passing between the lining cells. In the Talmage model, calcium eflux from the bone occurs by entering the osteocytes and osteoblasts whereupon it is actively transported through the cells and through the plasma membrane to reach the general ECF. Entry into the cell would not be difficult as a downhill gradient would exist, i.e., intracellular calcium levels are approximately 10-5. Extrusion from the cell would be an energy requiring activity as the concentration gradient would hinder eflux from the cell. Talmage has further postulated that PTH elevates plasma calcium levels by first increasing bone cell permeability to calcium allowing calcium to enter the cell more readily. It is then postulated that some "membrane pump" is activated that enhances the release of the cell calcium into the general ECF, but not into the bone ECF, a concept that would require the bone lining cells to be polarized such that the net result of the "pump" would be flow of calcium from the bone into the general ECF. Neuman and co-workers agree that calcium enters the bone fluid compartment by passive diffusion but they differ with the Talmage model in the explanation for the calcium eflux from the bone fluid compartment[3,4]. Their studies of aerobic glycolysis, ion fluxes, and bone membranes using an *in vitro* system indicate that significant changes in lactic acid secretion occur in bone cells as a consequence of PTH activity[6]. Presumably, CT would diminish the secretion of lactic acid. They suggest that the resultant changes in acid secretion are sufficient in magnitude to change the bone fluid pH to levels that would yield enough free calcium and phosphate in the bone fluid to produce a gradient that would let calcium escape from bone by passive diffusion through the same intercellular spaces through which it entered. Both models suffer some criticism as the Neuman model does not provide a basis for the significant differences in potassium concentration and also does not account for the non-stoichiometric release of calcium and phosphate from the bone. The Talmage model seemingly requires a large expenditure of cell energy to maintain a constant direct calcium pump. We have thus addressed ourselves to performing some experiments to determine: are there cell compartments for calcium and do their locations or concentrations change in response to PTH or CT? If the bone lining cells do serve to partition the two fluid compartments, do they show morphologic changes consistant with the physiologic responses to PTH or CT? Do tracers such as horseradish peroxidase, Lanthanum, etc., confirm the proposed fluid pathways? Do *in vitro* culture systems show cell change consistent with changes in ion concentrations in the accessable compartments? Does phosphate distribution correlate with calcium fluxes?

Rapid changes in bone lining cell morphology to PTH and CT have been reported by us[7,8]. These observations were made possible by the development of techniques for examining bone with the scanning electron microscope (SEM). With this instrument, large areas of bone cells can be viewed simultaneously so that large numbers of cells in different bone regions can be studied. This has the advantage of allowing the investigator to determine the extent of a given response without the tedious sampling required for transmission electron microscopy. With the SEM, the endosteal surface may be viewed following formalin fixation of the tissue and gentle washing away of the myeloid elements. Critical point drying and evaporative coating with gold-paladium are used following washing to preserve the cell integrity. With this technic the cells (bone lining cells) in immediate juxtaposition to the mineralized matrices may be viewed on their marrow aspect. The bone facing surface of these cells may also be viewed following micromanipulation as reported by Boyde[9]. Figure 1 shows the cell surface of the endosteal bone cells of a rat tibia. The cells appear to be separated by narrow intercellular channels that are artifactually wider by about 10% due to shrinkage artefacts. The cell surface is characterized by numerous microvilli. Using split rat tibia as a test model, SEM has been used to study the ultrastructure of these tibia from intact animals and also from split tibia cultured for several hours. The latter experimental condition permits intermittant analysis of the culture fluid to assess calcium and phosphate fluxes[10].

The endosteal lining cells show marked changes in morphology following PTH, assuming an ameboid, elongated appearance with the long axis of the cells coinciding with the longitudinal direction of the subjacent collagen fibrils. Zieosis and Blebbing also characterize the 1 hour post hormone response. Calcitonin (CT) produces changes in the lining cells within minutes following IV infusion of CT causing a shrinking of both osteocytes and a change in the intercellular distance between the lining cells. The responsiveness of bone lining cells have been further tested by exposing the cultured split tibia to cytochalasin B. This pharmacologic agent causes immediate changes in the cell configuration such that the cells assume a stellate appearance, a reaction that is readily reversible[12]. The responsiveness of these cells to cytochalasin B is indicative of a functional microfilament-membrane complex within these cells and suggests that they are adequately equipped to rapidly modify this cells configuration in response to stimuli.

We have used potassium pyroantimonate-osmium fixation as a histochemical tool for the study of calcium distribution as it has been shown that this compound forms electron dense precipitates with calcium[13]. Unfortunately, it will also precipitate with sodium and magnesium although it is more sensitive to calcium. Its pluripotential reaction has forced us to also use EGTA chelation and x-ray-spectroscopic technics to verify the predominant presence of calcium, which has been found valid in the results reported. Figure 2 is a transmission electron micrograph of an K-pyroantimonate-osmium fixed tibia from a TPTX rat. Because of the selective nature of the reaction, all parts of the cell are not readily demonstrated but rather, those parts of the cell that have a relatively high calcium concentration, i.e., plasma membranes, mitochondrial cristae, appear as dense black lines or precipitates. Plasma calcium levels fall within minutes post PTH prior to the rise in plasma calcium. This transient fall has been attributed to a possible rapid influx of calcium into bone cells as a consequence of changes in plasma membrane permeability. If that were the case, then one would expect the precipitate produced by the os-pyro tecnic to show increased deposits within bone cells shortly following PTH.

We used the ospyro-technique to follow the calcium distribution in bone cells from rats injected with 3 different dose levels of PTH with samples examined from a few minutes to hours following PTH[14]. Vehicle injected rats served as controls. The definitive membrane and mitochondrial distribution seen in figure 2 followed the same sequential change for all 3 dose levels. Generally, an initial diffuse increase in cytoplasmic precipitate was noted followed by loss of the diffuse pattern and an increase in organelle membrane precipitate. We interpret this increase in density to represent increased cell calcium. Corresponding determination of plasma calcium levels showed the initial dip in plasma calcium to be coincident with the increased diffuse pattern and the loaded organelle pattern to coincide with elevated plasma calcium levels. Isotopic technics have been used to establish that calcium mobilized from bone is not accompanied by a release of phosphate equivalent to the ratio of apatite, suggesting that the plasma calcium did not diffuse freely with phosphate into the general ECF. Interestingly, phosphate translocation from bone cell to bone fluid appears to be consequence of CT. Using phosphate depleted rats, normophosphate rats, and rats with supplemental phosphate, variation in the release of calcium from bone by calcitonin is effected[15,16]. Ultrastructural observations of calcitonin treated bone from those three groups indicate that an increase in bone fluid phosphate results from exposure to calcitonin. Fixation of these tissues in os-pyro shows an increased accumulation of calcium is also present here. Phosphate localization was demonstrated by aqueous incubations of the tissues in fixative such that apatite formation would occur, reflecting the presence of available phosphate. Non calcitonin treated animals did not produce apatite in these spaces when incubated while phosphate supplemented calcitonin treated rats showed the greatest accumulation of indicator crystals. Figure 3 shows an osteocyte bounded by crystal produced by aqueous incubation that indicates relative phosphate concentration.

The following model, figure 4, may summarize our present interpretations of the above data. Bone lining cells are separated by narrow channels through which fluids may enter the bone fluid compartment. Osteocytes are coupled to osteoblasts by gap junctions between their extended processes making a functional cell syncytium. Osteoclasts resorb bone and pass calcium through the cells to the ECF. Following CT, osteocytes release calcium into the pericellular space. Conversely, calcium enters the cells following PTH. The lining cells possess microfilaments and microtubules that enable these cells to change shape in response to hormonal stimulation. Shape changes would naturally effect the patency of the intercellular pathways. Because the plasma

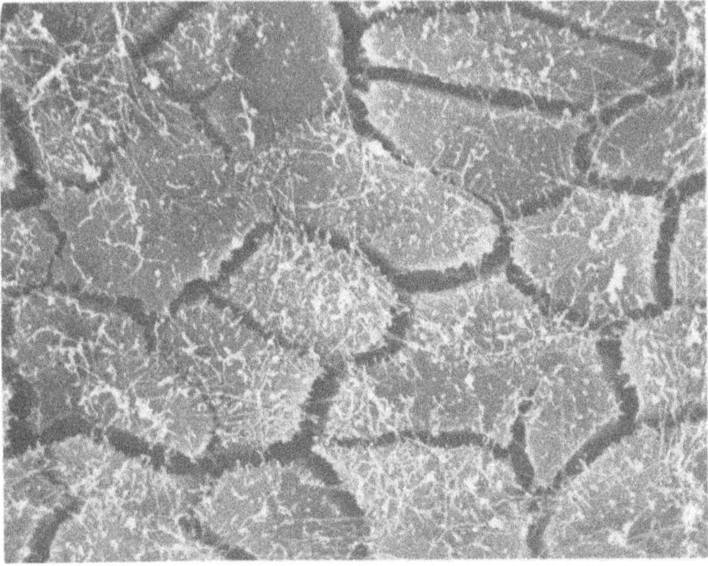

Fig. 1 - Scanning electron micrograph of endosteal bone lining cells showing surface microvilli and narrow intercellular spaces providing a diffusion pathway into bone fluid (x 1000).

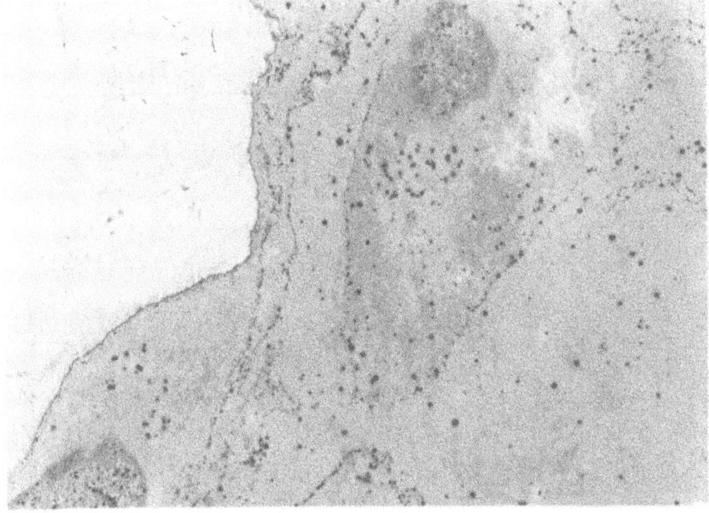

Fig. 2 - Transmission electronmicrograph of endosteal cells fixed in osmium-K-pyroantimonate for calcium localization. Plasma membranes and mitochondria show positive reactions (x 12,600).

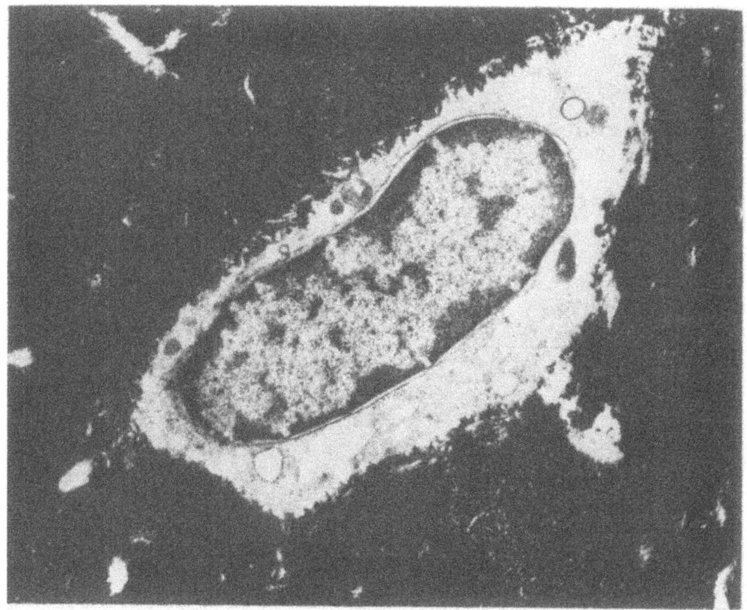

Fig. 3 - Transmission electronmicrograph of osteocyte from rat treated with 5 CT. Crystal deposition in the lacunae space following incubation indicates high calcium and phosphate (x 14,000).

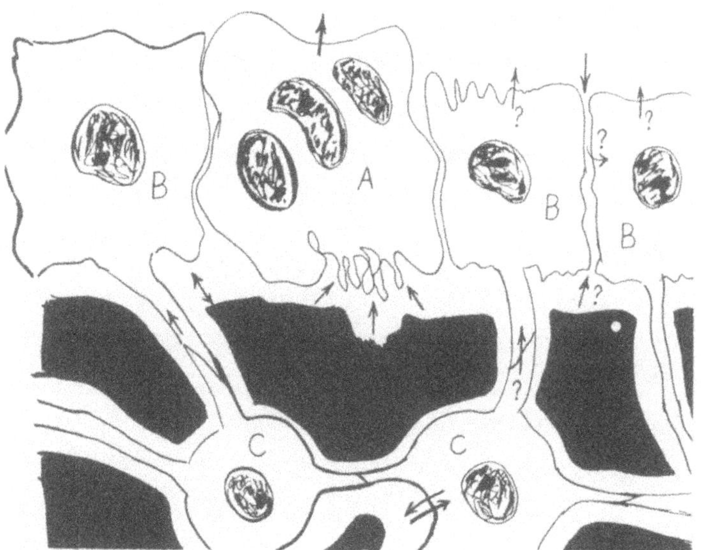

Fig. 4 - Diagram of bone cell organization. Osteoclasts (a), osteoblast (b), osteocyte (c). Arrows indicate presumed calcium fluxes.

changes in isotopically tagged calcium and phosphate do not indicate that they diffuse equally from the bone crystal to the ECF, and because the ospyro studies reflect significant bone cell calcium changes following PTH, movement of ions from bone likely involves movement primarily through the bone cells. Future studies should be directed towards assessing the possibility that this calcium movement may be achieved as an indirect benefit of the sodium pump acting as a carrier as occurs in nerve tissues, or some other transport system that does not require a continous expendition of cell energy solely for the purpose of calcium movement.

REFERENCES

1. Geisler, J.A., and Neuman, W.F.: The Membrane Control of Bone Potassium. Por. Soc. Exptl. Biol. Med. 130: 608, 1969.
2. Ramp, W.K., and Neuman, W.F.: Some Factors Affecting Mineralization of Bone In Tissue Culture. Am. J. Physiol. 220: 270, 1971.
3. Scarpace, P.J. and Neuman, W.F.: Quantitation of Ca Fluxes in Chick Calvaria. Biochem. Biophys. Acta (Amst).
4. Scarpace, P.J. and Neuman, W.F.: The Blood: Bone Disequilibrium. Calcif. Tiss. Res. 20: 151, 1976.
5. Talmage, R.V.: Calcium Homeostasis-Calcium Transport-Parathyroid Action. Clin. Orthop. 67: 210, 1969.
6. Neuman, W.F., Brommage, R.J., and Neuman, M.W.: Aerobic Glyeolysis, Ion Fluxes, and Bone Membranes, Proceedings of 6th Parathyroid Conference, 1977. in press.
7. Matthews, J.L., Martin, J.H., Collins, E.J., Kennedy, J.W., and Powel, E.L., Jr.: Immediate Changes in the Ultrastructure of Bone Cells Following Thyrocalcitonin Administration. In: Calcium, Parathyroid Hormone and the Calcitonins. Excerpta Medica. p. 375, 1972.
8. Davis, W.L., Matthews, J.L., Martin, J.H., Kennedy, J.W., and Talmage, R.V.: The Endostream as a Functional Membrane. In: Calcium Regulating Hormones, Excerpta Medica, p. 275, 1975.
9. Boyde, A.: S.E.M. Studies on Bone Cells in Culture, Proceedings of Sixth Parathyroid Conference. Excerpta Medica, in press.
10. Miller, G., Davis, W.L., Jones, R.G., Jones, J.L., and Matthews, J.L.: Intact Endosteal Membranes to Study Bone Cell Physiology: A Scanning Electron Microscopic and Metabolic Study of the Rat Endosteum. Anat. Rec., in press.
11. Jones, S.J., and Boyde, A.: Morphological Changes of Osteoblasts in vitro. Cell Tiss. Res. 166: 101, 1976.
12. Jones, J.L., Davis, W.L., Miller, G.W., Jones, R.G., and Matthews, J.L.: The Effect of Cytochalasin B on the Endosteal Lining Cells of Mammalian Bone: A Scanning Electron

Microscopic Study. Cell. Biol. in press.
13. Brighton, C.T., and Hunt, R.M.: Histochemical Localization of Calcium in Growth Plate Mitochondria and Matrix Vesicles. Fed. Proc. 35: 143, 1976.
14. Vander Wiel, C., Matthews, J.L., and Talmage, R.V.: Intracellular Calcium Localization in Cells Lining Bone Surfaces Following Parathyroid Hormone Injection. Proceedings of Sixth Parathyroid Conference. Excerpta Medica. in press.
15. Matthews, J.L., Davis, W.L., Martin, J.H., and Talmage, R.V.: The Endosteal Cell Response to Exogenous Stimuli, An Electron Microscope Study. In: Extracellular Matrix Influences on Gene Expression. Academic Press. p. 735, 1975.
16. Talmage, R.V., Matthews, J.L., Martin, J.H., Kennedy, J.W., Davis, W.L., and Roycroft, J.H.: Calcium, Phosphate and the Osteocyte-Osteoblast Bone Cell Unit. In: Calcium Regulating Hormones. Excerpta Medica, p. 284, 1974.

A NEW DIPHOSPHONATE: DISSOCIATION BETWEEN EFFECTS ON CELLS AND MINERAL IN RATS AND A PRELIMINARY TRIAL IN PAGET'S DISEASE

H.H.P.J.Lemkes, P.H.Reitsma, W.Frijlink, H.Verlinden-Ooms and Olav L.M.Bijvoet
Metabolic Unit, Dept. of Endocrinology and Metabolism, University Hospital, Leiden, The Netherlands

INTRODUCTION

Diphosphonates are of pharmacological interest because they act on bone (1). In animals they decrease the performance of osteoclasts and of osteoblasts and can hinder the mineralization of osteoid (2,3,4). The first two properties have been used to reduce bone turnover in patients with Paget's disease by treatment with Ethane-1-hydroxy-1,1-diphosphonate (EHDP) (5). But, whilst the desired decrement of activity of the disease was often achieved, the hindrance of mineralization has caused excesse of unmineralized osteoid in the diseased bones (6). This is probably why patients treated with EHDP have had an increased incidence of pathological fractures (7,8,9). Is undermineralization a necessary price to pay for reduction of bone formation and resorption in Paget's disease by diphosphonates?

Animal studies with another of the diphosphonates, Dichloromethylene-diphosphonate (Cl_2MDP), revealed that this substance at equimolar dose inhibits bone resorption more and matrix mineralization less than EHDP, but its effect on bone formation appears to be relatively poor (2,3). A diphosphonate which reduces resorption and formation without causing osteomalacia may be particularly useful in Paget's disease. We have therefore developed an experimental system which allows simultaneous measurement of bone formation, bone resorption and mineralization in young adult rats. In preliminary studies with a number of diphosphonates, 3-Amino-1-hydroxypropane-1,1-diphosphonate (ADP) was found to be particularly interesting and therefore selected for more extensive investigation and comparison with EHDP and Cl_2MDP. Results of these studies and of a preliminary clinical trial in Paget's disease are here reported.

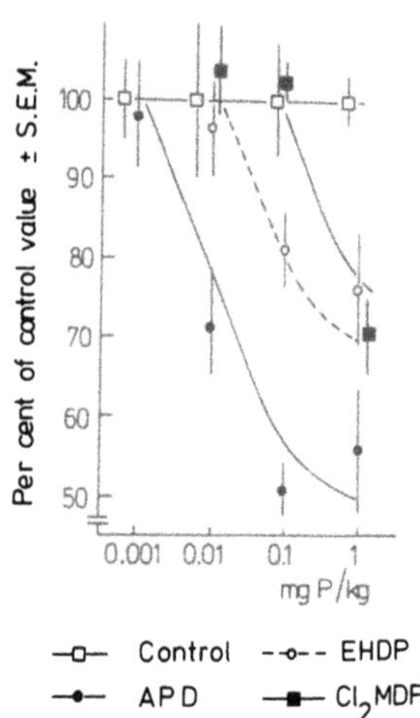

Fig. 1. Calcium uptake

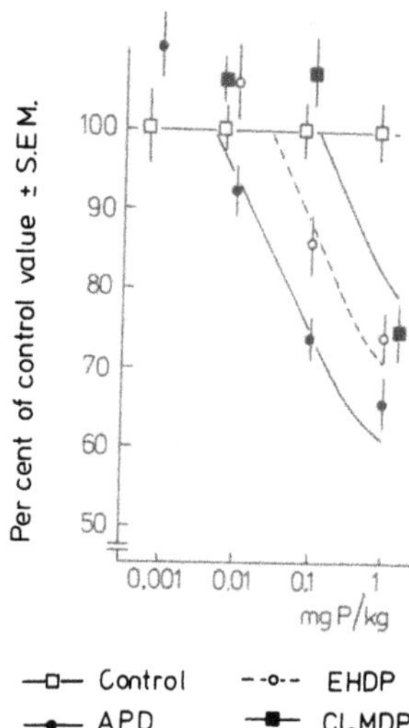

Fig. 2. Proline incorporation

To evaluate the importance of P-C-P bonds for diphosphonate action, a non-diphosphonate, Cyclohexacarboxylicacid (CHH), which like EHDP inhibits crystallization of apatite (Henkel GmbH, unpublished), was studied in the same system.

MATERIAL AND METHODS

The experimental design incorporates two important features: in-vivo administration of diphosphonates, enabling comparison with effects in human physiology and in-vitro incubation of bones of the same animals, allowing direct studies of aspects of bone metabolism. Histological studies (not reported here) were made to confirm conclusions derived from physical and biochemical data.

The male albino Wistar rat, weighing between 180 and 190 grams and bred in our laboratory, served as experimental animal. A single experimental sequence always consisted of 12 rats, divided into three groups of four per cage: (1) control, treated with 0.9% NaCl; (2) EHDP in isosmotic solution; (3) a solution of one of the other compounds. All compounds were administered daily by subcutaneous injection. The doses were equimolar to EHDP. The latter was given in a dose range of 1-10 mgP per kg body weight per day for 6 days when mineralization was studied and for 23 days in a dose range of 0.001-1 mgP/kg/day in all the other studies here reported. Four days before sacrifice the animals received 1 µCi of $^{45}CaCl_2$ sub-

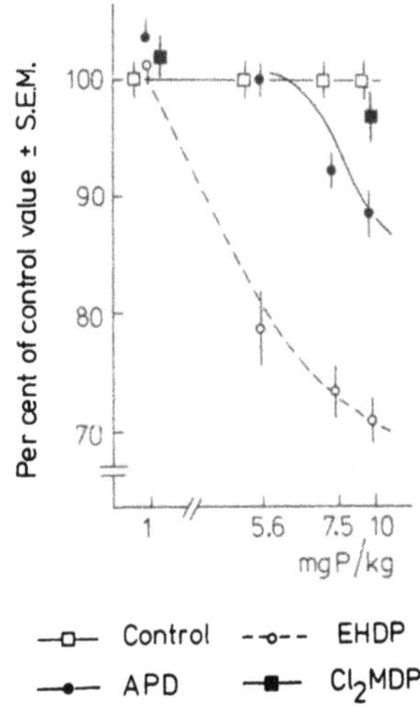

Fig. 3. Mineralization

cutaneously. The morning after the last treatment day, the animals were sacrificed by exsanguination under ether anaesthesia. Immediately after sacrifice the metaphyses of distal femur and proximal tibia were removed from both legs, cleaned from adjacent tissue and epiphyseal cartilage and from bone marrow, fragmented and incubated in 2 ml modified BCG medium in the presence of ^{3}H-proline. After 9 hours of incubation the fragments were analysed for Ca, ^{45}Ca, hydroxyproline (OHP) and ^{3}H-hydroxyproline (^{3}H-OHP) and the medium was assayed for lactate. Some experiments were performed in the presence of 1-^{14}C-, 6-^{14}C- or U-^{14}C-glucose to measure the lactate/$^{14}CO_2$ ratio. Both radii were removed for measurement of dry weight and one humerus for histological examination of undecalcified sections. All results were expressed as percent of control values $\pm$ one standard error of the mean (S.E.M.). Control values are represented in the figures by open squares and a horizontal line; EHDP by open circles and a interrupted line; APD by closed circles and Cl_2MDP by closed squares both with uninterrupted lines. Vertical bars are 2 S.E.M.

RESULTS

The uptake of labeled calcium, administered in-vivo, was measured as dpm ^{45}Ca per mole of cold calcium in the bone fragments (fig.1). The dose-response curves show that APD is the most potent inhibitor of calcium uptake and Cl_2MDP the least, the ratios of

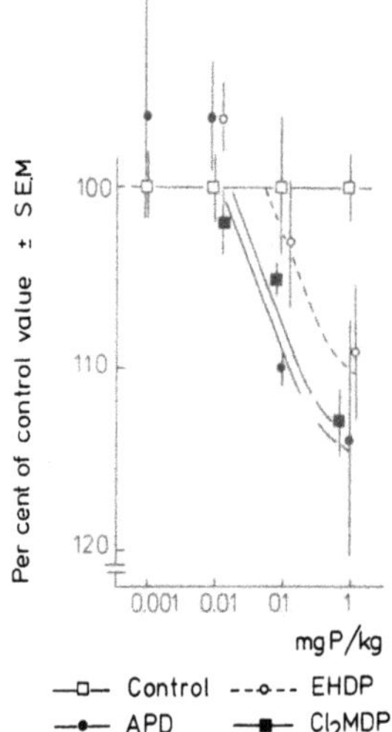

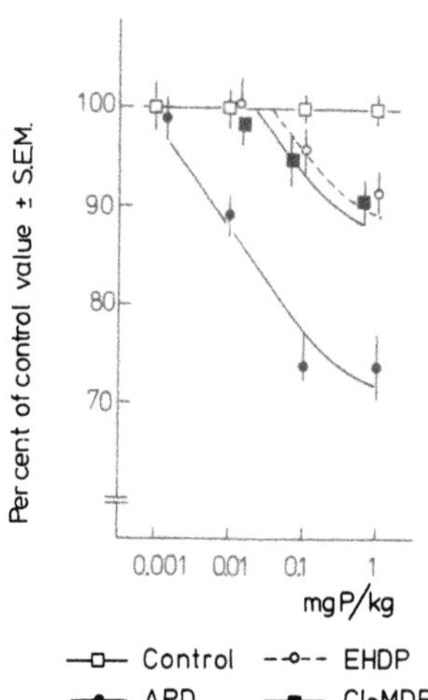

Fig. 4. Radius weight

Fig. 5. Hydroxyproline density

inhibitory activity with respect to EHDP (taken as 1 unity) being roughly 10:1:0.2.

The amount of labeled proline incorporated in-vitro as ^{3}H-OHP into collagen over 9 hours of incubation was measured as dpm ^{3}H-OHP per unit dry weight (fig.2). Again, the dose-response curves show APD to be the most potent inhibitor, followed by EHDP and then Cl_2MDP. Ratio's of inhibitory activity with respect to EHDP are in the order of 5:1:0.3.

Mineralization was measured as mole of cold calcium per mole of hydroxyproline (fig.3). Cl_2MDP had a minimal effect on mineralization, APD slightly more and EHDP produced the greatest disturbances at the doses employed. The ratio's of activity EHDP:APD: Cl_2MDP are 1:0.4:0.3.

The dry weight of the radii of diphosphonate treated rats relative to those of control rats was increased by all compounds (fig.4). After 23 days the highest weight was obtained with APD and Cl_2MDP, less net weight gain with EHDP, the ratio's of effectiveness being 5:5:1.

Whereas shortly after the start of treatment the calcium to OHP ratio decreased in a log-dose dependent fashion (Fig 3) the opposite happened when treatment was prolonged. Especially after

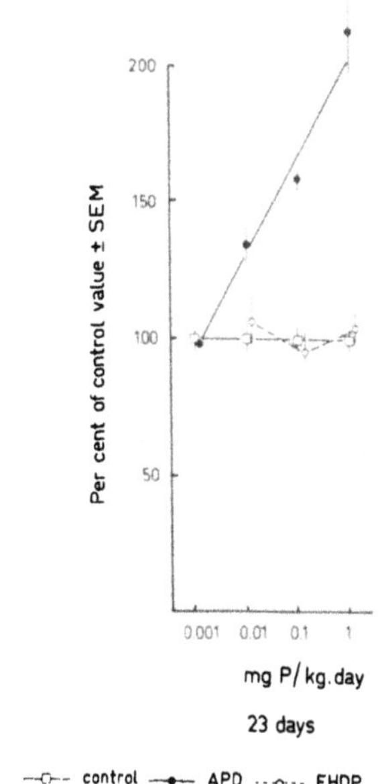

Fig. 6. Lactate production

APD treatment such ratios might even increase to 200 percent of control. After examination of histological sections it was realized that at that moment many of the metaphyseal trabecula consisted of unresorbed calcified cartilage. Since cartilage has a lower OHP density (10), the ratio of OHP to calcium then became a measure for the relative amount of calcified cartilage present in the metaphyses. The results are given in figure 5. The lower the OHP to Ca ratio, the more calcified cartilage has persisted. EHDP and Cl_2MDP had similar effects but APD had the same effect at only about one twentieth of the dose.

The effect on lactate production is an interesting point of difference between APD and EHDP (fig.6). After 23 days of treatment APD increased lactate production in a log-dose dependent fashion, contrary to EHDP. This increase cannot be due to an excess of cartilage cells (which are known to produce more lactate) in the metaphyseal bone fragments, since the same increase was found when solely diaphyseal bone was incubated in additional experiments.

In a first attempt to understand this effect, in another experiment the action of APD on the lactate/CO_2 ratio was measured using various glucose labels (table I). It appeared that the overall ratio increased, the increase being due to a large extent to an increase relative to 6-$^{14}CO_2$. This suggest qualitative changes in glucose breakdown, resulting in an enhanced glycolysis.

Table I. Effect of APD on lactate/CO_2 ratio

Period days	Dose mg P	Glucose label	Control	EHDP	APD
23	1	U-^{14}C-	100 $\pm$ 8	97 $\pm$ 5	208 $\pm$ 23
6	10	1-^{14}C-	100 $\pm$ 5	93 $\pm$ 11	82 $\pm$ 6
6	10	6-^{14}C-	100 $\pm$ 4	96 $\pm$ 8	240 $\pm$ 33

Table II shows the effect of CHH on the same system. At the given doses CHH had effects on bone mineralization, bone formation and bone resorption very similar to those of EHDP.

DISCUSSION

The results demonstrate that diphosphonates differ in the ratio between inhibition of bone turnover and inhibition of mineralization. Their effect on bone cells may therefore be due to a direct action instead of being secondary to a mineralization disturbance. The specificity of the effect on bone cells may depend on local high concentrations caused by the affinity of diphosphonates for hydroxy-apatite. In the next section the data are discussed in relation to relevant parameters.

Bone formation

Bone formation was measured as collagen formation and as calcium uptake (figs. 1 & 2). Collagen formation in our experiments is solely due to osteoblastic bone formation because the epiphyseal cartilage had been removed. Calcium uptake however, is not only due to osteo-blastic bone formation but also to short- and longterm exchange and calcification. This explains why inhibition of calcium uptake and collagen formation differ. Nevertheless, the data demonstrates that APD was far more potent than EHDP in reducing bone formation and that EHDP was more potent than Cl_2MDP.

Mineralization

Interestingly, the mineralization disturbance caused by APD, though somewhat greater than that from Cl_2MDP is less than that caused by EHDP (fig.3). This could be confirmed in histological

Table II. Comparison of effects on bone metabolism of EHDP, 1 mgP per kg body weight per day, subcutaneously, and of an equimolar dose of CHH, given for 23 days (see text)

	calcium uptake	proline incorp.	OHP density	radius weight	mineralization
EHDP	73 ± 3	78 ± 8	89 ± 3	108 ± 3	77 ± 3
CHH	71 ± 3	76 ± 8	85 ± 6	104 ± 2	71 ± 3

observations. When bone formation and mineralization are considered together one can conclude that a dose of APD which produces the same effect on bone formation as a given dose of EHDP, has less than one tenth the effect on mineralization.

Bone resorption

The effect of inhibition by diphosphonates of bone resorption could not be measured directly, but was derived from weight gain of radii of treated rats (fig.4). Despite reduction in bone formation these radii had gained more weight than those of the control rats. Therefore the inhibition of bone resorption must have exceeded that of formation. For the same effect as EHDP, five times less APD or Cl_2MDP was necessary. However APD was roughly ten times more active than Cl_2MDP in inhibiting bone formation and must therefore have been an even more potent inhibitor of bone resorption than Cl_2MDP, which in itself is more active than EHDP. This too was evident from histology. Rats treated with APD and Cl_2MDP showed persistence of great amounts of calcified cartilage, which, in the case of APD - which inhibits osteoblasts - was not covered by osteoblastic bone. This explains the high percentage of low-collagen bone found with APD, and to a less extent with Cl_2MDP and EHDP.

We conclude from the previous observations that APD is a far more potent inhibitor of bone formation and bone resorption than both Cl_2MDP and EHDP. Cl_2MDP, which is more active than EHDP on bone resorption, has less effect on bone formation. Both APD and Cl_2MDP are less damaging to mineralization than EHDP.

Lactate production

Bone formation and bone resorption can be considered as a performance of bone cells. Lactate production however, reflects the internal metabolic behaviour of these cells. APD increased lactate

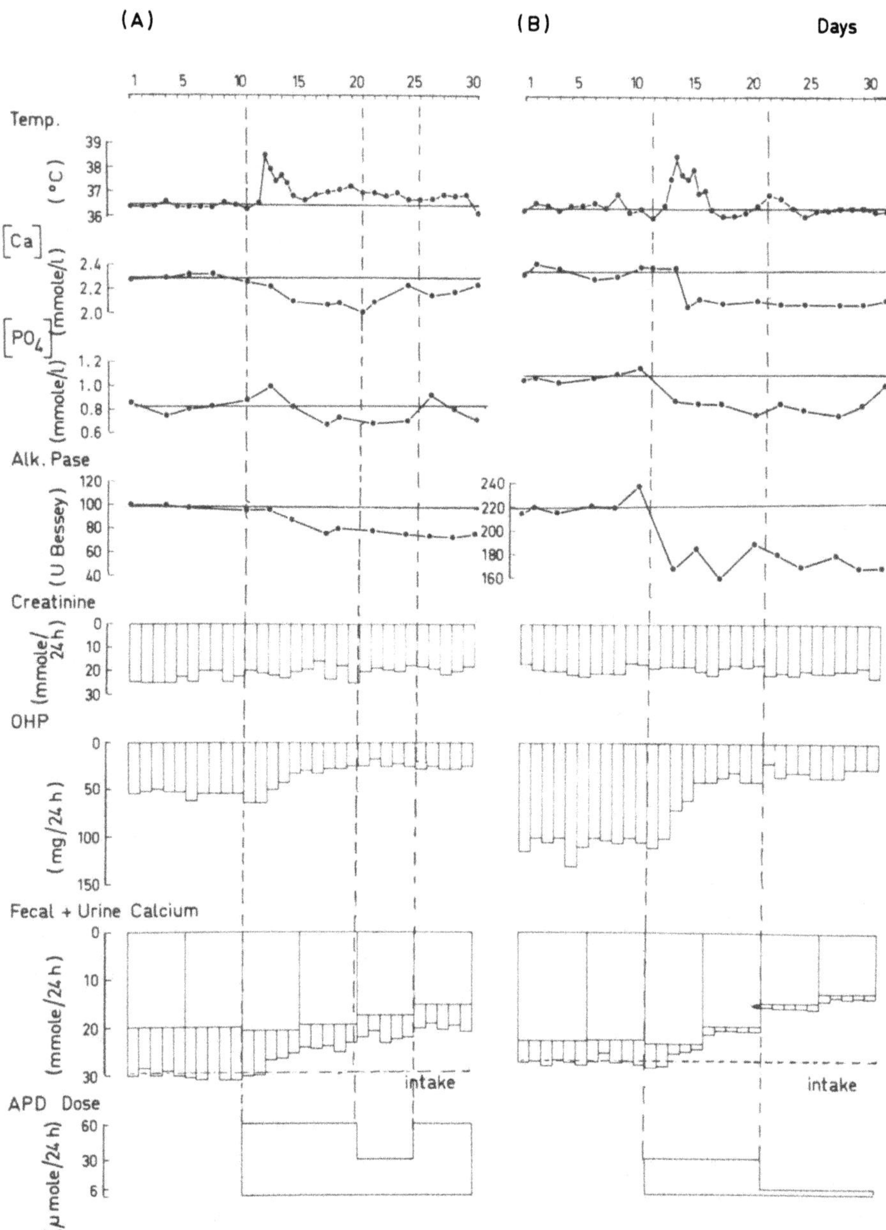

Fig. 7. Effects of APD on two patients with Paget's disease. From Bijvoet et al. (13), with permission.

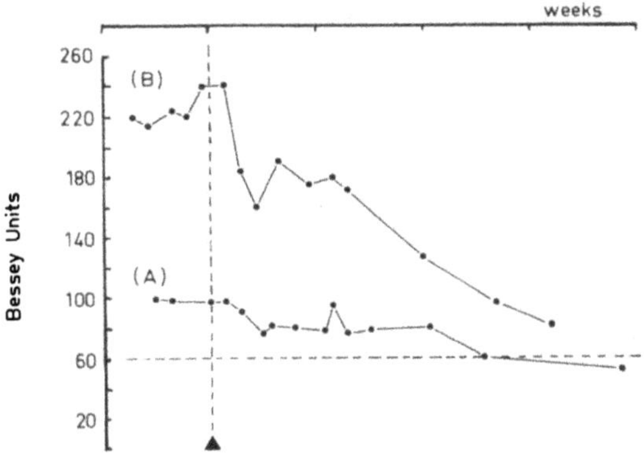

Fig. 8. Effect of APD on serum Alkaline Phosphatase in same patients. From Bijvoet et al. (13), with permission.

production and increased the lactate/6-$^{14}CO_2$ ratio. This suggests a qualitative change in glucose breakdown, that resulted in increased glycolysis. A possible explanation may be that APD influenced mitochondrial function by interference with calcium uptake and/or release.

P-C-P bonds not essential?

The non-diphosphonate CHH that resembles EHDP in its actions on hydroxylapatite _in-vitro_, had biological effects, which in all respects were _comparable to_ those of EHDP. It is therefore possible that the P-C-P bond is not essential to the effects of diphosphonates _in-vivo_ and that an action on intracellular calcium transport rather _than on_ the inhibition of pyrophosphatase (11,12), is responsible for their biological properties.

PRELIMINARY CLINICAL TRIAL

The results of this first part of this study showed APD to be more potent with respect to bone formation and resorption than EHDP, whereas it caused less disturbances of mineralization. In addition it inhibited bone formation as well as resorption and therefore seemed more suitable than Cl_2MDP for a clinical study in Paget's disease. Preliminary studies in rats and dogs (Henkel GmbH) let suppose that absorption after oral administration was comparable to that of EHDP. After acute and chronic toxicity studies had given sufficient assurance that no untowards effects had to be expected and after informed consent had been obtained from both the local ethical committee and patients, a preliminary clinical investigation was started. The results in the first two patients with Paget's disease are shown in figures 7 and 8.

The treatment with APD was started in a metabolic ward under balance conditions. After a suitable control period the patients received APD by oral route at a dose of 60 µmole/kg/day in the first patient and 30 µmole/kg/day in the second patient, divided over 3 doses and given half an hour before meals. The doses are equimolar to 15 and 7.5 mg EHDP/kg/day. After this initial period the patients were placed on a maintenance dose of 6 and 3 µmole APD/kg/day, which is only a tenth of the initial dose level.

There was a shortlasting rise of body temperature, not accompanied by other complaints or abnormal clinical findings. The temperature abated spontaneously. From the third day onwards serum calcium and phosphate were lowered by 0.2 mmol/l. The urinary output of creatinin remained constant during the whole study, but hydroxyproline excretion decreased to normal values within one week. Both urinary and faecal excretion of calcium decreased and the calcium balance became positive from the start of treatment. Serum alkaline phosphatase activity had decreased more slowly, but was also normal in both patients after the fifth treatment week. One patient had an increased temperature over an affected extremity and this decreased to normal. Both reported disappearance of bone pain. The second patient had a Pagetic lesion in the iliac crest. This lesion was biopsied. Before treatment the typical cellular lesion of Paget's disease were seen. After 6 months all abnormal osteoblasts and osteoclasts had disappeared and no unmineralized osteoid seams were visible. The patients are now seen in the outpatient clinic and are doing well, both clinically and biochemically.

These preliminary results demonstrate that normalization of abnormal bone turnover was obtained without any complication and that this effect developed much more rapidly than the usual effects of EHDP, calcitonin or a combination of both (13). The expectation, derived from animal studies, that APD may be of considerable pharmacological interest for the treatment of Paget's disease, is therefore justified.

ACKNOWLEDGEMENTS

All compounds were kindly donated by Henkel GmbH, Düsseldorf. The investigations were supported in part by the Foundation for Medical Research FUNGO, which is subsidized by the Netherlands Organization for the Advancement of Pure Research (Z.W.O.).

REFERENCES

1. Russell, R.G.G. and Fleisch, H.: Pyrophosphate and diphosphonates in skeletal metabolism. Clin.Orthop.Rel.Res. 108: 241, 1975.
2. Miller, S.C. and Jee, W.S.S.: The comparative effects of dichloromethylene diphosphonate (Cl_2MDP) and ethane-1-hydroxy-1,1-diphosphonate (EHDP) on growth and modeling of the rat tibia. Calc.Tiss.Res. 23:207, 1977.
3. Russell, R.G.G., Kislig, A.M., Casey, P.A., Fleisch, H., Thornton, J., Schenk, R. and Williams, D.A.: Effect of diphosphonates and calcitonin on the chemistry and quantitative histology of rat bone. Calc.Tiss.Res. 11:179, 1973.
4. Schenk, R., Merz, W.A., Mühlbauer, R., Russell, R.G.G. and Fleisch, H.: Effect of ethane-1-hydroxy-1,1-diphosphonate (EHDP) and dichloromethylene diphosphonate (Cl_2MDP) on the calcification and resorption of cartilage and bone in the tibial epiphysis and metaphysis of rats. Calc.Tiss.Res. 11:196, 1973.
5. Smith, R., Russell, R.G.G., Bishop, M.C., Woods, C.G. and Bishop, M.: Paget's disease of bone: Experience with a diphosphonate (disodium etidronate) in treatment. Quart.Med. 42:235, 1973.
6. Russell, R.G.G., Smith, R., Preston, C., Walton, R.J. and Woods, C.G.: Diphosphonates in Paget's disease. Lancet (i):894, 1974.
7. Fromm, G., Schajowicz, F. and Mautalen, C.A.: Disodium ethane-1-hydroxy-1,1-diphosphonate in Paget's disease. Lancet (ii): 666, 1975.
8. Reiker, M., Jong, A., Seiler, A., Schenk, R. and Fleisch, H.: Le traitement de la maladie de Paget par les diphosphonates. Schweiz.med.Wschr. 105:1701, 1975.
9. Finerman, G.A.M., Gronick, H.G., Smith, R.K., and Mayfield, J. Diphosphonate treatment of Paget's disease. Clin.Orthop. 120: 115, 1976.
10. Wuthier, R.E.: A zonal analysis of inorganic and organic constituents of the epiphysis during enchondral calcification. Calc.Tiss.Res. 4:20, 1969.
11. Russell, R.G.G. and Smith, R.: Diphosphonates - Experimental and clinical aspects. J.Bone Joint Surg.(Br) 55B:66, 1973.
12. Wöltgens, J.H.M., Bonting, S.L. and Bijvoet, O.L.M.: Inorganic pyrophosphatase in mineralizing hamster molars. III. Influence of diphosphonates. Calc.Tiss.Res. 13:151, 1973.
13. Bijvoet, O.L.M., Hosking, D.J., Lemkes, H.H.P.J., Reitsma, P.H. and Frijlink, W.: Development in the treatment of Paget's disease. To be published in: Proceedings of the Vth Parathyroid conference 1977. Elsevier, Amsterdam.

Topic on Vitamin D

CURRENT STATUS OF THE USE OF NEWER ANALOGS OF VITAMIN D IN THE MANAGEMENT OF RENAL OSTEODYSTROPHY

Jack W. Coburn and Arnold S. Brickman

Medical and Research Services, VA Wadsworth Hospital, Los Angeles, CA; Sepulveda VA Hospital, Sepulveda, CA; and Department of Medicine, UCLA School of Medicine, Los Angeles, CA.

In this discussion, the term renal osteodystrophy is used to denote a clinical syndrome observed in azotemic patients with a variety of skeletal lesions including osteitis fibrosa, osteomalacia, osteosclerosis, osteoporosis, and retardation of growth. The pathophysiologic alteration in advanced renal failure include hypocalcemia, hyperphosphatemia, hypermagnesemia, soft tissue calcification, and impaired intestinal calcium absorption. Secondary hyperparathyroidism is a major feature, and it is believed to have its onset early in the course of renal insufficiency. Parathyroid hyperplasia is thought to arise as a consequence of hypocalcemia produced in part by 1) phosphate retention and hyperphosphatemia, 2) from impaired renal conversion of 25-hydroxy-vitamin D_3 [25(OH)D_3] to 1,25-dihydroxy-vitamin D_3 [1,25(OH)$_2D_3$], and 3) reduced skeletal responsiveness to the calcemic action of PTH. Knowledge that the kidney is the sole organ capable of producing 1,25(OH)$_2D_3$, the most active known form of vitamin D, from 25(OH)D_3 (1) suggests a major pathogenic role of altered vitamin D metabolism in causing renal osteodystrophy. The observations that plasma levels of 1,25(OH)$_2D_3$ are low (2), the failure of conversion of radio-labeled 25(OH)D_3 to 1,25(OH)$_2D_3$ (3) and the restoration of intestinal Ca absorption to normal following treatment with 1,25(OH)$_2D_3$ (4,5) in patients with end-stage uremia support the concept that renal production of 1,25(OH)$_2D_3$ is impaired in advanced renal failure. Moreover, such observations have prompted numerous clinical trials employing newer vitamin D analogs to uremic patients with bone disease. It is our purpose to briefly review the present state of knowledge on the usefulness of these analogs in renal osteodystrophy.

Several reports have indicated that treatment with 1,25(OH)$_2D_3$ or its synthetic analog, 1-alpha-hydroxy-vitamin D_3 [1α(OH)D_3] can reverse many of the abnormalities of divalent ion metabolism observed in uremia (4,5,6). Thus, balance for calcium and phosphorus is improved (7), intestinal Ca absorption is enhanced, and hypocalcemia is corrected. Moreover, reports suggest that these sterols can reverse the skeletal manifestations of secondary hyperparathyroidism and improve osteomalacia in many uremic patients (6,8-11).

We have recently summarized our experience with managing overt renal osteodystrophy in uremic patients using $1,25(OH)_2D_3$ or $1\alpha(OH)D_3$ (12). In this study, 47 patients, 38 male and 9 female, were treated with $1,25(OH)_2D_3$ (44 studies) or $1\alpha(OH)D_3$ (7 studies). The major difference between $1,25(OH)_2D_3$ and $1\alpha(OH)D_3$ is pharmacologic and the latter must be 25-hydroxylated to $1,25(OH)_2D_3$ before it exerts its actions. Hence, the results with $1\alpha(OH)D_3$ and $1,25(OH)_2D_3$, which are similar, have been pooled.

Most of the patients were under treatment with maintenance hemodialysis for a mean duration of 4.0 years. Ten had stable, advanced renal failure, with creatinine clearances below 15 ml/min, and were not undergoing dialysis. Most patients were selected for treatment because of bone pain or muscular weakness in the presence of abnormal x-rays or skeletal biopsies. Elevated alkaline phosphatase levels, abnormal bone biopsies, and/or marked hypocalcemia existed in the 12 patients who lacked symptoms. Thus, the patients were highly selected and do not represent a cross section of osteodystrophy in patients with end-stage renal failure. In this regard, 25 patients were referred to us specifically because of their symptomatic bone disease, while the others represent only 7% of the patients treated with dialysis in our collaborating hospitals. Prior management of altered divalent ion metabolism include aluminum hydroxide or carbonate (95-100% of patients), oral Ca supplements (57%), treatment with pharmacological quantities of a vitamin D preparation (i.e. vitamin D_2, 1.25 mg/day or dihydrotachysterol 0.125-0.6 mg/day) in 41%, and/or parathyroidectomy (16%). The $1,25(OH)_2D_3$ was given as a single daily oral dose. Because of limited availability of the sterol at the outset of the clinical trails, initial doses were 0.14 to 0.28μg/day. Subsequently, the dose was 0.25μg/day for 1-2 weeks, with the dose slowly increased to 0.5 to 1.0μg/day. The dose of $1,25(OH)_2D_3$ averaged 0.62μg/day for the total group of patients, while the average dose of $1\alpha(OH)D_3$ was 1.60μg/day. The duration of treatment averaged 22 weeks.

Substantial symptomatic improvement was noted in a large fraction of the patients. Skeletal pain, present in 38 patients, began subsiding within 1-3 weeks after initiation of treatment and it totally disappeared in 55% of the afflicted patients. There was no improvement in 12 patients. Muscular weakness, typical of that reported in osteomalacia (12a) and present in 26 patients, improved in 19 was unchanged in 7. Among the 38 symptomatic patients, 23 noted improvement and 13 failed to improve. The latter group of patients,

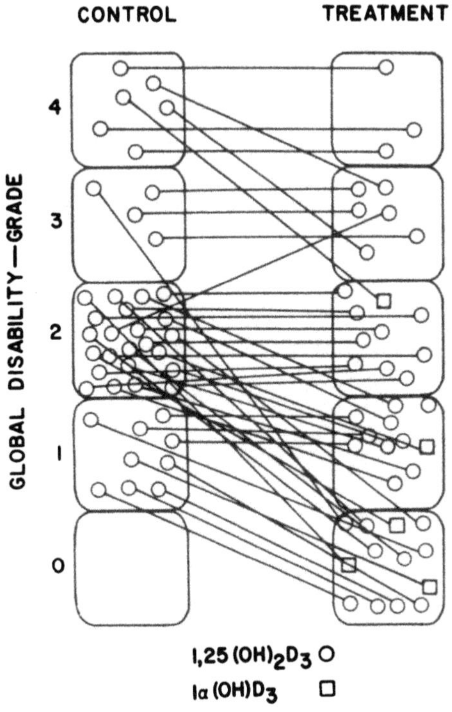

Figure 1

Global disability grade in patients treated with 1,25$(OH)_2D_3$ or 1α$(OH)D_3$ before and on completion of the treatment period. The scores for disability vary from 1, symptoms only with strenuous activity, to 5, totally disabled, restricted to bed or wheel chair (reproduced from Coburn et al (12) with permission of the publishers).

considered "treatment failures," are discussed below. The "Global Disability Score" (12), based on the degree of restriction of the patients' activities before and after treatment, is shown in figure 1.

Despite the arbitrary separation of patients on the basis of a clinical response, there were distinct biochemical differences between those who responded and the "treatment failure" group. Serum Ca increased from a mean of 9.00±0.26 (SE) to 9.90±0.19 mg/dl in those showing a response. In contrast, serum Ca averaged 10.6±0.20 mg/dl in the "treatment failure" group before treatment and was 11.9±0.40mg/dl after treatment. Alkaline phosphatase levels decreased in the responders and remained elevated in the other group (figure 2). The mean serum P was 4.59±0.18 before and 4.79±0.21 mg/dl after treatment, and there were no differences between the pretreatment serum P levels of the two groups.

In 14 instances, there was a decrease in serum P by 1 mg/dl or more during treatment: this generally occurred within the first 1-3 months of treatment and occurred in those exhibiting a favorable response (figure 3). This probably developed during a period of rapid skeletal remineralization. Serum P rose by 1.0 mg/dl or more

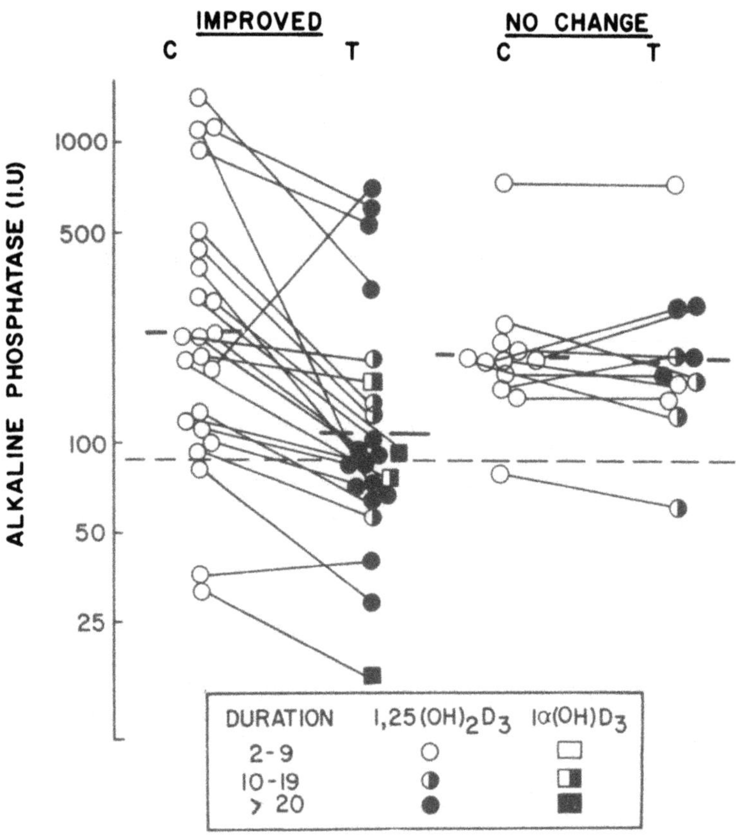

Figure 2. Serum alkaline phosphatase levels (log scale) in symptomatic patients separated according to clinical response. C = pretreatment, T = treatment. Duration of treatment is weeks; geometric means are indicated by horizontal lines. The "Treatment Failure" group is indicated as showing "No Change." (Modified from Coburn et al (12) with permission of the publishers).

in 22 patients; this usually occurred after 4-10 months of treatment was often coincident with a period of hypercalcemia (figure 4). This may be attributed, in part, to an action of $1,25(OH)_2D_3$ to stimulate intestinal absorption of P (7), as shown in figure 5.

In the patients responding to treatment, serum iPTH levels were 2-24 times the upper limit of normal before treatment, and they decreased by 25% or more in half the patients and returned to normal in many. Several of the patients classified as "treatment failures," showed "pure osteomalacia" on bone biospy with little or no increase in resorptive surface or osteitis fibrosa (13). Serum iPTH was

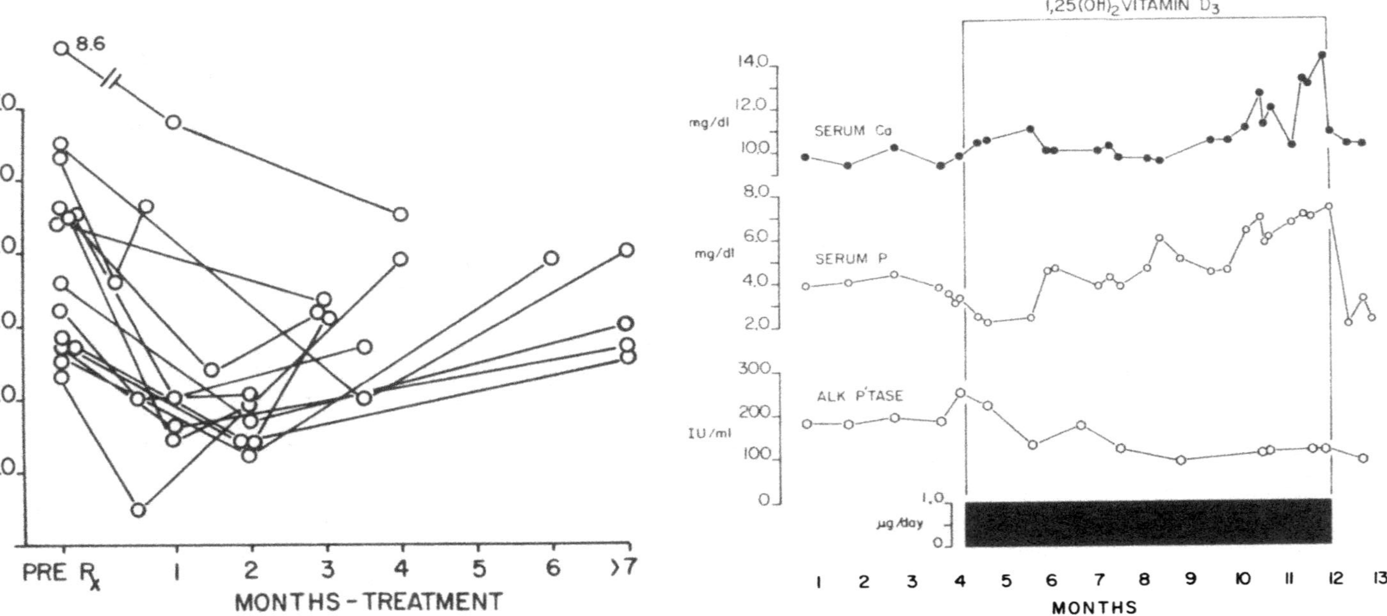

Figure 3. Levels of serum P in patients showing a fall in serum P by 1.0 mg/dl or more in relation to the duration of treatment with 1,25$(OH)_2D_3$. The final value represents the last observation during treatment.

Figure 4. Serial changes in serum Ca, P and alkaline phosphatase in a 56 year old dialysis patient with polycystic kidney disease. Serum iPTH fell from 1580 to 220 pg/ml. Notable are the early fall and the late rise in serum P. This occurred after alkaline phosphatase fell and coincident with an episode of hypercalcemia. (Reproduced from Coburn et al (12) with permission of the publisher).

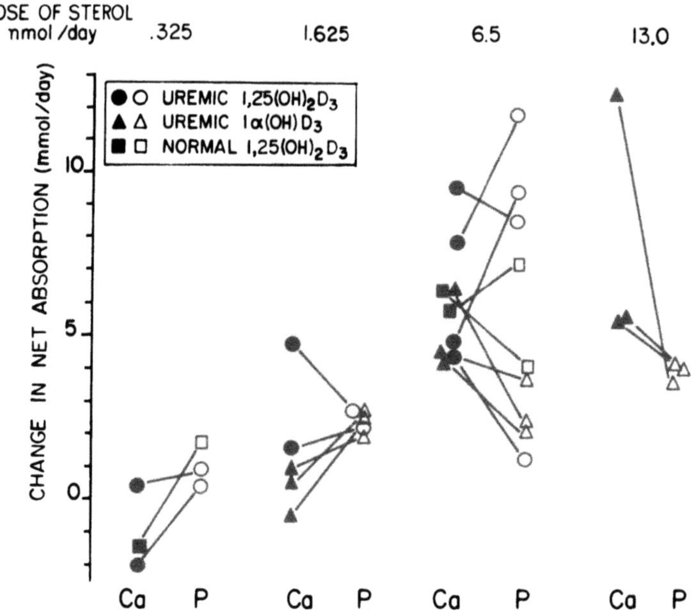

Figure 5. Relationship between changes in net absorption of phosphorus and calcium in 20 metabolic balance studies in subjects receiving either $1,25(OH)_2D_3$ or $1\alpha(OH)D_3$. Reproduced from Brickman et al (7) with permission of the publishers.

undetectable or normal in most of these. Serum P averaged 4.7 mg/dl, and there was no improvement following supplementation with oral phosphate. Thus, this group of patients showed no improvement in abnormal skeletal mineralization despite elevation of serum Ca and P and the administration of $1,25(OH)_2D_3$. The cause of this disorder is unexplained.

Thirty-three episodes of hypercalcemia occurred in 20 patients during the course of treatment. After withdrawal of treatment, serum Ca generally fell to normal within 1-3 days. Several patterns of hypercalcemia were seen: 23 episodes occurred in 11 patients within 8 weeks of starting treatment. Most patients were in the "treatment failure" group, and hypercalcemia often developed despite a daily dose of $1,25(OH)_2D_3$ less than 0.5 μg/day. In most of these patients, the pre-treatment level of serum Ca was normal or slightly elevated. Some had low levels of serum iPTH and bone biopsies showed a mineralizing defect; others had very high levels of iPTH and the bone biopsy showed osteitis fibrosa. In other patients, hypercalcemic episodes developed after treatment for 4-15 months of treatment. These patients had received higher daily doses of $1,25(OH)_2D_3$ and the hypercalcemia often occurred coincident with the return of serum alkaline phosphatase to normal levels (figure 4). Such hypercalcemia probably developed when remineralization of the skeleton was complete or greatly slowed. In several patients, treatment with a lower daily dose was resumed without difficulty.

Our observations point to the efficacy of $1,25(OH)_2D_3$ in improving symptoms and reversing many biochemical features of secondary hyperparathyroidism in patients with symptomatic renal osteodystrophy. In some instances, patients who were totally bedridden were able to walk, and the improvement of myopathy was prominent and gratifying. Clinical improvement correlated with a decline in serum alkaline phosphatase.

Other reports of trials with either $1\alpha(OH)D_3$ or $1,25(OH)_2D_3$ documents successful use of patients with secondary hyperparathyroidism and osteitis fibrosa and also in those with osteomalacia or defective mineralization (14-23). In such patients, treatment led to normalization of hypocalcemia, suppression of elevated levels of parathyroid hormone, and a fall in alkaline phosphatase levels (figure 6). Resolution of bone pain and tenderness often proceeded

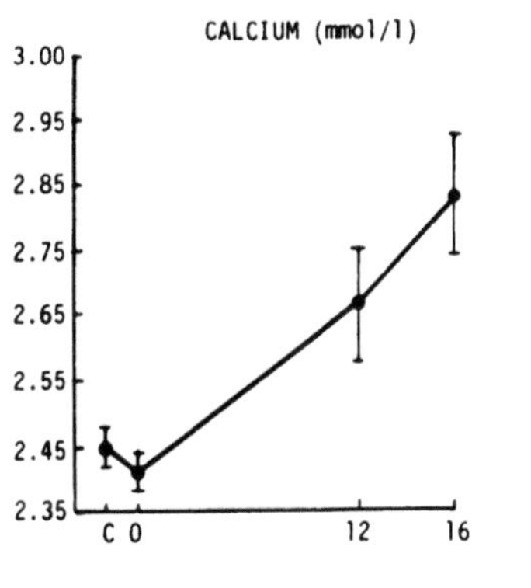

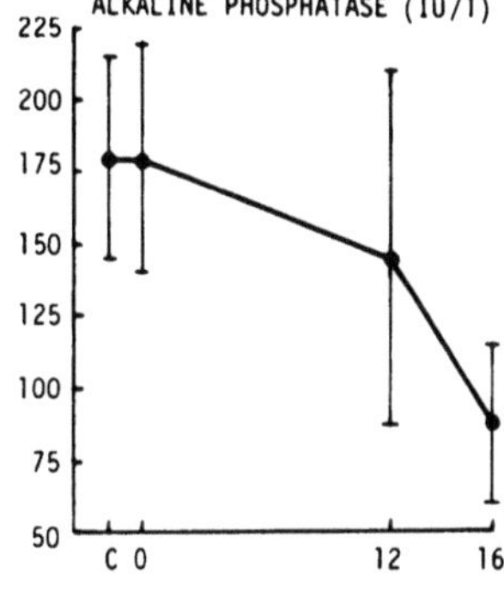

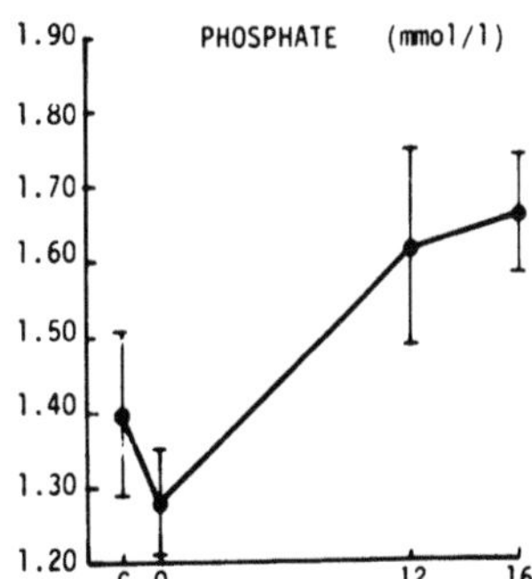

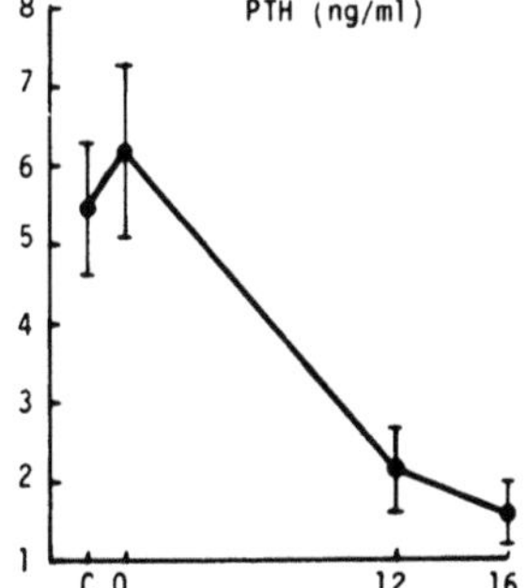

Figure 6

Mean values of plasma Ca,P, alkaline phosphatase, and serum immunoreactive PTH in 10 dialysis patients according to the duration of treatment with $1\alpha(OH)D_3$ shown in months. The initial dose was 1.0μg/day and the amount was adjusted in each patient during the trial. Reproduced from Papapoulus et al (23) with permission of the publishers.

the normalization of biochemical parameters, and improvement of proximal muscle weakness often occurred within 1-3 weeks.

The development of hypercalcemia during the early period of treatment may pose a problem as noted above. Patients with pre-existing, mild hypercalcemia as a manifestation of clinically overt secondary hyperparathyroidism are prone to develop hypercalcemia early in the course of treatment. Such patients may have such marked parathyroid hyperplasia that parathyroid surgery is indicated. It is possible that such patients might be effectively treated with a lower Ca concentration in dialysate and reduced dietary calcium intake so that continued treatment with $1,25(OH)_2D_3$ or $1\alpha(OH)D_3$ would be feasible.

Certain patients exhibiting a mineralizing defect of bone and failing to respond to $1\alpha(OH)D_3$ have been reported by Pierides et al (17). They attributed the failure response to phosphate depletion (24). However, we found no evidence for phosphate depletion in our "treatment failure"patients exhibiting a "mineralizing defect" (13). Tougaard et al observed a similar decrease in bone mineral content, as measured by photon absorption, in dialysis patients treated with either $1\alpha(OH)D_3$ and in those receiving placebo (25). It is possible that the heterogeneity of the patient population may account for some of the divergent results noted.

There does not appear to be a great difference between the effectiveness of $1,25(OH)_2D_3$ and $1\alpha(OH)D_3$ except in patients also receiving anticonvulsant drugs (19). The quantity of $1\alpha(OH)D_3$ needed may be 1.5 to 3-fold greater than the amount of $1,25(OH)_2D_3$ (12), and on cessation of treatment, the time required for dissipation of a pharmacologic effect is longer with $1\alpha(OH)D_3$ than with $1,25(OH)_2D_3$ (26,27).

Because of the known role of the kidney in the 1-hydroxylation of 25(OH)-vitamin D_3, early attention was directed to trials with $1,25(OH)_2D_3$ or $1\alpha(OH)D_3$ in renal osteodystrophy. However, a number of reports have documented the effectiveness of $25(OH)D_3$ in uremic patients with osteodystrophy (28-32). Eastwood et al have correlated the appearance of osteomalacia in patients seen in the United Kingdom with low plasma levels of 25(OH)D (33), and others have noted a reduction in plasma levels of 25(OH)D in uremic patients given a low protein diet (34). Thus, a deficiency of vitamin D, itself, or $25(OH)D_3$ could exist in a uremic patient and compound the defect in 1-hydroxylation of 25(OH)D to $1,25(OH)_2D_3$. The quantity of $25(OH)D_3$ given to stimulate intestinal Ca absorbtion in uremic patients was 500-1000μg/day (35). Also, Teitelbaum et al (30) observed significant healing of osteitis fibrosa and osteomalacia in 5 patients treated with $25(OH)D_3$, 40-100μg/day. Serum iPTH levels declined but hypercalcemia developed in 3 of 5 patients.

Witmer et al (28) reported improved mineralization and healing of osteitis fibrosa in children given $25(OH)D_3$, 25-300μg/day, for 3 to 16 months. In 4 patients hypercalcemia was observed. Also, preliminary findings on the efficacy of $25(OH)D_3$ in a 6 center study suggest there was significant healing of skeletal abnormalities of both secondary hyperparathyroidism and osteomalacia after 17 weeks of therapy (32). Such data document the efficacy of $25(OH)D_3$ in renal osteodystrophy. It should be noted that Colodro et al (36) found that the quantity of $25(OH)D_3$ necessary to augment urinary Ca absorption was 130-fold greater than the dose of $1,25(OH)_2D_3$; in contrast, the quantity of $25(OH)D_3$ needed in uremic patients was 400-fold greater. Clearly, the quantities of $25(OH)D_3$ necessary to produce an effect are pharmacologic and occur when plasma levels of 25(OH)D are substantially increased above normal. It remains uncertain whether $25(OH)D_3$ has advantages over the use of larger doses of vitamin D_2 or D_3, since optimal treatment with these drugs can lead to healing of renal osteodystrophy in many patients. Fournier et al (29) have suggested that $25(OH)D_3$ may have selective advantages over $1\alpha(OH)D_3$ in promoting bone formation and osteoid mineralization in patients with renal osteodystrophy $1,25(OH)_2D_3$. Similar conclusions were drawn by Bordier et al (37) when the 2 sterols were compared in patients with nutritional osteomalacia. Further observations comparing the effects of $25(OH)D_3$ or $24,25(OH)_2D_3$ with $1,25(OH)_2D_3$ in patients with renal osteodystrophy will be viewed with interest.

Results indicating the efficiacy of 5,6-trans-vitamin D_3 or 5,6-trans-25-hydroxycholecalciferol have also been reported (38-40). These sterols have a "pseudo-1α-hydroxyl" group due to the rotation of the A-ring (41). The quantities required to produce effects in uremic humans, 0.25 to 5mg/day, are similar to the amounts of dihydrotachysterol (DHT) given, and it is not clear that these compounds possess advantages over DHT or vitamin D_3. All in all, the presently available data provide evidence for the clinical usefulness of $1,25(OH)_2D_3$, $1\alpha(OH)D_3$, and $25(OH)D_3$ in reversing many severe manifestations of skeletal disease in uremia. In addition, evaluation of the therapeutic response to these agents may help separate and identify different "types" of bone disease that may arise from pathogenic processes different from those believed to be dominant. Further studies are necessary to identify the causes of bone disease in these patients.

ACKNOWLEDGMENT

Supported in part, by USPHS Grant AM 14750, Contract AM 5-2234, and VA Research Funds. Vickie Zomar, Karen Kanter and Patti Kentor provided assistance in preparing the manuscript.

REFERENCES

1. Fraser, D.R. and E. Kodicek: Unique biosynthesis by kidney of a biologically active vitamin D metabolite. Nature (London) 228: 764, 1970.

2. Haussler, M.R., D.J. Baylink, M.R. Hughes, P.F. Baumaugh, J.E. Wergedal, F.H. Shen, R.L. Nielsen, S.J. Counts, K.M. Bursac and T.A. McCain: The assay of 1-alpha-25-dihydroxyvitamin D_3; physiologic and pathologic modulation of circulating hormone levels. Clin. Endocrinol. 5: 151s, 1976.

3. Mawer, E.B., J. Backhouse and C.M. Taylor: Failure of formation of 1,25-dihydroxycholecaliferol in chronic renal insufficiency. Lancet 1: 626, 1973.

4. Brickman, A.S., J.W. Coburn and A. W. Norman: Effect of 1,25-dihydroxycholecalciferol, the active metabolite of vitamin D in uremic man. New Engl. J. Med. 287: 891, 1972.

5. Brickman, A.S., J.W. Coburn, S.G. Massry and A. W. Norman: 1,25-dihydroxy-vitamin D_3 in normal man and patients with renal failure. Ann. Intern. Med 80: 161, 1974.

6. Brickman, A.S., D.J. Sherrard, J. Jowsey, F.R. Singer, D.J. Baylink, N. Maloney, S.G. Massry, A.W. Norman and J.W. Coburn: 1,25-dihydroxycholecalciferol. Effect on skeletal lesions and plasma parathyroid hormone levels in uremic osteodystrophy. Arch. Intern. Med 134: 883, 1974.

7. Brickman, A.S., D.L. Hartenbower, A.W. Norman, J.W. Coburn: Actions of 1α-hydroxyvitamin D_3 and 1,25-dihydroxy-vitamin D_3 on mineral metabolism in man. I. Effects on net absorption of phosphorous. Amer. J. Clin. Nutr. 30: 1064, 1977.

8. Henderson, R.G., R.G.G. Russell, J.G.G. Ledingham, R. Smith, D.O. Oliver, R.J. Walton, D.G. Small, C. Preston, G.T. Warner and A.W. Norman. Effects of 1,25-dihydroxycholecalciferol on calcium absorption, muscle weakness, and bone disease in chronic renal failure. Lancet 1: 379, 1974.

9. Eastwood, J.B., M.E. Phillips, H.E. De Wardener, P.J. Bordier, P. Marie, C.D. Arnaud and A.W. Norman: Biochemical and histological effects of 1,25-dihydroxycholecalciferol in the osteomalcia of chronic renal failure, in Vitamin D and Problems Related to Uremic Bone Disease, edited by A.W. Norman, K. Schaefer, H.G. Grigoliet, D. Von Herrath and E. Ritz, W. de Gruyter, Berlin, pp. 595-601, 1975.

10. Silverberg, D.S., K.B. Bettcher, J.B. Dossetor, T.R. Overton, M.F. Holick and H. F. DeLuca: Effect of 1,25-dihydroxy-cholecalciferol in renal osteodystrophy. Canad. Med. Assn. 112: 190, 1975.

11. Pierides, A.M., M.K. Wards, F. Ude-Alvarez, H.A. Ellis, K.M. Peart, W. Simpson, D.N.S. Kerr and A.W. Norman: Long term therapy with $1,25(OH)_2D_3$ in dialysis bone disease. Proc. Europ. Dialysis. Transp. Assn.: 12: 237, 1975.

12. Coburn, J.W., A.S. Brickman, D.J. Sherrard, F.R. Singer, D.J. Baylink, E.G.C. Wong, S.G. Massry and A.W. Norman: Clinical efficacy of 1,25-dihydroxy-vitamin D_3 in renal osteodystrophy. In Vitamin D: Biochemical, Chemical and Clinical Aspects Related to Calcium Metabolism, edited by A.W. Norman, K. Schaefer J.W. Coburn, H.F. DeLuca, D. Fraser, H.G. Grigoliet and D. von Herrath; W. de Gruyter, Berlin, pp. 657, 1977.

12a. Schott, G.D. and M.R. Wills: Muscle weakness in osteomalacia, Lancet 1: 626, 1976.

13. Coburn, J.W., A.S. Brickman, D.S. Sherrard, E.G.C. Wong, F.R. Singer and A.W. Norman: Defective skeletal mineralization in uremia without relation to vitamin D, serum Ca or P. Abstract Book, 10th Annual Meeting, American Society of Nephrology, Washington D.C., p. 314, 1977.

14. Gatto, G.R.D., M. MacLeod, B. Pelc and E. Kodicek: 1α-Hydroxy-cholecalciferol: A treatment for renal bone disease. Brit. Med. J. 1: 12, 1975.

15. Chan, J.C.M., S.B. Oldham, M.F. Holick, H.F. DeLuca: 1α-Hydroxyvitamin D_3 in chronic renal failure. A potent analogue of the kidney hormone 1,25-dihydroxycholecalciferol. J.A.M.A. 234: 47, 1975.

16. Davie, M.D., T.M. Chalmers, J.D. Hunter, B. Pelc and E. Kodicek: 1α-hydroxycholecalciferol in chronic renal failure. Studies of the effect of oral doses. Ann. Intern. Med. 84: 281, 1976.

17. Pierides, A.M., H.A. Ellis, W. Simpson, J.H. Deward, M.K. Ward, and D.N.S. Kerr: Variable response to long-term 1α-hydroxy-cholecalciferol in hemodialysis osteodystrophy. Lancet 2: 1092, 1976.

18. Pierides, A.M., M.K. Ward, F. Alvarez-Ude, H.A. Ellis, K.M. Peart, W. Simpson, D.N.S. Kerr and A.W. Norman: Long term therapy with $1,25(OH)_2D_3$ in dialysis bone disease. Proc. Europ. Dialysis Transplant Assoc. 12: 237, 1976.

19. Pierides, A.M., D.N.S. Kerr, H.A. , Ellis, J.L.H. O'Riordan and H.F. De Luca: 1α-Hydroxycholecalciferol in hemodialysis renal osteodystrophy. Adverse effects of anticonvulsant therapy. Clin. Nephrol. 5: 191, 1976.

20. Madsen, S. and I. Olgaard: 1-alphacholecalciferol treatment of adults with chornic renal disease. Acta Med.Scand.200: 1, 1976.

21. Chan, J.C.M., S.B. Oldham and H.F. De Luca: Effectiveness of 1α-hydroxyvitamin D in children with renal osteodystrophy associated with hemodialysis. J. Pediatrics 90: 820, 1977.

22. Nielsen, H.E., F. Melsen, M.S. Christensen, H.E. Hansen, P. Rodbro and A. Johannsen: 1α-Hydroxycholecalciferol treatment of long-term hemodialyzed patients. Effects on mineral metabolism, bone mineral content and bone morphometry. Clin. Nephrol. 8: 429, 1977.

23. Papapoulos, S.E., A.M. Brownjohn, F.J. Goodwin, W. Haldey, F.P. Marsh and J.L.H. O'Riordan: The effect of 1α-hydroxycholecalciferol and secondary hyperparathyroidism of chronic renal failure. In Vitamin D: Biochemical, Chemical and Clinical Aspects Related to Calcium Metabolism (op.cit.) pp. 693, 1977.

24. Pierides, A.M., H.A. Ellis, M.K. Ward, Pl Aljama, J. Dewar and D.N.S. Kerr. The need and use of a phosphate enriched dialysate during regular hemodialysis. Trans.Am.Soc.Artif. Internal. Organs 23: 376, 1977.

25. Tougaard, L. E. Sorensen, J. Brochuer-Mortensen, M.S. Christiansen. P. Rodbro and A.W.S. Sorensen: Controlled trial of 1α-hydroxycholecalciferol in chronic renal failure. Lancet 1: 1044, May 15, 1976.

26. Brickman, A.S., J.W. Coburn, G.R. Friedman, W.H. Okamura, S.G. Massry and A.W. Norman: Comparison of effects of 1α-hydroxy-vitamin D_3 and 1,25-dihydroxy-vitamin D_3 in man. J. Clin. Invest. 57: 1540, 1976.

27. Kanis, J.A. and R.G.G. Russell: Rate of reversal of hypercalcaemia and hypercalciuria induced by vitamin D and its 1α-hydroxylated derivatives. Brit. Med. J. 1: 78, 1977.

28. Witmer, G., A. Margolis, O. Fontaine, J. Fritsch, G. Lenoir, M. Groyer, and S. Balsan: Effects of 25-hydroxycholecalciferol on bone lesions of children with terminal renal failure. Kidney Internat. 10: 395, 1976.

29. Fournier, A.E., P.H. Bordier, J. Gueris, J. Chanard, P. Marie, C. Ferriere, M. Osario, J. Bedrossian and H.F. De Luca: 1-alpha-hydroxycholecalciferol and 25 hydroxycholecalciferol in renal bone disease. Proc. Eur. Dial. Transplant Assoc 12: 227, 1976.

30. Teitelbaum, S.L., J.M. Bone, P.J., Stein, J.J. Gilden, M. Bates, V.C. Boisseau and L.V. Avioli: Calciferol in chronic renal insufficiency. Skeletal response. J.A.M.A. 235: 164, 1976.

31. Eastwood, J.B., T.C.B. Stamp, H.E. De Wardener, P.H. Bordier, C.D. Arnaud: The effect of 25-hydroxy vitamin D_3 in the osteomalacia of chronic renal failure. Clin. Sci. Molec. Med. 52: 499, 1977.

32. Recker, R.R., P. Schoenfeld, J. Litteri, E. Slatopolsky, K. Martin, L. Kleinman, D. Hartenbower, A. Brickman, R. Goldsmith, H. Frost, W. Hee, S. Teitelbaum, D. Kimmel, C. Arnaud, S. Arnaud and R. Heaney: 25- Hydroxyvitamin D in renal osteodystrophy: Results of a six-center trial. Preliminary report. In Vitamin D. Biochemical, Chemical and Clinical Aspects Related to Calcium Metabolism(op. cit.) pp. 649-655, 1977.

33. Eastwood, J.B., E. Harris, T.C.B. Stamp, H.E. De Wardener: Vitamin-D deficiency in the osteomalacia of chronic renal failure. Lancet 2: 1209, 1976.

34. Offermann, E., D. Van Herrath and K. Schaefer: Serum 25-hydroxycholecalciferol in uremia. Nephron 13: 269, 1974.

35. Rutherford, W.E., J. Blindin, K. Hruska, R. Kopelman, S. Klahr and E. Slatopolsky: Effect of 25-dydroxycholecalciferol on calcium absorption in chronic renal disease. Kidney Inter. 8: 320, 1974.

36. Colodro, I.H., A.S. Brickman, J.W. Coburn, T.W. Osborn and A.W. Norman: The Effect of 25-hydroxy-vitamin D_3 on intestinal absorption of calcium in normal man and patients with renal failure. Metabolism (in press).

37. Bordier, P. A Ryckwaert, P. Marie, L. Miravet, A. Norman and H. Rasmussen: Vitamin D metabolites and bone mineralization in man. In Vitamin D. Biochemical, Chemical and Clinical Aspects Related to Calcium Metabolism (op. cit), p. 897, 1977.

38. Gagnon, R., G.W. Ogden, G. Just and M. Kaye: Comparison of dihydrotachysterol and 5,6-trans vitamin D_3 on intestinal calcium absorption in patients with chronic renal failure. Can. J. Physiol. Pharmacol. 52: 272, 1974.

39. Rutherford, W.E., K. Hruska, J. Blondin, M. Holick DeLuca, S. Klahr and E. Slatopolsky: The effect of 5,6-trans vitamin D_3 on calcium absorption in chronic renal disase . J. Clin. Endocr. Metab. 40: 13, 1975.

40. Kraft, D. and G. Otterman: The effect of high doses of 5,6-trans-25-hydroxycholecalciferol on calcium metabolism in relative vitamin D resistance (hypoparathyroidism and chronic renal failure) in Vitamin D: Biochemical, Chemical and Clinical Aspects Related to Calcium Metabolism (op. cit.) ppl 679-680, 1977.

41. Holick, M.F., M. Garabedian and H.F. Deluca: 5,6-trans isomers of cholecalciferol and 25-hydroxycholecalciferol. Substitutes for 1,25-dihydroxycholecalciferol in anephric animals. Biochemistry 11: 2715, 1972.

PHYSIOLOGICAL AND PHARMACOLOGICAL ASPECTS OF 24,25-DIHYDROXY-CHOLECALCIFEROL IN MAN

R.G.G. Russell, J.A. Kanis, R. Smith, N.D. Adams,
M. Bartlett, T. Cundy, M. Cochran, G. Heynen & G.T. Warner
Renal Unit, Churchill Hospital, Oxford; Nuffield
Orthopaedic Centre, Oxford; Dept. Chemical Pathology,
University Sheffield Medical School, England

INTRODUCTION

It is now established that the biological activity of cholecalciferol (vitamin D_3) results from a series of metabolic conversions to more active compounds. (1-3) The first of these conversions is hydroxylation of D_3 to 25-hydroxycholecalciferol (25-HCC), which occurs in the liver. Further metabolism to dihydroxy metabolites (1,25-DHCC, 24,25-DHCC and 25,26-DHCC) then occurs. The synthesis of 1,25-DHCC probably takes place exclusively in the kidney (4), since its production becomes undetectable after nephrectomy. Synthesis of 24,25-DHCC also occurs in the kidney, but possibly also in other sites such as intestine (3) and cartilage (5), both of which can convert 25-HCC to 24,25-DHCC in vitro. The site of synthesis of 25,26-DHCC is unknown. The dihydroxymetabolite which has aroused the greatest interest is 1,25-DHCC, since it appears to be the major biologically active form of the vitamin. Thus at low doses it promotes the intestinal absorption of calcium and phosphate in vitamin D deficient animals or birds, and it increases mobilisation of calcium from bone and heals rickets. The rate of production of 1,25-DHCC is closely controlled by various factors, and it has therefore been considered a hormone derived from the kidney which acts in concert with parathyroid hormone (PTH) and calcitonin (CT) to regulate calcium metabolism. Defective synthesis of 1,25-DHCC, despite adequate supplies of the parent vitamin D_3, is thought to contribute to the abnormalities of mineral metabolism in a number of clinical disorders, including chronic renal failure (6), vitamin D-dependent rickets (7), hypoparathyroidism and pseudo-hypoparathyrodism (8).

In contrast to 1,25-DHCC the biological function of 24,25-DHCC is less clear. In the original animal studies the biological potency of 24,25-DHCC was less than that of 1,25-DHCC, and on the basis of such data it was reasonably supposed that, unlike 1,25-DHCC, 24,25-DHCC was of little physiological importance and may in some species, especially birds (9), represent a stage in the degradation of 25-HCC. However, the renal production of 24,25-DHCC is also regulated and in normal man, together with 25,26-DHCC, it is the major circulating dihydroxymetabolite of vitamin D. (10,11) Several recent reports derived from a variety of studies independently suggest that this metabolite may have specific effects of its own and may be more biologically active than formally appreciated. In this paper we describe in outline some of what is known about the biosynthesis and action of 24,25-DHCC and report some observations of our own which may help to elucidate the function of 24,25-DHCC in man.

Control of Biosynthesis of 1,25-DHCC and 24,25-DHCC

Observations from many laboratories indicates that the activity of the renal 1- and 24-hydroxylase are subject to regulation. Possible regulating factors include 1,25-DHCC itself (1,12) and the prevailing circulating concentrations of parathyroid hormone (PTH), calcium (1-3) and phosphate (2,13), prolactin (14) and oestrogens (14,33). Thus, under experimental conditions of deficiency of phosphate, calcium or vitamin D, 1,25-DHCC is a major dihydroxy metabolite in the blood. The effect of dietary deficiency of calcium, but not of phosphate or vitamin D, may be mediated by increased secretion of PTH. Prolactin and oestrogen may also stimulate 1,25-DHCC production under certain conditions, eg, during growth, lactation and egg-shell formation. In contrast, if the animal is made hyperphosphataemic, hypercalcaemic, or replete in vitamin D, production of 1,25-DHCC diminishes and that of 24,25-DHCC increases. Exogenous agents, such as strontium, cadmium or diphosphonates, may also influence the production of the renal metabolites. (1)

In general the capacity to produce 1,25-DHCC and 24,25-DHCC appears to be reciprocally related. For example, in vitamin D deficiency, 1α-hydroxylase activity is high and 24-hydroxylase activity is low, thereby favouring the synthesis of 1,25-DHCC. In contrast, in states of vitamin D sufficiency, 1α-hydroxylase activity is low and renal 24-hydroxylase activity is augmented. The naturally occurring form of 24,25-DHCC appears to be the 24R rather than the 24S epimer. (16,17) Further metabolism of 24R, 25-DHCC to 1,24R, 25-trihydroxy vitamin D_3 (1,24,25-THCC) can occur (9,17), especially in vitamin D deficient animals, but the importance of this pathway under physiological conditions is unclear (18).

In terms of the relative importance of these several regulating factors in controlling the biosynthesis of 24,25-DHCC, it is thought that 1,25-DHCC itself may be a major factor that raises 24-hydroxylase levels in the kidney (12). Rises in plasma calcium leading to a fall in PTH, or a rise in plasma phosphate, may be of lesser importance in enhancing the 24-hydroxylase. These experimental observations do not however explain the functional significance of 24,25-DHCC, unless one accepts the view that 24,25-DHCC has little biological potency, in which case this alternative pathway for 25-HCC metabolism could provide a means for regulating and reducing the biological activity of vitamin D-like compounds.

It must be emphasised, however, that knowledge of regulation of vitamin D metabolism is derived almost entirely from animal experiments, often under extreme conditions. There is too little comparable information available for man to assess which are the important factors in regulating the production of 1,25-DHCC and 24,25-DHCC. A simple illustration of this is the finding that levels of both 1,25-DHCC and 24,25-DHCC are high in patients with primary hyperparathyroidism (10,11), whereas the experimental data from animals would suggest that although 1,25-DHCC should be high, 24,25-DHCC should be low. The increasing availability of assays (19-22) for the dihydroxymetabolites should enable the control of vitamin D metabolism in man to be clarified.

Plasma Levels and Turnover of 24,25-DHCC

Several groups are now measuring plasma levels of the dihydroxymetabolites in man (8,11,19-22). Normal levels of 1,25-DHCC are in the order of 20-40 ng/l (8,19,20). In contrast, circulating concentrations of 24,25-DHCC may be a hundred-fold higher (11,21,22). Plasma 24,25-DHCC correlates with plasma levels of 25-HCC and may therefore reflect the nutritional status of the patient with regard to vitamin D. Although plasma levels of 24,25-DHCC are much higher than those of 1,25-DHCC it should **not be supposed** that in health the production rates of the two compounds necessarily differ, since plasma levels are also a function of metabolic clearance rates and these may be different.

It is of interest in this respect that under experimental conditions the amount of labelled 1,25-DHCC and 24,25-DHCC produced by the kidney from labelled 25-HCC can be of the same order of magnitude. For example the quantity of 24,25-DHCC produced in vitamin D deficient rats on a high phosphate intake is similar to the quantity of 1,25-DHCC produced under conditions of hypophosphataemia (2,13). Moreover, the "cross over point" where the two metabolites are produced in equal amounts from labelled precursors corresponds approximately to the plasma levels of calcium and phosphate found under physiological conditions. If the inferences made from these animal models are correct and if they apply to man, then in order to sustain plasma levels of 24,25-DHCC a hundred times greater than those for 1,25-DHCC, the half-life of 24,25-DHCC should be considerably longer than that of 1,25-DHCC. This appears to be the case, since radiolabelled 1,25-DHCC has a turnover time ($t\frac{1}{2}$) in plasma in the order of hours (23), whereas the half-life of 24,25-DHCC in rats (17) and in man (10,11) is considerably longer, probably days. Calculations based on such data suggest that the daily endogenous production of 24,25-DHCC in man may be as low as 0.5-1 μg daily, perhaps not greatly different from the production rate of 1,25-DHCC. (Table 1).

Table 1 - Vitamin D Metabolites

	Plasma concentration (μg/l)	Turnover rate $t\frac{1}{2}$ (days)	Production rate (estimated) (μg/day)
1,25-DHCC	0.02 - 0.04	1 - 3	0.5
24,25-DHCC	1 - 5	15 - 40	1.0
25-HCC	5 - 50	5 - 20	10

When comparisons are made between the biological activities of metabolites *in vivo*, more account should be taken of the possible importance of their respective plasma levels and clearance rates. If, for example, plasma levels are a major determinant of the amount of metabolite available to a target tissue, even if the affinity of target tissue receptor for these metabolites differ, apparently relatively inactive compounds such as 24,25-DHCC might assume physiological relevance.

Biological Effects of 24,25-DHCC

Vitamin D exerts its effects by actions on target tissues. These tissues include the intestine and bone and there is some evidence to suggest that muscle (24), parathyroid tissue (25,26, 27), C-cells and the kidney may all also respond to vitamin D. (Table 2). The target tissues that have been most thoroughly investigated are the gut and bone. In the case of 24,25-DHCC the results described below refer to the 24R rather than 24S form, since this is the naturally occurring compound.

(a) Gut. A variety of techniques have shown that 24,25-DHCC in sufficient concentration is able to promote the intestinal absorption of calcium and phosphate (1-3,16,17,28-30). Studies in intact animals suggest that its potency is approximately 20 times less than that of 1,25-DHCC. There seems to be considerable

Table 2 - Possible Biological Activities of 1,25-DHCC and 24,25-DHCC at Physiological Concentrations

	1,25(OH)$_2$vitamin D$_3$	24,25(OH)$_2$vitamin D$_3$
Intestine. -calcium and phosphate transport	stimulates	Stimulates (less potent but higher concentration in plasma)
Parathyroid -PTH secretion	Acute - stimulation chronic - suppression	Acute - suppression Chronic - ?
C-cells -CT secretion	?	Potentiates Secretagogues
Cartilage -Proteoglycan synthesis and sulphation	Inactive	Stimulates
Bone - resorption	Stimulates	Inactive
- formation and/ or mineralisation	Stimulates (? indirect)	Stimulates (? direct)
Muscle	Prevents myopathy	?
Kidney - phosphate reabsorption	? inhibits or promotes (? indirect)	?

variability among species, and the potency of 24,25-DHCC in rats is greater than in the chick. However, some of these studies have not been very extensive, utilising only single doses, so that proper dose-response relationships have not been worked out. Furthermore, potency camparisons can be misleading, unless they take account of differences in metabolism. For example, the effects of 24R, 25-DHCC on intestinal calcium absorption in vitamin D deficient animals appears to depend in part on conversion by the kidney to 1,24,25-HCC (17). Nephrectomy, therefore, reduces the apparent potency of 24,25-DHCC (16,17). Studies in which the metabolites are added to isolated gut systems <u>in vitro</u> (31,32) are less likely to be influenced by further metabolism and to allow a more direct measure of potency. The ability to enhance synthesis of the vitamin D-dependent calcium-binding protein by embryonic chick duodenum <u>in vitro</u> provides the basis for such an assay. In this system 24,25-DHCC is again about 20 times less active than 1,25-DHCC (31). This may seem a surprisingly high potency for 24,25-DHCC in view of the very large (more than 1,000-fold) difference in affinities of 1,25-DHCC and 24,25-DHCC for the isolated intestinal cytosolreceptor protein (8,20,34). Nevertheless, when the 100-fold difference in plasma concentrations of 24,25-DHCC and 1,25-DHCC is taken into account these measurements of potency *in vitro* suggest that both metabolites could be of comparable importance in maintaining intestinal transport of calcium.

(b) *Parathyroid tissue.* Several groups of workers (eg. 26,35) have shown that 1,25-DHCC may transiently augment, whereas 24,25-DHCC may inhibit, the release of PTH. The parathyroids contain a cytosol protein receptor for 1,25-DHCC comparable to that found in the intestine (25). The physiological significance of these findings is not yet known, particularly since *in vivo* it is unlikely that parathyroid cells are subject to abrupt changes in concentrations of the metabolites. Indeed long term studies in animals (27) and man (36) suggest that 1,25-DHCC leads to suppression rather than enhancement of parathyroid secretion. The effects of long-term administration of 24,25-DHCC are unknown.

(c) *C-cells and Calcitonin (CT) Secretion.* There are fewer studies of the effect on calcitonin (CT) secretion, but recently the secretion of CT by trout C-cells in culture in response to cholecystokinin (CCK) was shown to be markedly increased by prior exposure to low concentrations of 24,25-DHCC, whereas 1,25-DHCC had no effect (37).

(d) *Cartilage.* Low concentrations (10^{-13}-10^{-10}M) of 24,25-DHCC promote the synthesis and subsequent sulphation of proteoglycans synthesised by chondrocytes in culture, whereas 1,25-DHCC is without effect (5). This suggests specific effects on one of the target tissues of particular interest in skeletal metabolism. Moreover, cartilage appears to be a site of synthesis of 24,25-DHCC (5). It is also noteworthy that normal differentiation of epiphysial cartilage is maintained in chicks treated with high doses of ethane-1-hydroxy-1,1-diphosphonate (EHDP), whereas it is impaired in vitamin D deficiency (38). Chicks made deficient in vitamin D or treated with EHDP are both lacking in 1,25-DHCC, but with EHDP production of 24,25-DHCC can be maintained (39). These studies therefore indicate that 24,25-DHCC could be the major metabolite responsible for the cellular differentiation of the epiphysis prior to normal mineralisation.

(e) *Bone resorption.* 24,25-DHCC may increase bone resorption *in vitro* (40) but the doses required are several thousand-fold greater than those for 1,25-DHCC. In D-deficient animals the bone-resorbing potency appears to increase and possibly reflects its further metabolism, or longer half-life, or both. Although the effects of 24,25-DHCC on bone resorption in man has not yet been studied in detail, the animal studies would suggest that this is not a major function of 24,25-DHCC, in contrast to 1,25-DHCC.

(f) Bone Formation and Mineralisation. It is helpful to distinguish between factors that influence the formation of bone or cartilage by affecting the synthesis of matrix and the events which lead to their subsequent mineralisation. Surprisingly the role of vitamin D metabolites in the formation and mineralisation of bone and cartilage is still poorly understood. It is tempting to invoke their participation in mineralisation, since deficiency of vitamin D is associated with defective mineralisation. There is however no unequivocal evidence that vitamin D or its metabolites exert direct effects on mineralisation, although recent studies suggest that 1,25-DHCC can mimic many of the effects of PTH on isolated bone cells in culture (41). There is some evidence to suggest that many of the histological changes characteristic of D-deficiency are a function more of changes in extracellular levels of calcium and phosphate than of 1,25-DHCC deficiency (38,42). It is therefore possible that the major effect of vitamin D on mineralisation is mediated through changes in extracellular levels of calcium and phosphate. Certainly there are clinical situations in which levels of calcium and phosphate may be critical for mineralisation. Thus in vitamin D-resistant rickets due to a low renal threshold for phosphate reabsorption, skeletal mineralisation may be partly restored when phosphate levels are raised either by phosphate supplements (43), or indirectly by increasing intestinal absorption of phosphate with vitamin D. Similarly, there is an inverse relationship between phosphate and osteoid mineralisation in patients with chronic renal failure and in patients with Paget's disease (44).

It is clear, therefore, that comparison between the effects of metabolites of vitamin D on mineralisation may depend less on the direct actions of these agents and more on their effects on the extracellular environment. Indeed direct effects of 1,25-DHCC on mineralisation have not been demonstrated *in vitro*, possibly because current test systems are unsatisfactory. In rachitic animals, although larger doses of 24,25-DHCC are required than of 1,25-DHCC,both metabolites can restore skeletal mineralisation (9,15,17). Moreover, as mentioned above, cartilage cells may be a site of synthesis of 24,25-DHCC which, unlike 1,25-DHCC, may promote sulphate incorporation into proteoglycans (5). A further distinction between the effects of 1,25-DHCC and 24,25-DHCC on skeletal mineralisation may be inferred from the human disorder of vitamin D-dependent rickets. If, as is thought, this disease is due to renal 1α-hydroxylase deficiency (7,45), then 25-HCC and 24,25-DHCC may still be synthesised normally. The failure of skeletal mineralisation in this disease is therefore more likely to be the result of deficiency of 1,25-DHCC rather than of 24,25-DHCC or 25-HCC.

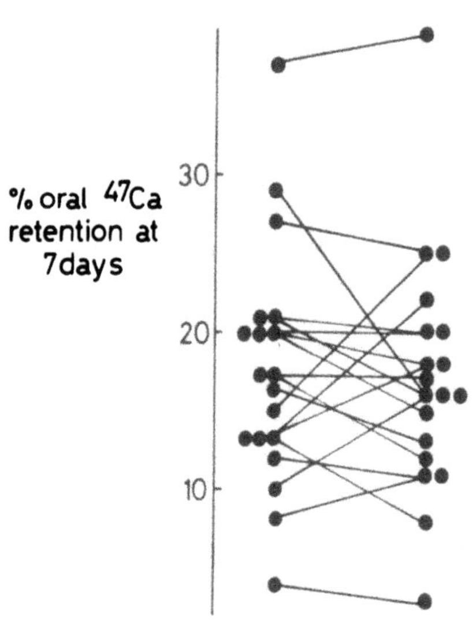

Fig. 1 - Intestinal absorption of calcium in healthy persons (on left) and in patients treated by haemodialysis for end-stage chronic renal failure (on right). None were receiving vitamin D or its derivatives. Calcium absorption was measured on a total body counter and was expressed as the % of an oral dose of ^{47}Ca given in 200 mg Ca (as Ca gluconate) retained after 7 days. Patients fasted for at least 4 hours before (usually overnight) and at least 2 hours after the test dose. ● denotes anephric patients. Note the lower absorption (P <0.001) in chronic renal failure with no obvious difference between patients with and without kidneys.

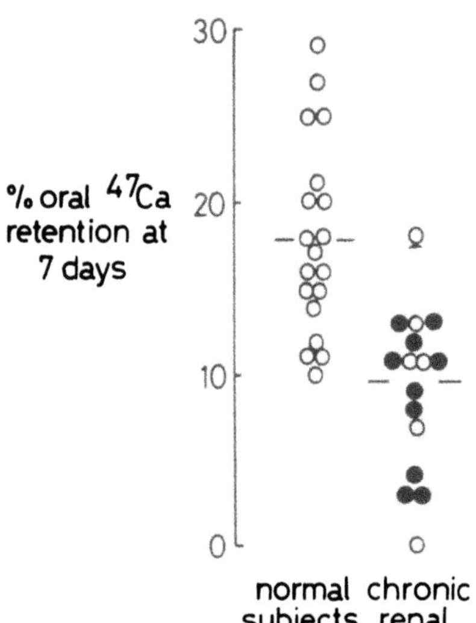

Fig. 2 - Reproducibility of measurements of intestinal absorption of calcium (total body counter method, see Fig. 1) in untreated subjects. The mean difference (±S.E.M.) between repeat tests was 0.5 ± 1.4%.

Studies with 24,25-DHCC Administered to Man

Our preliminary studies (4,6) in man suggest that intestinal absorption of calcium is increased by comparatively small oral doses (1-10 μg/day) of 24,25-DHCC (see figs. 3-5). Increases in retention of orally administered ^{47}Ca as measured by a total body counter (Figs. 3&4) have occurred both in normal subjects and in patients without kidneys maintained on haemodialysis. The interpretation of results of calcium absorption studies undertaken in this way depends upon considerations such as the total amount of calcium given and the unmeasured potential losses in dialysis fluid or urine. An apparent increase in ^{47}Ca retention does not necessarily reflect increased absorption through the gut nor increases in the net retention of calcium. Some of these uncertainties have been overcome by the use of traditional balance techniques, which confirm that 24,25-DHCC can increase the retention of calcium in patients with a variety of skeletal disorders (Table 3). Unfortunately, such techniques are difficult to apply to anephric patients and have not yet been done.

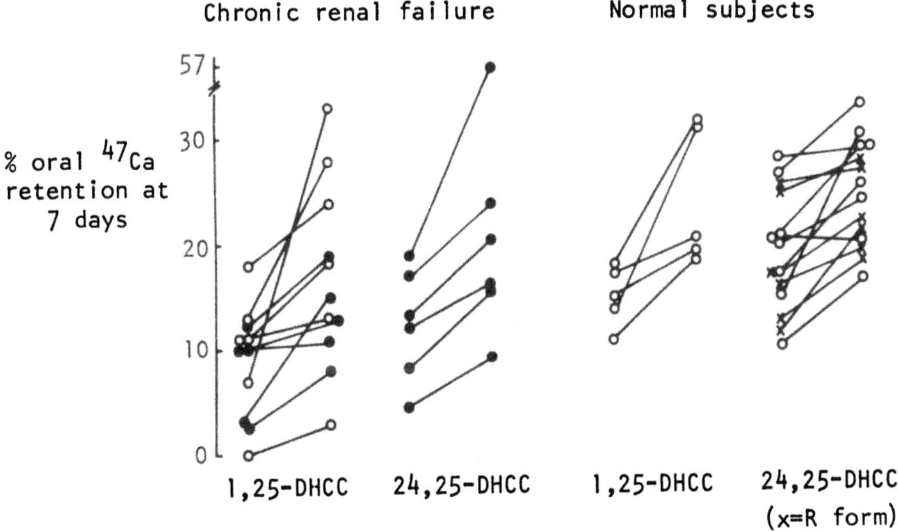

Fig. 3 - Intestinal absorption (see Fig. 1) of calcium before and on the 4th day of treatment with 1,25-DHCC or 24,25-DHCC, given by mouth at 1 μg/day (except one normal person given 2 μg/day) for a total of 7 days to healthy persons or patients with chronic renal failure on haemodialysis (● = anephric). The metabolites were chemically synthesised (52) and a kind gift from Hoffman La Roche, USA. Six of the normal subjects (denoted x) received a mixture of the R and S epimers of 24,25-DHCC (predominantly R), the remainder received the R form alone (46).

Table 3 - Metabolic Balance Studies

Patient M=male F=female	Age	Dietary calcium (mmol/day)	4-day study period	Dose of 24,25-DHCC (µg/day)	Urine calcium (mmol/day)	Balance of calcium (mmol/day
1. Idiopathic hypercalciuria	(M.34)	29.7	1	0	10.4	+ 1.6
			2	2	7.6	+ 13.1
2. Osteogenesis Imperfecta	(F.67)	9.1	1	0	1.8	- 1.7
			2	0	1.8	- 1.8
			3	2	2.0	- 0.1
			4	0	2.6	- 2.3
3. Type 1 Hypophosphataemic osteomalacia	(F.64)	15.2	1	0	1.5	- 3.1
			2	0	1.3	- 2.5
			3	2	1.2	- 0.5
			4	0	1.3	- 2.9
			5	10	1.3	- 0.1
4. Post-surgical Hypopara-thyroidism	(F.61)	37.3	1	0	3.7	+ 2.1
			2	1	3.3	+ 2.1
			3	10	3.2	+ 8.9
5. Idiopathic osteoporosis	(M.46)	22.5	1	0	3.7	- 3.4
			2	0	4.1	- 4.5
			3	2	4.6	- 5.0
			4	2	4.1	- 4.8
6. Idiopathic hypo-parathyroidism	(M.67)	49.3	1	0	1.4	+ 2.4
			2	4	2.0	+ 3.9

Balances were performed by standard techniques (51) using carmine as an external marker and copper thiocyanate as a continuous internal marker.

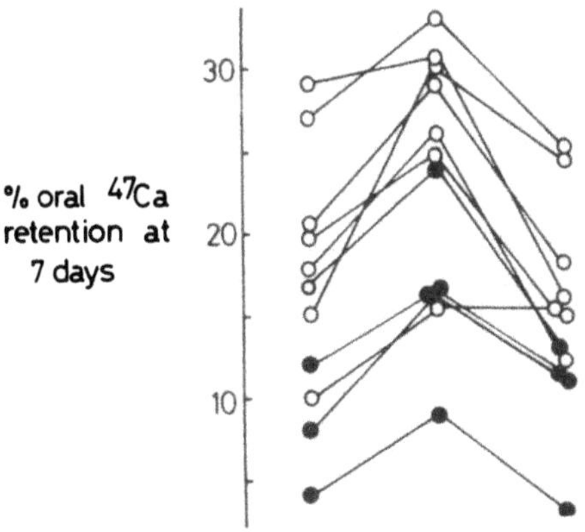

Fig. 4 - Intestinal absorption of calcium measured before and 4 days after starting a 7-day course of 1 μg/day of 24,25-DHCC. Absorption was measured again 4 days after stopping 24,25-DHCC in these 4 anephric and 7 normal subjects. Note return of absorption values towards baseline when treatment was withdrawn

The question arises whether the activity of 24,25-DHCC is a direct one or results from its further metabolism. It is also possible that 24,25-DHCC stimulates calcium transport indirectly by causing increased production of 1,25-DHCC or other hormones that act on the gut. Indeed, 24,25-DHCC may augment the synthesis of 1α-hydroxylase in experimental animals (1). If this were true in man, calcium absorption could be enhanced by the increased endogenous production of 1,25-DHCC or by the facilitated conversion of 24,25-DHCC to the potentially active 1,24,25-THCC.

In man it is unknown whether 1,24,25 THCC is formed at all under normal physiological conditions, either from 24,25-DHXX by 1α-hydroxylation, or from 1,25-DHCC by the 24-hydroxylase. In animals production of 1,24,25-THCC by either route is favoured when production of the respective immediate precursor is depressed. It seems less likely that formation of 1,24,25-THCC accounts for the apparent activity of 24,25-DHCC in man than in animal studies since the normal subjects studied (Figs. 3 & 4) were not deficient in vitamin D and therefore would be expected to have low 1α-hydroxylase activity. Moreover, responses to 24,25-DHCC occurred in a patient with hypoparathyroidism (Table 3), in whom 1α-hydroxylase activity would be expected to be suppressed, and also in the anephric patients (Figs. 3 & 4) in whom 1α-hydroxylase activity should have been absent, at least in the kidney. Further metabolism of 24,25-DHCC by other routes cannot however be excluded, even in anephric patients, since tracer studies have shown that 25-HCC can be metabolised to more polar metabolites in such patients (47).

If the metabolic clearance rates from plasma differ by as much as suggested (Table 1) then small doses of 24,25-DHCC might be expected to produce larger and longer-lasting increments in plasma levels than those achieved after equimolar doses of 1,25-DHCC. If this is an important consideration it is perhaps surprising that the biological effect of 24,25-DHCC on calcium absorption seemed to persist only for as long as the drug was taken (Fig. 4 and Table 3).

The increased intestinal absorption of calcium and positive calcium balances after 24,25-DHCC were not accompanied by an increase in either plasma or urine calcium (Table 3, Fig. 5). This is in striking contrast to the short-term effects of 1,25-DHCC or 1α-OHCC, which both increase plasma and urine calcium when given at doses sufficient to evoke comparable changes in intestinal absorption. It is probable that the calcium absorbed during treatment with 24,25-DHCC accumulates at different sites than during 1,25-DHCC so that it is not available to raise plasma calcium and thereby to increase the load of calcium filtered at the kidney. It is likely that after 24,25-DHCC the extra calcium is retained in bone. An alternative way of viewing the difference between 1,25-DHCC and 24,25-DHCC is to propose that the increase in intestinal absorption in the case of 1,25-DHCC, but not 24,25-DHCC, is accompanied by an increase in bone resorption, which contributes to the rise in urine calcium.

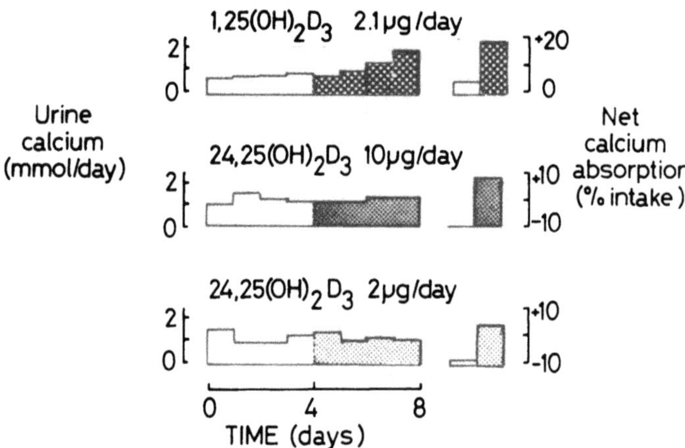

Fig. 5 - Response to 1,25-DHCC and 24,25-DHCC in a patient with type I hypophosphataemic osteomalacia (vitamin D-resistant rickets). Note substantial and similar increase in net calcium absorption (as % of intake measured during balance study) in all instances but that a rise in urine calcium occurs with 1,25-DHCC but not with 24,25-DHCC.

Quite independently, Bordier et al (48) have shown that, in patients with osteomalacia, administration of 25-HCC may restore defective mineralisation more effectively than either 1,25-DHCC or 1α-hydroxycholecalciferol (1α-HCC) alone. The more complete action of 25-HCC is reproduced by treating the patient with a mixture of 1,25-DHCC and 24,25-DHCC. These results may be criticised with regard to the adequacy of daily oral doses of 1,25-DHCC necessary to sustain effective plasma levels of the metabolite. However, the completeness of other responses such as the increase in calcium absorption and suppression of secretion of PTH suggests that metabolism of 25-HCC is a prerequisite for full remineralisation and that 24,25-DHCC, as well as 1,25-DHCC, could contribute to the eventual response.

If 24,25-DHCC is able to directly increase bone formation and mineralisation, it is conceivable that the increase in intestinal absorption of calcium is a secondary rather than a primary event brought about because enhanced bone mineralisation creates an additional need for calcium. The physiological mechanism that could produce this is unclear, but could be passive, or an example of a bone to gut homeostatic control system.

These various observations in man do not show unequivocally that 24,25-DHCC has a direct effect on mineralisation. They do however suggest that the metabolite has effects, direct or indirect, which clearly differ from those of 1,25-DHCC.

Physiological Role of 24,25-DHCC

The biological effects that follow exogenous administration of a hormone or naturally occurring metabolite do not necessarily represent the physiological action of the agent under normal conditions. There is an interesting analogy here with another calcium regulating hormone, calcitonin. Thus, whereas exogenous calcitonin, when given in large amounts, has a powerful inhibitory effect on bone resorption, the role of the endogenous hormone in the physiological control of skeletal homeostasis remains uncertain (49,50).

With these considerations in mind, it is difficult to ascribe physiological roles with any degree of confidence to the vitamin D metabolites. This is as true for 1,25-DHCC as for 24,25-DHCC. Although 1,25-DHCC has been more extensively studied, its production rate in rats and in man under physiological conditions is low and 24,25-DHCC is the major circulating dihydroxymetabolite. Since 24,25-DHCC is produced "electively" under physiological conditions and may exert biological effects, it is not unreasonable to suppose it has a function and that this may differ from that of 1,25-DHCC.

From a teleological point of view it is reasonable to suggest that 1,25-DHCC is involved in the maintenance of a constant extracellular concentration of calcium and phosphate. Its effects on intestinal absorption of calcium and phosphate and their resorption from bone, together with possible effects on secretion of PTH and CT, support this view. Since 1,25-DHCC is probably synthesised in greater amounts under non-physiological conditions not encountered in health, it may act principally as an emergency hormone to mobilise calcium and phosphate.

In contrast, 24,25-DHCC may be the metabolite produced naturally under physiological conditions, which favours accretion of calcium and phosphate into bone by its effects on gut, parathyroid tissue, the C-cells and possibly bone and cartilage itself. Both the accretion and resorption of skeletal calcium may therefore be controlled in part by different metabolites of vitamin D. Production of 1,25-DHCC may increase the availability of calcium or phosphate when calcium and phosphate are scarce and enhance bone resorption. Under physiological circumstances, where bone resorption may be controlled by other factors, the sustained secretion of 24,25-DHCC may ensure normal mineralisation.

Pathophysiological Role of 24,25-DHCC

The relationship between production of 24,25-DHCC and disorders of mineral metabolism in man has not yet been studied extensively, but, in hyperparathyroidism, high circulating levels of 24,25-DHCC have been found (10,11). In view of the possibility that 24,25-DHCC inhibits the secretion of PTH, this might be a compensatory response, but is curious since in animals PTH suppresses synthesis of 24,25-DHCC.

Furthermore, on the basis of tracer studies and direct measurement (10,11), it has been suggested that patients with severe impairment of renal function have low circulating levels or production rates of 24,25-DHCC. In chronic renal failure the association of defective production of 24,25-DHCC, the presence of renal bone disease, and the ability of 24,25-DHCC to augment calcium absorption and retention, might suggest that defective production of 24,25-DHCC and renal bone disease were causally related. Such associations have been used previously to argue causal relationships in the case of 1,25-DHCC, but should be interpreted with caution. Thus, a proportion of patients with renal bone disease do not respond favourably to 1α-hydroxylated metabolites, and in those who do respond, histological changes are often incomplete (44), suggesting that a simple deficiency of 1,25-DHCC is not necessarily a major cause of renal osteodystrophy. Since production of 24,25-DHCC may also be impaired in chronic renal failure, administration of 24,25-DHCC may permit more complete responses in patients with renal osteodystrophy. In this context the crucial question remains of whether the kidney is the sole site of production of both 1,25-DHCC and 24,25-DHCC. There is evidence from tracer studies in man that both metabolites might be produced in anephric patients (47), but these pathways may be relatively minor since both 1,25-DHCC and 24,25-DHCC are usually undetectable after nephrectomy (6,8,10,11). It is probably significant that nephrectomy is not associated with a worsening of renal bone disease and indeed may improve it (50). Possible explanations for this are either that the renal metabolites are relatively unimportant in maintaining the normal skeleton, or that 25-HCC can function alone to maintain the bone with or without conversion to other metabolites. However, not all groups agree that 24,25-DHCC disappears after nephrectomy (22). Continuing improvements in assay techniques should help to resolve these questions.

SUMMARY

The present study describes the response to small oral doses (1-10 μg/day) of 24,25-DHCC in man. Contrary to expectation, 24,25-DHCC was as potent as 1,25-DHCC in increasing intestinal absorption of calcium both in normal persons and in patients with a variety of disorders of calcium metabolism. Despite this increase in intestinal absorption, plasma and urine calcium did not increase after 24,25-DHCC as they did after 1,25-DHCC. Metabolic balance studies showed calcium balances to increase by 1.6 to 11.5 mmoles/day in 5 of the 6 patients studied.

24,25-DHCC increased intestinal absorption of calcium equally well in anephric patients, suggesting that conversion of 24,25-DHCC to 1,24,25-trihydroxycholecalciferol by the kidney cannot be the sole mechanism by which 24,25-DHCC expresses biological activity, even though in vitamin D deficient rats nephrectomy does abolish the ability of large doses of 24,25-DHCC to increase calcium absorption.

It is concluded that 24,25-DHCC may be a calcium-regulating hormone in man. In view of the effects demonstrated here and its relatively high concentration in plasma and slow turnover rate, 24,25-DHCC has the properties that might be ideal for a long-acting stimulator of bone mineralisation. Further work is needed to explain why 24,25-DHCC has effects in man which are not readily seen in other species.

Acknowledgments. We are grateful to the many patients and colleagues who have helped in this work and to the Wellcome Trust, The National Kidney Research Fund and the Peel Medical Trust, who have helped to support these studies.

REFERENCES

(1) DeLuca, H.F. and Schnoes, H.K.: Ann. Rev. Biochem. 45:631, 1976.
(2) Norman, A.W., Friedlander, E.J. and Henry, H.: In Phosphate Metabolism. Ed. Massry & Ritz. Adv. Exp. Med & Biol. vol 81 211, 1977.
(3) DeLuca, H.F.: In Proc. 6th Int. Parathyroid Conf. Excerpta Medica, in press, 1977.
(4) Fraser, D.R. and Kodicek, E.: Nature, 228:764, 1971.
(5) Garabedian, M. et al, In Proc. 6th Parathyroid Conference Excerpta Medica (in press).
(6) Mawer, E.B. et al: Lancet. 1:626, 1973.
(7) Fraser et al: New Eng. J. Med. 289:817, 1973.
(8) Haussler, M.R. et al: In Vit. D. Ed. Norman, A.W. et al. W. de Gruyter, Berlin & New York, p473, 1977.
(9) Holick, M.F. et al: J. Biol. Chem. 251:397, 1976.
(10) Mawer, E.B.: In Vit. D. Biochemical, chemical & clinical aspects related to calcium metabolism. Ed. Norman, A.W. et al. W. de Gruyter, Berlin & New York, 165-174, 1977.
(11) Taylor, C.M.: In Vitamin D. ed. Norman A,W. et al, W de Gruyter, Berlin & New York, 541-544, 1977.
(12) Tanaka, Y. and DeLuca, H.F.: Science. 183:1198, 1974.
(13) Tanaka, Y. and DeLuca, H.F.: Arch. Biochem. & Biophys. 151:566, 1973.
(14) MacIntyre, I.: In Vitamin D. Ed. Norman, A.W. et al. W. de Gruyter, Berlin & New York, 155-164, 1977.
(15) Tanaka, Y. et al.: Biochemistry, 14:3293, 1975.
(16) Tanaka, Y. et al.: Arch. Biochem. Biophys., 170:620, 1975.
(17) Boyle, I.T. et al.: J. Biol. Chem., 248:4174, 1973.
(18) Friedlander, E.J. and Norman, A.W.: Arch. Biochem. Biophys., 170:731, 1975.
(19) Haussler, M.R. et al: Clin. Endocr., 5:151s, 1976.
(20) Eisman, J.A. et al: Arch. Biochem. Biophys., 176:235, 1976.
(21) Taylor, C.M., Highes, S.E. and de Silva, P.: Biochem. Biophys. Commun., 70:1243, 1976.
(22) Haddad, J.G., Min, C. and Walgate, M.: In Vitamin D, ed. Norman, A.W. et al, W. de Gruyter, Berlin & New York, 463-472, 1977.
(23) Mawer, E.B. et al: Lancet, i:1203, 1976.
(24) Birge, S.J. and Haddad, J.G.: J. Clin. Invest., 56:1100, 1975.
(25) Brumbaugh, P.F., Hughes, M.R. and Haussler, M.R.: Proc. Nat. Acad. Sci. USA. 72:4871, 1975.
(26) Care, A.D. et al: In Vitamin D. Ed. Norman, A.W. et al. W. de Gruyter, Berlin & New York, 105-109, 1977.
(27) Capen, C.C., Henry, H.L. and Norman, A.: In Vitamin D. Ed. Norman, A.W. et al. W. de Gruyter, Berlin & New York, 101-104, 1977.
(28) Thomasset, M. et al: In Vitamin D. Ed. Norman, A.W. et al. W. de Gruyter, Berlin & New York, 619-622, 1977.
(29) Chen, T.C. et al: J. Nutrition, 104:1056, 1974.

(30) Boris, A., Hurley, J.F. and Trmal, T.: In Vitamin D. Ed. Norman, A.W. et al. W. de Gruyter, Berlin & New York, 553-563, 1977.
(31) Parkes , C.O.: In Proc. 6th Parathyroid Conference. Excerpta Medica (in press).
(32) Corradino, R.A.: Science, 179:402, 1973.
(33) DeLuca, H.: In Phosphate Metabolism. Ed. Massry, S.G. & Ritz, E. Adv. Expt. Med. & Biol. vol.81:195, 1977.
(34) Brumbaugh, P.F. and Haussler, M.R.: J. Biol. Chem., 250:1588, 1975.
(35) Canterbury, J.M. and Reiss, E.: In Proc. 6th Parathyroid Conference. Excerpta Medica (in press).
(36) Kanis, J.A. et al: Clin. Endocr. (in press).
(37) Roos, B.A. and Frelinger, A.L.: In Proc. 6th Parathyroid Conference. Excerpta Medica (in press)
(38) Bisaz, S. et al: Calc. Tiss. Res., 19:139, 1975.
(39) Baxter, L.A. et al: Arch. Biochem. Biophys., 164:655, 1974.
(40) Reynolds, J.J., Holick, M.F. and DeLuca, H.F.: Calc. Tiss. Res., 15:333, 1974.
(41) Cohn, D. and Wong, G.: In Proc. 6th Parathyroid Con. Excerpta Medica (in press).
(42) Baylink, D. et al: J. Clin. Invest., 59:1122, 1970.
(43) Glorieux, F.H. et al: New Eng. J. Med., 287:481, 1972.
(44) Kanis, J.A., et al: In Vitamin D. Ed. Norman, A.W. et al. W. de Gruyter, Berlin & New York. 671-674, 1977.
(45) Balsan, S. et al: Paed. Res., 9:586, 1975.
(46) Kanis, J.A., et al: In Vitamin D. Ed. Norman, A.W. et al. W. de Gruyter, Berlin & New York, 793-796, 1977.
(47) Gray, R.W., et al: J. Clin. Endocr. Metab., 39:1045, 1974.
(48) Bordier, P.J., et al: In Vitamin D. Ed. Norman, A.W. et al. W. de Gruyter, Berlin & New York, 897-909, 1977.
(49) Heynen, G., et al: Lancet, 2:1322, 1976.
(50) Kanis, J.A., et al: New Eng. J. Med., 296:1073, 1977.
(51) Smith, R., et al: Qrt. J. Med., 42:235, 1973.
(52) Uskokovic, M.R., et al: In Vitamin D. Ed. Norman, A.W. et al. W. de Gruyter, Berlin & New York, 279-293, 1975.

EFFECTS OF PARATHYROID HORMONE AND DIETARY PHOSPHORUS ON THE DECREASED SYNTHESIS OF 1,25-DIHYDROXYVITAMIN D_3 IN RATS WITH GRADED REDUCTION OF NEPHRON MASS

Y. Kawaguchi, Y. Kimura, M. Yamamoto, N. Imamura,
T. Endo, N. Horiuchi, T. Suda, S. Sakai, Y. Ogura, Y. Ueda
Department of Medicine, Tokyo Jikei-Kai University and
Department of Biochemistry, Tokyo Medical and Dental
University, Tokyo, Japan

Kidney plays a critical role for the metabolism of vitamin D_3 by converting 25-hydroxy-cholecalciferol (25-OH-D_3) to 1,25-dihydroxycholecalciferol (1,25-$(OH)_2$-D_3), an active metabolite of the vitamin. It has been suggested that the altered vitamin D metabolism is a major factor for the pathogenesis of renal osteodystrophy. Nevertheless, little data are available regarding the production of 1,25-$(OH)_2$-D_3 in chronic renal failure. We studied the effects of graded reduction of nephron mass on the renal conversion of 25-(OH)-D_3 to 1,25-$(OH)_2$-D_3 in rats. Furthermore, the roles played by parathyroid hormone and phosphorus on renal production of 1,25-$(OH)_2$-D_3 in experimental renal failure were evaluated.

Male Wistar rats were maintained on vitamin D-deficient diet with 0.45% Ca and 0.3% phosphorus for the entire course of the experiment ranging up to 6 weeks (normal P group). Reduction of renal mass was performed at two stages; in the first step, either 1/3 or 2/3 of the left kidney was removed at the end of the third week; a week later contralateral nephrectomy was performed as the second stage of surgery. Appropriate sham-operation was carried out, thus groups of animals with the reduced nephron ranging from 6/6K (intact), 3/6K, 2/6K, 1/6K and to 0/6K (anephric) were obtained. In some groups of rats, dietary content of phosphorus was altered from 0.3% to 0.1% (low P group) or 1.2% (high P group) following the second stage of nephrectomy. Two weeks later, thyroparathyroidectomy (TPTX) was carried out in some rats, and 12 hours later, ^{3}H-25-(OH)-D_3 was administered (see below). Successful TPTX was confirmed by a significant fall, at least 0.6 mg/dl, in plasma calcium level.

The rates of synthesis of 1,25-$(OH)_2$-D_3 were determined 48

Table 1

Nephron Mass	6/6K	3/6K	2/6K	1/6K	0/6K
Chronic Experiment			mean (SD)		
$1,25-(OH)_2-D_3$, %	12.0(2.6)	6.3(0.8)	3.6(1.5)	1.5(0.4)	0*
Plasma creatinine, mg/dl	0.5(0.1)	0.6(0.0)	0.7(0.2)	0.8(0.1	3.5(1.2)
Acute Experiment					
$1,25-(OH)_2-D_3$, %	14.0(2.8)	6.1(0.4)	4.2(0.6)	2.7(0.2)	0
Plasma creatinine, mg/dl	0.5(0.1)	0.5(0.0)	0.6(0.1)	2.0(1.0)	3.7(0.1)

*Anephric for 48 hours as a reference for the lack of 1-hydroxylation

hours (acute experiment) or two weeks (chronic experiment) after the second stage of nephrectomy. The animals received the intravenous injection of ^{3}H-25-OH-D_3, 0.5 μCi per animal, and sacrificed 6 hours later. Plasma samples were analyzed for ^{3}H-1,25-$(OH)_2$-D_3 after extraction and Sephadex LH-20 column chromatography. The conversion of ^{3}H-25-OH-D_3 to ^{3}H-1,25-$(OH)_2$-D_3 was expressed as percent of the latter in total radioactivity recovered. Results of acute and chronic experiments in normal P group are summarized in Table 1.

These data clearly demonstrated that the production of 1,25-$(OH)_2$-D_3 was decreased in proportion to the reduction in nephron mass. It is of note that plasma creatinine rose at 48 hours after 1/6K was produced but at two weeks it returnedto the levels not significantly different from control (6/6K) indicating the presence of compensatory mechanism for renal excretory function. By contrast, the capacity of the kidney to produce 1,25-$(OH)_2$-D_3 remained at a lower level with reduced nephron mass; the rates of 1,25-$(OH)_2$-D_3 production at 2 weeks of renal failure (3/6K,2/6K, 1/6K) never exceeded those at 48 hours at any given level of nephron loss. TPTX suppressed 1,25-$(OH)_2$-D_3 production to levels approximately 60% of control values at any given level of reduction in nephron mass. In rats fed with low P diet, 1,25-$(OH)_2$-D_3 was not higher than that in high P group. Furthermore, TPTX resulted in a marked reduction in 1,25-$(OH)_2$-D_3 production in high P group, while TPTX had little effect in low P group. These results suggest that 1) renal synthesis of 1,25-$(OH)_2D_3$ is closely related to the proportion of residual renal mass; 2) no compensatory increase in 1,25-$(OH)_2$-D_3 production by kidneys with reduced nephron mass, while compensatory mechanism may be operative for renal excretory function in chronic renal failure; 3) TPTX decreased renal production of 1,25-$(OH)_2$-D_3 at any level of reduced renal mass when animals were fed with normal or high P diet. Under these circumstances, PTH may be critical to stimulate renal 1,25-$(OH)_2D_3$ production; and 4) PTH has no significant effect on renal 1,25-$(OH)_2D_3$ production in renal failure when animals were fed with low P diet.

References

1. Bligh, E.G. and Dyer, W.J.: A rapid method of total lipid extraction and purification, Canad. J. Biochem. Physiol. 37; 911, 1957.
2. Holick, M.F. and DeLuca, H.F.: A new chromatographic technique for vitamin D_3 metabolite. J. Lipid Res. 12; 460, 1971.

EFFECTS OF 1,25-DIHYDROXYCHOLECALCIFEROL ON SERUM CALCIUM, PHOSPHATE, AND IMMUNOREACTIVE PARATHYROID HORMONE IN DOGS

S. B. Oldham, R. Smith, D. L. Hartenbower, H. L. Henry

Depts Med & Biochem, USC Sch Med, VA Wadsworth Hosp Ctr,

Dept Med, UCLA Sch Med, Dept Biochem, UC Riverside, CA

Parathyroid hormone (PTH) has been shown to stimulate the formation of 1,25-dihydroxycholecalciferol (1,25$(OH)_2D_3$), the most biologically active form of vitamin D_3, by the kidney (1, 2). It has been postulated that 1,25$(OH)_2D_3$ or other vitamin D_3 metabolites might directly influence the secretion of PTH. Receptors for 1,25$(OH)_2D_3$ have been identified in chick (3) and pig (4) parathyroid glands and in human parathyroid adenoma (5). Accumulation of 1,25$(OH)_2D_3$ by the parathyroid gland has been reported in the chick (6), and 1,25$(OH)_2D_3$ when administered together with 24,25-dihydroxycholecalciferol (24,25$(OH)_2D_3$), caused the size of the parathyroid glands in vitamin D-deficient chicks to regress (7). The effect of vitamin D metabolites on PTH secretion has been examined in several species. Studies several years ago by Oldham, *et al*, showed that the administration of pharmacological amounts of 25-hydroxycholecalciferol (25OH D_3) to vitamin D-deficient dogs appeared to decrease the circulating concentrations of immunoreactive parathyroid hormone (IPTH) before significant increases in serum calcium concentration occurred (8). Chertow, *et al*, reported a decrease in IPTH in rats administered 1,25$(OH)_2D_3$ and an inhibition of IPTH released from slices of bovine parathyroid tissue *in vitro* when 1,25$(OH)_2D_3$ was added to the culture medium (9). *In vivo* studies by Canterbury *et al* (10), and Care and his co-workers (11) in which IPTH was measured in thyroid venous effluent have shown that 24,25$(OH)_2D_3$ inhibited PTH secretion, whereas 1,25$(OH)_2D_3$ either stimulated PTH secretion or seemed to have little effect. Studies in normal man have shown no consistent direct effects of 1,25$(OH)_2D_3$ on IPTH concentrations in the peripheral circulation (12). The present study was undertaken to examine the acute effects of 1,25$(OH)_2D_3$ on peripheral levels of IPTH in the vitamin D-deficient dog and the effects of 1,25 $(OH)_2D_3$ on the response of PTH secretion to changes in serum calcium.

EXPERIMENTAL PROCEDURES

Littermate weanling mongrel puppies were fed a diet deficient in both calcium and vitamin D (13) for at least 3 months and until their serum calcium concentrations had decreased by at least 2.0 mg/dl. To study the acute effects of $1,25(OH)_2D_3$, 1 μg of this vitamin D metabolite was injected i.v. and blood samples were obtained sequentially for 12 hrs. Control experiments were also performed in which an equal volume of 50:50 ethanol:1,2 propanediol vehicle alone was administered. To study a possible effect of $1,25(OH)_2D_3$ on the response of the parathyroid glands to elevations in serum calcium concentration, calcium infusions were performed in vitamin D deficient animals beginning 4 hrs after the injection of either vehicle alone or 1 μg of $1,25(OH)_2D_3$. Rates of calcium infusion were 6-18 mgCa/kg/hr.

Serum IPTH was determined by radioimmunoassay (14). The anti-PTH antiserum used was AS 211/32, obtained from Burroughs-Wellcome Laboratory, London U.K. Bovine PTH was used both for iodination and as a reference standard. Crystalline $1,25(OH)_2D_3$ was obtained from Hoffman La Roche Laboratories. Serum concentrations of calcium were determined by EGTA titration, serum concentrations of phosphorus were determined by the method of Hohenwallner and Wimmer (15).

RESULTS

Acute Effects of $1,25(OH)_2D_3$

A total of nine vitamin D-deficient dogs were administered 1 μg of $1,25(OH)_2D_3$. This had either no acute effect on the peripheral concentration of IPTH (2 dogs) or, as in the example shown in Figure 1, caused an increase in IPTH within the first hour following the injection, (7 dogs). By 12 hrs following $1,25(OH)_2D_3$ the mean serum IPTH had decreased by approximately 30% from the basal value ($P < 0.05$). The animal whose response is shown in Figure 1 appears to have decreased serum IPTH levels at 3 hrs. This was not typical of most animals and may reflect the large amount of PTH released during the initial hour of the experiment. The increase in serum calcium concentration seen at 8 hrs in this animal was seen in the other animals as well. The mean serum calcium was significantly above the basal value during the last 4 hrs of the experiment ($P < 0.05$). There was no significant change in serum phosphorus concentration throughout the experiment. Ad-

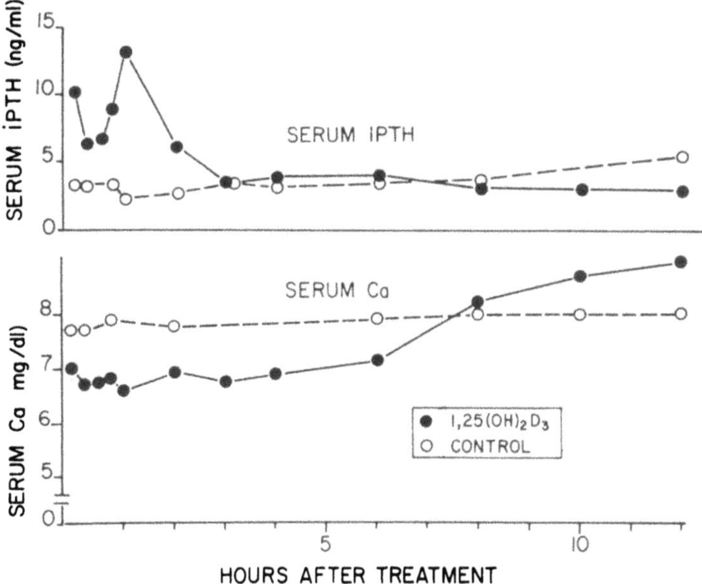

Figure 1. Effect of $1,25(OH)_2D_3$ on Serum IPTH and Serum Calcium in a Vitamin D-deficient Dog. At the beginning of the experiment, 1 ml of either vehicle alone (o control) or vehicle containing 1 µg of $1,25(OH)_2D_3$ (o $1,25(OH_2)D_3$) were injected i.v.

ministration of vehicle alone resulted in no significant change in either IPTH, serum calcium, or serum phosphorus.

Effect of $1,25(OH)_2D_3$ on Parathyroid Response to Calcium Infusions

When calcium was infused rapidly, 10-18 mgCa/kg/hr, serum IPTH concentrations rapidly decreased. There appeared to be no difference in the response of the parathyroid glands to a rapidly increasing serum calcium 4 hrs after receiving either vehicle alone or 1 µg of $1,25(OH)_2D_3$. In both cases, IPTH concentrations became undetectable within 60 min, and there was no significant difference in the mean $\pm$ SEM calcium concentration at which this occurred, 9.84 ± 0.25 mg/dl before $1,25(OH)_2D_3$ and 9.98 ± 0.34 mg/dl after $1,25(OH)_2D_3$. The response of one dog in which serum IPTH was measurable in several blood samples taken during the initial hr of each calcium infusion is shown in Figure 2. As can be seen, the IPTH decreased similarly with an increase in serum calcium both before and after $1,25(OH)_2D_3$.

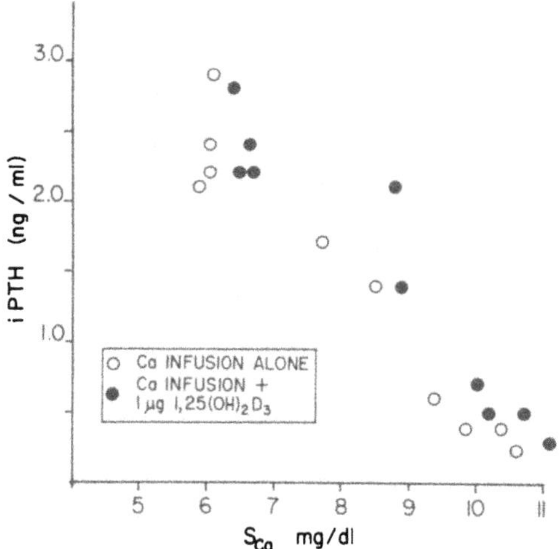

Figure 2. Effect of a Rapid Calcium Infusion on Serum IPTH in a Vitamin D-deficient Dog. Rate of calcium infusion was 15 mg Ca/kg/hr. Infusion was begun 4 hrs after injection of vehicle alone (o) or 4 hrs after injection of 1 μg of $1,25(OH)_2D_3$ (o).

When calcium was infused more slowly, 6-8 mgCa/kg/hr, a different response was observed. The changes in serum calcium, phosphorus, and IPTH during the calcium infusions performed before and after $1,25(OH)_2D_3$ observed in one dog are shown in Figure 3. During the calcium infusion which followed injection of vehicle alone, IPTH failed to change significantly, despite an increase of serum calcium concentrations to within the normal range. During the calcium infusion which was begun 4 hrs following injection of 1 μg of $1,25(OH)_2D_3$, serum IPTH tended to decrease only moderately during the initial 1-1½ hrs of the calcium infusion, but then showed a progressive decrease until the end of the infusion.

DISCUSSION

The results of this study indicate that $1,25(OH)_2D_3$ does not directly suppress PTH secretion in hypocalcemic, vitamin D-deficient dogs. There was, in fact, some evidence for a stimulatory effect of the bolus i.v. injection of $1,25(OH)_2D_3$ on PTH secretion. The stimulus of PTH release caused by an acute injection of 1,25 $(OH)_2D_3$ has been previously observed (10). It seems to be somewhat

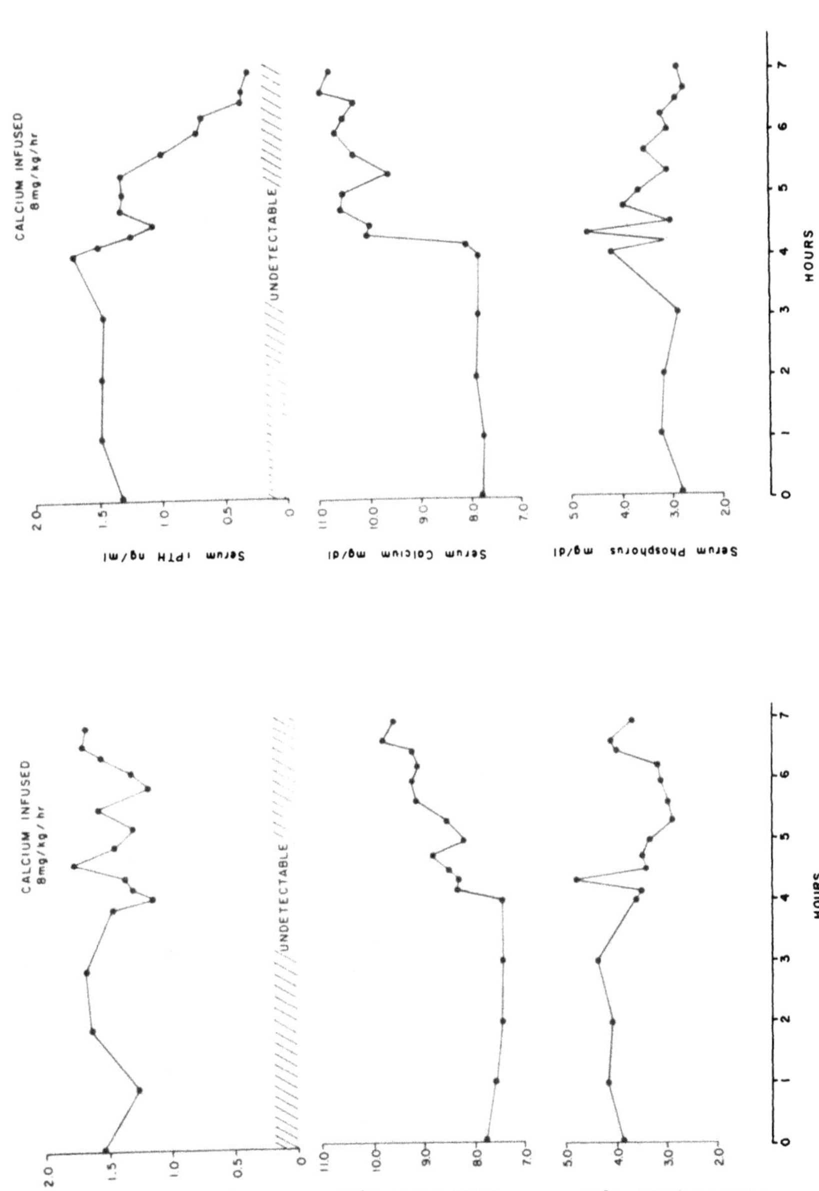

Figure 3. Effect of a Slow Calcium Infusion on Serum IPTH, Calcium and Phosphorus in a Vitamin D-deficient Dog. Rate of calcium infusion was 8 mgCa/kg/hr. Left Panel: infusion begun 4 hrs after injection of vehicle. Right Panel: infusion begun 4 hrs after injection of 1 µg of 1,25(OH)2D3.

specific since 24,25$(OH)_2D_3$ has the opposite acute effect (10, 11). However, the response is so rapid it is unlikely that the process by which these sterols acutely influence PTH release involves a nuclear mechanism. A suppression of serum concentrations of IPTH below basal levels was observed only at 12 hrs, at which time the serum calcium concentration had increased 1-2 mg/dl. These results differ from those of Chertow et al (9) who found significantly decreased serum IPTH levels at 4 hrs following the i.p. administration of 130 pmole of 1,25$(OH)_2D_3$ to 140g normal rats. The dosage we used on the basis of animal weight was approximately 1/5 that used by Chertow and his collaborators. Since both experiments were performed in vivo, it is difficult to be sure in either case whether the response seen was a direct effect of 1,25$(OH)_2D_3$. 1,25$(OH)_2D_3$ can be converted to 1,25,24$(OH)_2D_3$ and presumably other metabolites which may have inhibitory effects on PTH secretion. Another perhaps significant difference is that the rats used by Chertow et al were normocalcemic, whereas the vitamin D-deficient dogs used in our study were hypocalcemic. The serum calcium concentrations have been shown to influence the relative amounts of the different immunoreactive species of PTH in the circulation (16). Since antisera with different immunological specificities were employed to measure serum IPTH in these studies, the different response may reflect altered secretion or metabolism of different species of IPTH. In addition, our calcium infusion studies indicate that the response of the parathyroid gland to 1,25$(OH)_2D_3$ may be influenced by the serum calcium concentration.

The results of our calcium infusion studies indicate that the response of the parathyroid gland depends on the rate and magnitude of the change in serum calcium concentration.. In response to a rapid calcium infusion and a rapidly increasing serum calcium concentration, the parathyroid glands appeared to suppress equivalently before treatment and at 4 hrs following 1,25$(OH)_2D_3$. In contrast, with a slow calcium infusion, the parathyroid glands appeared to resist suppression in the vitamin D-deficient state, but appeared to show increased sensitivity to calcium at 5-6 hrs after treatment with 1,25$(OH)_2D_3$. Parathyroid gland responsiveness to calcium infusions have been previously studied in vitamin D-deficient humans (17, 18). In a study by Fischer et al in which calcium was infused very slowly, serum IPTH was poorly suppressed (17), whereas in a study by Lumb et al, in which calcium was infused more rapidly, IPTH appeared to decrease normally (18). Our results would be consistent with these previous findings. It appears from these studies that there may be two calcium sensitive regulatory mechanisms in the parathyroid gland. One is rapidly responsive to large changes in serum calcium and is not vitamin D-dependent. The second responds more slowly to the steady-state concentration of calcium in the circulation and is affected by 1,25$(OH)_2D_3$. It would, therefore, appear that both the serum calcium concentration and vitamin D status may be involved in determining the functional activity of the parathyroid gland.

REFERENCES

1. De Luca, H.F. and Schnoes, H.K., "Metabolism and Mechanism of Action of Vitamin D", Ann. Rev. Biochem. 45:631, 1976.

2. Norman, A.W. and Henry, H., "1,25-Dihydroxycholecalciferol - A Hormonally Active Form of Vitamin D", Rec. Prog. Horm. Res. 30:431, 1974.

3. Brumbaugh, P.F., Hughes, M.R. and Haussler, M.R., "Cytoplasmic and Nuclear Binding Components for 1α,25-dihydroxyvitamin D_3 in Chick Parathyroid Glands", Proc. Nat. Acad. Sci. USA 72: 4871, 1975.

4. Cloix, J.F., Ulmann, A., Bachelet, M. and Funck-Brentano, J. L., "Cholecalciferol Metabolites Binding in Porcine Parathyroid Glands", Steroids 28:743, 1976.

5. Haddad, J.G., Walgate, J., Min, C. and Hahn, T.J., "Vitamin D Metabolite-Binding Proteins in Human Tissue", Biochim. Biophys. Acta 444:921, 1976.

6. Henry, H.L. and Norman, A.W., "Studies on the Mechanism of Action of Calciferol. VII. Localization of 1,25-Dihydroxy-Vitamin D_3 in Chick Parathyroid Glands", Biochem. Biophys. Res. Commun. 62:781, 1975.

7. Henry, H.L., Taylor, A.N. and Norman, A.W., "Effect of the Vitamin D Metabolites, 1,25-Dihydroxyvitamin D_3 and 24,25-Dihydroxyvitamin D_3 on Chick Parathyroid Gland Size", J. Nutr. in press.

8. Oldham, S.B., Arnaud, C.D., Jowsey, J., "The Influence of Vitamin D on the Parathyroid", in Endocrinology, 1973, Taylor, S., Ed., L. Heinemann, London, 1974, p. 261.

9. Chertow, B.S., Baylink, D.J., Wergedal, J.E., Su, M.H.H., and Norman, A.W., "Decrease in Serum Immunoreactive Parathyroid Hormone in Rats and in Parathyroid Secretion in vitro by 1, 25-Dihydroxycholecalciferol", J. Clin. Invest. 56:668, 1975.

10. Canterbury, J.M., Claflin, A.J., Lerman, S., Henry, H.L., Norman, A.W., and Reiss, E., "In Vivo Effects of Vitamin D_3 Metabolites on Parathyroid Hormone (PTH) Secretion", The Endocrine Society, 58th Annual Meeting, 1976, pg. 65.

11. Care, A.D., Bates, R.F.L., Pickard, D.W., Peacock, M., Tomlinson, S., O'Riordan, J.L.H., Mawer, E.B., Taylor, C.M., De Luca, H.F., and Norman, A.W., "The Effects of Vitamin D Metabolites

and Their Analogues on the Secretion of Parathyroid Hormone", Calc. Tiss. Res. 21(S):142, 1976.

12. Llach, F., Coburn, J.W., Brickman, A.S., Kurokawa, K., Norman, A.W., Canterbury, J.M., and Reiss, E., "Acute Actions of 1,25-Dihydroxy-Vitamin D_3 in Normal Man: Effect on Calcium and Parathyroid Status", J. Clin. Endocrinol. Metab., 1977, in press.

13. Kelly, P.J., "Bone Remodeling in Puppies with Experimental Rickets", J. Lab. Clin. Med. 70:94, 1967.

14. Arnaud, C.D., Tsao, H.S., and Littledike, T., "Radioimmunoassay of Human Parathyroid Hormone in Serum", J. Clin. Invest. 56:21, 1971.

15. Hohenwallner, W. and Wimmer, E., "The Malachite Green Micromethod for the Determination of Inorganic Phosphate", Clin. Chim. Acta 45:169, 1973.

16. Fischer, J.A., Hunziker, W., and Dambacher, M., "Distribution of Circulating Parathyroid Hormone Forms in Normal Subjects and in Patients with Hyperparathyroidism", Clin. Res. 25:390A, 1977.

17. Fischer, J.A., Binswanger, U., Fanconi, A., Illig, R., Baerlocher, K., and Prader, A., "Serum Parathyroid Hormone Concentrations in Vitamin D Deficiency Rickets of Infancy: Effects of Intravenous Calcium and Vitamin D", Horm. Metab. Res. 5:381, 1973.

18. Lumb, G.A. and Stanbury, S.W., "Parathyroid Function in Human Vitamin D Deficiency and Vitamin D Deficiency in Primary Hyperparathyroidism", Amer. J. Med. 56:833, 1974.

Topics on Parathyroid Hormone

CALCIUM-INDUCED MODULATION OF THE TUBULIN POOL IN PARATHYROID GLANDS

C.A. BADER, J.D. MONET and J.L. FUNCK-BRENTANO

INSERM U.90, Hôpital Necker, 161, rue de Sèvres

75730 - PARIS CEDEX 15

Participation of cytoplasmic microtubules has been implicated in various secretory processes such as release of hormone from secretory cells and secretion or movement of granular products (see ref. 1, 2 for review). The great bulk of these works is based on the inhibitory effects of colchicine (3) and vinca-alkaloids (4). The mechanism of action has been attributed to the ability of these agents to bind to tubulin, the protein subunit of the cellular microtubules, and as a consequence, to prevent microtubule assembly. With these techniques it has been shown that colchicine and vinca-alkaloids may affect Parathyroid Hormone (PTH) secretion in *in vitro* culture of Parathyroid Glands (PTG) (5, 6). It has been suggested that these effects may indicate a role of microtubules in the sequence of events leading to release of PTH. Nevertheless although ultrastructural studies of PTG have demonstrated the presence of microtubules (6, 7, 8, 9), anatomical evidence to support a mechanism by which microtubules might affect intracellular processing of PTH are rare. On the other hand in *in vivo* studies the precise site of action of colchicine is difficult to ascertain because it has been shown that this product may produce hypocalcemia (10) and may inhibit bone resorption (11). Moreover recent studies have shown that the renal handling of phosphate and its regulation by PTH may depend on cytoplasmic microtubules, which have been described in proximal renal tubule cells (12). To further assess the presence of a microtubular system (MTS) in PTG and its possible functional significance, we initiated the following studies which extend previous work in our laboratory (13) in order to demonstrate tubulin in PTG on a biochemical basis. After demonstration of a specific Colchicine Binding Protein (ColBP) in PTG, the tubulin pool size level in PTG slices incubated *in vitro* in various extracellular calcium concentrations was assayed.

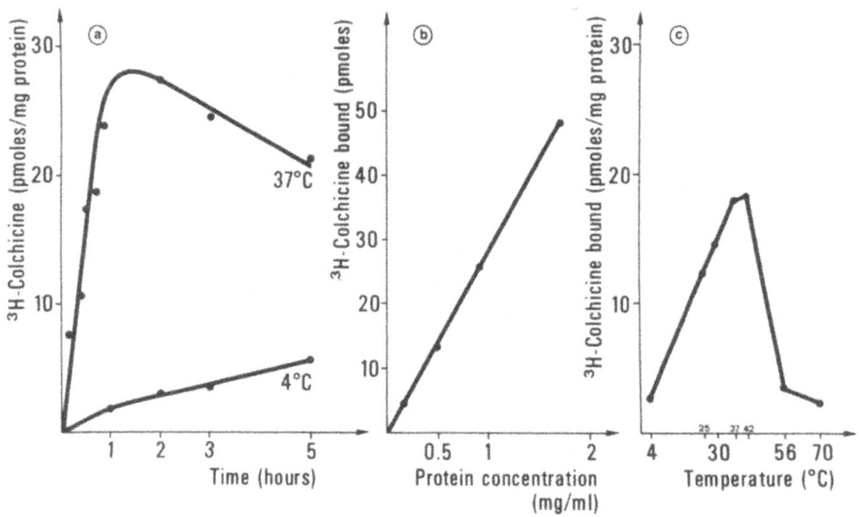

Figure 1 : Kinetic parameters of (^3H) colchicine binding to 48 000 g supernatant of bovine PTG homogenized in SPMG buffer : 100 µl of supernatant aliquots were incubated with 4.5 10^{-6} M (^3H) colchicine. The tubulin - colchicine complex was separated from free colchicine by adsorption of the complex on DEAE-cellulose filter (27). a) final protein concentration 0.86 mg/ml, b) incubation 1h30 at 37°C, c) incubation 1h30 protein concentration 0.86 mg/ml.

TUBULIN IDENTIFICATION

This study was performed by observing the well-known colchicine binding properties of this protein (3) in high speed supernatants of bovine PTG homogenates. Details of experiments are given in figure captions.

Lability of the Colchicine Binding Site

Preliminary experiments showed that the ability to bind colchicine decreases rapidly when high speed supernatants of PTG homogenates in phosphate buffer 10^{-4} M were incubated with (^3H) colchicine. Addition of sucrose, magnesium and GTP to the buffer (SPMG buffer) result in a good stability. Thus the following experiments were performed using homogenates of PTG in this buffer stored in liquid nitrogen. Under these conditions, no significant loss of binding capacity was observed during a three month period.

Abbreviations : SPMG buffer : 0.25 M sucrose ; 0.5 mM $MgCl_2$; 0.1 mM GTP in 10 mM phosphate buffer, pH 6.95. DMSO : Dimethylsulfoxide.

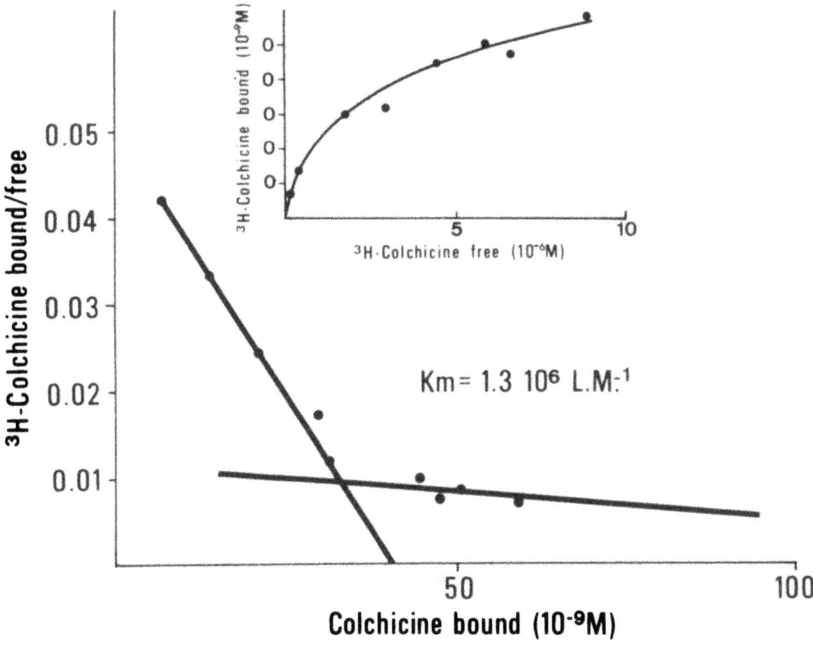

Figure 2 : Scatchard plot of colchicine binding to PTG 48 000 g supernatant fraction. Saturation curve is shown in the insert.

Kinetic Parameters of ^{3}H-Colchicine Binding

The following parameters of the binding of ^{3}H colchicine were investigated. The binding is dependant on cytosolic protein concentration and is linear in all the range of values assayed (Fig 1a). Time course of binding shows that the binding is complete in about 60 min. after which there is a plateau followed by a decline in binding (Fig 1b). Binding is strongly temperature dependant : minimal at 4°C, it is maximal at 37°C after which binding falls off sharply (Fig 1c). Colchicine binding capacity is a saturable process with a binding constant of 1.3 10^6 $L.M^{-1}$. (Fig 2).

Specificity of the Colchicine Binding Site

Proof of the specificity of the colchicine binding was obtained using lumicolchicine -a photoisomere of colchicine- which lacks antimitotic activity and does not bind to tubulin (4). Figure 3 shows that lumicolchicine neither had affinity nor effects upon colchicine Binding Activity (Col BA) in PTG homogenates. Another evidence which can be used to ascertain the specificity of the

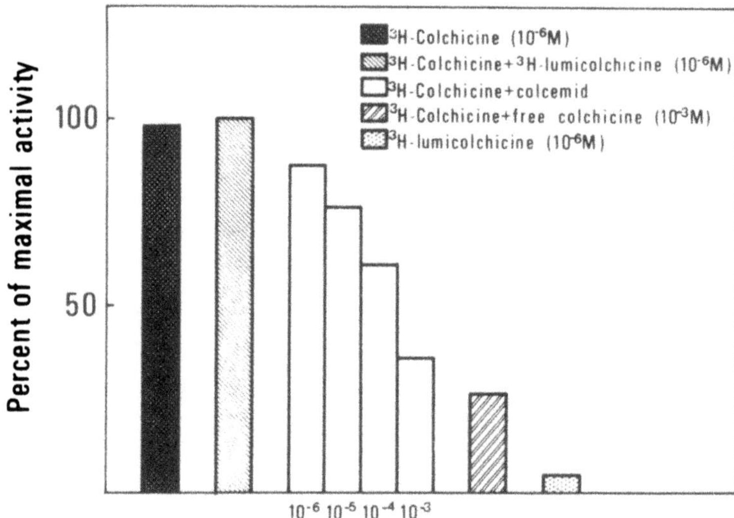

Figure 3 : Specificity of the colchicine binding site : No effect of lumicolchicine and competitive inhibition of colcemid upon colchicine binding to tubulin.

colchicine binding was obtained using colcemid, a chemical analogue of colchicine (14). This compound competitively inhibits colchicine binding (Fig 3).

Purification of Tubulin in PTG

As the preceding properties, i.e., kinetic parameters, specific colchicine binding activity as well as biochemical characteristics we have previously studied (13) -Molecular Weight of 110 000 and Sedimentation Constant 6.1 S- strictly resemble that of the well-known neurotubulin (15), we will refer to it in the following sections as tubulin.

Purification of this tubulin was attempted by chromatography of PTG supernatants on Sepharose 6B followed by DEAE - A25 ion-exchange chromatography (Fig 4). This results in a purification of 22 to 25 times as compared to the initial specific Col BA in the homogenate. All these experiments showed a low content of tubulin in the cytosolic fraction of PTG which was estimated as 1 - 2 % of total soluble protein.

This tubulin was found in porcine and bovine PTG as well as in human PTG tissues.

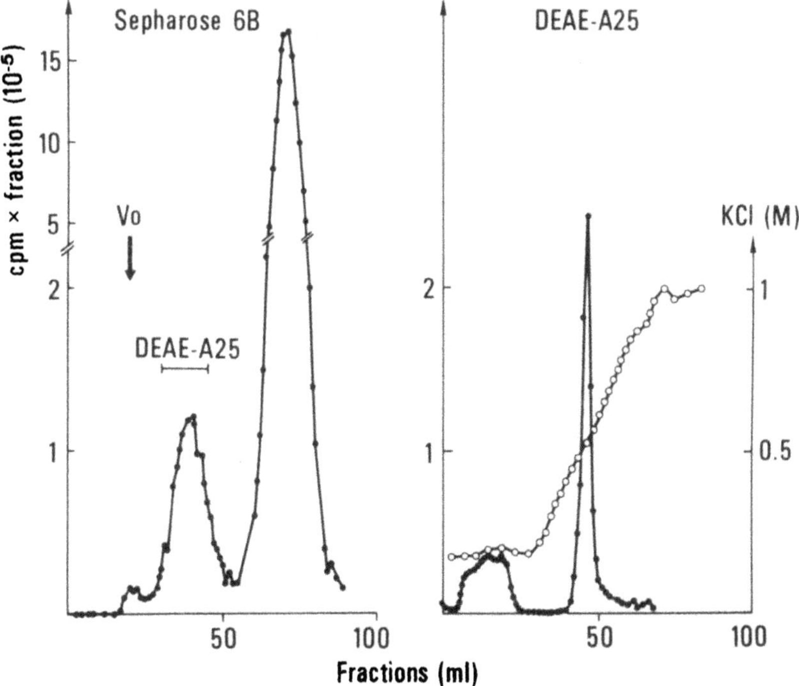

Figure 4 : Chromatography on Sepharose 6B followed by ion-exchange chromatography on DEAE A 25 of PTG supernatant. 1.5 ml in buffer SPMG was incubated with 4 µM (^3H) colchicine final concentration for 1 hour at 37°C and then chromatographied on a 2.6 cm x 38 cm column of Sepharose 6B. The fractions eluting between 32-45 ml were combined and applied to a 0.9 x 5 cm column of DEAE A 25 cellulose previously equilibrated with buffer SPMG. The column was first eluted with 20 ml of buffer SPMG containing 0.2 M KCl and then by a linear gradient from 0.2 to 1 M KCl in the same buffer. The tubulin peak appeared between 0.50 and 0.55 M KCl.

EXTRACELLULAR CALCIUM AND THE MTS IN PTG

In the second part of this paper we present evidence for the regulation of the tubulin pool in PTG slices incubated *in vitro* in various calcium concentrations.

This was performed using bovine PTG slices from freshly-killed animals. They were incubated at 37°C in Minimum Essential Medium (Eagle) with calcium free Earle's salt (GIBCO). Calcium concentrations were adjusted using the required quantity of $CaCl_2$. Quantification of the tubulin pool was performed using the specific colchicine binding assay described above.

Results of this study show that the tubulin pool is both depen-

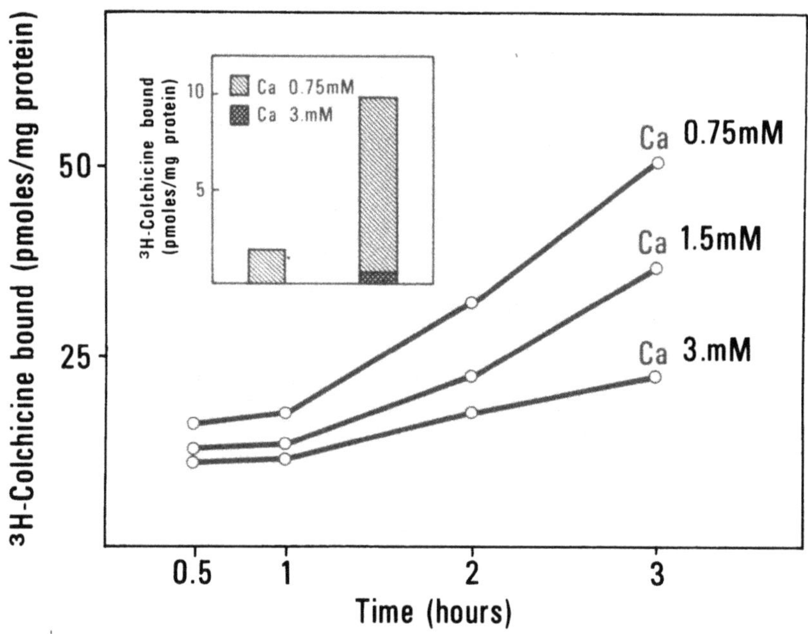

Figure 5 : Soluble tubulin pool as a function of extracellular calcium concentration and incubation time : bovine PTG slices (10 - 20 mg) were incubated in 2 ml MEM at the indicated calcium concentration and time. After incubation slices were rapidly frozen and tubulin was extracted by homogenization in SPMG. Assay of Col BA in supernatants was used to quantitate the total tubulin pool. Insert shows result of an experiment in which after having incubated in an hypocalcemic media for 1 h30, the slices were further incubated partly in the same media and partly in an hypercalcemic media.

dant on the incubation time as well on the extracellular calcium concentration (Fig 5) : 1) There is an inverse relationship between the amount of the soluble tubulin pool and the calcium concentration in the media. 2) There is a continuously increasing pool of tubulin during a 3 hour incubation period. It was also shown (Fig 5 insert) that when PTG slices, after having been incubated in low calcium concentration (0.75 mM), are further incubated in high calcium concentration (3 mM), the tubulin pool is strongly reduced as compared to slices which have been left for the same incubation time in an hypocalcemic media. These results suggest that the tubulin pool in PTG may be a calcium dependant protein.

To obtain at least an insight into the ratio between the free tubulin and the portion which is polymerized as microtubules, the same experiments were performed by separating free and polymerized tubulin. This was done using a temperature dependant process combined with the use of glycerol and DMSO as microtubules stabi-

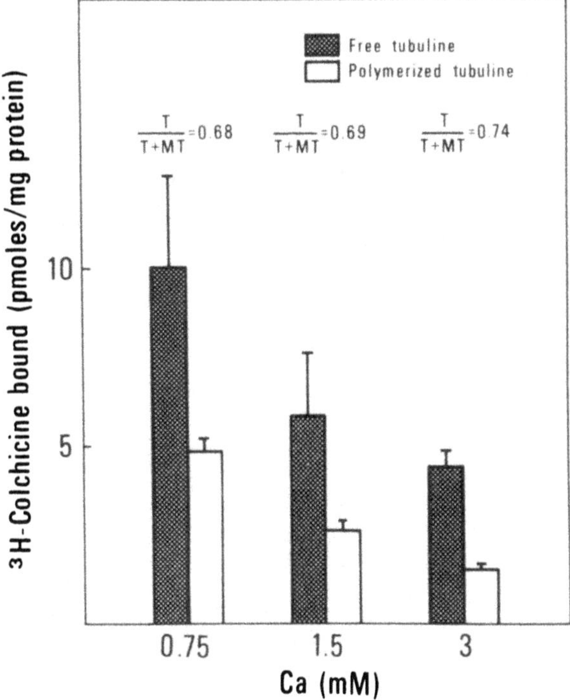

Figure 6 : Free and polymerized forms of tubulin in PTG as a function of extracellular calcium concentrations. Separation of the two forms was achieved by extracting slices first in SPMG buffer containing glycerol 4 M and DMSO 5 % at room temperature 15 min. 12 000 g (supernatant I). Pellets were depolymerized by cooling at 4°C - 30 min., centrifuged 15 min. 12 000 g (supernatant II). Assay of Col BA was performed in supernatant I (Free tubulin T) and supernatant II (Microtubules MT). The ratio T/T + MT were computed and were found not significantly different ($p > 0.05$).

lizing agents and differential centrifugation (16). Figure 6 shows that the two forms of tubulin decrease when calcium concentration in the media were increased, but the ratio between free tubulin (T) and total pool of tubulin (T + MT) are not significantly altered and remain about 70 %.

DISCUSSION

Participation of a microtubular system in the secretory process of PTH has been previously demonstrated using the inhibition of PTH secretion by vinca-alkaloids (5 - 6). Using colchicine and vinblastine the precise site of action was ascribed to the conversion step of proparathyroid hormone to PTH (17). Ultramicroscopic examination of rat (8 - 9), bovine (7) and human (6) PTG reveal the presence of a few organized microtubules in these tissues. Our study demonstrates unambiguously the presence of a tubulin in PTG whose properties are very similar to the most studied form of tubulin, i.e., neurotubulin (15). This then provides the possibility of a biochemical study concerning the possible role of MTS in PTG.

This functional role was at first investigated by measuring the tubulin pool size in PTG slices incubated in vitro in various extracellular calcium concentrations. Our results suggest that calcium may modulate the tubulin pool at least during short incubation periods, but whithout modifying the equilibrium between free tubulin subunits and microtubules.

The mechanism by which external calcium may affect the MTS in PTG is difficult to explain on the basis of present knowledge. Nevertheless, the following hypothesis can be suggested by comparison with other systems : a) MTS may act in the ionic transfer between extracellular and cellular media and/or in the intracellular ionic transfer. Such a possibility is supported by studies showing interrelationships between ionic fluxes and MTS in bone (11) kidney (12) and the gill of seawater teleost fish (18). b) Tubulin and calcium have been shown to have many interactions : tubulin has calcium binding properties (19), and calcium as well as magnesium, have been shown to be able to regulate the dynamic equilibrium between the free tubulin subunits and the polymerized form both in cellular (20) and in in vitro systems (21). c) calcium may act on the MTS via the cAMP system. In fact calcium is a potent inhibitor of the adenylate cyclase enzyme in PTG (22). On the other hand cAMP has been demonstrated to be implicated in the secretion process of PTH (23) and to participate in the regulation of MTS (24). d) calcium may act directly on tubulin synthesis in PTG as to adjust in the endocrine cells the proper amount needed the synthetic and/or secretion process. In this context it has been previously shown that calcium regulates PTH synthesis and secretion as well as those of other proteins (25 - 26).

In conclusion it is worthwhile to note the close interrelationships between factors which are implicated both in the PTH secretion process and in the properties of the cytosolic microtubules. Among these factors calcium seems to be essential.

REFERENCES

1 - The Biology of Cytoplasmic Microtubules. D. Soifer (Ed.), Annals of the New York Academy of Sciences, Volume 253, 1975.

2 - Wolff, J. and Williams, J.A. : The Role of Microtubules and Microfilaments in Thyroid Secretion. Rec. Prog. Horm. Res. 29 : 229, 1973.

3 - Borisy, G.G. and Taylor, E.W. : The Mechanism of Action of

Colchicine. J. Cell. Biol. 34 : 525, 1967.

4 - Wilson, L. : Properties of Colchicine Binding Protein from Chick Embryo Brain. Interactions with Vinca-Alkaloids and Podophyllotoxin. Biochemistry : 9, 4999, 1970.

5 - Chertow, B.S, Williams, G.A., Kiani, R, Stewart, K.L., Hargis, G.K. and Flayter, R.L. : The Interactions Between Vitamin A, Vinblastine, and Cytochalasin B in Parathyroid Hormone Secretion. Proc. Soc. Exp. Biol. Med. 147 : 16, 1974.

6 - Chertow, B.S., Manke, D.J., Williams, G.A., Baker, G.R., Hargis, G.K. and Buschmann, R.J. : Secretory and Ultrastructural Responses of Hyperfunctioning Human Parathyroid Tissues to Varying Calcium Concentration and Vinblastine. Lab. Invest. 36 : 198, 1967.

7 - Chertow, B.S., Buschmann, R.J. and Henderson, W.J. : Subcellular Mechanisms of Parathyroid Hormone Secretion. Lab. Invest. 32 : 190, 1975.

8 - Reaven, E.P. and Reaven G.M. : A Quantitative Ultrastructural Study of Microtubule Content and Secretory Granule Accumulation in Parathyroid Glands of Phosphate- and Colchicine- Treated Rats. J. Clin. Invest. 56 : 49, 1975.

9 - Reaven, G.M, Reaven, P.D. and Reaven, E.P. : Hypercalcemia in Acute Uremia and Following Citric Acid Administration : Differential Effect on Parathyroid Gland Microtubule Content. Metabolism, 25 : 203, 1976.

10 - Heath, D.A., Palmer, J.S. and Aurbach, G.D. : The Hypocalcemic Action of Colchicine. Endocrinology, 90 : 1589, 1972.

11 - Raisz, L.G., Holtrop, M.E. and Simmons, H.A. : Inhibition of Bone Resorption by Colchicine in Organ Culture. Endocrinology, 92 : 556, 1973.

12 - Dousa, T.P., Duarte, C.G. and Knox, F.G. : Effect of Colchicine on Urinary Phosphate and Regulation by Parathyroid Hormone. Amer. J. Physiol. 231 : 61, 1976.

13 - Bader, C., Monet, J.D., Chanard, J. and Funck-Brentano, J.L. : Mise en évidence d'une protéine microtubulaire (Tubuline) dans le cytosol de la parathyroïde de porc. C.R. Acad. Sc. Paris, 282 : 2099, 1976.

14 - Zweig, M.H. and Chignell, C.F. : Interaction of some Colchicine Analogs, Vinblastine and Podophyllotoxin with Rat Brain Microtubule Protein. Biochem. Pharmacol. 22 : 2141, 1973.

15 - Eipper, B.A. : Rat Brain Microtubule Protein :Purification and Determination of Covalently Bound Phosphate and Carbohydrate. Proc. Nat. Acad. Sci. U.S.A. 69 : 2283, 1972.

16 - Pipeleers, D.G., Pipeleers-Marichal, M.A. and Kipnis, D.M. : Microtubule Assembly and the Intracellular Transport of Secretory Granules in Pancreatic Islets. Science, 191 : 88, 1976.

17 - Kemper B., Habener J.F., Rich, A and Potts, J.T., Jr. : Microtubules and the Intracellular Conversion of Proparathyroid Hormone to Parathyroid Hormone. Endocrinology, 96 : 903, 1975.

18 - Maetz, J. and Pic, P. Microtubules in the "Chloride Cell" of the Gill and Disrupting Effects of Colchicine on the Salt-Balance of the Sea-Water Adapted Mugil Capito. J. Exp. Zool. 199 : 325, 1976.

19 - Solomon, F. : Binding Sites for Calcium on Tubulin. Biochemistry, 16 : 358, 1977.

20 - Schliwa, M. : The Role of Divalent Cations in the Regulation of Microtubule Assembly. J. Cell. Biol. 70 : 527, 1976.

21 - Olmsted, J.B. and Borisy, G.G. : Ionic Nucleotide Requirements for Microtubule Polymerization in Vitro. Biochemistry, 14 : 2996, 1975.

22 - Matsuzaki, S. and Dumont, J.E. : Effect of Calcium Ion on Horse Parathyroid Gland Adenyl Cyclase. Biochim. Biophys. Acta. 284 : 227, 1972.

23 - Williams, G.A., Hargis, G.K., Bowser, E.N., Henderson, W.J. and Martinez, N.J. : Evidence for a Role of Adenosine 3', 5'-Monophosphate in Parathyroid Hormone Release. Endocrinology, 92 : 687, 1973.

24 - Gillespsie, E. : Microtubules, Cyclic AMP, Calcium, and Secretion. In Ref. 1, p. 771.

25 - Raisz, L.G. : Effects of Calcium on Uptake and Incorporation of Amino Acids in the Parathyroid Glands. Biochim. Biophys. Acta. 148 : 460, 1967.

26 - Kemper, B., Habener, J.F., Rich, A. and Potts, J.T., Jr. : Parathyroid Secretion : Discovery of a Major Calcium-Dependent Protein. Science, 184 : p. 167, 1974.

27 - Weisenberg, R.C., Borisy, G.G. and Taylor, E.W. : The Colchicine-Binding Protein of Mammalian Brain and its Relation to Microtubules. Biochemistry, 7 : 4466, 1968.

PARATHYROID HORMONE METABOLISM IN NORMAL AND UREMIC MAN

N.Lustenberger, R.Hehrmann, H.Jüppner and R.D.Hesch

Department Innere Medizin, Medizinische Hochschule

Hannover, W. Germany

For low-molecular weight proteins, the kidney is regarded to be a primary organ of catabolism by means of glomerular filtration and tubular metabolism (1). In chronic renal failure increased plasma levels of low-molecular weight proteins ("middle molecules", MW 350-2.000) are assumed to be toxic, contributing to the "uremic syndrome" (2).

High levels of circulating immunoreactive parathyroid hormone (iPTH) is a constant finding in uremic patients despite the fact that in some cases there is litte evidence for the presence of hyperparathyroidism (3).

Plasma level of PTH (Figure 1.) results from 1) secretion of the intact (1-84) hormone molecule (4,5,6) by the glands and 2) metabolic turnover by binding to receptors in its main target organs: bone, kidney, liver (7,8,9) and cleavage of the intact hormone to its degradation products, known to take place in the liver (10,11) and in the kidney (11-16).

Influence of impaired kidney function on parathyroid hormone metabolism has been tested in man after parathyroidectomy (17,18) and in dogs before and after nephrectomy (18,20).

The present study was undertaken to evaluate the role of the kidney in PTH turnover in man, using specific assays for intact PTH (1-84), carboxyl-terminal and amino-terminal fragment.

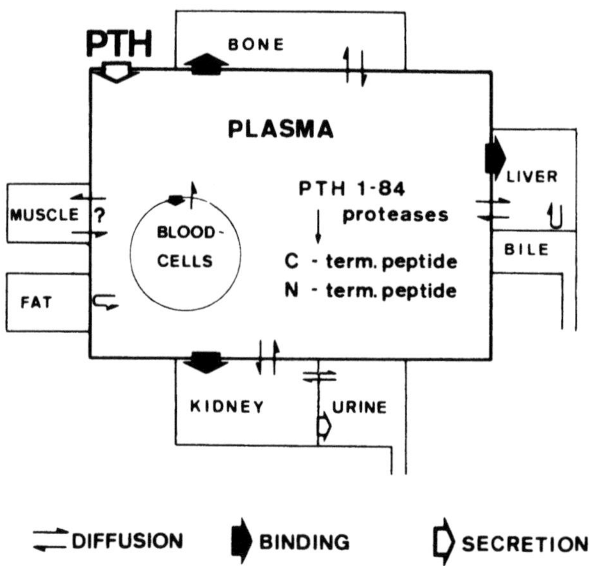

Figure 1. Regulation of plasma PTH level.

CLINICAL MATERIAL

Studies were performed in randomly selected patients suffering from chronic renal diseases with moderate reduction of glomerular filtration rate (GFR 15-30 ml/min; 4 patients) and severe chronic renal failure (GFR $\leq$ 10 ml/min; 36 patients (17 female, 19 male); age: 46.7 $\pm$ 9.8 years (mean $\pm$ S.D.) including 3 anephric, bilateral nephrectomized patients, the others not needing dialysis treatment then). No selection was done for signs or symptoms of overt secondary hyperparathyroidism. Most of the patients were treated with phosphate binding drugs. Vitamin D - treated patients were excluded. 12 healthy volunteers served as controls.

EXPERIMENTAL PROCEDURE

Kinetics of PTH turnover were examined by following plasma levels before and after a 20 min-infusion of 400 U of bovine parathyroid hormone (bPTH) (obtained from Hormon-Chemie,

Munich, W.-Germany). Blood samples were drawn at the time: 0; 10; 20; 25; 30; 35; 45; 60; 90; and 120 min.

METHODS

PTH-assays for intact bPTH (1-84), carboxyl-terminal and (1-34) amino-terminal peptide fragment were performed as described by us previously (21,22).

Inulin (Inutest R, obtained from Deutsche Laevosan-Gesellschaft) having about the same molecular size (MW 5.200) as C-terminal PTH fragment was infused simultanously, thus enableing us to separate the periods of distribution and glomerular filtration.

RESULTS

Disappearance curves of inulin, when transferred into a semilogarithmic plot, exhibit a two compartment open system (see Figure 2.) with a rapid component representing distribution processes and equilibration with interstitial fluid, followed by a slow component representing glomerular filtration.

Half-lives were calculated from the mean values for all substances under study (half-life -1-: 20.-30. min; half-life -2-: 35.-120. min) (see Table 1.).

Intact bPTH (1-84) shows a most rapid decline of plasma levels, half-life -1- being 1.9 min in controls. Cleavage is complete within the period of distribution in controls, whereas in uremia, disappearance of the hormone is slightly impaired and a second component (half-life: 25 min) becomes detectable.

Carboxyl-terminal peptide fragment (bPTH - C-RIA) is of most interest because it is the object of standard radioimmuno assay in most laboratories. Plasma levels detected in our experiments are found to be ten times higher than those of intact (1-84) hormone or (1-34) amino-terminal fragment. In controls disappearance rate of C-terminal fragment for the first time period ("distribution phase") is more rapid and more pronounced than in uremic patients, and cleavage is complete at the end of the second time period ("metabolic phase"), whereas this is not the case in uremia, despite the fact that half-lives do not differ as much in this period.

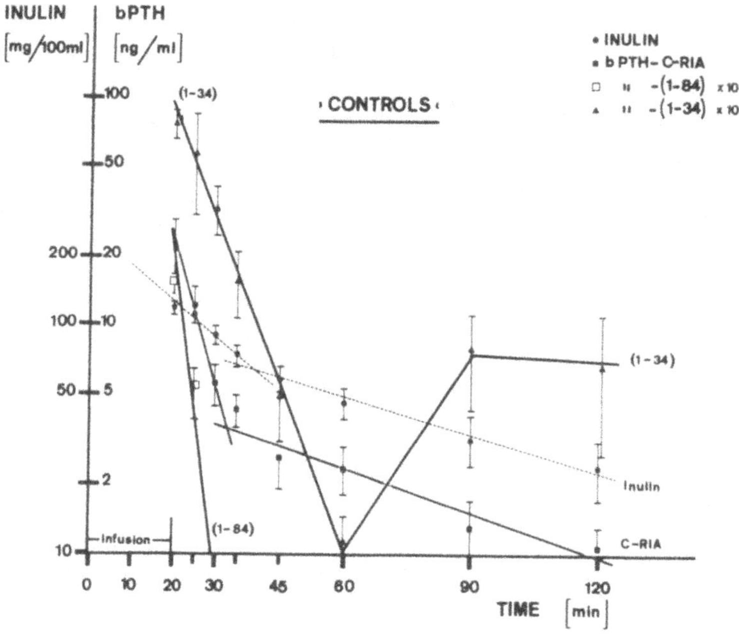

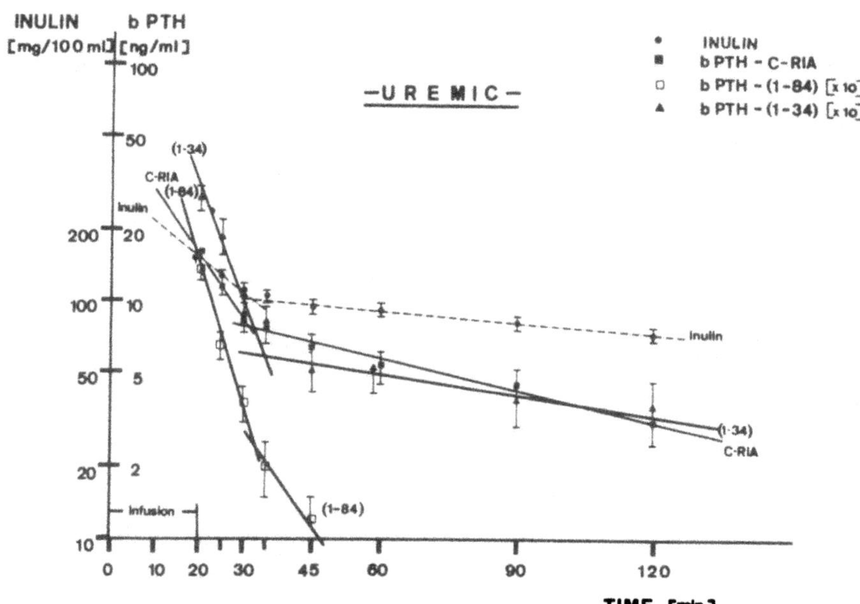

Figure 2. Disappearance curves of bovine parathyroid hormone, C- and N-terminal fragments and inulin (mean values ± SE). (Upper panel: controls; lower panel: chronic renal failure)

Table 1. Half-lives of inulin and parathyroid hormone for groups of different renal function (values calculated from the curves of figure 2.). BNX= bilateral nephrectomized patients.

	HALF-LIFE -1- (20.-30. min)				HALF-LIFE -2- (35.-120. min)			
		bPTH				bPTH		
	INULIN	(1-84)	C-RIA	(1-34)	INULIN	(1-84)	C-RIA	(1-34)
Con-trols (n=12)	24.7	1.9	5.2	8.0	56.4	n.d.	46.2	2nd peak
GFR 15-30 ml/min (n=4)	31.5	5.5	11.7	6.1	121.6	55.0	50.6	231
GFR ≤ 10 ml/min (n=36)	21.4	5.1	11.8	6.1	173.3	24.4	71.5	86.6
BNX (n=3)	32.8	2.7	12.2	11.0	182.4	27;2	41.3	36.1

Amino-terminal peptide fragment in controls exhibits a second peak in 7 out of 12 experiments that is seen only in a few of the uremic patients, whose half-lives are found to be in the same range as those of C-terminal fragment.

Disappearance curves of parathyroid hormones exhibit shortened half-lives when compared to inulin for the period of distribution, indicating additional active binding and metabolism.

Disappearance rates of carboxyl- and amino-terminal peptide fragment are compatible with mere glomerular filtration in controls in the second time period. In uremic patients correlation between half-lives of inulin and parathyroid hormones is poor and not significant

DISCUSSION

In the present study, kinetics of distribution and degradation of parathyroid hormone is examined in man. By testing bovine PTH using sequence specific assays for intact PTH (1-84), carboxyl- and amino- terminal peptide fragments, interference of circulating endogenous PTH is avoided. Previous studies of PTH metabolism in man after parathyroidectomy (17,18) have to take into account peripheral generation of peptide fragments by rediffusion from the receptor sites into the blood. Different behaviour of the alien bovine PTH in man compared to human PTH is not known by now, but may be objected.

The data presented here show a most rapid cleavage of the intact (1-84) hormone with little influence of kidney function, suggesting degradation taking place mainly at extrarenal sites. No significant difference between anephric patients and others suffering from chronic renal failure is found, but degradation is not as fast as in controls.

Half-lives of peptide fragments are similar to those described by Slatopolsky and collaborators (19,20) for dog experiments, but influence of renal failure on PTH turnover is less pronounced in man.

ACKNOWLEDGEMENTS

This work was supported in part by the Deutsche Forschungsgemeinschaft (He 593/3).

The authors wish to thank Mrs. Angelika Prahst and Mrs. Ulrike Ley for their excellent technical assistance.

REFERENCES

1. Strober,W., and Waldmann,T.A.: The Role of the Kidney in the Metabolism of Plasma Proteins. Proc. 6th int. Congr. Nephrol., Florence 1975, pp. 392-405 (Karger, Basel 1976)

2. Babb,A.L., Farrell,P.C., Krelli,D.A., and Scribner,B.H.: Hemodialyzer evaluation by examination of solute molecular spectra. Trans. Amer. Soc. Artif. Int. Organs 18: 98-105, 1972

3. Reiss,E., and Canterbury, J.M.: Genesis of Hyperparathyroidism. Amer. J. Med. 50: 679-685, 1971

4. Arnaud, C.D., Sizemore,G.W., Oldham,S.B., Fischer,J.A., Tsao,H.S., and Littledike,E.T.: Human parathyroid hormone: Glandular and secreted species. Amer. J. Med. 50: 630, 1971

5. Silverman,R., and Yalow,R.S.: Heterogeneity of Parathyroid Hormone, Clinical and Physiologic Implications. J. Clin. Invest. 52: 1958-1971, 1973

6. Segre,G.V., Niall,H.D., Habener,J.F., and Potts,Jr.,J.T.: Metabolism of Parathyroid Hormone. Physiologic and Clinical Significance. Amer. J. Med. 56: 774-784, 1974

7. Nordquist,R.E., and Palmieri,G.M.A.: Intracellular Localization of Parathyroid Hormone in the Kidney. Endocrinology 95: 229-237, 1974

8. Zull,J.E., Shriver,J., and Chuang,J.: in: Vitamin D and Problems Related to Uremic Bone Disease (Norman,A.W., Schaefer,K., Grigoleit,H.G., Herrath,V.D., and Ritz,E., eds.), pp. 431-438, Walter de Gruyter, Berlin, New York, 1975

9. Goltzman,D., Peytremann,A., Callahan,E.N., Segre,G.V., and Potts,Jr.,J.T.: Metabolism and Biological Activity of Parathyroid Hormone in Renal Cortical Membranes. J. Clin. Invest. 57: 8-19, 1976

10. Canterbury,J.M., Bricker,L.A., Levey,G.S., Kozlovskis,P.L., Ruiz,E., Zull,J.E., and Reiss,E.: Metabolism of Bovine Parathyroid Hormone. Immunological and Biological Characteristics of Fragments generated by Liver Perfusion. J. Clin. Invest. 55: 1245-1253, 1975

11. Martin,K., Hruska,K., Greenwalt,A., Klahr,S., and Slatopolsky, E.: Selective Uptake of Intact Parathyroid Hormone By the Liver. Differences between Hepatic and Renal Uptake. J. Clin. Invest. 58: 781-788, 1976

12. Orimo,H., Fujita,T., Morii,H., and Nakao,K.: Inactivation in vitro of parathyroid hormone activity by kidney slices. Endocrinology 76: 255, 1965

13. Kleeman,C.R., Better,O., Massry,S.G., and Maxwell,M.H.: Divalent ion metabolism and osteodystrophy in chronic renal failure. Yale J. Biol. Med. 40: 1, 1967

14. Martin,T.J., Melick,R.A., and De Luise, M.: Metabolism of parathyroid hormone. Degradation of radioiodinated hormone by a kidney enzyme. Biochem. J. 111:509, 1969

15. Okano,K., Fujita,T., Orimo,H., Ohata,M., and Yoshikawa, M.: Effekt of Renal Injury on the Activity of Enzymes Preferentially Hydrolyzing Parathyroid Hormone. Endocrinol. Japon. 18: 327-333, 1971

16. Catherwood,B., and Singer,F.R.: Generation of a Carboxyl-Terminal Fragment of Bovine Parathyroid Hormone by Canine Renal Plasma Membranes. Biochem. Biophys. Res. Commun. 57: 469-475, 1974

17. Melick,R.A., and Martin,T.J.: Parathyroid hormone metabolism in man: Effect of nephrectomy. Clin. Sci. 37: 667, 1969

18. Massry,S.G., Coburn,J.W., Peacock,M., and Kleeman,C.R.: Turnover of endogenous Parathyroid Hormone in Uremic Patients and Those undergoing Hemodialysis. Trans. Amer. Soc. Artif. Int. Organs 18: 416-421, 1972

19. Slatopolsky,E., Hruska,K., and Rutherford,W.E.: Current concepts of parathyroid hormone and vitamin D metabolism: Perturbations in chronic renal disease. Kidney Int., S-90 - S-96, 1975

20. Hruska,K.A., Kopelman,R., Rutherford,W.E., Klahr,S., and Slatopolsky,E.: Metabolism of Immunoreactive Parathyroid Hormone in the Dog: The role of the kidney and the effects of chronic renal disease. J. Clin. Invest. 56: 39-48, 1975

21. Hesch,R.D., McIntosh,C.H.S., and Woodhead,J.S.: New Aspects of Radioimmunochemical Measurement of Human Parathyroid Hormone Using the Labelled Antibody Technique. Horm. Metab. Res. 7:347-352, 1975

22. Hehrmann,R., Wilke,R., Nordmeyer,J.P., and Hesch,R.D.: Hochsensitiver, C-terminal-spezifischer Radioimmunoassay für menschliches Parathormon als Routinemethode. Dtsch. Med. Wschr. 101: 1726-1729, 1976

PARATHYROID HORMONE RECEPTORS AND STIMULATION OF RENAL CYCLIC 3', 5' AMP *IN VITRO*: PHYSIOLOGICAL RELEVANCE?*

N. Kugai, L. Dorantes, R. Nissenson and C. D. Arnaud

Endocrine Research Unit, Mayo Clinic and Medical School,

Rochester, MN, 55901

INTRODUCTION

Few would challenge the concept that parathyroid hormone (PTH) action on the kidney, at least in part, depends upon the ability of the hormone to stimulate increased production of intracellular cyclic 3', 5' adenosine monophosphate (cyclic AMP) by activating membrane bound adenylate cyclase.

In vivo, PTH administration to a variety of hypoparathyroid mammals stimulates the urinary excretion of cyclic AMP as much as 5 - 100 fold and administration of dibutyryl cyclic AMP faithfully reproduces the changes in urinary ion excretion which accompanies PTH administration. *In vitro*, PTH stimulates cyclic AMP production in renal slices and isolated renal tubules and activates adenylate cyclase in renal homogenates and renal cortical membranes.

However convincing and consistent these observations are, they have never been scrutinized from the point of view of their relevance to normal physiology. The present communication is concerned with this problem and attempts to explain an important discrepancy which, taken at face value, tends to undermine the importance of cyclic AMP as a second messenger in PTH action under physiological conditions.

---

* This work was presented in part at the 1977 Annual Meeting of the American Society for Clinical Investigation.

RENAL RECEPTOR AND CYCLIC AMP INVESTIGATIONS *IN VITRO*

We have studied both the binding of biologically active, electrolytically labeled ^{125}I synthetic bPTH 1-34 (bPTH 1-34) and bPTH 1-34 stimulation of cyclic AMP production in isolated chicken renal tubules. Inhibition of binding of ^{125}I bPTH 1-34 occurred over a range of unlabeled bPTH 1-34 concentrations from $10^{-9}M$ to $10^{-6}M$ and half maximal inhibition of binding (K_d) was achieved at $5.4 \times 10^{-8}M$. Stimulation of cyclic AMP production occurred over the same range of bPTH 1-34 concentrations and the half-maximal (K_m) value was $5.5 \times 10^{-8}M$. The similarity in these kinetic values for binding and stimulation of cyclic AMP production provides strong evidence for the coupling of the binding and adenylate cyclase activation processes in this system and suggests that the binding component we have studied probably represents a true receptor for PTH *in vivo*.

PLASMA [bPTH 1-34] NEEDED TO SUPPORT MINERAL HOMEOSTASIS IN THE CHICKEN

To determine the concentration of bovine PTH 1-34 in the plasma required to support mineral homeostasis in the chicken, we perfused 4-week-old thyroparathyroidectomized (TPTX) and ultimobranchialectomized (UBX) chickens intravenously over 24 hours with a physiologic solution containing varying concentrations of bPTH 1-34 but no calcium. Blood was obtained before and after TPTX - UBX and at 16 and 24 hours of infusion for the measurement of plasma calcium and immunoreactive PTH (using an antiserum produced against synthetic PTH 1-34 and ^{131}I PTH 1-34 as labeled ligand). Serum calcium decreased from 9.5 mg/dl to 6.5 mg/dl within six hours of TPTX - UBX. Plasma calcium increased during the bPTH 1-34 infusion and achieved a steady-state after 12 hours. As expected, plasma iPTH correlated with plasma calcium ($r = 0.763$, $p < 0.001$). Most important, plasma calcium was restored to normal at concentrations of plasma iPTH in the range of $10^{-10}M$. These results are clearly at odds with those we obtained in our studies *in vitro*. The concentration of plasma bPTH 1-34 required to support mineral homeostasis in the chicken appears to be as much as 2 orders of magnitude lower than that required to stimulate renal cyclic AMP production or inhibit the binding of ^{125} I bPTH 1-34 in isolated chicken renal tubules half maximally.

POSSIBLE EXPLANATIONS FOR "THE DISCREPANCY"

Our observation of this discrepancy is not new. Others (1,2,3,4) have commented upon the fact that so-called physiologic concentrations of PTH were lower than the concentrations of PTH required to produce activation of renal adenylate cyclase *in vitro*. However, the focus of discussion of the discrepancy has, in general, avoided direct confrontation of the issues involved.

In our view, the possible explanations for the discrepancy include:

1. Under physiologic conditions, PTH supported renal ion transport does not depend upon PTH induced changes in renal tubule cell cyclic AMP.

2. The *in vitro* systems available for the study of renal receptor binding of PTH and PTH induced changes in cyclic AMP or adenylate cyclase are altered in some way so that they are markedly less sensitive to PTH than under physiologic conditions *in vivo*.

3. The values of kinetic constants derived from the study of bPTH 1-34 induced changes in cyclic AMP and the binding of ^{125}I bPTH 1-34 in isolated renal tubules *in vitro* (and probably all renal systems *in vitro* reported to date) accurately reflect the initial events in the molecular *pharmacology* of parathyroid hormone *in vivo*.

4. Under physiologic conditions, a very limited number of renal PTH receptors are occupied (too few to detect by classical displacement experiments) and only small, PTH induced oscillations in intracellular cyclic AMP (too small to detect by classical measurements) are required to maintain PTH dependent renal ion transport.

Clearly, all of these possible explanations have important implications from both practical and theoretical points of view. On the one hand, it would be foolish to continue to use available systems in vitro for the study of the initial molecular events in PTH action if these systems carried with them large artifactual components. On the other hand, it would be extremely important to know if the kinetic parameters generally derived from the study of systems *in vitro* and used to describe the initial molecular events in hormone action reflected pharmacologic and not physiologic phenomena in the case of PTH.

PLASMA [bPTH 1-34] NEEDED TO STIMULATE RENAL CYCLIC AMP AND PRODUCTION *IN VIVO*

As far as we are aware, the relationship between the concentrations of plasma PTH and renal cyclic AMP *in vivo* has never been studied. We administered varying doses of bPTH 1-34 intravenously to 4-week-old lightly anesthetized chickens 12 - 14 hours after they had been TPTX - UBX'd. Exactly 1.5 minutes after PTH administration, plasma was obtained from the inferior vena cava through an abdominal incision for the measurement of plasma iPTH (radioimmunoassay employing an antiserum to synthetic PTH 1-34). Exactly two minutes after PTH administration, liquid nitrogen was poured into the abdominal wound on one exposed kidney. The rapidly frozen kidney was excised and processed (TCA extraction) for the measurement of cyclic AMP. Plasma containing relatively high concentrations of immunoreactive PTH (1 μg/ml) were bioassayed in the cultured bone explant system described by Raisz and coworkers(5).

The concentrations of biologically active PTH in plasma samples were exactly as predicted by radioimmunoassay of the same samples supporting the contention that the iPTH measurements we made accurately reflected the plasma concentration of biologically active PTH to which kidneys were exposed _in vivo._ No significant change in renal cyclic AMP content was observed over a range of plasma iPTH concentrations from 10^{-10}M to 10^{-9}M. With further increases in plasma iPTH, renal cyclic AMP content increased in a "dose dependent" fashion and the curve described by a plot of these variables was essentially superimposable on the curve of isolated chicken renal tubule cyclic AMP content plotted as a function of medium concentration of bPTH 1-34.

DISCUSSION AND COMMENT

The results of these latter experiments are key to sorting out the alternatives we have listed (see above). Possibility number 2 (artifactual insensitivity of _in vitro_ systems) can probably be eliminated. The concentrations of PTH which are required to stimulate renal cyclic AMP production significantly appear to be the same _in vivo_ (plasma iPTH) as they are _in vitro_ (medium PTH). However, it is important to recognize that the technology employed in both _in vivo_ and _in vitro_ experiments would not have permitted the detection of changes of renal cyclic AMP of as much as 10%. Therefore, it is possible and indeed quite likely that small increases in renal cyclic AMP were produced by very low doses or plasma concentrations (probably in the physiological range) of PTH. Unfortunately the technical difficulties encountered in collecting urine from chickens prevented us from obtaining crucial data concerning the lowest plasma concentration of administered bPTH 1-34 which would elicit changes in the renal handling of ions (Ca^{++}, Mg^{+}, $PO_4^{=}$, Na^{+}, K^{+}, H^{+} and HCO_3^{-}).

On the surface, the alternative to which our data says "yes" is number 1, that is, PTH supported renal ion transport does not depend upon PTH induced changes in renal tubule cell cyclic AMP under physiologic conditions. However, for reasons already cited, we would prefer to think that the changes of renal tubule cyclic AMP at physiologic plasma or medium concentrations of PTH for which we were looking were too small to detect with the methodology we used. The important point to be made here is that in normal physiology, the oscillations of renal cell cyclic AMP concentration caused by PTH are probably very small and certainly not of the degree observed in classical dose response curves generated *in vitro* using various preparations of renal tissue.

Our comments regarding the technical difficulty in detecting changes in renal cyclic AMP at physiologic concentrations of PTH probably relate equally well to our inability to detect significant inhibition of binding of ^{125}I bPTH 1-34 to chicken renal tubules at physiologic concentrations of PTH. This would mean that, in normal physiology, only a small number of the available renal cell receptors for PTH would be occupied.

Therefore, although certain crucial data are not at hand at the present time, we favor excluding alternative #1 and strongly endorsing alternative #4, which states that "under physiologic conditions, a very limited number of renal PTH receptors are occupied and only small, PTH induced oscillations in intracellular cyclic AMP (perhaps large in certain intracellular compartments) are required to maintain PTH dependent renal ion transport".

Finally, the question of the biological meaning of the kinetic values obtained from our own studies of PTH stimulated cyclic AMP production and ^{125}I bPTH 1-34 binding in isolated chicken renal tubules should be addressed. It is clear that these values are derived primarily from cyclic AMP or binding data generated at a medium bPTH 1-34 concentration range which is between 10 and 1000 times the plasma concentration of bPTH 1-34 capable of supporting mineral homeostasis. But, as noted above, the plasma concentration range of administered bPTH 1-34 required to stimulate renal cyclic AMP *in vivo* is not substantially different than the required medium concentration range of bPTH 1-34 *in vitro*. Therefore, since the measured response (tissue cyclic AMP) can only be detected *in vivo* and *in vitro* at concentrations of plasma or medium PTH which are in the unphysiologic range, these responses must be pharmacologic by definition. Thus, we would also subscribe to alternative #3 which states that "The values of kinetic constants derived from the study of PTH induced changes in cyclic AMP and the binding of labeled PTH in isolated chicken renal tubules *in vitro* (and probably all renal systems *in vitro* reported to date) accurately reflect those initial events involved in the molecular *pharmacology* of parathyroid hormone *in vivo*. We would therefore caution that inferences about the renal *pharmacology* of this naturally occurring and critically important hormone can be justifiably derived from the results of classical cyclic AMP stimulation or labeled PTH binding experiments, but not necessarily about its renal *physiology*.

ACKNOWLEDGMENTS

This work was supported by USPHS project grant AM 12302 and the Mayo Foundation. Dr. Kugai was supported by a National Kidney Foundation Fellowship, Dr. Dorantes by a Fogarty Foundation Fellowship and Dr. Nissenson by USPHS training grant AM 7147. We greatly appreciate the excellent technical assistance rendered by Ms. Kathy Zawistowski, Julianna Gilkinson and Linda Zitzner, and we thank Ms. Marylee Fair for providing superior secretarial help and typing the manuscript under deadline circumstances.

REFERENCES

1. Zull, J.E., Malbon, C.C. and Chuang, J.: Binding of Tritiated Bovine Parathyroid Hormone to Plasma Membranes from Bovine Kidney Cortex. J. Biol. Chem., 252:1071-1078 (1977).

2. Parsons, J.A., Rafferty, B., Gray, D., Reit, B., Zanelli, J. M., Keutmann, H.T., Tregar, G. W., Callahan, E. N. and Potts, J.T., Jr.: Pharmacology of Parathyroid Hormone and Some of its Fragments and Analogues. *In* Calcium Regulating Hormones (Parsons, J.H., Talmage, R.V. and Owen , M., editors) pp. 33-39, Excerpta Medica, Amserdam, 1975.

3. Heath, D.A. and Aurbach, G. D.: Studies on the Binding of ^{125}I-Parathyroid Hormone to Renal Cortical Membranes. *In* Calcium Regulating Hormones (Parsons, J.H., Talmage, R.V. and Owen , M., editors) pp. 159-162, Excerpta Medica, Amsterdam, 1975.

4. Chabardes, D., Imbert, M. and Morel, F.: Localization of PTH Action Sites Along The Rabbit Nephron. *In* Phosphate Metabolism of Kidney and Bone (Avioli, L., Bordier, Ph.,Fleisch, H., Massry, S., and Slatopolsky, E., editors) pp. 123-130, Nouvelle Imprimerie Fournie, France, 1975.

5. Raisz, L.G. and Niemann, I.: Effect of Phosphate, Calcium and Magnesium on Bone Resorption and Hormonal Responses in Tissue Culture. Endocrinol., 85:446-452, (1969).

INDEX

GPSR Compliance
The European Union's (EU) General Product Safety Regulation (GPSR) is a set of rules that requires consumer products to be safe and our obligations to ensure this.

If you have any concerns about our products, you can contact us on

ProductSafety@springernature.com

In case Publisher is established outside the EU, the EU authorized representative is:

Springer Nature Customer Service Center GmbH
Europaplatz 3
69115 Heidelberg, Germany

www.ingramcontent.com/pod-product-compliance
Ingram Content Group UK Ltd.
Pitfield, Milton Keynes, MK11 3LW, UK
UKHW050919270726
13967UKWH00014B/2987
* 9 7 8 1 4 6 8 4 7 7 5 9 7 *